D1263065

Encyclopedia of
DISEASES AND DISORDERS

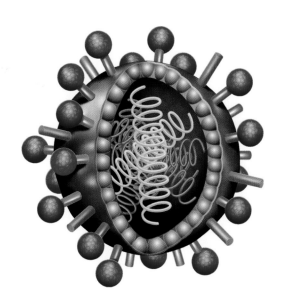

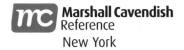 **Marshall Cavendish**
Reference
New York

Library of Congress Cataloging-in-Publication Data
Encyclopedia of diseases and disorders.
      p. ; cm.
   Includes bibliographical references and index.
   ISBN 978-0-7614-7941-3 (alk. paper)
   1. Medicine--Encyclopedias. 2. Diseases--Encyclopedias. I. Marshall Cavendish Reference.
   [DNLM: 1. Medicine--Encyclopedias--English. 2. Physiological Phenomena--Encyclopedias--English. WB 13 E56281 2011]
   R125.E565 2011
   610.3--dc22
                                        2010023903

Printed in Malaysia

14 13 12 11 10 1 2 3 4 5

Marshall Cavendish
Publisher: Paul Bernabeo
Project Editor: Brian Kinsey
Production Manager: Michael Esposito
Indexer: Cynthia Crippen, AEIOU, Inc.

Foreword

The *Encyclopedia of Diseases and Disorders* provides authoritative information on a wide variety of diseases and health disorders. Although the focus in planning this collection of articles was on subjects of interest to young readers, the information provided here is valuable to users of any age. More than two hundred articles are categorized in three major areas of interest: infections, noninfectious diseases, and mental disorders. The prevalence of infections and their periodic outbreaks make headlines, especially when the news concerns new and emerging infectious diseases, but reports on the resurgence of old scourges such as tuberculosis and up-to-date information about everyday health issues are also important. Articles on noninfectious diseases cover a broad spectrum of illnesses, including heart attacks, diabetes, and kidney stones, among others. Mental illness is common worldwide, and depression, eating disorders, and anxiety are particularly common in adolescents. It is important to note that many diseases are preventable; therefore, knowledge of these diseases, how they are transmitted, and the effectiveness of prevention strategies could help reduce disease transmission in particular populations, including young people. While this encyclopedia is not a substitute for obtaining advice and treatment from a licensed medical practitioner, the knowledge about disease offered in this reference work can help promote good health.

All articles were written and edited by experts in the field, including specialists in mental health, medicine, infectious disease, and microbiology. The content of these articles can be accessed and enhanced in a variety of ways because of their structured organization, cross-referencing, the simple A-Z format, and the provision of glossaries and resources for further reading. Valuable information is also conveyed through photographs, charts, graphs, and artworks with clear descriptive captions.

Understanding diseases and disorders

Infections are caused by bacteria, fungi, other microorganisms, viruses, and prions. From the beginning of time, infections have been a major cause of illness and death. Powerful infectious diseases that sometimes give rise to epidemics like smallpox, influenza, tuberculosis, and plague have had a major impact on large numbers of people in the world for centuries. The types of infections that affect humans include common bacterial diseases, such as pneumonia, as well as viral disorders, such as chicken pox.

Noninfectious diseases include all the medical and surgical conditions that are not mental disorders or infections. This is a broad category that includes muscular and skeletal conditions, cardiovascular disease, autoimmune diseases, kidney diseases, lung diseases, and diseases affecting the gastrointestinal tract.

Mental disorders are conditions that affect thinking, behavior, personality, judgment, and brain function. Examples of mental disorders include anxiety, depression, eating disorders, mood disorders, schizophrenia, and personality disorders. Mental disorders are often underdiagnosed and may not be publicly disclosed because of fear of the stigma associated with mental illness or because of a lack of knowledge about its causes, diagnostic methods of detection, or available therapies and treatments.

Some diseases that run in families are categorized as *genetic diseases*; these include depression, diabetes, and some cancers. In some cases, risk factors and the causes of these diseases are known. However, for many diseases, the exact causes are still unknown.

Bacteria, viruses, and other microorganisms cause infections by penetrating into human or animal organs, tissues, and cells and then replicating to cause disease. Microorganisms can cause disease by damaging and killing human cells, producing toxins, and creating an inflammatory response. Some microorganisms are harmless in normal healthy individuals, but many microorganisms can cause disease if they penetrate the body's normal host defenses and immune system. Certain organisms that are less virulent and do not normally cause disease are capable of causing opportunistic infections in individuals who have weakened immune systems.

One of the unique characteristics of infectious diseases is the variety of mechanisms by which these diseases are transmitted or acquired. Some infectious diseases are considered *communicable diseases* and can be transmitted person to person through direct contact with infected persons or a contaminated environment, large droplets that are shed in close proximity when infected people cough or sneeze, and airborne transmission, especially in contained environments with limited air circulation.

There are also a number of infectious diseases that are transmitted through exchange of body fluids or as sexually transmitted diseases. Some are transmitted as blood-borne pathogens through transfusions or they are spread when people share contaminated needles or when they have unprotected intercourse with infected persons. Still other infections occur through fecal-oral contamination, when food or water become contaminated with bacteria or viruses, or both, causing vomiting and diarrhea. Infections such as rabies can be acquired from animals; this is called *zoonotic* transmission.

Prevention and treatment

Prevention of some mental illnesses is possible with early diagnosis and treatment of mild disorders or underlying conditions. Recognition of risk factors and preexisting conditions can also allow for support, education, counseling, and therapy to prevent complications.

Many noninfectious diseases can be prevented with regular exercise, good nutrition, avoidance of alcohol and substance abuse, avoidance of smoking, and in some cases, use of medications. For example, aspirin can reduce the incidence of heart attacks and weight loss can reduce the risk of developing diabetes.

Many communicable diseases can be prevented with good infection control measures. Proper sanitation and reducing contamination of the food and water supply are essential elements to prevent infections and promote good health. Primary measures to limit infections transmitted by direct contact include hand washing or use of alcohol preparations to disinfect hands. Acquisition of many cold viruses and respiratory illnesses can be reduced with frequent hand washing. Infections spread by droplet and through airborne transmission can be contained with isolation measures to limit the spread of these illnesses. Vaccinations to prevent infections have been developed for many common childhood diseases including measles, mumps, rubella, and chicken pox. Broad implementation of vaccinations against hepatitis A and B has reduced the incidence and prevalence of these infections. Smallpox has been virtually eliminated because of worldwide vaccination campaigns. Other diseases such as polio and tetanus have been reduced thanks to the use of effective vaccination programs. Vaccines against other pathogens continue to emerge from medical laboratories.

Not all diseases require treatment. Many diseases resolve without specific treatment, particularly in healthy people. Serious diseases need to be treated with appropriate medical and or surgical therapy. For several mental illnesses, therapy and counseling are used along with medications. Medications are used to treat mental conditions, noninfectious diseases, and infections to restore normal function and to facilitate healing. Medications, physical therapy, occupational therapy, behavioral therapy, and surgery can all be used to control symptoms, improve function, and reduce the burden of diseases. Bacterial infections are treated with antibiotics, which interfere with bacterial replication or kill the bacteria. Advances have occurred in antiviral therapies and drug regimens to treat viruses such as HIV/AIDS, herpes, hepatitis B and C, and influenza. Treatments for mental illness, noninfectious diseases, and infections have improved outcomes for patients throughout the world.

This encyclopedia covers a broad range of diseases and disorders. Despite significant increases in scientific and medical knowledge, medical disorders remain a significant cause of illness and death throughout the world. Providing information about health and disease is vital for students and the general public in order to increase knowledge of conditions likely to affect them, their friends, and their families. Increased awareness of disease may foster healthier behaviors and risk reduction strategies. An understanding of disease can also promote earlier diagnosis and treatment, resulting in improved health outcomes. It is also hoped that use of these articles will inspire readers to study science, medicine, and public health and even to seek careers in health-related professions.

Victoria Fraser, MD
J. William Campbell Professor of Medicine
Co-Director Infectious Diseases Division
Washington University School of Medicine
Saint Louis, Missouri

Additional related information on these health topics is available in the online *Diseases and Disorders* database at *www.marshallcavendishdigital.com*.

Consultants and contributors

CONSULTANTS

Robert S. Ascheim, MD, Associate Professor of Medicine, Weill Cornell College of Medicine, New York Presbyterian Hospital, New York

Dorothy P. Bethea, EdD, MPA, OTR-L, Chair and Associate Professor, Department of Occupational Therapy, Winston-Salem State University, North Carolina

Laurence Burd, MD, Associate Professor of Clinical Obstetrics and Gynecology, Department of Obstetrics and Gynecology, Division of Maternal Fetal Medicine, University of Illinois at Chicago, Chicago, Illinois

Viki Christopoulos, MD, Assistant Clinical Professor of Ophthalmology, Eye and Ear Institute, University of Pittsburgh, Pennsylvania

Maria Descartes, MD, Associate Professor of Genetics and Pediatrics, Department of Genetics, University of Alabama at Birmingham, Birmingham, Alabama

Victoria J. Fraser, MD, Professor of Medicine, Division of Infectious Diseases, Washington University School of Medicine, St. Louis, Missouri

Barry L. Gruber, MD, Professor of Medicine and Dermatology, Division of Rheumatology, State University of New York at Stony Brook, Stony Brook, New York

Jennifer L. Hall, PhD, Assistant Professor of Medicine, Director, Cardiovascular Genomics Division of Cardiology, Department of Medicine, Lillehei Heart Institute, University of Minnesota, Minneapolis

Michael Kalos, PhD, Director, Clinical Immunobiology Correlative Studies Laboratory, Division of Cancer Immunotherapeutics and Tumor Immunology, Division of

Hematology and Hematopoietic Cell Transplantation, City of Hope National Medical Center, Duarte, California

Elizabeth Liebson, MD, Staff Psychiatrist, McLean Hospital, Belmont, Massachusetts

Gregg Y. Lipschik, MD, Clinical Associate Professor of Medicine, University of Pennsylvania School of Medicine, Philadelphia, Pennsylvania; Director, Medical Intensive Care Unit, Philadelphia Veterans Affairs Medical Center, Philadelphia, Pennsylvania

Kathleen McKee, PhD, RD, Co-Chair, Department of Nutrition and Dietetics, Marywood University, Scranton, Pennsylvania

Steven W. Mifflin, PhD, Professor of Pharmacology, Department of Pharmacology, University of Texas Health Science Center, San Antonio, Texas

Antoinette Moran, MD, Division Head of Pediatric Endocrinology, Division of Endocrinology, Department of Pediatrics, Medical School, University of Minnesota, Minneapolis, Minnesota

Guy W. Neff, MD, Associate Professor of Medicine, Department of Medicine, University of Cincinnati, Cincinnati, Ohio

Amy S. Paller, MD, Professor of Dermatology, Feinberg School of Medicine, Northwestern University, Chicago, Illinois

C. Matthew Peterson, MD, John A. Dixon Professor and Chair, Division of Reproductive Endocrinology and Infertility, University of Utah Health Sciences Center, Salt Lake City, Utah

David Relling, PT, PhD, Instructor, University of North Dakota, School of Medicine and Health Sciences, Department of Physical Therapy, Grand Forks, North Dakota

Jaclyn B. Spitzer, PhD, Director of Audiology and Speech-Language Pathology, Department of Otolaryngology, Columbia

University Medical Center, New York

Alexander Urfer, PT, PhD, Department Chair and Professor of Physical Therapy and Physiology, Department of Physical and Occupational Therapy, Idaho State University, Pocatello, Idaho

Robert M. Youngson, MD, Fellow of the Royal Society of Medicine, Officer of the Order of St. John of Jerusalem, Diploma in Tropical Medicine and Hygiene, Fellow of the Royal College of Ophthalmologists, UK

CONTRIBUTORS

Monica S. Badve, DNB, Clinical Fellow, Department of Medicine (Neurology), University of Ottawa, Ottawa, Ontario, Canada

Kim E. Barrett, PhD, Professor of Medicine, University of California San Diego Medical Center, Division of Rheumatology, San Diego, California

Daniel Bausch, MD, MPH, TM, Associate Professor, School of Public Health and Tropical Medicine, Tulane University, New Orleans, Louisiana

Richard C. Beatty, MA (University of Cambridge), London, UK

Kathleen Becan-McBride, EdD, MT (ASCP), Professor, Department of Family Medicine, University of Texas Medical School at Houston, Texas

Patti J. Berg, MA, MPT, Assistant Professor, Department of Physical Therapy, University of South Dakota, Vermillion, South Dakota

Nisha Bhatt, MD, New York

Halvard B. Boenig, MA, MD, Acting Assistant Professor of Medicine/Hematology, Department of Medicine, Division of Hematology, University of Washington, Seattle, Washington

Richard N. Bradley, MD, Associate Professor of Emergency Medicine, University of Texas Health Science Center at Houston, Medical

5

School, Department of Emergency Medicine, Houston, Texas

Matthew D. Breyer, MD, Senior Medical Fellow II, Biotechnology Discovery Research, Lilly Research Laboratories, Eli Lilly and Company, Indianapolis, Indiana

Amanda J. Brosnahan, BA, University of Minnesota Medical School, Department of Microbiology, Minneapolis, Minnesota

Brian C. Brost, MD, Associate Professor of Maternal Fetal Medicine, Department of Obstetrics and Gynecology, Mayo Clinic College of Medicine, Rochester, Minnesota

Edward R. Cachay, MD, Fellow, Division of Infectious Diseases, University of California, San Diego

Bernard C. Camins, MD, MSCR, Assistant Professor of Medicine, Division of Infectious Diseases, Washington University, St. Louis, Missouri

Corrado Cancedda, MD, Division of Infectious Diseases and Internal Medicine, Washington University School of Medicine, St. Louis, Missouri

William E. Cayley, MDiv, MD, Assistant Professor, University of Wisconsin, Department of Family Medicine, Eau Claire, Wisconsin

Eliza Farmer Chakravarty, MD, Division of Immunology and Rheumatology, Stanford University School of Medicine, Palo Alto, California

Jonathon Cross, MS, CCC-SLP, Speech-Language Pathologist, Baltimore, Maryland

Christine P. Curran, MS, University of Cincinnati, Department of Environmental Health, Cincinnati, Ohio

Robert B. Daroff, MD, Professor and Interim Chair of Neurology, Case School of Medicine, University Hospitals of Cleveland, Department of Neurology, Cleveland, Ohio

Robyn Davies, BHScPT, MAppScPT, FCAMT, Department of Physical Therapy, Faculty of Medicine, University of Toronto, Ontario, Canada

Chadrick E. Denlinger, MD, Department of Surgery, University of Virginia, Charlottesville, Virginia

Antonette T. Dulay, MD, Yale University School of Medicine,

Department of Obstetrics and Gynecology, Section of Maternal-Fetal Medicine, New Haven, Connecticut

Christopher Duncan, MD, Division of Digestive Diseases, University of Cincinnati, Cincinnati, Ohio

Randi Ettner, PhD, New Health Foundation Worldwide, Evanston, Illinois

Josephine W. Everly, BS, Director of Research Support and Communications, Department of Ophthalmology, Louisiana State University Health Sciences Center, New Orleans, Louisiana

Mark S. Freedman, MD, Professor of Medicine (Neurology), University of Ottawa, Ottawa, Ontario, Canada

Gary N. Frishman, MD, Associate Professor, Department of Obstetrics and Gynecology, Women and Infants Hospital, Brown Medical School, Providence, Rhode Island

Joseph M. Fritz, MD, Fellow, Division of Infectious Diseases, Washington University, St. Louis, Missouri

Arun K. Gadre, MD, Heuser Professor of Otology and Neurotology, Medical Director, Louisville Deaf Oral School, Heuser Hearing Institute; Director of Otology, Neurotology, and Skull Base Surgery, Associate Professor of Otolaryngology/Head and Neck Surgery, University of Louisville, Louisville, Kentucky

Medley O'Keefe Gatewood, MD, Clinical Instructor, Division of Emergency Medicine, University of Washington Medical Center, Seattle, Washington

Diana M. Gitig, PhD, White Plains, New York

Isaac Grate Jr., MD, FACEP, Clinical Assistant Professor, Department of Emergency Medicine, University of Texas Health Science Center at Houston, Houston, Texas

Sonia Gulati, BA, Graduate School of Arts and Science, College of Physicians and Surgeons, New York

Stephen Higgs, BSc, PhD, FRES, Professor, Director, Experimental Pathology Graduate Program; Leon Bromberg Professor for Excellence in Teaching; Department of Pathology, Center for Biodefense and Emerging

Infectious Diseases, Sealy Center for Vaccine Development, WHO Collaborating Center for Tropical Diseases, University of Texas Medical Branch, Galveston, Texas

Ramona Jenkin, MD, Science Director, TalkingScience, New York

Sonal Jhaveri, PhD, Massachusetts Institute of Technology, Department of Brain and Cognitive Sciences, Cambridge, Massachusetts

Andreas M. Kaiser, MD, Associate Professor of Clinical Colorectal Surgery, Department of Colorectal Surgery, Keck School of Medicine, University of Southern California, California

Richard S. Kalish, MD, PhD, Professor of Dermatology and Acting Chair, Department of Dermatology, State University of New York at Stony Brook, Stony Brook, New York

Herbert E. Kaufman, MD, Boyd Professor of Ophthalmology and Pharmacology and Experimental Therapeutics, Louisiana State University Health Sciences Center, New Orleans, Louisiana

Evelyn B. Kelly, PhD, Ocala, Florida

Nigar Kirmani, MD, Associate Professor of Medicine, Division of Infectious Diseases, Washington University, St. Louis, Missouri

Bonnie Klimes-Dougan, PhD, Assistant Professor, Department of Psychiatry, University of Minnesota, Minneapolis, Minnesota

Maya Kolipakam, MD, Department of Dermatology, State University of New York at Stony Brook, Stony Brook, New York

Adam Korzenko, MD, Department of Dermatology, State University of New York at Stony Brook, Stony Brook, New York

David M. Lawrence, MS, Mechanicsville, Virginia

Alan M. Levine, PhD, RD, Co-Chair and Professor, Department of Nutrition and Dietetics, Marywood University, Scranton, Pennsylvania

Lori M. Lieving, PhD, Carolinas College of Health Sciences, Carolinas HealthCare System, Charlotte, North Carolina

Debby A. Lin, MD, Department of Medicine, Harvard Medical School; Division of Rheumatology, Immunology, and Allergy, Brigham and Women's Hospital, Boston, Massachusetts

Joanna C. Lyford, BSc, London, UK

Julie A. McDougal, RRT, MAE, Pediatric Pulmonary Centre, University of Alabama, Birmingham, Alabama

Julie McDowell, Senior Editor, *Clinical Laboratory News and Strategies*, American Association for Clinical Chemistry, Washington DC

Sanjay Mehta, MD, Fellow, Division of Infectious Diseases, University of California, San Diego

Ian H. Mendenhall, BS, Doctoral Student, Department of Tropical Medicine, Tulane School of Public Health and Tropical Medicine, New Orleans, Louisiana

Kirk D. Moberg, MD, PhD, Clinical Associate Professor of Medicine, University of Illinois College of Medicine at Urbana-Champaign, Illinois; Medical Director, Carle Addiction Recovery Center, Carle Clinic Association, Urbana, Illinois; Medical Director, New Choice Center for Addiction Recovery, The Pavilion, Champaign, Illinois

Rashmi V. Nemade, PhD, BioMedText, New Albany, Ohio

Diana Nurutdinova, MD, Staff Physician, Infectious Diseases, St. Louis Veterans Affairs Medical Center, St. Louis, Missouri

Joanne L. Oakes, MD, FACEP, Associate Residency Director, Department of Emergency Medicine, University of Texas Health Science Center at Houston, Houston, Texas

Martin L. Pall, PhD, School of Molecular Biosciences, Washington State University, Pullman, Washington

Moeen K. Panni, MD, PhD, Associate Professor of Anesthesiology, Director of Obstetric Anesthesia, University of Texas Medical School at Houston, Houston, Texas

Kevin D. Pereira, MD, MS (ORL), Professor of Otolaryngology and Pediatrics, Vice Chair, Otolaryngology/Head and Neck Surgery, University of Texas Health Science Center at Houston, Houston, Texas

Mary Quirk, BSc, Golden Valley, Minnesota

Mary D. Ruppe, MD, Assistant Professor, University of Texas Medical School at Houston, Department of Internal Medicine, Division of Endocrinology, Diabetes, and Metabolism, Houston, Texas

Linda A. Russell, MD, Assistant Professor of Clinical Medicine, Weill Cornell Medical College, Hospital for Special Surgery, New York

Gregory S. Sayuk, MD, Instructor, Division of Gastroenterology, Washington University School of Medicine, St. Louis, Missouri

Patrick M. Schlievert, PhD, Professor of Microbiology, University of Minnesota Medical School, Department of Microbiology, Minneapolis, Minnesota

Nance A. Seiple, CRNA, MEd, Medical Communications, Park Ridge, Illinois

Laurel B. Shader, MD, Pediatric Department Chair, Fair Haven Community Health Center, New Haven, Connecticut

Janet Yagoda Shagam, PhD, RhizoTech, Albuquerque, New Mexico

Nurun N. Shah, MD, MPH, Associate Professor of Psychiatry and Behavioral Sciences, University of Texas Medical School at Houston, Houston, Texas

Pravani Sreeramoju, MD, MPH, Department of Medicine, University of Texas Health Science Center at San Antonio, San Antonio, Texas

Manakan Betsy Srichai, MD, Clinical Instructor of Medicine, Department of Medicine, Division of Nephrology, Vanderbilt University Medical Center, Nashville, Tennessee

Graeme Stemp-Morlock, BSc, Waterloo, Ontario, Canada

Lise M. Stevens, MA, Brooklyn, New York

Kristi L. Strandberg, BA, University of Minnesota Medical School, Department of Microbiology, Minneapolis, Minnesota

Sharon Switzer-McIntyre, PhD, MEd, BScPT, BPE, Assistant Professor and Vice-Chair, Education, Department of Physical Therapy, Faculty of Medicine, University of Toronto, Ontario, Canada

Oleg V. Tcheremissine, MD, Behavioral Health Center, Research; Department of Psychiatry, Carolinas Health Care System, Charlotte, North Carolina

M. David Ullman, PhD, Associate Research Professor, University of Massachusetts Medical School, Worcester, Massachusetts; Research Biochemist, VA Hospital, Bedford, Massachusetts

Roxanne A. Vrees, MD, Clinical Instructor, Department of Obstetrics and Gynecology, Women and Infants Hospital, Brown Medical School, Providence, Rhode Island

David J. Wainwright, MD, Associate Professor, Division of Plastic and Reconstructive Surgery, University of Texas Medical School at Houston, Houston, Texas

Yanni Wang, PhD, International Biomedical Communications, Frederick, Maryland

Rita M. Washko, MD, MPH, Physician, NHANES (National Health and Nutrition Examination Survey), Westat Research Corporation, Rockville, Maryland

Y. Etan Weinstock, Resident in Otolaryngology/Head and Neck Surgery, University of Texas at Houston, Health Science Center, Houston, Texas

Emily M. White, MD, Clinical Instructor, Department of Obstetrics and Gynecology, Women and Infants Hospital, Brown Medical School, Providence, Rhode Island

Tonya White, MD, Assistant Professor, Division of Child and Adolescent Psychiatry, University of Minnesota, Minneapolis, Minnesota

Michael Windelspecht, PhD, Blowing Rock, North Carolina

Euson Yeung, BScPT, MEd, FCAMT, Department of Physical Therapy, Faculty of Medicine, University of Toronto, Ontario, Canada

Jon H. Zonderman, AB, MS, Orange, Connecticut

Stephen D. Zucker, MD, Associate Professor of Medicine, Director, Gastroenterology Training Program, Division of Digestive Diseases, University of Cincinnati, Cincinnati, Ohio

Contents

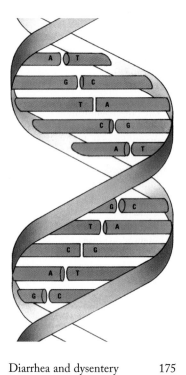

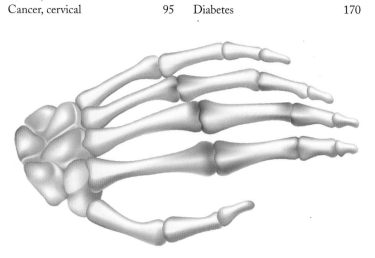

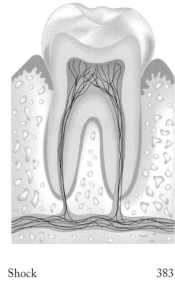
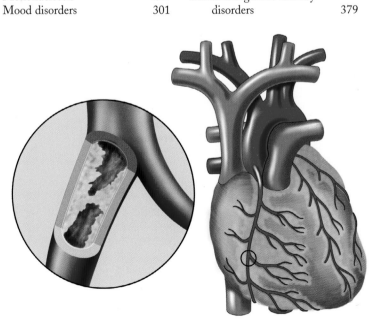

9

Thematic contents

Each article in the *Encyclopedia of Diseases and Disorders* falls into one of three categories: infections; noninfectious diseases and disorders; and mental disorders. Articles in these three categories are color coded:

INFECTIONS	NONINFECTIOUS DISEASES AND DISORDERS	MENTAL DISORDERS

Infections include systemic, local, contagious, and noncontagious infections by bacteria, viruses, protists, parasites, and other pathogens.

The category of infections includes disorders such as acne, a localized bacterial infection, which is not contagious, as well as infectious diseases such as the common cold, which is highly contagious.

The category of noninfectious diseases and disorders includes any medical disorder not defined as an infection.

The category of mental disorders includes conditions that manifest behavioral, psychological, or biological dysfunction in the person.

Infections

Noninfectious diseases and disorders

Mental disorders

Acne

The most common skin disorder in the United States, acne is related to the activity of the skin's oil glands. Overactivity of the glands clogs hair follicles in the skin, resulting in pimples or acne. Although not life threatening, severe acne can lead to disfiguring and permanent scarring as well as emotional distress.

Acne is a disorder of the body's pilosebaceous units. Each unit consists of a sebaceous gland and a canal or follicle, which is lined with cells called keratinocytes and which contains a fine hair. Most numerous in the skin of the face, upper back, and chest, sebaceous glands manufacture an oily substance called sebum, which is released onto the skin's surface through the follicle's opening, or pore.

All the constituents of the narrow follicle—the hair, sebum, and keratinocytes—may form a plug that prevents the sebum from reaching the surface of the skin through the pore. The plug allows a strain of bacterium, called *Propionibacterium acnes*, to multiply in the plugged follicle. As bacteria build up, white blood cells accumulate, causing inflammation. The wall of the plugged follicle eventually breaks down, and the bacteria form a pimple at the skin's surface.

Causes

Although the cause of acne is currently unknown, researchers link its development to several related factors. One important factor is an increase in hormones called androgens. The levels of androgens in the body increase during puberty in both boys and girls, causing the sebaceous glands to enlarge and produce more sebum. Genetics, or heredity, is also thought to be a factor, as well as environmental irritants such as pollution and high humidity, which can plug the follicles.

Symptoms

Acne can appear in a variety of forms. The most basic form is called the comedo, which is simply an enlarged hair follicle that has become plugged. If the comedo stays below the skin's surface, it forms a white bump called a whitehead. If the comedo reaches the surface of the skin and opens up, it forms a blackhead. Other types of acne include inflamed bumps called papules; pus-filled pimples called pustules; solid bumps lodged in the skin called nodules; and deep, pus-filled bumps called cysts, which often result in scarring. Acne can affect people of all ages and races. However, the disorder is most common in young people—nearly 80 percent of people between the ages of 12 and 24 develop acne.

Treatments and prevention

Many people with acne seek treatment from dermatologists (doctors who specialize in skin disorders). Over-the-counter and prescription medications are helpful in treating existing pimples, as well as preventing new ones from forming. Doctors may prescribe a combination of oral and topical medications that reduce inflammation and clumping of cells in the follicles, or that kill bacteria. These medications come in a variety of forms: antibiotics or

CAUSE OF SKIN SPOTS

Skin spots can form when an excessive amount of sebum becomes trapped and clogs the pores on the surface of the skin. The trapped sebum forms a plug that is raised at the top. The plug forms a blackhead when exposed to the air. Around the plug the skin becomes inflamed and infected; the result is a pimple or spot filled with pus. The pimple may become red and swollen and painful to touch.

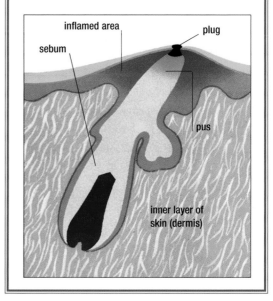

inflamed area
plug
sebum
pus
inner layer of skin (dermis)

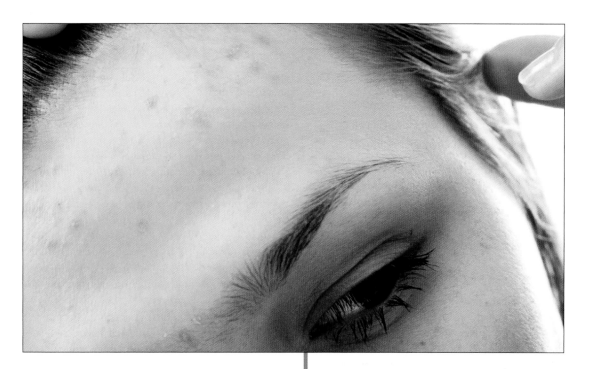

KEY FACTS

Description

A skin disorder related to the overproduction of sebum in the skin's glands, resulting in outbreaks of pimples, pustules, or nodules.

Causes

Exact cause is unknown, although it is linked to the increased production of hormones called androgens, which cause the sebaceous glands to enlarge and produce more sebum.

Symptoms

Any of various types of pimples on or in the skin.

Diagnosis

Serious cases may need examination by a dermatologist, a doctor who specializes in skin disorders.

Treatments

Medications including benzoyl peroxide and antibiotics reduce bacteria and inflammation. Retinoids unblock pores.

Pathogenesis

Blockage of hair follicle leads to a buildup of sebum, bacteria, and pus, forming a pimple.

Prevention

Medication can prevent outbreaks, and acne can be controlled by proper care of the skin.

Epidemiology

People of all ages and races can get acne. However, it is most common in adolescents.

benzoyl peroxide to kill bacteria, or retinoids (chemically related to vitamin A) to unblock pores. Niacinamide (nicotinamide) cream reduces inflammation, though it is available only by prescription in the United States. Early treatment is important to prevent scarring. Pimples should be left alone to heal—squeezing and picking can cause scarring.

Because the underlying cause of acne is unknown, there are currently no preventive measures, although many medications are successful in preventing new pimples. In addition, proper care of the skin may help prevent outbreaks. Skin should be cleaned gently with a mild cleanser. Strong detergent soaps and rough scrubbing often worsen rather than improve acne.

Epidemiology

Acne is a worldwide skin condition that is most common in adolescents, particularly males. The condition can also run in families. Drug-induced acne or occupational acne is more rare.

Julie McDowell

See also
• Dermatitis

Adrenal disorders

The adrenal glands secrete hormones that have widespread effects on the body. Adrenal disorders usually involve either over- or underproduction of hormones. Overproduction is often the result of an adrenal tumor. Underproduction may have various causes, including tumors, autoimmune diseases, and infections. Sometimes adrenal disorders result from disorders of the pituitary gland or hypothalamus, other endocrine organs that influence the adrenal glands.

The adrenal glands form part of the body's endocrine system, which is a network of glands that produce interacting hormones. The hormones affect numerous body functions, and sometimes hormones from one endocrine gland can affect other endocrine organs; for example, the adrenal glands are influenced by hormones produced by both the pituitary gland and the hypothalamus.

The body has two adrenal glands, one near the top of each kidney. The gland's main function is to produce hormones. The adrenal cortex (outer layer) produces the corticosteroids cortisol, aldosterone, and adrenal androgens (male sex hormones). The adrenal medulla (inner layer) produces epinephrine and norepinephrine. Cortisol plays a role in the body's metabolism of carbohydrates, lipids, and proteins, helps the body cope with stress, influences growth and development, and is involved in the healthy functioning of the immune system. Aldosterone helps regulate levels of sodium and potassium in the body, two minerals that influence blood pressure. Adrenal androgens affect the development of secondary sexual characteristics, such as body hair. Epinephrine and norepinephrine play a key role in the body's immediate reaction to stress by triggering the "fight-or-flight" response.

Causes and types

Adrenal disorders are often caused by nonmalignant tumors called adrenal adenomas. Adenomas arise from the adrenal cortex and can occur at any age, although they are more common with increasing age. The reason adenomas develop is not known, but it is thought they may arise from genetic mutations that have not yet been identified. Rarely, a malignant tumor may arise in the adrenal cortex; this type of tumor is called an adrenocortical carcinoma. More commonly, malignant tumors in the adrenal glands result from the metastasis (spread) of cancer from elsewhere in the body. Malignant melanoma (a type of skin cancer), lung cancer, and breast cancer are the types most commonly associated with adrenal metastases.

Tumors may cause symptoms by growing so large that they press on surrounding organs or by affecting the production of adrenal hormones. A tumor that produces hormones is described as functioning; one that does not produce hormones is nonfunctioning. Both adenomas and adrenocortical carcinomas may be functioning or nonfunctioning; metastatic tumors are nonfunctioning. Functioning tumors cause various disorders depending on the hormone produced.

Overproduction of cortisol is known as Cushing's syndrome, and this may result from a functioning tumor or from excess pituitary hormones overstimulating the adrenal gland. Cushing's syndrome can also result from long-term treatment with corticosteroid medications such as prednisone. Overproduction of aldosterone is called hyperaldosteronism, and it is usually caused by a functioning tumor. Overproduction of adrenal androgens is also usually caused by a functioning tumor and may result in virilization (the development of masculine characteristics) in women or feminization in men. Overproduction of epinephrine and norepinephrine is caused by functioning tumors of the adrenal medulla called pheochromocytomas.

Underproduction of the adrenal hormones is known as adrenal insufficiency. Addison's disease results from an adrenal insufficiency in which the adrenal cortex produces too little corticosteroids. It may be caused by an autoimmune disorder (in which the immune system attacks the adrenal glands), by infections such as tuberculosis, by insufficient stimulating hormones from the pituitary gland or hypothalamus, or by large metastatic cancers or nonfunctioning adrenocortical carcinomas. Suddenly stopping corticosteroid medication can cause a rapid fall in the body's natural level of corticosteroids, which is a potentially fatal event known as an Addisonian crisis.

Symptoms and signs

Most adrenal adenomas do not produce symptoms. However, adenomas and other nonfunctioning tumors that grow very large may press on other organs, producing abdominal pain and weight loss. Symptoms also occur when hormone production is affected, either as a result of a functioning tumor or other causes.

Symptoms and signs of Cushing's syndrome include acne, weight gain around the chest and abdomen, abdominal stretch marks, facial changes, which may become rounded and red, deposits of fat between the shoulder blades, excessive hair growth, diabetes mellitus, muscle weakness, and high blood pressure. Adrenal insufficiencies can cause fatigue, muscle weakness, thirst, excessive urination, and high blood pressure. Tests often reveal low levels of sodium and high levels of potassium in the blood. Overproduction of adrenal androgens may produce exaggerated male secondary sexual characteristics, which often go unnoticed in men but may produce virilization in women.

Symptoms of virilization include excessive hair growth, acne, deepening of the voice, muscularity, reduction in breast size, and menstrual abnormalities. In some men excess androgens are converted to estrogens (female sex hormones), which may cause gynecomastia (breast enlargement). Symptoms of overproduction of epinephrine and norepinephrine include high blood pressure, palpitations, excessive sweating, and headaches.

Adrenal insufficiency and Addison's disease may produce weakness, fatigue, dizziness, weight loss, nausea, darkening of the skin, sensitivity to cold, and low blood pressure. An Addisonian crisis, an acute episode that can sometimes result from an infection, can cause dehydration, extreme weakness, abdominal pain, confusion, and very low blood pressure; without prompt treatment it may be fatal.

Diagnosis, treatments, and prevention

Adrenal disorders are usually diagnosed from their symptoms, through blood and/or urine tests to measure the levels of hormones and sodium and potassium, and by computed tomography (CT) or magnetic resonance imaging (MRI) scans. However, the majority of adrenal adenomas are discovered incidentally when scans are done for other reasons.

The treatment for adrenal disorders depends on the specific disorder. Small, nonfunctioning adrenal adenomas usually require only regular follow-up scans. Large adenomas and functioning tumors that cause hormone overproduction may be treated by surgery to remove the tumor or the entire affected gland. Chemotherapy may also be used, and it is also the principal treatment for metastatic tumors. Treatment of adrenal overproduction may additionally include medications to block hormone production. If the underlying cause of adrenal overproduction is a pituitary or hypothalamus disorder, the treatment is directed primarily at the underlying cause. Adrenal insufficiency and Addison's disease are both treated with hormone replacement medications. An Addisonian crisis requires urgent hospital treatment, including intravenous fluids, glucose, and corticosteroid injections.

There is no known way of preventing adrenal disorders or reducing the risk of developing them because the fundamental causes have not been established.

Mary Ruppe

KEY FACTS: ADENOMAS

Description
Noncancerous tumor of the adrenal glands.

Cause
The cause of adrenal adenomas is unknown, although they may be related to genetic mutations not yet identified.

Risk factor
Increasing age.

Symptoms and signs
Most adenomas do not cause symptoms. When symptoms occur they vary according to which hormone is overproduced as well as the size of the adenoma.

Diagnosis
CT or MRI scan. Laboratory tests on blood or urine samples.

Treatments
Adenomas that are small or are not producing hormones usually require only clinical follow-ups with periodic scans. Large or hormone-producing adenomas may be treated by surgery or hormone-blocking medication, or both.

Pathogenesis
The origination of adenomas is not known and their development is variable: they may remain small and/or nonfunctioning or they may grow and/or produce hormones.

Prevention
There are no known ways of preventing adenomas.

Epidemiology
An estimated 2 to 10 percent of people in the United States have adenomas. In those older than 60 the estimated prevalence is 6 percent.

See also
• Cancer, breast • Cancer, lung
• Cancer, skin

AIDS

AIDS is the acronym for acquired immune deficiency syndrome, a chronic life-threatening disease caused by the human immunodeficiency virus (HIV). AIDS is described as chronic because it persists over a long period of time. This virus attacks the immune system, allowing diseases and certain cancers to develop that would otherwise be thwarted by a healthy immune response. First recognized in 1981, AIDS has progressed from a disease considered to be uniformly fatal to one in which, with targeted treatment, prolonged survival is now a possibility.

First identified in the United States in 1981, this life-threatening disease is thought to date back to the mid-1970s and possibly earlier. It is believed that the virus was transmitted to humans from exposure to the blood of monkeys in Africa. Since the recognition of AIDS, it has gone from a disease perceived to affect only homosexual men to a pandemic that knows no age, gender, racial, or geographic barrier. Availability of therapy for AIDS, however, is a different story. Despite the development of new drugs that have revolutionized the treatment of AIDS—decreasing opportunistic infections and prolonging lives—only about 15 percent of those in need of treatment have access to these drugs.

According to the Joint United Nations Programme on HIV and AIDS, the area most affected by the pandemic is sub-Saharan Africa, where, in 2007, there were 22.5 million people living with HIV and 1.7 million new HIV infections. The magnitude of the AIDS pandemic in Africa has had a profound impact on families, society, and life expectancy. In several African countries, life expectancy at birth has dipped below 40 years.

Also in 2007, there were 2.1 million people living with AIDS and 78,000 new infections reported in the combined region of North America and Western and Central Europe. In these countries, affected people have access to AIDS treatment, unlike the affected people who are living in less developed areas of the world.

Causes

HIV, identified as the causative agent of AIDS in 1983, belongs to a family of viruses called retroviruses. HIV attacks cells that have a CD4 receptor on their surface. Such cells include a type of white blood cell called a CD4 lymphocyte. This type of cell plays a major role in coordinating the body's immune defenses against foreign substances, such as harmful bacteria and viruses.

HIV is found in the blood, semen, vaginal fluid, and breast milk of infected people. It is also present in their saliva and tears. However, saliva and tears have not been shown to facilitate HIV infection.

Risk factors

Unprotected sexual intercourse with an HIV-infected partner can result in contracting HIV by contact with the infected blood, semen, or vaginal secretions. Transmission can occur via vaginal, anal, or oral sex. Infected blood and blood products can also transmit the virus. However, this type of transmission is much less likely since the United States began screening its blood supply for the presence of antibodies to HIV in 1985. Additionally, a heat treatment to kill HIV was also implemented, further ensuring a safer blood supply. Intravenous drug users can contract HIV by using needles that are contaminated with HIV-infected blood. Health care workers can be infected with HIV as a result of accidental needlestick injuries, although this risk of infection is low. HIV can be transmitted from mother to child during pregnancy, childbirth, or through breast feeding. Ninety percent of children with HIV are infected in this manner.

Other reported ways in which the virus is known to have been transmitted are through surgical instruments that are contaminated with HIV and through tissue and organ transplants.

AIDS cannot be spread through casual contact such as shaking hands, coming into contact with sweat or tears, or sharing food, utensils, or other items such as a toilet seat with someone who has HIV infection or AIDS. There also is no evidence that HIV infection can be transmitted by kissing. The virus requires a human host to replicate and therefore cannot be transmitted by insects.

Symptoms and signs

The symptoms and signs of HIV infection and AIDS depend upon the stage of the illness. Initially, a person infected with the virus may have no symptoms at all or may have a brief flulike illness. This stage is referred to as primary HIV infection. Common complaints are headache, fever, sore throat, swollen lymph nodes, and rash. About one-fifth of these people seek evaluation by a physician; however, the diagnosis is often missed at this time because the symptoms are nonspecific and resolve spontaneously. The HIV-infected person is nevertheless highly infective during this time and can transmit the disease to others. This transmission is all the more possible because he or she may be unaware of his or her infection with HIV.

After a few weeks of rapid replication by the virus, B lymphocytes begin to produce antibodies to HIV. The process of production of antibodies is known as seroconversion and usually occurs within four to ten weeks after exposure to HIV. The presence of antibodies to HIV is the basis for HIV testing. A negative result could occur if testing for HIV happens before seroconversion. By six months after contracting the virus, at least 95 percent of people infected with HIV test positive for HIV.

Following primary infection, the individual may remain free of symptoms for several years. During this stage, which is called latency, the only abnormality an HIV-infected person may present, on physical examination, is persistent enlargement of the lymph nodes. However, the virus is anything but dormant. It remains active in the lymph nodes, where it continues to attack the immune system, producing large quantities of virus and killing CD4 T cells. The small amount of HIV found outside of the lymph nodes and in the bloodstream can be detected by a viral load test, a procedure that measures the virus's RNA.

Eventually, the number of CD4 T cells (CD4 count) begins to fall and the individual is now in the early stage of symptomatic HIV infection. "Class B" diseases, as defined by the Centers for Disease Control and Prevention (CDC), occur during this period. Rapid weight loss is common along with other persistent symptoms including fatigue, diarrhea, headache, night sweats, and fevers. Dry cough and shortness of breath, sores of mucous membranes, and blurred vision or other visual defects may develop. These disorders are not AIDS-defining illnesses because they can occur in people without AIDS; however, they tend to be more severe and persistent in those who are infected with HIV.

KEY FACTS

Description

Chronic, life-threatening, infectious disease that affects many body systems.

Cause

Infection with human immunodeficiency virus (HIV), a virus that attacks and weakens the immune system.

Risk factors

Unprotected sexual intercourse (oral, vaginal, or anal) with someone infected with HIV or exposure to HIV-contaminated blood or breast milk. Babies born to HIV-positive mothers are at increased risk; transmission also has occurred from organ and tissue transplants, blood transfusions, and from unsterilized surgical instruments.

Symptoms

Depend on stage of disease but in general involve fatigue, weight loss, sweating, diarrhea, enlargement of lymph nodes, coughing, and problems with the nervous system such as memory loss. Initial symptoms, if present, mimic a flulike illness. As the disease progresses, opportunistic infections and cancers, which afflict persons with a weakened immune system, occur.

Diagnosis

HIV infection: blood test or oral test for antibodies to the virus. AIDS: HIV infection and presence of an AIDS-defining illness.

Treatments

Antiretroviral drugs have had a dramatic impact on progression but do not cure AIDS.

Pathogenesis

The virus infects white blood cells called CD4 cells, which help fight infection. It inserts its own genetic material into the CD4 T cells, making copies of itself. The CD4 T cells die, and viruses infect more of these cells. Although the body responds by increasing its production of CD4 T cells, the virus ultimately prevails. As the number of CD4 T cells falls, the body becomes susceptible to opportunistic infections and certain cancers.

Prevention

No vaccine is available. Avoidance of behaviors that would allow infected blood, semen, vaginal secretions, or breast milk into the body.

Epidemiology

In 2007 an estimated 33 million people worldwide—31 million adults and 2 million children—had HIV infection or AIDS; almost 2.7 million people acquired HIV infection; and 2 million people died from AIDS. In 2007 about 1.2 million people in the United States had HIV infection or AIDS, and about 22,000 people died from AIDS.

Conditions that define a diagnosis of AIDS have been set forth by the CDC. They include certain opportunistic infections, for example, *Pneumocystis carinii* pneumonia, and cancers such as Kaposi's sarcoma, as well as a CD4 count that is less than 200 cells/mm^3. (A normal CD4 count is 600 to 1,500 cells/mm^3.) As AIDS progresses, advanced HIV infection results, with a CD4 count that is less than 50 cells/mm^3 and an expected survival of only 12 to 18 months without antiretroviral therapy. Most people who contract HIV infection and AIDS die within 10 years without treatment. A small proportion of 4 to 7 percent of those infected survive for 13 or more years without treatment. These long-term nonprogressors are thought to produce robust immune responses to the virus.

In children, similar signifiers are applied to define various stages of HIV infection or AIDS. Opportunistic diseases of children are used as indicators of AIDS. In developing countries, where access to standard testing is often lacking, a more general definition is used. This AIDS-defining definition includes signs of immune deficiency with the exclusion of other known causes of immunosuppression, such as cancer and kidney disease.

Diagnosis

A diagnosis of HIV infection usually is made by detecting HIV-specific antibodies in a blood sample. The test most commonly used is an enzyme-linked immunosorbent assay (ELISA) test, which, if positive, is then confirmed by a blood test called a Western blot. This test detects the presence of specific antibodies to HIV proteins and is a necessary step in ELISA-positive samples because some ELISA-test results are falsely positive. It may take up to 2 weeks to get the results for these tests. Diagnosis can also be made by checking for the HIV viral p24 antigen or, less commonly, by culturing HIV.

More recently, rapid HIV testing has become available. One such test uses a drop of blood from a finger prick and another uses secretions collected from a pad rubbed against the gums. This oral test has a sensitivity of detecting the presence of HIV that is very close to that for blood testing. Results are available within 20 to 60 minutes. In addition, there is currently a Food and Drug Administration (FDA) home test available to check for HIV. In this test, a drop of blood placed on the specified testing media is mailed, and the results are available by calling a toll-free number. However, the CDC recommends confirmation of positive test results with standard laboratory tests for HIV infection.

Once a diagnosis is made, a viral load test is done to determine the amount of HIV present. Results are used to decide when to initiate treatment and when to make changes in treatment regimens. The affected person should be counseled to practice behaviors that prevent transmission of HIV to others, such as abstaining from sex or using condoms if they choose to continue sexual activity, and refraining from donating blood, semen, or body tissues (although most countries now screen such donations). A diagnosis of AIDS occurs with a positive test result for HIV infection and the presence of an AIDS-defining illness, such as Kaposi's sarcoma.

Treatments

Early treatment is important because it helps preserve immune function, reduces the frequency and severity of opportunistic infections, improves well-being, and prolongs survival. Antibiotics, antifungal drugs, and antiviral drugs for opportunistic infections play a major role in therapy, but more important, there are antiretroviral drugs available to fight HIV. The first of the antiretroviral drugs became available in 1987. Nine years later, highly active antiretroviral therapy (HAART) was introduced, a process involving treatment with three or more drugs active against HIV. This "cocktail" more readily suppresses the virus because HIV has the capacity to mutate (change) and become resistant to drug therapy. HAART can be used in all stages of HIV infection or AIDS. Although there is a risk of toxicity with HAART, the benefits are remarkable. During the first three years of HAART, a 60 to 80 percent reduction was noted in AIDS-defining diagnoses, deaths, and AIDS-related hospitalizations. In other countries where these medicines are available, similar results have been seen. However, HAART treatment is prohibitively expensive for most people with HIV infection or AIDS, costing upward of $12,000 per year. Although treatment provides great benefit—people living with HIV are able to lead longer, healthier lives—it is not a cure and may be needed lifelong.

Pathogenesis

Once an HIV particle enters a CD4 cell, it inserts its own genetic material into the host cell. The genetic material of retroviruses is RNA (ribonucleic acid); transcription (conversion) of the HIV genes from RNA to DNA (deoxyribonucleic acid) is made

HUMAN IMMUNODEFICIENCY VIRUS (HIV)

The human immunodeficiency virus (HIV) can invade many different cells in the body but appears to mainly target certain types of white cells of the human immune system. These cells are called CD4 lymphocytes and they are responsible for fighting infection in the body. The genetic information of the virus is in the form of ribonucleic acid (RNA), but this is altered by enzymic action into DNA (deoxyribonucleic acid) so that the viral DNA can invade the host cell's chromosomes. The virus multiplies in the infected cells, which then die. More virus is released into the blood stream. To begin with, the immune system fights against the virus, but if the infection remains untreated and more CD4 lymphocytes are destroyed, the immune system is unable to cope.

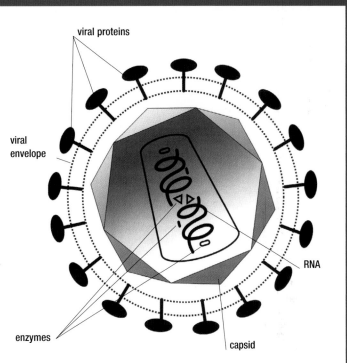

possible by the enzyme reverse transcriptase. This process allows HIV to integrate into the host cell's genetic material and begin to produce copies of itself. Billions of new HIV particles can be produced daily in this manner, a process that the human immune system tries to counteract by producing more CD4 cells. Initially, the number of viruses (viral load) in the body is high because no antibodies (proteins that attack specific targets) have yet been formed to the virus. Later, different types of white blood cells called B lymphocytes begin to produce antibodies to the virus. These HIV-specific antibodies cause a fall in the viral level, but the virus progressively reaches higher levels, the host's CD4 level falls, and a severe immune deficiency results. The infection progresses to AIDS when the individual begins to suffer from certain cancers or infections of disease-causing bacteria and viruses. Often these are infectious agents that do not cause illness in healthy persons and are referred to as opportunistic infections.

Without treatment, a person with HIV infection lives about 10 years after becoming infected. With treatment, this interval is different. However, data to project accurate estimates are not yet available. The

viral load has been found to be the main predictor of how quickly HIV progresses in the early stages, whereas CD4 counts are important in this regard during later stages. Without treatment, the viral load stabilizes around six months after HIV infection and then slowly but steadily increases. CD4 counts do the opposite, with a decline of about 50 cells per mm^3 per year.

Prevention

Various successes have been achieved in preventing HIV infection and in treating people with HIV infection or AIDS. Educational programs have raised awareness of issues central to HIV prevention, providing people with the tools necessary to reduce individual risk.

Treatment of HIV-infected mothers with zidovudine (ZDV) has reduced the transmission of HIV infection to babies. The AIDS Clinical Trial Group Protocol—a study involving prevention of perinatal HIV infection—showed that treatment of HIV-infected mothers with ZDV reduced HIV infection in the child from 25.5 to 8.3 percent. Treatment of people after recent contact with an

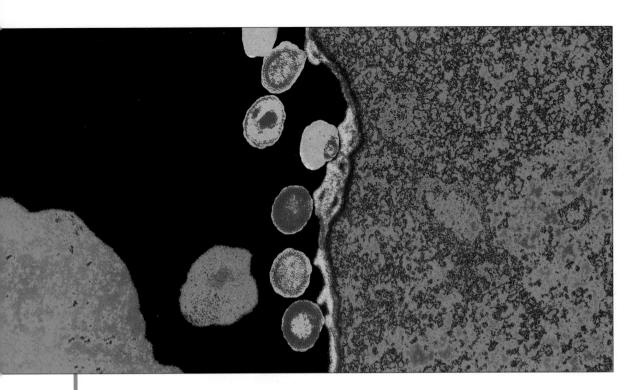

An electron micrograph shows human immunodeficiency virus particles bursting from an infected CD4 lymphocyte. The infected cell is part of the immune system; once cells are destroyed and numbers fall, the immune system starts to fail.

HIV-infected person or after exposure to the virus—for example, after an accidental needlestick injury—is called postexposure prophylaxis. This involves giving two or three antiretroviral drugs, and it has prevented many new infections. Although improved survival has been achieved with recent therapies, it has had the adverse effect, in some cases, of an increase in risky sexual behavior.

An area of ongoing concern in prevention of HIV transmission involves the estimated 25 percent of HIV-infected people who are unaware of their infection. Given this situation, they may not take appropriate precautions, making it more likely that they spread the disease. However, anonymous testing has most likely increased the number of people tested for HIV and thus may have decreased the pool of those unknowingly carrying the virus.

Preventive efforts are challenged by the shifting patterns of HIV transmission. In many areas, patterns of infection have been changing, further taxing the preventive efforts of aid agencies and governments alike. In recent times, heterosexual transmission has become the primary mode of transmission with more than 80 percent of new HIV infections resulting from unprotected heterosexual contact. Now, half of all HIV and AIDS cases are identified in women. In many parts of Asia, the area with the world's second largest number of HIV infections, injection of drugs is fueling the pandemic.

To keep up with effective public health measures—such as free condoms—requires ongoing surveillance of the HIV infection and AIDS pandemic and a system that can respond in an efficient, effective manner. Data that allow accurate predictions of public health needs, such as determining at-risk groups and risk factors, must be available. Even so, future projections can be very difficult to make owing to many of the previously mentioned factors. As an example, the worldwide prevalence of HIV infection reported in 2004 was more than 50 percent higher than WHO (the World Health Organization) predicted in 1991.

Until a vaccine is developed to prevent HIV infection, educational and public-health strategies will continue to be the mainstay of preventive interventions and control of the pandemic.

Rita Washko

See also
• Pneumonia

Albinism

Albinism refers to a rare condition in which there is a lack of the pigment melanin. Albinism is an inherited defect, which results in little or no pigment in hair, eyes, or skin. It also causes significant visual problems.

Albinism refers to a group of related genetic conditions affecting melanin production. People with albinism have little or no pigment in their eyes, skin, or hair; they can also suffer from visual problems. Some are legally blind; other affected people have vision good enough to drive a car. There are different kinds of albinism, but the most common and severe form, oculocutaneous albinism, causes people to have white hair and skin and pink irises, the normally colored part of the eye. Albinism occurs in people of all races.

Causes and risk factors

Albinism is a genetic disorder caused by a defect in the genes that are involved in the production of the pigment melanin. Almost all types of albinism result from both parents carrying the gene for the condition. Everybody carries two copies of most genes (except for the sex chromosome genes)—one set from each parent. If a person carries one gene for normal pigmentation and one gene for albinism, he or she will have enough genetic material to produce normal pigmentation and therefore will not have albinism. However, if a person has inherited two albinism genes (one from each parent) and therefore has no gene for normal pigmentation, she or he will have albinism. When both parents carry an albinism gene, even though neither parent has the disorder, there is a one in four risk that any baby of theirs will have albinism.

The visual problems associated with this condition result from the abnormal development of the retina and abnormal patterns of nerve connections between the eyes and the brain.

Diagnosis

Albinism is often obvious at birth from the symptoms—lack of pigmentation. It can be confirmed with a DNA test to determine the presence of the albinism gene. Associated visual problems can be detected through eye examinations.

Treatments

Treatment for albinism focuses on easing symptoms. The skin is more sensitive to the sun's ultraviolet (UV) rays; because extended exposure to UV increases the risk of skin cancer, any exposed skin must be protected from the sun by the use of sunscreens with a high sun protection factor (SPF). The eyes should be protected by sunglasses with high UV protection.

Vision problems associated with albinism can be treated with surgery. One common visual problem that can be corrected with surgery is strabismus, a muscle imbalance of the eyes resulting in "crossed eyes" or a "lazy eye." However, surgery cannot correct the misrouting of nerves from the eyes to the brain, which severely impairs vision, and optical aids such as contact lenses, bifocals, or other bioptics are often worn.

Julie McDowell

KEY FACTS

Description
Albinism is an absence of pigment from the hair, skin, or iris of the eyes.

Causes
Albinism results from a lack of the pigment melanin because of a genetic defect.

Symptoms and signs
Little or no pigment in the hair, eyes, or skin; decreased vision or blindness; skin cancer.

Diagnosis
DNA test to determine the presence of the albinism gene.

Treatments
Visual aids, such as prescription glasses and contact lenses, for visual problems. To prevent damage from the sun, protection such as sunglasses and high sun-protection-factor sunscreen, or avoidance of sun exposure.

Pathogenesis
Because albinism is a genetic condition, it emerges at birth and remains for life.

Prevention
Testing for abnormal genes, genetic counseling.

Epidemiology
Albinism can affect people from all races.

See also
- Cancer, skin

Alcohol-related disorders

While many people consume alcohol without deleterious effects, there are a significant percentage of individuals who experience serious adverse consequences. Both alcohol intoxication and withdrawal can be life threatening. Alcohol is a toxin that affects nearly all organ systems, and the medical consequences from heavy alcohol use are legion. Alcohol dependence is an addictive disorder that has significant social, financial, psychological, and physical consequences.

Ethyl alcohol is a small and rather simple molecule that is found in many beverages that are consumed by people throughout the world. Indeed, alcoholic beverages have been used in social and religious settings for thousands of years. The ability of alcohol to access the brain accounts for its intoxicating and addictive properties.

Alcohol intoxication

The degree of alcohol intoxication is proportional to the amount of alcohol in the bloodstream (blood alcohol level; BAL), which is easily measured directly or inferred from a measurement of an exhaled breath. Alcohol is a depressant, although the depression of inhibitions may make it appear as if an individual is under the influence of a stimulant, especially at lower levels. Coordination impairment as well as mood and behavior changes occur with levels as low as 20–30 milligrams (mg) per 100 milliliters (ml), the equivalent of one to two standard drinks. A standard drink is defined as approximately 12 ounces (350 ml) of beer, 5 ounces of table wine, or 1½ ounces of 80 proof spirits (hard liquor). Further mental and physical impairment occur as blood alcohol levels rise. At levels above 200 mg/100 ml, individuals are clearly intoxicated. Amnesia, severe slurred speech, loss of coordinatory function, and hypothermia can occur at levels of 300 mg/100 ml. Coma is induced at levels above 400 mg/100 ml, and levels above 600 mg/100 ml can be fatal. Individuals who have a tolerance for alcohol due to frequent and heavy exposure may require a higher BAL before experiencing these symptoms.

Alcohol withdrawal

Alcohol withdrawal is a syndrome that results after the abrupt cessation or decrease in intake of alcohol. Risk factors include the amount and duration of drinking.

Symptoms and signs generally appear within 24 hours after the last drink. The manifestations of alcohol withdrawal can be grouped into three categories: neurological subjective complaints, neurological objective findings, and the hyperadrenergic state. Subjective complaints include anxiety, agitation, and hallucinations. Objective signs include hyperactive reflexes, tremor, elevated body temperature, confusion, delirium, and seizures. Findings characteristic of a hyperadrenergic state are rapid heart rate, elevated blood pressure, sweating, and dilated pupils.

The American Society of Addiction Medicine has identified three stages of alcohol withdrawal. These include mild reactions (Stage I), alcoholic hallucinosis (Stage II), and delirium tremens (Stage III). Stage I is characterized by mild elevations in blood pressure, heart rate, and temperature. Patients are usually anxious and agitated and often manifest a tremor. They remain aware of their surroundings, however, and do not hallucinate or lose consciousness. Hallucinations are the hallmark of stage II withdrawal. However, patients have insight into their hallucinations, that is, they know they are hallucinating. In addition, they may have a greater degree of stage I findings. Delirium tremens is a medical emergency and is characterized by significant elevations in heart rate and blood pressure, which can eventually lead to cardiovascular collapse and death. Patients do not have insight into their hallucinations and may become terrified by them. They are unaware of their surroundings and lapse in and out of consciousness. Although the staging system is a helpful way to conceptualize withdrawal, the stages constitute a continuum of the same disease process.

Seizures may occur in any stage of alcohol withdrawal without any warning. They are usually grand mal seizures and occur within 48 hours of the last drink. The most significant risk factor for an alcohol withdrawal seizure is a prior alcohol withdrawal seizure. Alcohol withdrawal is a treatable disorder. Those at risk should be monitored and treated with medications if needed. Sedatives such as barbiturates and benzodiazepines have been used for decades to treat alcohol withdrawal. Benzodiazepines have a greater safety profile and are preferred. The goal of treatment is to prevent the progression to delirium tremens and to prevent seizures.

Alcohol dependence

Alcohol dependence is a serious public health problem affecting up to 10 percent of men and 5 percent of women. Studies show that it is often unrecognized. It affects not only the alcoholic but also has significant consequences for the alcoholic's family and the rest of society. It is a disorder characterized by the persistent, compulsive, and maladaptive use of alcohol. Individuals who suffer from this disease continue to drink alcohol despite the negative consequences they experience from doing so. These consequences are financial, social, familial, job-related, psychological, and physical. *The Diagnostic and Statistical Manual*, which lists diagnostic criteria for all recognized psychiatric disorders, provides the following criteria for alcohol dependence. Three or more of the following need to be present over a 12-month period: tolerance; withdrawal; substance taken often in larger amounts or over a longer period than intended; persistent desire or attempts to cut down, or both; increased time acquiring, using, and recovering from the substance; giving up of important social and occupational, or recreational responsibilities, or both; continued use despite knowledge that there is a persistent physical or psychological problem that is likely to have been caused or exacerbated by the substance.

Like other chronic diseases, such as hypertension and diabetes mellitus, alcoholism is characterized by relapses and remissions. It is also a separate and distinct disorder—not a symptom of another psychiatric illness such as depression or anxiety. The seat of addiction is in the unconscious portion of the brain in an area of the midbrain known as the nucleus accumbens. The normal function of the nucleus accumbens is to reinforce life-sustaining or species-sustaining behaviors—for example, food and water intake and sexual behavior. Normally, when an individual engages in these behaviors a neurotransmitter called dopamine is released in the nucleus accumbens. The behavior that stimulated the release of dopamine is interpreted by the brain as a behavior that should be repeated again and again. There is evidence that addictive drugs of all classes activate the dopamine system. In the alcoholic brain, therefore, alcohol exposure causes the release of dopamine in the nucleus accumbens, and the brain interprets alcohol ingestion as a behavior that is just as important as food or water intake. Thus, alcohol alters the normal functioning of the nucleus accumbens.

Obviously, not everyone who is exposed to alcohol becomes an alcoholic, so there must be differences among individuals concerning the susceptibility of their brains to alcohol dependence. This susceptibility or predisposition has both genetic and environmental (exposure) components.

Research continues in both the areas of genetics (to identify the actual genes involved) and neurochemistry (to determine the effects of alcohol exposure on the brain). Variation in predisposition may explain why some individuals are alcoholics early in life with little alcohol exposure, while others manifest symptoms much later and only after significant exposure.

KEY FACTS

Description
A compulsive, maladaptive use of alcohol.

Causes
Believed to be an interpretation by the brain that alcohol is necessary to the system.

Risk factors
Amount of alcohol ingested and the frequency and duration of drinking.

Symptoms and signs
Continued use of alcohol despite negative consequences.

Diagnosis
There are criteria established in *The Diagnostic and Statistical Manual*.

Treatments
Alcoholics Anonymous, psychotherapy, medications.

Pathogenesis
Neurotransmitter dysregulation in the nucleus accumbens, a structure in the midbrain. Untreated, alcoholism has a high morbidity and mortality.

Prevention
Medication that modifies the release in the brain of dopamine; other drugs that have a deterrent effect; group or individual counseling.

Epidemiology
Up to 10 percent of men and 5 percent of women will suffer from alcohol dependence.

Treatments for alcohol dependence

There are many treatments for patients with alcohol dependence. Alcoholics Anonymous provides a supportive, confidential group setting where alcoholics can receive help from peers. In addition, individuals are encouraged to identify a sponsor who serves as a mentor for the alcoholic. Many alcoholics seek treatment in formal treatment centers, in an outpatient or inpatient setting, where they learn to identify triggers, learn about the disease, and develop skills to avoid relapse following treatment.

Medications are also used to treat alcoholism. Disulfiram is a drug that causes very unpleasant symptoms, including flushing, rapid heart rate, headache, nausea, and vomiting, when interacting with alcohol. The idea behind this treatment is that the alcoholic will avoid alcohol to prevent this interaction. Disulfiram does not have good evidence supporting its efficacy, but it is thought that it might help selected patients, especially those for whom observed dosing is possible. Naltrexone acts in the addiction circuitry in the brain and therefore modulates dopamine release in the nucleus accumbens. It has been shown to reduce relapse and to decrease craving. A new injectable form of the drug has been developed. This form facilitates compliance because it needs to be administered only once a month. Acamprosate is another drug that has been shown to reduce relapse and to decrease craving. It acts through a different neurotransmitter system. Multiple medications are currently being studied to assess their effectiveness.

There is some evidence that alcohol taken in moderation (generally defined as no more than two drinks a day for a man and one for a woman) is associated with some health benefits. There are studies that suggest a that moderate alcohol intake may result in a reduction in the risk of strokes, heart attacks, dementia, and decreased incidence in diabetes mellitus. Nevertheless, alcohol consumed in greater amounts than this carries with it significant health risks.

Perhaps the most serious consequences involve the cardiovascular system. Greater than moderate alcohol consumption is associated with increased risk of high blood pressure, stroke, and coronary heart disease. In addition, alcohol is a heart muscle toxin and causes a condition known as alcoholic cardiomyopathy. This condition is characterized by a gradual thinning of the heart wall, leading to congestive heart failure. It is possible to observe some improvement in this condition if caught early enough and sobriety is initiated, but this is not guaranteed.

Effects on the liver and other organs

Alcohol also has toxic effects on the liver. Fatty liver is the earliest stage of alcoholic liver disease. It results from the accumulation of fat in the liver because the liver preferentially uses alcohol as its fuel source. Much of the time the condition is reversible once sobriety is achieved; however, in some patients this deposition of fat in the liver can lead to inflammation (hepatitis) and scarring (cirrhosis). Alcoholic hepatitis is a noninfectious inflammatory process in the liver that is caused by alcohol. It can present in a variety of ways. In its most benign form it is evident only in the form of mild blood chemistry abnormalities. However, it may take a chronic, progressive course that leads to cirrhosis or it may be present as acute liver failure. Individuals who have liver failure may require an emergency transplant. Cirrhosis is the end stage of alcoholic liver disease. The liver cells become in-

---

PHYSICAL DISORDERS ASSOCIATED WITH ALCOHOL USE

1. Although moderate drinking may confer some health benefits, heavier drinking is associated with myriad health problems.
2. Greater than moderate consumption of alcohol increases the risk of heart attack and stroke.
3. Alcohol has a toxic effect on the liver. The presentation of alcoholic liver disease can range from the fairly benign fatty liver to serious conditions such as alcoholic hepatitis and cirrhosis. Some of these patients will eventually require a liver transplant.
4. There is a significant association between traumatic injuries and alcohol consumption.
5. Wernicke-Korsakoff syndrome is caused by a vitamin deficiency that, if not recognized and treated, can result in permanent brain damage.
6. Neurological syndromes can result from chronic, excessive alcohol intake, causing chronic pain syndromes, cognitive, and gait disturbances.
7. Several cancers are associated with alcohol consumption.
8. Alcohol is a bone marrow toxin that can lead to anemia, immune system impairment, and an increased bleeding tendency.
9. It is important to recognize and treat patients who may also have a psychiatric illness.

flamed, die, and are replaced by scar tissue, which affects the blood vessels servicing the cells. Compression of the blood vessels leads to a host of problems including esophageal varices, splenomegaly, and ascites. All three conditions are related to obstruction of normal blood flow through the liver.

Esophageal varices are abnormal dilatations in certain blood vessels in the esophagus. These vessels are stretched very thin and are prone to bleed, sometimes resulting in death. Splenomegaly is the enlargement of the spleen and is associated with sequestration and increased destruction of red blood cells in the spleen leading to anemia. Ascites is the accumulation of fluid in the abdominal cavity. The presence of this fluid can increase pressure in the abdomen to the point that breathing is compromised. These patients require aspiration of fluid on a regular basis. The fluid is also a rich medium for bacterial growth, and as a result these patients are susceptible to intra-abdominal infections. In addition, various metabolic processes are impaired, such as blood clotting and immune function.

Other organs in the digestive system are also vulnerable to the toxic effects of alcohol. Pancreatitis in both its acute and chronic forms can be caused by alcohol ingestion. Patients who present with acute pancreatitis have severe abdominal pain. A severe complication is necrotizing pancreatitis, which carries with it a significant morbidity and mortality. Chronic pancreatitis presents as a chronic pain syndrome. Esophagitis can result from the reflux of stomach acid, which increases with alcohol consumption. In the stomach, alcohol disrupts the mucosal barrier, resulting in alcoholic gastritis. Esophagitis and gastritis cause pain, which is sometimes severe, and may result in bleeding.

Traumatic incidents are much higher in the setting of alcohol consumption. Up to 10 percent of all traumatic deaths are alcohol related. Nearly half of all auto accidents and up to two-thirds of all deaths from domestic injuries, drownings, fires, and occupational injuries involve alcohol.

Multiple neurological syndromes are associated with alcohol use. The Wernicke-Korsakoff syndrome is actually a thiamine (Vitamin B_1) deficiency syndrome that is due to poor nutrition, which is a risk for alcoholics. Thiamine is a necessary cofactor in the normal metabolism of glucose in multiple organs, including the brain. Altered metabolism of glucose in the brain is thought to be the cause of the Wernicke-Korsakoff syndrome. Wernicke's encephalopathy is an acute disorder characterized by paralysis of the eye

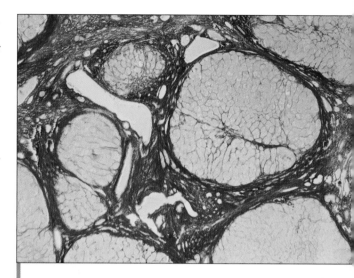

A light micrograph of a section through liver tissue shows alcohol-induced liver cirrhosis. Fibrous scar tissue (pink) is shown around oval liver lobules. Heavy alcohol consumption is the most common cause of cirrhosis in developed countries.

muscles, gait disturbance, and mental status changes. It is usually quickly reversed with the administration of thiamine but may progress to Korsakoff's syndrome, a chronic condition characterized by the inability to lay down new memories and by confabulation. Thiamine administration in this setting may or may not be successful in reversing this condition.

Pathogenesis

Other significant neurological disorders include alcoholic dementia, cerebellar degeneration, and peripheral neuropathy. Alcohol consumption adversely affects learning and memory; however, the deficits often improve with sobriety. Prolonged nutritional deficiency often results in alcoholic dementia. This can sometimes be reversed by a healthy diet and sustained abstinence from alcohol. Cerebellar degeneration presents as a significant gait disturbance and is thought to be due to nutritional deficiencies. Alcoholics are also prone to alcoholic neuropathy which has sensory (tingling, numbness, burning, and pain) and motor (weakness) components. The exact cause is unknown but is thought to be due to the toxic effects of alcohol or nutritional deficiency, or a combination of both.

Alcoholics constitute a high risk group for certain cancers. Malignancies of the head and neck, esophagus, stomach, breast, liver, pancreas, and colon are all associated with alcohol consumption. There are also a

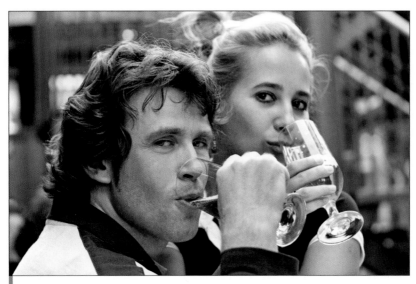

Many young people are encouraged to drink because of peer-group pressure. Gradually increasing consumption can lead to addiction; drinking heavily may result in an increased risk of accidental injury or alcohol poisoning.

Epidemiology

In 2000, in the United States, 85,000 deaths were directly attributable to drinking alcohol, either excessively or in a risky way. Deaths caused by alcohol vary from state to state, but all are directly related to the quantity of alcohol consumed and the pattern of consumption. In 2002 more than 17,000 people died in automobile accidents that were alcohol related. These motor vehicle crashes accounted for 41 percent of all traffic-related deaths. Around 30 percent of people who died of unintentional alcohol-related injuries had a BAL of 0.10 grams per deciliter or greater. People who are brought into an emergency room for treatment for an unintentional injury are 13 times more likely to have consumed at least five alcoholic drinks a few hours before they became injured.

Forty percent of violent crimes in the late 1990s were committed under the influence of alcohol. The consumption of alcohol appears to exacerbate the incidence of crimes such as rape, partner violence, child abuse, and neglect, and 23 percent of suicides were associated with alcohol.

Binge drinking of five or more drinks at one time during the first trimester of pregnancy is associated with an eightfold increase in the incidence of the infant dying of SIDS (sudden infant death syndrome). Other problems in pregnancies exposed to alcohol are miscarriage, premature birth, low birth weight, fetal alcohol syndrome, and alcohol-related neurodevelopmental disorders. Alcohol use is also related to earlier sexual activity and a higher risk for sexually transmitted diseases. The risk of various cancers also increases with increasing consumption of alcohol.

Kirk Moberg

variety of hematological abnormalities that are associated with alcoholism. Alcohol acts as a direct bone marrow toxin, and deficiencies can arise in all three types of cells as a result. Red blood cell counts may be decreased, causing anemia. The anemia may be further worsened by nutritional deficiencies.

Alcohol not only causes a decrease in the number of white blood cells, it also impairs their function, leading to an impairment of the immune system and placing the alcoholic at higher risk of infection. Decreased platelet counts and impaired platelet function are associated with alcohol intake and increase the risk of bleeding.

Other psychiatric disorders are also common in the alcoholic. About one-third of alcoholics suffer from a coexisting psychiatric disorder. The greatest difficulty in the approach to these patients is in differentiating whether their symptoms are due to alcohol use or whether they constitute a separate disorder.

Those who have experienced symptoms prior to the onset of their alcoholism or those whose symptoms persist despite continued sobriety are likely to have a separate diagnosis. They are said to be "dually diagnosed." It is important to recognize those with a dual diagnosis because untreated psychiatric symptoms can serve as a trigger for relapse. Treatment consists of psychiatric medications, although prescribing drugs that have addictive potential should be avoided.

See also

- Cancer, breast • Cancer, colorectal
- Cancer, liver • Cancer, pancreatic
- Cancer, stomach • Cirrhosis of the liver
- Coronary artery disease

Allergy and sensitivity

Allergy, also known as hypersensitivity, is an inappropriate immune response to a harmless substance, called an allergen, which leads to a characteristic set of symptoms that range from mild to potentially life threatening. An allergic reaction, suggesting a sensitivity, occurs in contrast to an appropriate, protective response to infectious organisms, which is known as immunity. Allergic diseases affect millions of people in the form of allergic rhinitis, asthma, atopic and contact dermatitis, and allergic reactions to foods, medications, and venoms.

Allergic responses are thought to be determined by both genetic and environmental factors, although it is often difficult to prove a direct cause-and-effect relationship between a risk factor and the disease. An allergic reaction occurs when a specific type of antibody called immunoglobulin E (IgE) is produced in response to an otherwise harmless substance, known as an allergen. *Atopy* is the term used to describe the predisposition to produce this reaction, for which there appears to be a strong genetic influence; personal or family history of allergies is a risk factor in developing asthma and other allergies.

Although genetic factors play a role in atopy and allergic conditions such as asthma and allergic rhinitis, environmental factors are also important. For example, where some individuals are atopic and suffer several allergies, other people may develop an allergy to just one allergen, such as the house dust mite, due to high-level exposure. A theory known as the hygiene hypothesis supports the claim that environment influences the development of allergies and believes that life in the developed world increases the likelihood of the development of allergies due to overly high standards of hygiene. The theory suggests that decreased exposure to disease-causing microorganisms in the early years of life may increase the risk of developing allergies because exposure to microorganisms stimulates a type of cell called the T helper cell (TH1), which provides an immune response. In support of this theory is the observation that European children raised on farms had a lower risk of allergic diseases compared to their nonfarming peers who lived in more sterile conditions and had less exposure to microorganisms.

Types of allergies

There are four main types of allergic reactions. Some allergens can induce more than one type of immunologic reaction, whereas some reactions do not fit any of the four classifications.

Type I hypersensitivity reactions are classical, immediate allergic reactions in which exposure to an allergen leads to the production of IgE antibodies specifically against that allergen, a process called sensitization. The IgE antibody binds to the surface of specialized cells of the immune system, called mast cells and basophils. Reexposure to the allergen activates the mast cells to release the substances that produce allergic reactions, the most well-known being histamine; other substances include leukotrienes and cytokines. Histamine increases the permeability of blood vessels, allowing the leakage of fluid, which accumulates and causes swelling, called edema. Histamine is also responsible for allergic symptoms such as nasal itching, sneezing, watery eyes, and the raised, itchy welts called hives. In the lungs, histamine and leukotrienes cause contraction of the smooth muscle lining the airways, which can result in acute asthmatic symptoms. Cytokines help recruit other cells in the immune system that promote allergic inflammation and can contribute to the symptoms of an allergic reaction.

Type II hypersensitivity reactions result from the production of antibodies called IgG or IgM, which are produced in response to an allergen and which attack blood cells. This type of reaction can be caused by a reaction to certain drugs such as penicillin. The symptoms of the reaction depend on the type of cell involved. For instance, in a type of anemia known as hemolytic anemia, antibodies are directed against red blood cells, which are broken down and destroyed faster than they can be replaced. In contrast to type I reactions, type II reactions typically occur hours to days after exposure to the allergen.

Type III hypersensitivity results from the development of antibodies against a soluble allergen that in turn leads to an immune response. An example of a type III reaction is serum sickness, in which an individual has an allergic reaction to an injected antiserum such as penicillin. Serum sickness is characterized by fever, rash, joint pains, and swollen lymph nodes, and symptoms generally occur days to weeks after exposure.

In contrast to the previous antibody-dependent allergic reactions, type IV hypersensitivity reactions involve the T lymphocyte cells of the immune system—the so-called helper cells, which destroy abnormal organisms. The classic example is a delayed-onset contact allergy. A contact allergen, such as that in poison ivy, penetrates the skin barrier, and the T cells become sensitized to the allergen. Reexposure to the allergen results in activation of the sensitized T cells, which secrete substances that lead to the typical rash. However, some compounds that cause irritant contact

dermatitis do not require previous exposure or sensitization of the immune system.

Causes and risk factors

Allergic reactions occur in response to a variety of substances, including environmental agents, food, medication, venom, and contact agents. Common inhaled allergens are pollen from trees, grasses, and weeds, which provoke seasonal allergy symptoms. Year-round inhaled allergens include dust mites, molds, feathers, and dander from animals such as cats, dogs, and horses. Cockroaches are also thought to cause allergic reactions and are believed to play a role in inner-city asthma. Venoms from stinging insects, including honey bees, wasps, hornets, yellow jackets, and fire ants can also provoke type-I allergic reactions.

Allergic contact dermatitis occurs through a type IV hypersensitivity reaction. Common contact allergens include the resin of poison ivy, nickel in inexpensive jewelry, topical antibiotics, rubber chemicals, and fragrances. Latex can cause type I and IV reactions, and latex sensitivity is most common in people with high-level, repetitive exposure to rubber latex, such as health care workers who use latex gloves. Irritant contact agents cause dermatitis on contact with the skin rather than through an immunologic response. Many substances can cause an irritant dermatitis if there are sufficiently high levels of the substance or repeated exposure. Common irritants include alcohol, rubber products, soap, and solvents. Chronically wet or dry skin can also lead to the development of dermatitis.

In the United States the most common type I food allergies involve milk, egg, wheat, soy, peanuts, tree nuts, shellfish, and fish. Allergies to peanuts, tree nuts, shellfish, and fish are generally considered to be lifelong and can also develop in adulthood, whereas the other food allergies occur predominantly in children and are usually outgrown by school age. For these classic IgE-mediated types of food allergies, even trace quantities of exposure to the allergen can provoke a reaction. Adverse food reactions can also occur through nonallergic mechanisms. For instance, lactose intolerance is commonly mistaken for a food allergy, but the gastrointestinal symptoms result from an inability to digest lactose. Some reactions are described as oral allergy syndrome in which plant-based foods, such as fruits or tree nuts, cause symptoms such as an itchy mouth in people with pollen allergies.

In contrast to predictable side effects such as gastrointestinal upset from antibiotics, medications can cause immunologically based allergic reactions. The

KEY FACTS

Description

Allergy is an inappropriate immune response to an allergen, which is normally harmless.

Cause

Allergens, which trigger hypersentivity reactions.

Risk factors

Both genetic and environmental factors are important, especially production of IgE antibodies and decreased early exposure to microbes.

Symptoms

Common symptoms of allergic rhinitis are sneezing, watery eyes, itching of the nose. Asthma may present with shortness of breath, wheezing, chest tightness, or a cough. There are many types of allergic skin rashes, but they are all typically itchy.

Diagnosis

The diagnosis is usually made based on a typical history and symptoms. When allergy testing can be done, these tests may show the presence of a specific IgE antibody against a particular allergen.

Treatments

Various drugs such as antihistamines and steroids; allergy shots.

Pathogenesis

Allergies usually first develop in childhood and may be lifelong.

Prevention

Exclusive breast-feeding, delayed introduction of highly allergenic foods, and allergy shots may reduce the risk of developing allergies or asthma in children.

Epidemiology

The highest rates of all allergic diseases are present in affluent, industrialized countries.

THE CAUSE OF A TYPE I ALLERGIC REACTION

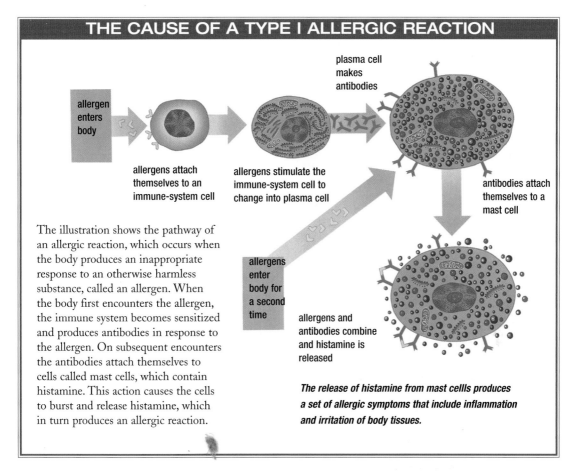

plasma cell
makes
antibodies

allergen
enters
body

allergens attach
themselves to an
immune-system cell

allergens stimulate the
immune-system cell to
change into plasma cell

antibodies attach
themselves to a
mast cell

allergens
enter
body for
a second
time

allergens and
antibodies combine
and histamine is
released

The illustration shows the pathway of an allergic reaction, which occurs when the body produces an inappropriate response to an otherwise harmless substance, called an allergen. When the body first encounters the allergen, the immune system becomes sensitized and produces antibodies in response to the allergen. On subsequent encounters the antibodies attach themselves to cells called mast cells, which contain histamine. This action causes the cells to burst and release histamine, which in turn produces an allergic reaction.

The release of histamine from mast cellls produces a set of allergic symptoms that include inflammation and irritation of body tissues.

beta-lactam class of antibiotics, which includes penicillin, is the most common cause of IgE-mediated drug allergies. About 10 percent of penicillin-allergic patients also react to another class of antibiotics known as cephalosporin antibiotics. Sulfonamide antibiotics are a common cause of a rash, particularly in HIV-positive patients. Aspirin and other nonsteroidal anti-inflammatory drugs (NSAIDs) can cause a range of allergy symptoms, including exacerbation of asthma and rhinitis in some patients who have a combination of asthma, nasal polyps, and aspirin/NSAID intolerance. Other causes of adverse drug reactions include local and general anesthetic agents, anti-seizure medications, narcotic pain medications, and substances used in contrast X-rays.

Symptoms

Allergic symptoms commonly occur in three conditions: allergic rhinitis, asthma, and atopic dermatitis. Symptoms of allergic rhinitis include nasal congestion, sneezing, and a watery nose, while allergic conjunctivitis presents with symptoms of itchy, watery eyes.

Symptoms can occur year-round or seasonally (also known as hay fever). Chronic inflammation of the nasal and sinus passages due to allergies can also predispose to the development of sinus infections. Rhinitis can occur unrelated to allergies, such as with exposure to irritants or as a side effect from chronic use of topical decongestants.

Asthma is a condition in which the airways become inflamed, leading to symptoms such as wheezing, shortness of breath, chest tightness, or a repetitive cough. Asthma is classified according to the frequency and severity of symptoms and the degree of airway obstruction as measured by a lung function test. Asthmatic symptoms can be provoked by both allergic and nonallergic triggers. For example, animal proteins or pollens commonly induce allergic asthma, while viral infections, pollutants, cold air, or exercise may also precipitate attacks of asthma. Occupational asthma is defined as asthma that occurs due to an allergen in the workplace. Symptoms for this type of asthma typically occur during the workday and are absent when away from work. A classic example

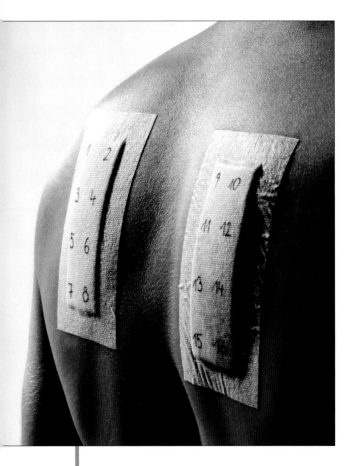

Patch tests are used to identify allergy-causing substances. Small amounts of substances are placed on a disk and then stuck to the skin. After a certain period of time the disks are removed, and a red patch signals a positive allergic reaction.

The most common allergic drug reaction is known as the morbilliform rash, which is a red, flat, itchy skin rash that typically begins days after exposure to the culprit medication. Serious, but rare, drug allergy syndromes may involve ulceration of the mouth, skin reactions, fever, or hepatitis. Anaphylaxis is a potentially life-threatening allergic reaction that can produce respiratory, cardiovascular, skin, or abdominal symptoms and is caused by the IgE antibody and mast cells triggering a type I hypersensitivity reaction.

Diagnosis

Blood tests may reveal an increase in certain cell types associated with TH2 or IgE immune responses, which suggest the presence of an allergic disease. In anaphylaxis there may be an elevation in the level of histamine and tryptase, which are released from activated mast cells during an allergic reaction. Allergy prick skin tests are used in the evaluation of type I hypersensitivity reactions and involve the introduction of an allergen through the skin. In a sensitized individual the allergen is recognized by the IgE antibodies and triggers local activation of mast cells, which leads to the immediate release of histamine and the development of a localized hive. Some allergy skin tests are commercially available to check for environmentally inhaled allergens, foods, and venoms. A type of antibiotics known as beta lactam antibiotics, which include penicillin, are the only antibiotics for which allergy skin testing can be routinely done. Levels of allergen-specific IgE can be quantified through commercially available tests, known as the RAST or immunoCAP tests, but these are less sensitive than skin allergy tests. Patch testing is performed to assess for type IV hypersensitivity reactions to contact allergens. A panel of common allergens, including metals, rubber, chemicals, antibiotics, and fragrances, is placed directly onto the skin, and a localized skin response is assessed at both 48 and 72 hours. Types II and III hypersensitivity reactions can be evaluated by measuring levels of IgG or IgM antibodies. The diagnosis of allergic diseases such as asthma is based on the patient's history, results of lung function testing, and response to asthma medications.

is baker's asthma, which occurs as a result of sensitivity to allergens from fine white wheat flour.

Atopic dermatitis, commonly referred to as eczema or simply dermatitis, is a chronic skin condition characterized by itchy, dry patches of skin in locations such as the face, neck, and creases of the elbows and knees. Atopic dermatitis often occurs in early childhood and may be exacerbated by food or environmental allergies. Contact dermatitis occurs when the skin responds to contact with an irritant and produces intensely itchy papules or vesicles.

Urticaria, also known as hives, appears as itchy welts on the skin that typically come and go over the course of hours. Angioedema is swelling that occurs deeper in the skin and is typically not itchy. Urticaria and angioedema can occur in response to a specific allergen as part of a type I hypersensitivity reaction, or they can result from nonallergic mechanisms.

Pathogenesis

The "atopic march" describes the common progression of allergic sensitization and disease. Atopic dermatitis often begins in infancy, with the development of asthma and allergic rhinitis occurring later in childhood. With specific allergies, infants may produce IgE antibodies against certain food proteins, which leads to a food allergy. As children become exposed to environmental allergens, they may develop indoor allergies such as dust mite sensitivity. In subsequent years the child is exposed to more outdoor allergens and may develop environmental allergies to pollens.

Treatments

The most effective treatment for allergies is strict avoidance of the allergen, such as a culprit food or medication. When this is not possible the symptoms can be controlled with medications. Antihistamines block the action of histamine and are effective in controlling symptoms such as itching, sneezing, and a watery discharge from the eyes. Corticosteroids are medications that inhibit the production of cytokines that cause inflammation and are useful in treating many types of allergic diseases. Systemic steroids are reserved for severe allergies or asthma symptoms due to their potential side effects. Topical steroids are available in nasal, inhaled, and skin preparations to treat chronic symptoms of allergic rhinitis, asthma, and atopic dermatitis. Inhaled medications called beta-agonists, or relievers, relax the smooth muscle of the airways and are useful for both immediate relief and long-term control of asthma symptoms. Drugs known as leukotriene modifier drugs, used in the treatment of asthma and allergic rhinitis, work by preventing inflammation. Cromolyn is a mast cell stabilizing agent, which is effective for allergy and asthma symptoms, but its use is limited by the need for frequent dosing, and a drug called theophylline treats asthma but is now rarely used due to potential toxicities. Epinephrine is a potentially life-saving treatment for anaphylaxis, a sometimes fatal allergic reaction, as it counteracts the contraction of the airways and cardiovascular shock. Patients with an IgE-mediated food allergy should be instructed to self-administer epinephrine early in the course of anaphylaxis, and then to call for immediate medical attention.

For IgE-mediated reactions, desensitization can be performed. During desensitization an allergen is given repeatedly over several hours in gradually increasing doses until tolerance of the allergen is achieved. As the procedure carries a risk of causing anaphylaxis, it is only performed when medically necessary and under the supervision of an experienced allergist. Allergy shots, also called immunotherapy, involve giving increasing doses of a specific allergen in order to change the immune response against that allergen. Immunotherapy is a very effective treatment for allergic

---

PREVENTION

Repeated allergic reactions can be prevented by strictly avoiding the relevant allergens. Avoiding allergic diseases altogether is called primary prevention and is more controversial. Exclusive breast-feeding for at least the first 4–6 months of life has been shown to reduce the risk of developing allergies. In infants at high risk for food allergy, the American Academy of Pediatrics recommends that breast-feeding mothers avoid eating peanuts and that children delay eating peanuts, tree nuts, fish, and shellfish until the age of three. However, these interventions do not conclusively prevent food allergy. Allergy shots, when given for the treatment of allergic rhinitis in young children, can reduce the future risk of developing asthma.

---

rhinitis, allergic asthma, and venom allergy, but has not proved effective in treating food allergies or atopic dermatitis and also carries the potential risk of causing anaphylaxis. Anti-IgE injections target IgE molecules to prevent them from binding to the surface of mast cells and basophils. Anti-IgE is currently used to treat moderate-to-severe asthma and is being investigated as a treatment for other allergic conditions.

Epidemiology

Allergic diseases are common, and rates have increased dramatically in the past 20 years in the United States. Allergic rhinitis affects up to 50 million Americans and asthma affects 20 million. An estimated 1–2 percent of adults and 2–4 percent of children in the United States have a food allergy.

The prevalence of allergies varies significantly throughout the world and is generally more common in affluent, industrialized countries compared to developing nations. In the International Study of Asthma and Allergies in Childhood, the highest prevalence rates for allergic diseases of more than 30 percent were found in the United Kingdom, New Zealand, and Australia. This was followed by rates of 20 to 25 percent in Canada, the United States, South America, and continental Europe. The lowest rates for allergies, less than 15 percent, were found in Africa and Asia.

Debby Lin

See also
- Asthma • Conjunctivitis • Dermatitis
- Food intolerance • Hay fever

Alopecia

Alopecia is the partial or complete loss of hair. There are different types of alopecia, but the most common form of significant localized hair loss is alopecia areata, which is an autoimmune disorder. Alopecia areata can be limited to just a few patches or be more extensive. Although there is no cure or an approved drug for the disorder, different therapies, including topical treatments and steroid injections, may help hair grow back.

The average person has around five million hairs on the body, growing almost everywhere apart from the lips, palms of the hands, and soles of the feet. Some hair loss accompanies normal growth; about 100 hairs fall from the scalp every day. Significant hair loss, however, might indicate an autoimmune condition called alopecia areata.

The most common type of hair loss is male-pattern baldness (androgenetic alopecia), which affects one-third of all men and women. This is usually permanent hair loss. Alopecia areata is temporary, but there is no way of predicting regrowth.

Causes

Although the immune system protects the body from foreign invaders, such as viruses and bacteria, in alopecia the immune system's white blood cells attack the rapidly growing cells in the hair follicle—the tiny cup-shaped structures from which hair grows. The follicles shrink and hair production slows.

Other causes of temporary hair loss include diseases such as diabetes, lupus, and thyroid disorders. Poor nutrition, such as protein or iron deficiency, can cause hair loss. Medical treatments such as chemotherapy or radiation therapy, or flu or high fever, can cause temporary hair loss. After the treatment or illness ends and recovery commences, hair will typically begin to regrow. Hair loss is also not uncommon following childbirth. During pregnancy, hair shifts into an active growth state, which returns to normal once the baby is delivered. Again, this hair loss usually corrects itself.

Androgenetic alopecia is caused by heredity; a history of the disorder on either side of the family increases the risk of balding. Heredity also affects the rate of hair loss, as well as pattern and extent of baldness.

Diagnosis and treatments

Diagnosis of alopecia is usually based on appearance and pattern of hair loss. A skin biopsy may also be needed to diagnose any other reasons behind hair loss.

Some medications may help hair grow back, at least temporarily. However, none of these treatments have been found to prevent hair loss. Treatments include locally applied corticosteroids, anti-inflammatory drugs that suppress the immune system.

Other treatments include causing an irritant or allergic reaction to promote hair growth; drug treatments; and photo-chemotherapy, in which a person is given a light-sensitive drug, then is exposed to an ultraviolet-light source. This treatment has been found to promote hair growth, but it carries a risk of skin cancer.

Julie McDowell

KEY FACTS

Description

Significant hair loss that can be a few bald patches or total hair loss on the head or complete loss of hair on the head, face, and body.

Causes

Alopecia areata is an autoimmune disease in which the immune system attacks hair follicles, slowing or halting hair production.

Risk factors

No known risk factor for alopecia areata.

Symptoms

Hair loss.

Treatments

Various treatments may help hair grow back, at least temporarily.

Pathogenesis

Often emerges in childhood and is incurable.

Epidemiology

Male and females of all ages and ethnic backgrounds can be affected by alopecia areata.

See also
• Male-pattern baldness

Alzheimer's disease

Alzheimer's disease is a progressive neurodegenerative disease that is rarely seen before the age of 60. It is characterized by memory loss, poor judgment, and the inability to cope with everyday life. Alzheimer's care is very expensive; it costs about $100 billion a year in the United States.

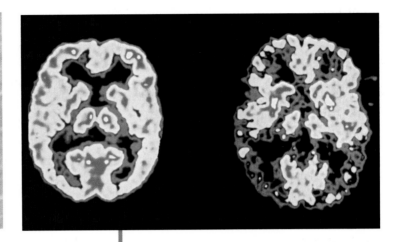

These PET scans are of a normal brain (left) and one from a patient with Alzheimer's disease. High brain activity shows as red and yellow; low brain activity is blue and black, indicating a reduction of function and blood flow.

Alzheimer's disease is an incurable neurodegenerative disease and the most common form of dementia (deterioration of brain function). It normally occurs after the age of 65. However, there is also an early onset form of the disease. Both forms have similar symptoms, and neither one can be prevented or cured. Alzheimer's disease causes an enormous burden on those affected, their families, and society. Affected people may live for 8 to 20 years after their diagnosis, which explains the high cost of caring for the 4.5 million people diagnosed with Alzheimer's in the United States. The costs will continue to increase as the world's population ages and life expectancies increase. The number of people with Alzheimer's in the United States could top 11 million by 2050. The disease was first recognized and described by medical doctor Alois Alzheimer in 1906 after closely analyzing the brain tissue of a woman who exhibited signs of dementia before her death. In the brain, Alzheimer discovered two telltale signs of the disease, which are still used to diagnose it today. These indicators are: aggregates of protein called plaques between nerve cells, and fibrous tangles inside the neurons.

Causes and risk factors

The cause of Alzheimer's in most people with the disease is unknown. However, a clear genetic component has been found in a small number of families with the early onset form of the disease. In these families, the disease is much different from most Alzheimer's cases. The disease strikes earlier in life—well before retirement age—occasionally in a person's 30s or 40s. Three different genes have been identified that contribute to this form of the disease.

The first Alzheimer's gene discovered produces a large protein called amyloid precursor protein (APP), which can be broken down into smaller pieces. When a tiny fragment of APP called amyloid-beta is formed, it can clump together between nerve cells and block the normal signals that move through the brain. These are the plaques described by Alzheimer. Eighteen different mutations or variants of the normal protein have been identified. It is believed that the mutations lead to excessive amyloid production and eventual nerve cell death. The gene is located on chromosome 21. Having three copies of this chromosome causes Down syndrome, and many people with Down syndrome have brain damage similar to that found in Alzheimer's.

The other two early onset genes that have been identified are presenilin-1 and presenilin-2. Scientists are still trying to understand how they cause disease. It is thought that they might affect the way the large APP protein is broken down. What is clear is that having just one copy of any early onset gene is enough to cause Alzheimer's. That means that children of someone with early onset Alzheimer's have a 50 percent chance of developing the disease themselves.

Late onset Alzheimer's is the most common form of the disease, and it is closely associated with age.

A 65-year-old has a 10–15 percent risk of developing the disease, and the risk further increases with ages above 65. One study estimated that the risk might be as high as 50 percent once a person reaches 85 years. However, it is important to note that Alzheimer's disease is not a normal part of aging.

Several genes have been linked with late onset Alzheimer's. The most studied gene is called APOE and is on chromosome 19. There are three common forms, or alleles, of the gene. A person's risk depends on which allele of APOE he or she has. Someone with two copies of APOE*4 is at the highest risk of developing late onset Alzheimer's disease.

Several environmental factors have been linked to the development of Alzheimer's, including solvents and head injuries. Boxers have long been recognized as having a certain kind of dementia—called dementia pugilistica—linked to their sport. However, this

dementia is not the same as Alzheimer's. In the same way, many chemicals damage neurons, but they do not necessarily cause Alzheimer's. Because Alzheimer's takes a long time to develop, it is difficult to find out what an affected person may have been exposed to earlier in life. Studies on exposure to aluminum, which occurs in higher concentrations in the brain of Alzheimer's patients, have proved inconclusive.

Symptoms and diagnosis

In the early stages, a person may experience forgetfulness and difficulty with common tasks such as paying bills. In the later stages, the affected person loses the ability to cope with nearly all functions of daily life. But the death of brain cells is rarely the actual cause of death in Alzheimer's disease. Most people with Alzheimer's die from infections such as pneumonia that become established once they lose the ability to breathe and swallow normally.

In the earliest stages, it can be easy to confuse Alzheimer's disease with many other conditions. For example, depression can cause similar mood and behavior changes, and stress can impair memory. Alzheimer's disease is diagnosed by elimination. A complete mental and physical assessment must be performed, which is important because, unlike Alzheimer's, many other disorders can be treated effectively. Newer imaging techniques are being developed to help doctors look for pathological changes in the brain. Ninety percent of cases are diagnosed correctly while the patient is still alive. The only absolute diagnosis is after death, when the brain can be studied for signs of plaques and tangles.

A common expression is, "It's not Alzheimer's if you forget where you put your car keys. It's Alzheimer's when you forget how to use them." The progression of Alzheimer's begins with symptoms most people have experienced to a certain degree, but as a patient moves through the various stages, there is no question that Alzheimer's is more than a few misplaced memories.

The disease begins with a mild cognitive impairment (MCI) that involves memory lapses, difficulty remembering familiar words, and misplacing common objects. It is uncertain whether everyone who develops mild cognitive impairment will progress to Alzheimer's, but MCI clearly increases a person's risk of Alzheimer's. In stage three, the impairment worsens, and occasionally a person can be diagnosed with Alzheimer's at this point. More likely, the diagnosis will occur in a later stage. Stage four is mild or early Alzheimer's. By now, family and friends

KEY FACTS

Description
A debilitating neurodegenerative disease.

Cause
Both genetic and environmental factors appear to play a role.

Risk factors
Age, family history, obesity, and a less active lifestyle.

Symptoms
Appear gradually as an affected person's memory and ability to think and reason deteriorate.

Diagnosis
A complete physical and mental examination is required to rule out other possible disorders. An absolute diagnosis requires examination of damaged brain tissue after death.

Treatments
Some drugs reduce symptoms, but no drug can prevent the ongoing death of brain cells.

Pathogenesis
Patients often live several years after the initial diagnosis, but the later stage disease is marked by the loss of most mental and bodily functions.

Prevention
Staying active mentally and physically appears to be the most effective way to delay or avoid symptoms.

Epidemiology
About 4.5 million people in the United States have Alzheimer's disease. The number is expected to increase dramatically by 2025.

TRANSMISSION OF NERVE IMPULSES

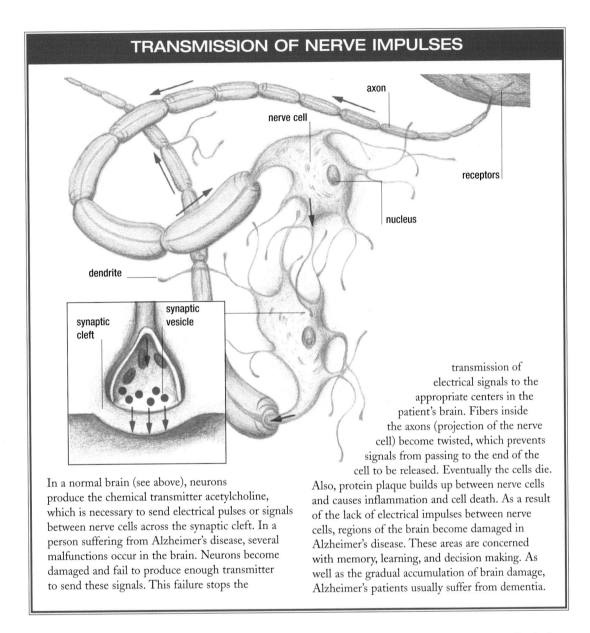

In a normal brain (see above), neurons produce the chemical transmitter acetylcholine, which is necessary to send electrical pulses or signals between nerve cells across the synaptic cleft. In a person suffering from Alzheimer's disease, several malfunctions occur in the brain. Neurons become damaged and fail to produce enough transmitter to send these signals. This failure stops the transmission of electrical signals to the appropriate centers in the patient's brain. Fibers inside the axons (projection of the nerve cell) become twisted, which prevents signals from passing to the end of the cell to be released. Eventually the cells die. Also, protein plaque builds up between nerve cells and causes inflammation and cell death. As a result of the lack of electrical impulses between nerve cells, regions of the brain become damaged in Alzheimer's disease. These areas are concerned with memory, learning, and decision making. As well as the gradual accumulation of brain damage, Alzheimer's patients usually suffer from dementia.

recognize that the affected person's brain and behavior have changed. A simple test—counting backward by sevens—becomes a daunting challenge to a person with Alzheimer's. Inappropriate words may be substituted for the correct ones. Affected people have trouble recalling recent events and may become depressed or withdrawn. Others become combative or hostile. In the ensuing stages, there are major memory lapses. A person may not realize which day it is or how to dress properly. With moderate Alzheimer's, some assistance is needed with daily activities. However, even at this stage someone with Alzheimer's can continue to participate in sports or other physical activities he or she has enjoyed in the past. In the later stages (stages 6 and 7), the damage to the brain is so severe that even motor circuits are damaged. By this time, it may be impossible to care for affected people in their own home. They have difficulty in walking and sitting up without help and are unable to feed themselves. Eventually, they can no longer speak or smile normally. Impaired swallowing often leads to respiratory infections as food or saliva enters the trachea instead of the esophagus, and many people with Alzheimer's eventually die of pneumonia. They are at higher risk for infections, and it is more difficult for them to recover from an infection.

Treatments

There is no effective treatment or cure for Alzheimer's disease, but researchers are finding ways to improve the quality of life for those affected. This is important, because there is such a long time between diagnosis and death. Finding a way to delay the more serious symptoms not only lowers the costs of the disease but also reduces the emotional burden on families and other caretakers.

The first medicines approved to treat Alzheimer's focused on the neurotransmitter acetylcholine. The drugs inhibited the enzyme that breaks down acetylcholine. In theory, this helps nerve cells make the most of the acetylcholine still available. However, the drugs are only effective at delaying symptoms for a time and do not stop the ongoing cell death. Other novel therapies are in development, but none has proved effective in clinical trials on humans yet. For example, a vaccine was developed against the amyloid plaques, and early experiments looked promising. The vaccines created an immune response that destroyed plaques in genetically modified mice. However, when the first vaccines were tested on humans, some developed a dangerous brain inflammation and the tests were stopped.

New findings on Alzheimer's and new ideas about the causes of the disease are published almost every day. Researches have even found a potential new treatment in cyanobacteria—the blue-green "algae" commonly called pond scum. However, new findings must be considered cautiously. Like the aluminum hypothesis that frightened many people into throwing away their beverage cans and pots and pans, it takes many years before new ideas and treatments are confirmed or discarded.

Nevertheless, progress is being made. In the future, there will be more effective techniques to diagnose the disease and to identify those at highest risk. Drugs are being developed that may slow the progression of the disease even further. Behavioral scientists are finding better ways to care for people with Alzheimer's, to nurture remaining memories, to control their erratic behavior, and to help them remain in their homes and with their families as long as possible.

Pathogenesis

Alzheimer's disease targets very specific regions of the brain, whereas other areas function normally almost until an affected person's death. Not surprisingly, the brain regions damaged in Alzheimer's are involved in learning, memory, and making decisions. The neurons most damaged are in an area called the nucleus basalis of Meynert.

These neurons produce the neurotransmitter acetylcholine. Without enough neurotransmitter to send signals between nerve cells, the memory circuits begin to fail. Other brain regions affected include the hippocampus, which is crucial for short-term memory and memory storage; the amygdala, which is associated with behavior; and the frontal cortex, which is the major information-processing center of the brain.

At a finer scale, the damage is a result of plaques and tangles. Dense protein plaques form between nerve cells, causing inflammation and cell death. The tangles are abnormally twisted fibers inside a neuron's long fiberlike process, or axon. In healthy neurons, packets of neurotransmitters can move from the cell body down the axon to the end of the cell where they are released. Obviously, there can be no signaling when the axon is blocked with a tangled mess. Eventually, these cells die as well.

Other forms of dementia cause different patterns of damage, which can be identified during an autopsy. Mini-strokes can temporarily disrupt the flow of blood in the brain, leading to brain damage and dysfunction. But this type of dementia, called multi-infarct dementia, can be distinguished from Alzheimer's because the affected person deteriorates in a notable stepped fashion, following each small stroke. Alzheimer's damage accumulates more gradually.

Prevention

Preventive measures can reduce the risk of developing Alzheimer's. Increasingly, it has become clear that a healthy lifestyle pays off in old age. Obesity, high blood pressure and cholesterol, and a lack of exercise all increase the risk of dementia. In addition, exercising the mind, such as by doing puzzles, playing chess, learning a new word game, or reading, may reduce the risk. Vitamin E was once thought to be protective, but new research indicates that it is not effective at preventing or slowing the course of Alzheimer's disease.

Chris Curran

See also
• Pneumonia • Stroke and related disorders

Amnesia

Amnesia is the inability to retain new information or to recollect information already stored in the memory. The ability to recall past events in life is an intricate process orchestrated by various parts of the brain. The mechanisms by which memories are processed or recalled are not completely understood. However, by studying amnesiacs, science is gaining some insight into these complex processes.

Memory loss may occur after damage to part of the brain called the temporal lobe, which is essential for processing, memory storage, and recall. Such brain damage results in the loss of irreplaceable brain cells. Most significant brain damage usually occurs as a result of physical trauma, disease, drug or alcohol abuse, malnutrition, or reduced blood flow to the brain, which is called vascular insufficiency. Infections, such as herpes, and inflammation, such as encephalitis can cause brain damage and also contribute to the onset of amnesia. Mental disorders, such as depression and schizophrenia, may also impair the ability to remember personal details. This disorder is called psychogenic amnesia. Amnesia is also commonly associated with disorders in which the brain degenerates, such as Alzheimer's disease.

Amnesia is often subdivided into three categories, each differing in its cause and symptoms. Anteriograde amnesia is often caused by brain trauma and presents itself as the inability to lay down new memories acquired after the trauma. Therefore, recall of recent events and short-term memory are poor, but events prior to the trauma are recalled with clarity. Conversely, retrograde amnesia is the inability to recall events that occurred prior to the trauma. Retrograde and anteriograde amnesia can occur together in the same patient.

The third category is transient global amnesia, which is assumed to be caused by ischemia. Research suggests that it may be triggered by migraines or transient ischemic attack, which occurs when a blockage in an artery temporarily blocks off blood supply to part of the brain. Transient global amnesia can last anywhere from an hour to a day, but patients lose all memory of recent events and have difficulty remembering new information.

Diagnosis

There is no diagnostically conclusive test for establishing the cause of amnesia. Information that may prove helpful includes recent traumas or illness, drug and medication history, and an affected person's general health. A neuropsychological examination is often done to determine the extent of amnesia and the memory system affected. Magnetic resonance imaging (MRI) may be helpful in finding out whether the brain has been damaged. In addition, blood and urine tests may be done to determine exposure to environmental toxins or recent consumption of alcohol or drugs of abuse. Blood tests may also exclude treatable metabolic causes or chemical imbalances.

Treatments

If the amnesia is associated with neuronal death, it is likely to be irreversible. Depending on the cause of

---

KEY FACTS

Description
Loss of memory.

Causes
Brain damage either through injury or the degeneration of brain cells as a result of dementia or infection.

Risk factors
Physical trauma, disease, malnutrition, infection, drug and alcohol abuse, or reduced blood flow to the brain all increase the risk of amnesia.

Symptoms
Loss of the ability to retain new information or recall information already stored in memory.

Diagnosis
Both a physical examination and an imaging test such as magnetic resonance imaging; blood and urine tests.

Treatments
Depends on cause. Regardless of cause, cognitive therapies may help.

Pathogenesis
Develops as a result of brain damage.

Prevention
Minimizing or preventing brain injury. Brain infections should be treated swiftly and aggressively to reduce the damage due to swelling. Strokes, brain aneurysms, and transient ischemic attacks should be treated immediately.

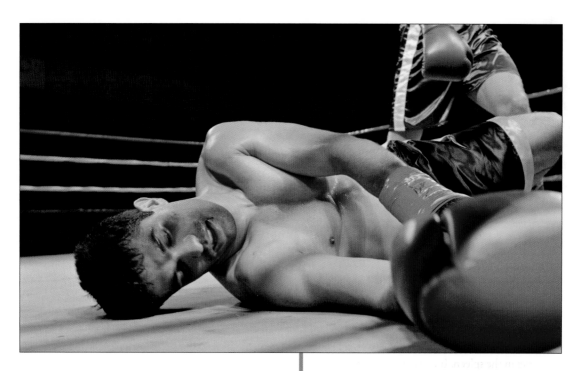

If a competitor is knocked out during a boxing match, there is a risk of brain injury. The physical trauma can cause amnesia, resulting in a loss of memory of events before or after the blow. In severe injury, amnesia may be permanent.

amnesia, the brain may be able to recover many of its previously lost functions, or conversely may get worse. Those who suffer amnesia as a result of a brain injury may see some improvement in their cognitive (mental processing) function over a period of time as the brain attempts to heal itself. However, when amnesia is associated with a neurodegenerative disorder such as Alzheimer's, improvement is unlikely.

Treatment varies with the type of amnesia and is often case specific. Cognitive rehabilitation, a form of guided therapy to help people learn or relearn ways to concentrate, is helpful regardless of cause, in that it helps patients learn strategies to cope with their memory loss, such as keeping a memory notebook or putting notes around the house as reminders of important events or tasks. Depending on the degree of amnesia and its cause, amnesiacs may be able to lead relatively normal lives.

Prevention

By preventing or minimizing brain injury, the risk of developing amnesia is reduced. Such interventions include wearing a helmet when bicycling or when participating in potentially dangerous sports and using automobile seat belts. Avoiding excessive alcohol or drug use also reduces the risk of brain damage. Furthermore, viral brain infections that cause encephalitis should be treated immediately and aggressively to minimize the damage that results from

inflammation of the brain. People who have had a stroke, brain aneurysm, or transient ischemic attacks should also seek immediate medical treatment. People with vascular risk factors or a family history of cerebrovascular events may benefit from prophylactic treatment with aspirin under the supervision of a primary care physician.

Epidemiology

In the United States, amnesia caused by head injuries affects mainly young men. Alcohol-induced amnesia is most common in people over the age of 40 with a history of prolonged heavy alcohol use. Drug-abuse induced amnesia is most common in people between the ages of 20 and 40. Transient global amnesia usually appears in people over 50. Only 3 percent of people who experience global transient amnesia have symptoms that recur within a year.

Sonia Gulati

See also
• Alcohol-related disorders • Alzheimer's disease • Aneurysm • Stroke and related disorders

Anemia

Anemia, or "tired blood" as it is often called, is one of the most common blood disorders in the United States, affecting an estimated 3.4 million adults. It is characterized by a deficit of red blood cells, which contain the protein hemoglobin that is necessary to carry oxygen to the body's tissues. Many of the common symptoms associated with anemia, such as fatigue, heart palpitations, and dizziness, are due to a decrease in the transport of oxygen to the vital organs. There are many types of anemia—over 400—each stemming from a unique cause and varying in treatment.

Anemia is a condition in which the concentration of red blood cells (erythrocytes) or hemoglobin—the oxygen-carrying pigment—is below normal. This reduction in red blood cells may be caused by blood loss, a decrease in the production of red blood cells, or their accelerated destruction.

A vital balance exists in the body between the production of red cells in the bone marrow and their destruction in the spleen. If this balance mechanism fails, anemia will be the result.

Types of anemia

There are over 400 different types of anemia. The most common types are described below.

Iron deficiency anemia is one of the most common forms of anemia; it affects about one in five women, 50 percent of pregnant women, and 3 percent of men in the United States. Iron is essential for the bone marrow to produce hemoglobin. Depletion of iron stores may occur as a result of prolonged or heavy menstruation, chronic blood loss due to an ulcer, erosive gastritis (inflammation of the stomach lining), colorectal cancer, pregnancy (in which the fetus takes maternal iron), or eating an iron-deficient diet. Hemorrhoids (swollen veins in the lining of the anus) can also steadily cause blood loss. Using certain medications, such as aspirin and various nonsteroidal anti-inflammatory drugs (NSAIDs) can result in bleeding in the gastrointestinal tract. Sometimes, although rarely, bleeding may occur because of kidney tumors and bladder tumors.

Diets may be deficient in food sources of iron. Healthy sources of iron are legumes, such as lentils and beans, green leafy vegetables (such as spinach), egg yolks, whole grains, dried fruits, and organ meats. In the case of celiac disease, in which the lining of the small intestine has been damaged, malabsorption of iron may be the cause of the anemia.

Megaloblastic anemia is a major form of anemia. In addition to iron, both folate and vitamin B_{12} are vital for maintaining a sufficient number of healthy red blood cells. A deficiency in either or both of these vitamins may result in megaloblastic anemia, in which the production of red blood cells is badly affected. In this form of anemia, the bone marrow produces large, abnormal red blood cells. Those suffering from intestinal disorders that affect the absorption of nutrients, such as Crohn's disease, are prone to this type of anemia.

Pernicious anemia is a type of anemia in which there is impaired absorption of vitamin B_{12}, owing to an autoimmune disorder, in which the body's immune system attacks the body's own tissues, destroying the parietal (wall) cells of the stomach. The stomach lining then fails to produce a substance called intrinsic factor, which is necessary to promote the absorption of vitamin B_{12} from food. A deficiency of vitamin B_{12} stops the production of normal red blood cells in the bone marrow.

Aplastic anemia is a life-threatening type of anemia that develops as result of the inability of the bone marrow to produce not only red blood cells but also white blood cells (leukocytes) and platelets. Although the exact cause of aplastic anemia is unknown, it is believed that genetics or injury to the bone marrow incurred by chemotherapy, radiation therapy, environmental toxins, or infection can contribute to its onset. These factors may prevent the bone marrow from producing stem cells, which are the initial versions (progenitors) of all cells in the body.

Thalassemia is a group of inherited blood disorders that vary in severity, depending on how many defective genes are inherited. Anemia occurs because the red blood cells cannot mature and grow properly. They are fragile and tend to break up as a result of a defect in the production of oxygen-carrying hemoglobin in the cell. Thalassemia is an inherited condition typically affecting people of the Mediterranean, African, Middle Eastern, and South Asian descent.

Sickle-cell anemia is another inherited genetic disorder, which is characterized by sickle-shaped red blood cells. These abnormal red blood cells die prematurely, resulting in a chronic shortage of red blood cells. Sickle-shaped red blood cells can also block blood flow through small blood vessels in the body, producing other, often painful, symptoms.

Hemolytic anemia develops as result of premature and excessive destruction of red blood cells in the bloodstream. There are various causes that contribute

KEY FACTS

Description

A blood disorder characterized by a decrease in red blood cells, which are the primary transporters of oxygen to the body's tissues.

Causes

Physiological causes of anemia include blood loss as well as inadequate production or excessive destruction of red blood cells.

Risk factors

Prolonged menstruation, poor diet, pregnancy, genetic susceptibility, medicinal side effects, cancer, and certain diseases associated with chronic bleeding can all contribute to anemia.

Symptoms

Most common symptoms include fatigue, shortness of breath, dizziness, heart palpitations, and difficulty concentrating. Symptoms may vary with the cause of anemia.

Diagnosis

A medical history, a physical examination, and a blood test are all necessary to confirm a diagnosis of anemia. One of the most basic and commonly utilized blood tests is a complete blood count, which determines the hemoglobin content and number of red blood cells. Additional blood tests may be ordered depending on the suspected cause of anemia.

Treatments

The treatment of anemia is cause specific. Treatment for one type of anemia is not only deleterious for another type of anemia but may actually exacerbate its symptoms.

Pathogenesis

Develops as a result of a reduction of red blood cells.

Epidemiology

Anemia affects about 3.4 million people in the United States.

to this type of anemia. Hemolytic anemia may stem from an autoimmune disorder in which the body produces antibodies to red blood cells, destroying them prematurely. It may also be triggered by infections, certain medications (such as antibiotics), some foods, and incompatible blood transfusions. It can be acquired later in life when the cause of the hemolysis (process of breaking down red cells) is outside the blood cells. People who have hemolytic anemia will have the usual symptoms of anemia, such as fatigue and breathlessness, but often they will look jaundiced (yellowing of the skin and whites of the eyes) as a result of the constant breakdown of red blood cells. A by-product of the breakdown of red cells is an excess of bile pigments, which gives the person jaundice. Treatment for hemolytic anemia is dependent on the cause of the anemia. Blood transfusions may be indicated for severe cases.

There are many other forms of anemia, some of which have no identifiable cause. However, most can be broadly categorized into three classes: anemia caused by blood loss, anemia caused by decreased or faulty red blood cell production, or anemia caused by the destruction of red blood cells.

Symptoms and signs

The symptoms and signs of anemia will vary according to the type of anemia and its underlying cause. However, there are some symptoms that are common to most types of anemia. These include fatigue, shortness of breath, dizziness, heart palpitations, and difficulty concentrating. Sometimes there are symptoms of angina pectoris, such as chest pain, as a result of insufficient oxygen reaching the heart muscle, and palpitations because the heart is overworking in an attempt to compensate for a lack of oxygen.

Each anemia will also exhibit a set of unique symptoms. For example, iron deficiency anemia is often associated with peculiar cravings to eat substances such as paper, ice, or dirt. Also, there may be the signs of koilonychia, which is the upward curvature of the nails, or soreness of the mouth with cracks at the corners.

People suffering from anemia caused by vitamin B_{12} deficiency may experience peripheral neuropathy (nerve damage), clumsiness, or dementia, as well as hallucinations. Anemia associated with abnormal red blood cell production, such as sickle-cell anemia, is often characterized by delayed growth and development in children and episodes of severe joint, abdominal, or limb pain.

Types of anemia that are caused by the excessive destruction of red blood cells are accompanied by symptoms such as jaundice, brown or red urine, failure to thrive in infancy, and leg ulcers.

Diagnosis

A complete medical history, a physical examination, and blood tests are all essential to diagnose anemia. A complete blood count (CBC) is usually performed, which determines the number, size, volume, and hemoglobin content of red blood cells. Once a diagnosis of anemia is confirmed, additional tests are given to ascertain the specific underlying cause. If initial studies point to iron deficiency, then the blood levels of iron and the serum levels of ferritin—the principal form in which iron is stored in the body—are measured, because these are the best indicators of the body's total iron stores. However, if vitamin deficiency is suspected, then blood levels of vitamin B_{12} and folate are measured. Specific blood tests are used to detect rare causes of anemia, such as an autoimmune disorder directed against the red blood cells, or red blood cell fragility.

Hemolytic anemia can be identified by measuring the by-products of red blood cell degradation in the urine and blood. In some rare cases, a bone marrow biopsy (sample of the bone marrow) may be removed for analysis in order to determine whether the cause of the anemia is a result of defective red blood cell production.

Treatments

Treatment of anemia is cause specific. Anemias caused by the deficiency of nutrients such as iron or B_{12} are treated with long-term supplementation of the depleted nutrient by injection or tablet form.

Aplastic anemia may be treated by a blood transfusion, a bone marrow transplant, or a course of immunosuppressant drugs to suppress the immune system. Currently there are no treatments for inherited anemias, such as thalassemia and sickle-cell anemia, which is caused by the production of abnormal red blood cells. The administration of oxygen, pain-relieving drugs, and oral and intravenous fluids are provided to improve the symptoms. Treatment is sometimes with blood transfusions, but regular transfusions can cause a buildup of iron in the body. Bone marrow transplant is another possibility.

Management of hemolytic anemia includes avoiding suspect medications, treating related infections, and taking drugs that suppress the immune system.

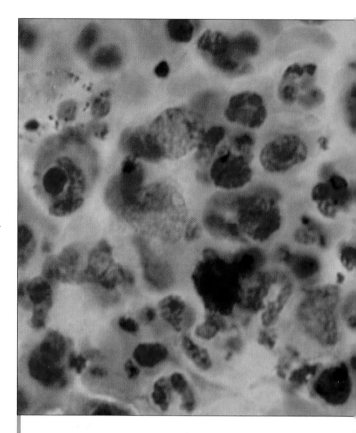

This photomicrograph of a bone marrow smear shows normal iron stores. The smear was stained with Prussian blue. Normal iron stores in the bone marrow are seen as dark blue stained material. In iron deficiency anemia these stores are depleted for reasons such as heavy blood loss, pregnancy, or lack of iron in the diet.

Prevention

Most types of anemia cannot be prevented. However, anemia caused by a nutrient deficiency can be prevented by eating a healthy and varied diet. To avoid iron deficiency, people should eat a diet rich in iron-containing foods such as meat, beans, lentils, and dark green leafy vegetables. In addition, supplementing the diet with vitamin C helps prevent iron deficiency anemia because vitamin C helps increase iron absorption, especially iron from plant sources.

Eating iron-rich foods is particularly important for people who have high iron requirements, such as children (iron is needed during growth spurts) and pregnant and menstruating women. Adequate iron intake is also crucial for infants, strict vegetarians, and long-distance runners. Folate and vitamin B_{12} deficiency may also be prevented by eating a diet rich in these B vitamins. Folate can be found in such foods as citrus

TYPES OF ANEMIA

TYPE	CAUSES	TREATMENTS
Iron deficiency	Menstruation, blood loss, iron-deficient diet	Supplementation with iron
Megaloblastic	Deficiency of folic acid and vitamin B_{12}	Short course of B_{12} injections or folic acid, suitable diet
Aplastic	Inability of the bone marrow to make blood cells; may be a result of radiation therapy	Blood transfusion, bone marrow transplant, or immunosuppressant drugs
Thalassemia	Inherited condition in which red blood cells are unable to grow and mature	Blood transfusions, sometimes removal of spleen
Sickle-cell	An inherited anemia in which red blood cells are typically sickle-shaped and die early, leaving a shortage of red blood cells	Blood transfusion, penicillin, supplements of folic acid, immunization against infection
Hemolytic	Various causes, such as autoimmune disorder, infections, certain drugs	Removal of the spleen, immunosuppressant drugs, red blood cell transfusion
Pernicious	A deficiency of vitamin B_{12}	Vitamin B_{12} injections for life
Anemia caused by other diseases	Bleeding caused by kidney and bladder tumors	Treatment of the tumors may resolve the anemia

juices, fortified breakfast cereals, and vegetables. Vitamin B_{12} is found in meat and dairy products.

Parents or relatives of a child with thalassemia may be advised to undergo genetic counseling to find out their risk of having another child with this inherited type of anemia.

Epidemiology

Iron deficiency anemia is one of the most common disorders worldwide; it is more prevalent in children and women of childbearing age.

The prevalence of iron deficiency anemia is around 50 percent in the developing world and 10 percent in developed countries. Around 3 to 4 million people in the United States have some form of anemia. The condition affects about 12 percent of women and about 7 percent of men. The prevalence increases with age, being around 45 percent in men who are more than 85 years old. Although older people are more likely to develop iron-deficiency anemia, it is not necessarily because of their age. A huge percentage of the population in developing countries have iron-deficiency anemia; in Africa, about 206 million people have anemia.

Sonia Gulati

See also
- Cancer, bladder • Cancer, colorectal
- Cancer, kidney • Celiac disease
- Eating disorders • Menstrual disorders
- Sickle-cell anemia • Stomach ulcer
- Vitamin deficiency

Aneurysm

An aneurysm is a cardiovascular disorder in which the walls of an artery are distorted by bulging. An aneurysm may be due to deterioration of the vessel wall and fatty deposits called atherosclerotic plaques.

An aneurysm is an abnormal dilation of a weakened artery. There are two major types of aneurysms: saccular, or berry, aneurysms, which are more common, develop on one side of an artery, and may be attached via a stem; and fusiform aneurysms, in which there is no stem and the arterial wall bulges on all sides. Aneurysms commonly form along the aorta. Abdominal aortic aneurysms are the most common, but aneurysms can also develop in the thorax, or chest, region. Cerebral aneurysms are dilatations of arteries that supply the brain. Ventricular aneurysms result from a weakened left ventricle (upper chamber) of the heart.

Causes and symptoms

Exact causes are generally unknown, although Marfan's syndrome and syphilis are both known to cause aneurysms. Aneurysms form in regions where proteins in the vessel wall are degraded. Atherosclerotic plaques (cholesterol deposits) are often present, but it is unknown which comes first: the plaque or the aneurysm. Risk factors for aneurysm include smoking, high blood pressure, and a family history of aneurysm. It is most common in Caucasian men more than 60 years of age.

Small aneurysms remain undetected, but larger ones tend to bleed and rupture. Fast-growing aneurysms can press on nearby organs. Lower-back or abdominal pain or a tender, pulsating mass indicates an abdominal aneurysm; massive loss of blood from a rupture leads to collapse of the blood pressure. A cerebral aneurysm causes headache and loss of sensation or vision, depending on its location; when it ruptures, the headache becomes severe, there may be nausea, fainting, stroke, permanent disability, or death.

Diagnosis and treatments

Aneurysms are often detected during tests for other conditions. Ultrasound imaging, which uses sound waves, is a noninvasive detection technique. X-rays, such as CT scans or angiograms, use a contrast-enhancing dye in blood vessels, or magnetic resonance imaging (MRI) is used before surgery to locate the aneurysm.

Aortic aneurysms occur in 5 to 7 percent of Americans over 60. Aneurysms more than $2\frac{1}{2}$ inches (6 cm) in diameter have a 20 percent risk of rupturing, with mortality rates up to 80 percent. Ruptures occur in about 5 in 10,000 people suffering from aneurysms.

If the aneurysm is more than 2 inches (5 cm) wide, surgical intervention is indicated. Aneurysms can be bypassed using vascular grafts in which a blood vessel from the patient is used to shunt the blood away from the weak area of the vessel wall. Blood then flows through the graft, relieving pressure on weakened walls. Nonsurgical repair involves insertion of stent grafts in the vessel at the site of the aneurysm. Prevention includes quitting smoking and reducing blood pressure.

Sonal Jhaveri

KEY FACTS

Description

A balloonlike expansion of an artery.

Causes

No cause is known.

Risk factors

High blood pressure, smoking, family history, age.

Symptoms

No symptoms if the aneurysm is slow-growing. Localized pain if large. Headaches if in brain. If ruptured, severe headache, nausea, fainting, permanent disability, or instant death.

Diagnosis

Imaging tests such as ultrasound, X-rays, or MRI.

Treatments

Surgery if large and rapidly growing; stent graft.

Pathogenesis

Weak vessel wall, often with atherosclerotic plaque formation, leads to dilatation. Large aneurysms bleed, rupture with massive blood loss.

Prevention

Managing risk factors can help prevent aneurysms.

Epidemiology

Most common in Caucasian men of 60 and above.

See also
- Stroke and related disorders

Anthrax

A bacterial disease occurring naturally in the environment and usually transmitted among herbivorous animals, anthrax can be spread to humans by contact with infected animals or animal products.

Anthrax is a disease caused by the spore-forming soil bacterium *Bacillus anthracis*; it occurs mainly in herbivores, such as goats, camels, antelope, and sheep. The bacterium occurs naturally in the environment, and anthrax is common in animals worldwide, especially in Africa, Asia, and South America. Prior to the 22 cases of human illness—five of which were fatal—resulting from bioterrorism in 2001, the most recent human case of the deadliest form of the disease in the United States was in 1976, when a weaver contracted pulmonary anthrax from yarn imported from Pakistan. There have been no cases of human anthrax in the United States since 2001.

Symptoms

Contact with infected animals or animal products can lead to human illness. Symptoms depend on the site of infection and are caused by toxins produced by the bacterium. In cutaneous anthrax, a swollen, painless black eschar (area of dead tissue) forms at the site of infection within 1 to 12 days; lymph glands in the area near the sore may enlarge. Up to 20 percent of cutaneous anthrax cases are fatal if untreated.

Gastrointestinal anthrax occurs within seven days after ingesting the anthrax bacterium and is marked by nausea, loss of appetite, bloody diarrhea, fever, and abdominal pain. Pharyngitis and neck pain may occur. Death occurs in 20 to 60 percent of cases.

The most deadly form of the disease is pulmonary anthrax. Within 1 to 42 days after inhaling airborne anthrax spores, the individual develops common-cold or flulike symptoms followed by pain in the chest, shortness of breath, and respiratory failure. Septicemia and toxemia are common; meningitis may develop and is usually fatal. Death occurs in 45 to 90 percent of cases of pulmonary anthrax.

Diagnosis and treatments

Anthrax can be diagnosed by isolating *Bacillus anthracis* from blood, skin lesions, or respiratory secretions;

KEY FACTS

Description

Acute, potentially fatal infection that can spread from livestock to humans.

Cause

Infection with the spore-forming bacterium *Bacillus anthracis*.

Risk factors

Contact with infected animals or animal products.

Symptoms and signs

Depend on site of infection.

Diagnosis

Isolation of the *B. anthracis* from skin lesions, blood, or respiratory secretions; measurement of antibodies in the blood; tests using polymerase chain reaction (PCR) to identify anthrax spores.

Treatments

Antibiotics; antibiotics and a vaccine for those exposed to anthrax but not yet ill.

Pathogenesis

In the body, swelling. Toxins released impair immunity and cause bleeding, tissue death, and further swelling. Lymph nodes are affected and destroyed and septicemia develops. In pulmonary anthrax, meningitis and respiratory failure are common and often cause death.

Prevention

Antibiotic prophylaxis for up to 60 days after exposure to prevent the disease. A vaccine is available for military personnel and laboratory workers who may be exposed to anthrax.

Epidemiology

Apart from a bioterrorist attack in 2001, there have been no cases of pulmonary anthrax in the United States since 1976.

measuring specific antibodies to the bacterium in the blood; or by using polymerase chain reaction (PCR) techniques to identify anthrax spores.

Treatment is with antibiotics, usually ciprofloxacin or doxycycline. Preventive treatment, or prophylaxis, involves injections of a vaccine in six doses. This vaccine is primarily given to laboratory workers with potential exposure to the bacterium and to military personnel.

Rita Washko

See also
• Throat infections

Antibiotic-resistant infections

Antibiotics were discovered in the 1940s and have been used to successfully treat infections caused by bacteria. For decades, these miracle drugs have prevented serious illness and death from bacterial diseases. Unfortunately, antibiotic use also promotes the development of antibiotic-resistant bacteria. According to the U.S. Centers for Disease Control and Prevention (CDC), almost all significant bacterial infections affecting humans are becoming resistant to commonly prescribed antibiotics.

Doctors can no longer rely on their first or second choice of antibiotics to fight many human infections. Scientists are concerned that physicians will lose these essential infection-fighting tools. The majority of the most serious antibiotic-resistant infections occur in hospitalized people, but these infections are becoming more frequent in healthy people. Public health officials are sounding the alarm about antibiotic resistance because of the emergence of "superbugs" in the last decade. These germs are resistant to many antibiotics, including powerful drugs such as vancomyin, which is reserved by physicians to fight the most stubborn infections.

Causes and risk factors

Antibiotic-resistant infections are caused by bacteria that survive treatment with commonly prescribed antibiotics. When bacteria reproduce, slight changes occur in their genetic material. Some of these changes allow bacteria to evade certain antibiotics.

Each person carries more microorganisms on the skin than there are people in the world. Bacteria that coexist on our skin and in our bodies without causing disease are called healthy bacterial flora. When antibiotic-resistant bacteria develop, they compete with our own flora, becoming a trivial member of our bacterial melting pot. However, in the presence of an antibiotic drug, the resistant bacteria can magnify their population a thousandfold to a millionfold. The resulting infection is harder to treat and often requires a more powerful antibiotic drug.

Both viruses and bacteria cause common infections. However, antibiotics fight only those infections caused by bacteria, not those caused by viruses. Viruses and bacteria are distinct. Bacteria are one of the smallest life-forms and occur as single cells. Many bacteria are not harmful, and some are actually beneficial. Disease-causing bacteria can grow on the skin or inside the body and cause illness. For example, strep throat is caused by bacteria called *Streptococcus pyrogenes*.

KEY FACTS

Description
Hard-to-treat infections caused by bacteria that survive treatment with common antibiotics.

Causes
Repeated and improper use of antibiotics.

Risk factors
In hospital settings, antibiotic use and underlying health conditions. In the community, close contact with people who have antibiotic-resistant infections. Use of antibiotics in livestock.

Symptoms and signs
Bacterial infection that does not improve after treatment with antibiotics.

Diagnosis
Laboratory tests of blood or infected tissues.

Treatments
Laboratory testing determines which antibiotics will be most effective.

Pathogenesis
When bacteria survive treatment with antibiotic, they continue to multiply. The bacterial infection becomes more severe and harder to treat. Doctors must prescribe more powerful and toxic antibiotics.

Prevention
Only take antibiotics for bacterial infections. Take antibiotics as prescribed by your health care provider, and finish the course.

Epidemiology
Antibiotics were discovered in the 1940s. Unfortunately, antibiotic use also promotes the development of antibiotic-resistant bacteria. For example, MRSA was first isolated in the 1960s.

Viruses are even smaller than bacteria. They are mostly genetic material—DNA or RNA—and often have a protective coat surrounding their genes. A virus cannot reproduce outside the body's cells. Viruses invade healthy cells. They use the machinery of the body's cells to make copies of themselves. Typically, newly formed viruses destroy the cell as they leave it to infect new cells. Viruses rather than bacteria are the more frequent culprits of respiratory illnesses such as colds, sore throats, and coughs. Most stuffy noses are caused by viruses called rhinoviruses.

Symptoms

During the early days of a cold or upper respiratory infection, the nose produces clear mucus. The mucus helps wash the germs from the sinuses (air-filled spaces in the skull) and nose. Immune cells then join in to fight the infection, and the mucus changes from clear to a whitish or yellowish color. During recovery from a stuffy nose, the bacteria that live normally in the nose grow back, which can change the mucus to a greenish color, which experts say is normal.

According to the CDC, doctors feel pressure to prescribe antibiotics for respiratory infections. Respiratory infections such as sore throat, cold, and coughs are usually caused by viruses. Tens of millions of antibiotics prescribed in doctors' offices are for viral infections. Using antibiotics for a viral infection offers no benefit to the affected person and could possibly cause harm. Taking unnecessary antibiotics increases the risk of antibiotic resistance developing in bacteria.

Staphylococcus aureus, commonly called staph bacteria, is found on human skin and in the nose. Staph bacteria are one of the most common causes of skin infections in the United States. Most of these skin infections are minor. However, staph bacteria can also cause serious blood infections and pneumonia, which can be fatal. Hospitalized patients are particularly at risk for antibiotic-resistant infections, including infections caused by staph bacteria. Often, these infections are introduced by urinary or intravenous catheters, and can be serious. Certain underlying health conditions increase the risk of infection. Such conditions include diabetes, kidney disease, and immune-system problems. Also, antibiotic use—for example, to prevent infection after surgery—increases a patient's risk of developing a resistant infection. Staph superbugs are often referred to by their abbreviations: for example, MRSA (methicillin-resistant *Staphylococcus aureus*),

VRSA (vancomycin-resistant *Staphylococcus aureus*), and VISA (vancomycin-intermediate *Staphylococcus aureus*). MRSA infections are becoming more common in various communities and are affecting healthy people. No longer confined to health care settings, MRSA outbreaks have occurred among children, athletes, and military recruits.

In the last decade, doctors are seeing more cases of antibiotic resistant infections in healthy adults and children. Close contact with people who have antibiotic-resistant infections is an important risk factor in healthy people. In one outbreak among high-school athletes, sharing of towels, sports equipment, and uniforms were important factors in transmitting MRSA from one athlete to another.

The use of antibiotics in livestock on farms is also under scrutiny by government agencies. There appears to be a link to the development of antibiotic resistance in humans, especially when the same class of drugs (for example, fluoroquinolones) are used in both livestock and to treat humans.

Prevention and treatments

To help prevent antibiotic-resistant infections, antibiotics should be taken as prescribed by a health care provider. A course of antibiotics should not be stopped at the first sign of improvement. To help prevent resistant bacteria from gaining an upper hand, it is very important to take every dose of the prescribed antibiotic until it is finished. Antibiotics should not be saved for use at a later time.

Experts on the subject of infections maintain that many bacterial infections get better on their own and that physicians should only prescribe antibiotics when it is likely to benefit the patient. Viral infections, such as cold or flu, do not respond to antibiotics.

Frequent hand washing is one of the easiest ways to reduce transmission of infectious diseases. Sometimes an antibiotic is needed. A health care provider should be consulted if a respiratory illness gets worse or lasts a long time. To treat an antibiotic-resistant infection, clinicians perform laboratory tests to find the antibiotic or combination of drugs that will beat the superbug. Providing clinicians with better tools to distinguish a viral illness from a bacterial infection will help prevent unnecessary antibiotic use.

Mary Quirk

See also
• Diabetes

Anxiety disorders

An anxiety disorder is any of several mental disorders that fills an individual's life with overwhelming fear, dread, or worry. The person may suffer from shortness of breath, pounding heartbeat, dizziness, or other symptoms. An anxiety disorder can cripple a person's ability to lead a normal life; if left untreated it can become progressively worse.

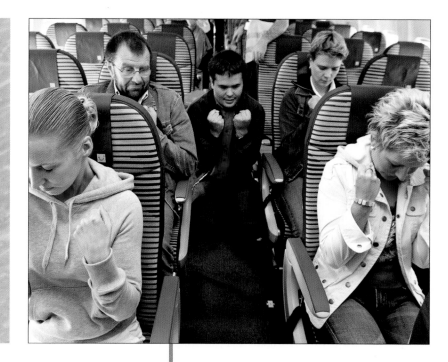

One of the most common fears is fear of flying. A workshop on an airplane at Hanover airport is conducted by a therapist who specializes in treating this debilitating fear, which sometimes causes panic attacks. During the session, the therapist tries to help passengers overcome their anxiety and fear of the airplane crashing.

Everyone has feelings of fear, dread, and worry. To feel nervous or anxious before a chemistry exam or before making an important decision, such as purchasing a car, is normal and may even be adaptive. However, anxiety disorders are not normal. All anxiety disorders have the common theme of excessive, irrational, and uncontrollable fear and dread.

Types and causes

Six types of anxiety disorders are identified: panic disorder, obsessive-compulsive disorder (OCD), post-traumatic stress disorder (PTSD), social anxiety disorder, specific phobias, and generalized anxiety disorder (GAD). Each disorder has unique features.

Although each of the disorders has different characteristics, a chemical imbalance of serotonin appears to be a common factor. Serotonin is a neurotransmitter, a chemical messenger that helps move information from one nerve cell to another. If serotonin is out of balance, messages cannot get through and can alter the way the brain acts in certain stressful situations. Scientists working with brain imaging have added another part to the puzzle. They have uncovered a network of interacting structures that control thoughts and fears. The amygdala, an almond-shaped structure deep within the brain, is the communications center between the brain and incoming signals from the senses. Certain emotional memories stored in the amygdala are involved in fears and phobias. The hippocampus, another structure in the brain, plays a key role in encoding information into memory and is responsible for processing threatening stimuli. Improper functioning of these brain parts are related to abnormal fears.

Anxiety disorders tend to run in families. Studies of twins suggest that heredity plays a role in anxiety disorders, but experience and environment are also contributory factors.

Symptoms of panic disorder

Sudden and repeated terror strikes people with panic disorder. There is no warning of an impending attack, and the fear experienced is out of proportion to the situation. Difficulty breathing, palpitations, dizziness, trembling or shaking, even thoughts of dying and losing one's mind are typical symptoms. Fearing future panic attacks, the person may avoid certain places where the attack may occur. Panic attacks can occur at any time, even during sleep, and usually peak within 1 minute, lasting up to 1 hour. This disorder affects about 6 million adults in the United States, is twice as common in women as men, and often begins during late adolescence. About 90 percent of people with panic disorder can be treated. However, many do not seek treatment, which can lead to serious consequences. For example, an affected person may avoid essential activities, like driving or shopping; this avoidance makes normal work and home life impossible.

Symptoms of obsessive-compulsive disorder

This anxiety disorder has two components: obsession and compulsion. An obsession is a persistent thought that a person cannot suppress. Compulsions are actions that someone does again and again, sometimes hundreds of times. An individual may realize that the obsession and compulsion are irrational and make life difficult. For example, a boy may think that his father is going to die and that counting every step he takes may save his father. The boy knows that this is not true, but he still must do it. In another example, a woman is convinced that germs and dirt are taking over her life, and she must wash her hands repeatedly.

Senseless rituals plague the person, and aggressive thoughts are common. OCD traps people in repetitive thoughts or behaviors. Some of the most common obsessions are contamination, persistent doubts about having locked the door or turned off the stove, extreme need for orderliness, and aggressive thoughts such as the urge to yell "Fire!" in a crowded building. The most common compulsions are cleaning, checking for something that might be forgotten, repeating words or actions, slowness, or hoarding things, such as old newspapers. In the United States, OCD affects about 3.3 million adults and strikes men and women in equal numbers. About one-third of affected adults first experienced symptoms as children.

Symptoms of post-traumatic stress disorder

Although the plight of Vietnam War veterans brought post-traumatic stress disorder (PTSD) to the public's attention, the condition may also occur after a person experiences a criminal assault, serious accident, natural disaster, or anything that interferes with normal life. More people appear to experience PTSD after large-scale violence than other types of terrible events. For example, one study showed that 8 percent of people

---

KEY FACTS

Description

A serious mental disorder that fills the person's life with overwhelming anxiety and fear.

Causes and risk factors

Exact cause is unknown, but changes in the brain and environmental stresses are involved.

Symptoms

Vary with the type of anxiety disorder, but general symptoms include fear, uneasiness, and uncontrollable, irrational thoughts.

Diagnosis

Evaluation by a psychiatrist from the patient's reports of the symptoms.

Treatments

Drugs such as antidepressants, psychotherapy, and behavior therapy.

Pathogenesis

Emerges in childhood, teen years, or early adulthood. Left untreated, it will become worse.

Epidemiology

In the United States, about 40 million adults have anxiety disorders; about 6 million have panic attacks. They occur slightly more often in women than in men and occur with equal frequency in Caucasians, African Americans, and Hispanics.

---

living in a certain area of Manhattan—about 67,000 people—experienced PTSD after 9/11. Whatever the source, people with PTSD relive the trauma in nightmares or during the day. The person may have a general feeling of numbness and detachment from surroundings. Ordinary events may trigger flashbacks in which the person reenacts the experience. Other symptoms include startling easily, irritability, and outbursts of anger. Symptoms usually begin within three months after the event, although some may not appear until years later. About 5.2 million adults in the United States have PTSD, which can occur at any age, including childhood. Women are more likely than men to have the condition.

Symptoms of social phobia

Also called social anxiety disorder, social phobia is a condition in which the person has an unreasonable fear of everyday social situations. For example, a man may be excessively self-conscious and think others are watching and judging him. As a result, he hates social situations and may avoid them completely. In addition, he may anticipate or worry about being in the situation weeks before it is to happen. This condition can negatively interfere with his normal daily routine, including school, work, social activities, and relationships. The phobia may occur in one type of situation, such as a fear of public speaking or speaking to strangers, or it may have a broad severe form that the person experiences anytime people are around. Physical symptoms include heart palpitations, shaking, sweating, diarrhea, confusion, and blushing. This disorder is the most common anxiety disorder. In any year, some 5.3 million people in the United States may have the disorder, which often begins in early adolescence or in childhood.

Specific phobias and GAD

These phobias may plague an individual with an abnormal fear of certain objects or situations. There are hundreds of fears or phobias. The most common fear is that of animals, such as dogs, cats, snakes, or insects. Others include situational phobias, such as heights or being in a closed-in place, fears of storms or water, seeing blood or injections, and even fear of a costumed clown. These phobias are not just being afraid but are irrational fears of something that poses no harm. For example, one may not like snakes, but someone with a phobia may experience the symptoms of a panic attack, and the condition interferes with normal activities.

The National Institute of Mental Health estimates that about 19 million people, or 8.7 percent of the adult population, in the United States have phobias, which usually appear in adolescence but can occur in people of all ages. Diagnosis is based on reported symptoms and if the phobia interferes with daily routine. People with generalized anxiety disorder (GAD) worry about many things, even those that would be insignificant to most people. They expect impending disaster in health, family, work, or school, disproportionate to the situation.

Worry causes muscular tension, sweating, nausea, irritability, and a host of other anxiety symptoms. About 6.8 million adults in the United States suffer from GAD during the course of a year. Often beginning in childhood or adolescence, it is more common in women than men.

Diagnosis

To diagnose an anxiety disorder, a psychiatrist evaluates the affected person from a report of his or her symptoms. For example, to make a diagnosis of OCD, the obsession or compulsions must take up at least an hour every day and interfere with normal routines, and in PTSD the affected person must exhibit symptoms for more than a month.

Treatments

Researchers are developing effective treatments for each of the anxiety disorders. Two types of treatment are generally available: medication and psychotherapy, including cognitive-behavioral therapy. Drugs can be used for general treatment of anxiety disorders. Certain antidepressants, called selective serotonin reuptake inhibitors or SSRIs, act on the chemical neurotransmitter serotonin. These SSRIs are especially prescribed for panic disorder, OCD, PTSD, and social phobia. Benzodiazepines, types of high-potency tranquilizers, relieve symptoms quickly and may be effective in panic attacks. Other drugs, for example beta blockers, may target symptoms such as rapid heartbeat.

The second treatment, psychotherapy, involves the care of a mental health professional, such as a psychiatrist, psychologist, or counselor, trained in dealing with anxiety disorders. A form of psychotherapy, cognitive behavioral therapy (CBT), helps people change their thinking patterns, overcome fear, and understand the irrationality of their fears. The behavioral part seeks to change the person's reactions to the anxiety-provoking situation by confronting the thing that he or she fears. For example, in treating someone who fears dirt or germs, the therapist encourages dirtying the hands and even going without washing them for a certain period of time. Behavior therapy alone has been used to treat certain specific phobias by making the person face the source of that fear. The goal of CBT is to eliminate the irrational beliefs or behaviors that help maintain the anxiety disorders. Some people with these disorders benefit from joining a self-help group. By sharing their problems and achievements with others, they learn techniques of coping with anxiety disorders.

Epidemiology

Around 6 million people in the United States, 2.7 percent of adults, are affected by panic attacks. About 1.5 percent of the world's population, around 89 million people, have an anxiety or panic disorder.

Evelyn Kelly

See also
• Depressive disorders • Post-traumatic stress disorder

Appendicitis

The severe abdominal pain of appendicitis is a result of acute inflammation of the appendix. Anyone who is suspected of having appendicitis must be examined and treated rapidly to prevent the appendix rupturing, which can lead to a potentially fatal condition, peritonitis.

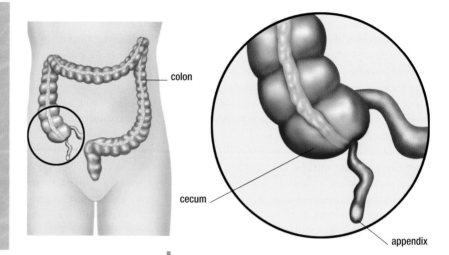

colon

cecum

appendix

The appendix is a small, narrow tubelike structure attached to the cecum (first part of the large intestine) at one end and closed at the other end. The appendix is usually located in the right lower portion of the abdomen. The inner lining of the appendix produces mucus that flows into the cecum.

Causes

Appendicitis is an inflammation of the appendix. It may be caused by mucus or fecal material blocking the opening of the appendix. Other causes of appendicitis include swelling of lymphatic tissue within the appendix or infection by bacteria.

Symptoms

The main symptom of appendicitis is abdominal pain. At first the pain is felt around the navel. Most people will indicate the location with a circular motion of the hand around the central portion of the abdomen. Appendiceal inflammation increases the spread to its outer covering and then to a thin membrane on the inside of the abdomen called the peritoneum. Once the peritoneum becomes inflamed, the pain becomes localized in one small area in the lower right abdomen.

There is usually loss of appetite, fever, nausea, vomiting, constipation, or diarrhea, inability to pass gas, and abdominal swelling associated with appendicitis. Not everyone will have all of the symptoms, which are more likely to be seen in younger patients. Older patients may present with only one or two symptoms. The pain intensifies and worsens with

The appendix projects in front of or behing the cecum, which is the beginning of the colon or large intestine. An inflamed appendix is a common cause of pain and peritonitis, which is inflammation of the abdominal cavity.

movement, breathing deeply, coughing, or sneezing. People may experience tenesmus, a feeling that a bowel movement will relieve their discomfort, but laxatives and pain medication should not be taken.

Pathogenesis

If appendicitis is not diagnosed or goes untreated, and rupture occurs, it can lead to an infected abscess and peritonitis, which is difficult to treat and can often prove fatal. If the appendix ruptures, the infection spreads into the abdominal cavity, where it can attack other tissues. Occasionally, the body is able to fight off the infection, and inflammation does not spread throughout the abdomen. Infants, young children, and older adults are at highest risk of appendicitis.

A lesser complication of appendicitis is intestinal obstruction. Obstruction occurs when the inflammation surrounding the appendix stops the intestinal muscles from working, thereby preventing the contents of the bowel from passing. A life-threatening complication of appendicitis is sepsis, a condition in which bacteria enter the blood and travel to other parts of the body, causing organ failure and death. Because signs and symptoms vary widely, delays before operating can be hazardous.

Diagnosis

The diagnosis is based on the history and physical examination and supported by blood tests and imaging. There will be pain, which becomes localized to the right lower abdomen region (peri-umbilical area) when the inflamed appendix comes in contact with the peritoneum. Other signs include rebound tenderness (pain that occurs when the abdomen is pushed in by the examining hand of the physician and then quickly released). The pain becomes sudden but then transiently worse. Right-sided tenderness on digital rectal examination implies an increased likelihood that the patient has appendicitis since the appendix normally lies on the right. Other signs used in support of diagnosis are the psoas sign (pain on flexion of the hips), the obturator sign (pain on internal rotation of the hip), and Rovsing's sign (pain on the right side when pressing on the left). These signs are all indicators of inflammation, although not all patients have them.

X-rays, ultrasounds, and computed tomography (CT) scans can produce images of the abdomen. Plain X-rays can show signs of obstruction, perforation (free air in abdomen), and a foreign body, but rarely an appendicolith (calcified deposit). The most common test is the CT scan, used when the clinical examination is in doubt. A CT scan with modern equipment has a sensitivity of over 95 percent and specificity of greater than 95 percent for diagnosing appendicitis. The white blood cell count (WBC) in the blood is usually elevated with infection. However, appendicitis is not the only condition that causes an elevated WBC count; almost any infection or inflammation can cause an elevated count. Urinalysis usually is abnormal if there is an inflammation, infection, or stone in the kidney or bladder, which sometimes can be confused with appendicitis. Confusion can also occur when the inflamed appendix lies in close proximity to the ureter, spreading inflammation to that area, resulting in pyuria (pus in the urine) or increased WBC in the urine.

KEY FACTS

Description

An inflammation of the blind-ended tubelike structure attached to the cecum (large intestine).

Causes

Blockage of opening of appendix by thick mucous buildup or a hard mass of fecal material. Obstruction of the appendix results in increased pressure buildup that leads to reduced blood flow. Bacteria invade the appendix, causing inflammation, tissue death, and perforation.

Symptoms

Abdominal pain that migrates from around the navel to the right lower abdomen. Associated with loss of appetite, fever, nausea, vomiting, constipation, or diarrhea.

Diagnosis

Based primarily on clinical examination supported by blood test and imaging studies (X-rays of abdomen, ultrasound scans, computed tomography).

Treatment

By surgical removal of the appendix; either by open laparotomy or closed laparoscopic approach using a camera.

Epidemiology

Overall incidence of appendicitis is approximately 1 case per 1,000 population per year in the United States. There is a 28–57 percent failure to diagnose appendicitis in patients under 12 years old; and there is a 70–94 percent perforation rate in young children who are under 2 years of age.

Treatments

Appendicitis is treated by removal of the appendix through a surgical procedure called an appendectomy. The operation has historically involved an open surgical incision in the right lower part of the abdomen. The operation can be performed by laparoscopy, which involves small incisions and a camera to visualize areas of interest. The appendix is usually removed, even if it is normal, since it is an evolutionary organ that has no current function in humans. This practice eliminates the appendix from future episodes of pain. Antibiotics are often given prior to surgery to reduce inflammation and help kill remaining bacteria. No single test can diagnose appendicitis.

Epidemiology

Anyone can develop appendicitis, but it occurs most often in those between the ages of 10 and 30 years. The overall incidence of appendicitis is estimated at 1 case per 1,000 population each year. About 6 percent of the U.S. population will experience appendicitis at some point in their life. Patients under the age of 6 years and elderly patients have higher rates of failed diagnosis of appendicitis. In the United States around 700,000 people are hospitalized each year with acute appendicitis.

Isaac Grate

See also
• Peritonitis

Arrhythmia

Any irregularity of the normally steady, rhythmic beating of the heart is called arrhythmia. It may be temporary, intermittent, continuous, or immediately life-threatening, resulting in cardiac arrest (cessation of the pumping action of the heart). Known causes are as diverse as caffeine and cardiovascular disease. Before treatment, the cause of the arrhythmia usually needs to be identified. However, in a life-threatening emergency, intravenous medication or electrical conversion is necessary to return the heartbeat to a normal rhythm. Arrhythmias with a cause that cannot be identified are referred to as idiopathic arrhythmias, and the symptoms of these, rather than the cause, must be treated.

Arrhythmia is the result of a disturbance that alters the transmission of electrical impulses within the heart, affecting the normal rhythm or rate of the heartbeat. There are two main types of arrhythmias: tachycardias, in which the heart rate is too high, and bradycardias, in which it is too low.

Tachycardias vary in severity. Sinus tachycardia presents a fast but regular heart rate, similar to the heart rate of someone under stress or during exercise. Supraventricular tachycardia is regular but much faster. Ventricular tachycardia is a fast, irregular heartbeat. Atrial fibrillation is very fast, irregular beating of the atria (the upper chambers of the heart), which leads to rapid, irregular beats of the ventricles (the lower chambers of the heart). During ventricular fibrillation, the very fast twitching movements of the ventricles prevent the heart from pumping blood. This type of arrhythmia is very serious and requires emergency treatment.

Bradycardias, such as sinus bradycardia, produce a slow but regular beat as a result of reduced electrical activity. A slow, regular beat is often normal in fit people, such as athletes, but it can also occur in people with hypothyroidism (an underactive thyroid gland) or those who are taking antidepressant drugs.

Heart block is another type of bradycardia in which there is a slow, irregular heartbeat as a result of complete or partial blockage of electrical impulses through the heart.

Causes

The causes of arrhythmia can be divided into two categories. Primary rhythm disturbances, which are not associated with any underlying heart disease, may be triggered by factors such as alcohol, smoking, or drug side effects. Secondary rhythm disturbances arise from existing heart conditions, such as coronary artery disease, cardiomyopathy, hyperthyroidism, rheumatic heart disease, or heart valve problems.

Risk factors

Risk factors include coronary artery disease; high blood pressure (hypertension); high blood cholesterol levels; unhealthy lipid or triglyceride blood levels; atherosclerosis, diabetes, thyroid-gland disorders; and damaged heart valves. People who have had a heart attack and those who have undergone heart surgery are also at risk of developing arrhythmia.

Over-the-counter (OTC) drugs can produce heartbeat irregularities, although these rarely become serious. OTC medications include cold, cough, and sinus medications and decongestants, which should be avoided by people with high blood pressure, heart disease, diabetes, or the eye disorder glaucoma.

Weight loss products, such as diet pills and powders, can also produce slight arrhythmia. Recent widespread publicity on the danger of ephedrine alkaloids, which are found in some herbal medicines, such as ma huang, has raised public awareness of the dangers of these compounds, although stimulants found in "pep" pills or beverages are also a danger.

Smoking, obesity, and high fat intake may increase the likelihood of developing arrhythmia. A long-term follow-up study of the well-known Framingham Heart Study has established that both overweight and obese individuals are at greater risk of developing serious, dangerous abnormal heart rhythms.

Symptoms and signs

A common symptom of arrhythmia is palpitations, which may be described by the person experiencing them as skipped beats, although no heartbeat is skipped—only the time interval between heartbeats is altered. Fluttering, pounding, racing, and flip-flopping feelings are other common descriptions. However, palpitations do not necessarily indicate a serious arrhythmia; they can also be caused by caffeine, nicotine, alcohol, anxiety, fatigue, or infections.

If the heart irregularities recur frequently, or are associated with fainting, shortness of breath, pain in the chest or neck, or light-headedness, a physician should be consulted because unrecognized heart disease, lung disease, or heart-valve malfunctions may be present. Another major concern is an increase in the pulse rate at the same time, which requires immediate medical attention to prevent sudden death.

Diagnosis

If the symptoms of arrhythmia are present, a physician will usually check the patient's pulse, listen to the heart with a stethoscope, and arrange for the patient to have electrocardiography (ECG), which involves attaching electrodes to the chest and measuring the electrical activity in various sites in the heart.

The results of the ECG are recorded on a tape, on which abnormal heartbeats can be seen. If the arrhythmia occurs only infrequently, patients are sometimes monitored for 24 hours, or they may be fitted with an ambulatory ECG, also called a Holter monitor, which is worn for 24 hours.

Treatments

Some types of arrhythmias can be treated with anti-arrhythmic drugs, such as beta blockers, ion channel blockers, and drugs that prolong repolarization. Defibrillation or cardioversion, which involves administering a short electric shock to the heart, can sometimes be used to restore the heartbeat back to normal.

If a patient continually experiences tachycardia, radiofrequency ablation—a nonsurgical technique that uses energy from electromagnetic waves—can be carried out to remove diseased tissue and restore a normal rhythm. In cases of a low heart rate, a cardiac pacemaker may be fitted.

Prevention

Maintaining a healthy lifestyle is the best way to eliminate the risk of cardiovascular disease or arrhythmias. Regular exercise and a low-fat diet with the emphasis on vegetables and fruits are preventive measures that can easily be implemented into daily life. Other healthy lifestyle choices include quitting smoking; cutting down on caffeine and alcohol intake; avoiding stressful situations; and having regular health checkups, which can detect the early signs of cardiovascular disease.

Epidemiology

The incidence of two types of arrhythmias, atrial fibrillation and ventricular fibrillation in particular, is on the rise worldwide and is projected to increase in coming years. Both of these types of arrhythmias are most often associated with cardiovascular disease. The more chronic type, atrial fibrillation, which increases the risk of heart failure and stroke, now affects more than 2 million people in the United States.

The American Heart Association estimates that the immediately life-threatening arrhythmia—ventricular fibrillation—is responsible for more than 400,000 deaths in the United States alone each year. Worldwide, more than 100 million people suffer from arrhythmia.

Nance Seiple

KEY FACTS

Description
Abnormalities of the heartbeat.

Risk factors
Heart disease, congenital heart defects, being overweight, caffeine, and some drugs.

Symptoms
Palpitations experienced by the individual as a fluttering, pounding, or racing. More serious irregularities may be light-headedness, shortness of breath, chest pain, or fainting.

Diagnosis
Checking the pulse; listening to the heart with a stethoscope; electrocardiogram.

Treatments
Depends on the cause. Goal is to restore the heart to beating regularly and rhythmically as quickly as possible.

Pathogenesis
Depends on type of arrhythmia; ventricular fibrillation is potentially fatal without immediate treatment. Supraventricular tachycardia is not usually a serious disorder.

Prevention
Avoiding substances and situations that may affect heartbeat; having existing health problems properly treated and controlled; maintaining a healthy lifestyle involving regular exercise.

Epidemiology
The incidence of arrhythmias is on the rise worldwide and projected to increase substantially.

See also
• Heart attack • Thyroid disorders

Arthritis

The term *arthritis* simply means inflammation of a joint and may be used to refer to more than 100 inflammatory or degenerative conditions that can vary in severity, causing swelling, pain, and stiffness in the joints. Arthritis can affect any age group, although it is more common in older people. Each type of arthritis may have different associated symptoms and treatments.

Arthritis is one of the most common chronic health problems in the United States and the leading cause of disability, affecting about 43 million adults. The most common form is osteoarthritis (OA), which affects about 21 million mostly older people in the United States.

Osteoarthritis is characterized by degeneration of joint cartilage, which causes pain and restriction of movement. It typically develops gradually and usually begins after the age of 40.

Other forms of arthritis can appear at any age including the autoimmune disorder rheumatoid arthritis, the metabolic disorder gout, and septic arthritis. Almost any joint may be affected, although the knees, hips, spinal, hand, and finger joints are most commonly affected.

Causes and risk factors

Many different disorders can cause arthritis, and the risk factors are similarly diverse. In some cases, arthritis may occur without an identifiable cause.

In osteoarthritis cartilage covering the ends of the bones at joints becomes eroded and the bones rub together, producing pain, swelling, and stiffness; over time, joints may become deformed. The affected joints flare up periodically and become inflamed. In many cases the underlying cause of the degeneration is not known, although weakness of the joint cartilage can sometimes be inherited. Excessive stress, repeated injuries, being overweight, and wear and tear as a result of increasing age may also contribute to osteoarthritis.

Rheumatoid arthritis (RA) is an autoimmune disease in which the immune system attacks the body's joints, causing inflammation. The disease can affect almost any joint, including those in fingers, wrists, shoulders, elbows, hips, knees, ankles, feet, and neck, however, the fingers are most commonly affected. The joints become swollen, inflamed, stiff, and eventually, deformed. Rheumatoid arthritis may also affect the heart, blood vessels, muscles, nervous system, and eyes. Rheumatoid arthritis is more common in women and may occur at any age. The exact cause of the condition is unknown, although there may be a genetic factor. Other immune disorders, such as systemic lupus erythematosus, may also produce arthritis.

Some infections may produce arthritis as a symptom or complication. Such infections include Lyme disease, tuberculosis, staphylococcal infection, gonorrhea, hepatitis B and C, and rubella. Septic arthritis occurs when a pathogen (an infectious agent such as a bacterium) directly attacks a joint. The infection can spread from elsewhere in the body, or the joint may be infected by a penetrating injury or in surgery. People at greatest risk of septic arthritis include intravenous drug users and people with joint implants, suppressed immune sys-

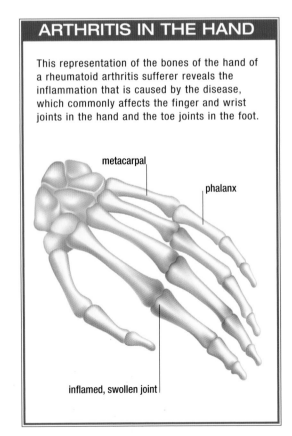

ARTHRITIS IN THE HAND

This representation of the bones of the hand of a rheumatoid arthritis sufferer reveals the inflammation that is caused by the disease, which commonly affects the finger and wrist joints in the hand and the toe joints in the foot.

metacarpal

phalanx

inflamed, swollen joint

KEY FACTS

Description

Inflammation of one or more joints.

Causes and risk factors

Arthritis may occur for various reasons. It may result from degeneration of the joint lining, an underlying autoimmune disease, an infection, or a metabolic disorder. In some cases the underlying cause is not known. Risk factors generally include increasing age, excess weight, past joint injuries, and a family history of arthritis.

Symptoms and signs

Swelling, pain, stiffness, redness, and heat in one or more joints. The location, pattern, and severity of symptoms vary depending on the type and cause of the arthritis. Septic arthritis may produce fever.

Diagnosis

Physical examination, medical history, and possibly various other tests depending on the type and/or suspected cause. Such tests may include X-rays, scans, blood tests, urine tests, tissue biopsies, tissue typing, and testing of fluid from inside an affected joint.

Treatments

Treatment depends on the type and cause of arthritis. Treatments may include medication, exercise, diet modification, and surgery.

Pathogenesis

Arthritis can affect almost any joint. The onset and course of the condition vary according to its type and cause.

Prevention

Preventive measures include maintaining a healthy body weight, exercising appropriately, and protecting joints from overuse or injury. Early diagnosis and treatment of all types of arthritis and any associated diseases may help limit symptoms.

Epidemiology

About 43 million adults in the United States (about one in five of the adult population) have some form of arthritis. It affects more women than men and is more common in older people.

exacerbated by drinking alcohol, being overweight, and taking certain medications.

Symptoms and signs

Symptoms of arthritis include pain, stiffness, swelling, tenderness, heat, and redness in or around one or more joints.

Almost any joint can be affected; the principal exceptions are fixed joints, like the sutures between the skull bones. The pattern, severity, and location of symptoms vary, and they can come on gradually or suddenly. Septic arthritis may also produce fever. If the cause of the arthritis is an immune disorder, infection, or metabolic disorder there may also be symptoms of the underlying disorder.

Diagnosis

Arthritis is diagnosed from the symptoms, a detailed medical history, and a physical examination. Various investigations may be carried out to try to determine an underlying cause. These investigations can include X-rays and scans such as computed tomography (CT) or magnetic resonance imaging (MRI), blood and urine tests, muscle or skin biopsies, tissue typing, and testing fluid samples from inside affected joints.

Treatments

The specific treatment depends on the type and cause of the arthritis; however, treatment generally involves a combination of therapies. Medication may be prescribed to relieve pain and inflammation, and exercises may be recommended to reduce stiffness, increase flexibility, and help in the reduction of body weight. Applying heat or cold to the affected joints may help reduce inflammation, and wearing splints or braces on the affected joints can also be helpful. Surgery is sometimes recommended to repair or replace damaged joints, restore function, or relieve pain.

Prevention

Achieving and maintaining a healthy body weight and protecting joints from overuse or injury can help reduce the risk of osteoarthritis.

Early diagnosis and prompt treatment of all types of arthritis, as well as the associated diseases, may help limit joint damage.

Ramona Jenkin

tems, or sickle-cell anemia. Septic arthritis can occur at any age and usually affects the knee and hip joints.

The metabolic disorder gout can produce one of the most painful forms of arthritis. Gout occurs when crystals of uric acid (a normal waste product) are deposited in the joints or connective tissues. The crystals cause inflammation and stiffness in the affected joints, most commonly in the big toe. Gout is more common in men and sometimes runs in families. It is sometimes associated with eating certain foods and may be

See also
• Dislocation

Asbestosis

A progressive lung disease that cannot be cured, asbestosis is an occupational disease that strikes workers who have been exposed to airborne asbestos fibers for many years. The dangers of asbestos are now better understood, and workers can be protected from the devastating effects of the disease.

Asbestos mining and production began in the 1800s, and the fibrous mineral's ability to resist heat and fire quickly turned it into a valuable commodity. By the 1970s, more than five thousand products containing asbestos were being made, from hair dryers to giant ships. At that same time, it was becoming clear that inhaling asbestos fibers could damage the lung in several ways, including causing the deadly disease asbestosis. Today, almost all asbestos usage has been banned.

Causes and risk factors

When needlelike asbestos fibers penetrate deeply into the lung, white blood cells try to destroy them. But the body cannot break down asbestos or remove it, so inflammation occurs. Ultimately, the lungs become scarred and are unable to transport oxygen efficiently.

Asbestos has been used in so many building materials and products that almost everyone is exposed to it. The levels in cities are 10 times higher than in the country, but even these levels are considered too low to cause disease. The risk of asbestosis is almost entirely limited to workers exposed to high levels for many years. These include miners, construction workers, shipbuilders, and factory workers. Because asbestos fibers can be carried home on workers' clothes, family members are also at risk. Smoking increases the risk of asbestosis ninetyfold over nonsmokers.

Symptoms, diagnosis, and pathogenesis

Symptoms usually appear decades after the initial exposure and include shortness of breath, cough, and tiring easily. A history of asbestos exposure, chest X-ray, physical examination, and lung function tests are used to make a diagnosis, which is confirmed by a computed tomography (CT) scan that reveals the characteristic scarring. In rare cases a biopsy of the lung may be necessary to prove the diagnosis.

Asbestosis increases the risk of both lung cancer and a rare cancer of the lungs called mesothelioma. Almost all cases of mesothelioma are caused by asbestos.

Treatments and prevention

The number of people with asbestosis is expected to rise in the coming years, even though the dangers are now well known, because so many workers have already been exposed. Most treatments for asbestosis focus on maximizing remaining lung capacity. For severe cases, a patient may use a portable oxygen tank that delivers gas via a tube in the nose.

Handled by professionals who use proper protective equipment, asbestos removal is the most common preventive measure.

Chris Curran

KEY FACTS

Description
A chronic lung disease that worsens over time.

Cause
Prolonged exposure to airborne asbestos fibers.

Risk factors
Long-term exposure to asbestos fibers.

Symptoms
Difficulty breathing, cough, chest pain, and fatigue.

Diagnosis
History of exposure, chest X-ray, physical examination, lung function tests, CT scan.

Treatment
Oxygen therapy can help breathing. In extreme cases, lung transplants may be done.

Pathogenesis
Asbestos fibers trapped deep inside the lung cannot be destroyed or removed. Scar tissue builds up, leading to reduced lung capacity.

Prevention
Using proper protective gear when working with asbestos; not smoking; hiring professionals to remove asbestos-containing building materials.

Epidemiology
Around 9 million people in the United States are at risk of asbestosis because of prior exposure.

See also
• Cancer, lung • Radiation sickness

Asian influenza

Within the past 50 years, two influenza pandemics struck, taking millions of lives worldwide. Influenza virus A H2N2, the "Asian flu" of 1957–1958, did what all influenza viruses have the capacity to do: it evolved into a new virus, unrecognizable to the human immune system. Another virus, H3N2, or the "Hong Kong flu," hit about a decade later. Because of the ability of influenza viruses to change, there will always be yearly "flu-season" epidemics and the potential for future pandemics.

Influenza is a highly infectious virus that attacks the respiratory system, leading to an abrupt fever and, in some cases, serious health complications and death. There are three types of influenza viruses: A, B, and C. The most important is A, the type associated with pandemics (worldwide epidemics). The most recent pandemics occurred in 1957–1958 ("Asian flu") and 1968–1969 ("Hong Kong flu"), in which millions of people died. In 2003–2005, an influenza A virus circulating in Southeast Asia struck mostly birds but also caused sporadic human illness and death. This virus, called H5N1, is an avian or bird flu virus and was initially mostly confined to Asian countries. Some reports have thus erroneously referred to H5N1 as Asian flu.

Causes and risk factors

Influenza is spread by respiratory droplets created through sneezing and coughing. The illness can also be contracted by touching surfaces contaminated with secretions containing flu virus and then touching one's mouth or nose. Young children, elderly people, and those with underlying chronic (long-term) health problems are at highest risk of complications from infection with influenza virus.

Symptoms and signs

After an incubation period of 1 to 4 days, people infected with influenza virus develop an abrupt fever, headache, sore throat, and dry cough that can in some cases progress to viral pneumonia, respiratory failure, and death. Severe fatigue and muscle aches are also commonly reported. Symptoms resolve within three to seven days, although a cough may last for more than two weeks. In some cases, complications develop, including bacterial pneumonia and worsening of underlying chronic medical disorders, such as heart and lung disease. In children, symptoms may include stomach upset, nausea, vomiting, and diarrhea as well as sinus problems and ear infections. As a result of infection with influenza virus, children can suffer febrile seizures, nervous-system disorders, and heart problems. Adults with influenza are infectious to others from about one day prior to the onset of symptoms to five days after becoming ill. In children, this period of infectivity can last 10 or more days after developing symptoms.

KEY FACTS

Description
An acute viral infection of the respiratory system.

Causes
Infection with type A influenza virus.

Risk factors
Contamination with the virus from droplets sneezed or coughed; touching surfaces contaminated by secretions containing virus.

Symptoms
Fever, cough, sore throat, muscle aches, and severe fatigue. Pneumonia, severe respiratory distress, and death can result.

Diagnosis
Blood tests; tests of infected tissues.

Treatments
Antiviral medicines such as Tamiflu and Relenza reduce severity of symptoms.

Pathogenesis
Influenza viruses change over time. Humans are very susceptible to these evolved viruses because they have no immunity to novel flu viruses, which invade cells in the respiratory passages.

Prevention
Flu vaccine.

Epidemiology
Every year, 5 to 10 percent of the U.S. population contract flu; more than 200,000 people are hospitalized with complications from flu, and about 36,000 die from the infection.

Diagnosis and treatment

Diagnosis of influenza A can be made using seven rapid tests that can be carried out in a physician's office by individuals who do not need special laboratory training, or by testing blood or swabs of infected tissue in a laboratory. During flu epidemics, diagnoses of flu are also made by clinical criteria alone, because a clinician is aware that flu is prevalent in the community and sees very many patients with the same symptoms. Viral culture, which takes three to 10 days, plays an important public health role because it identifies the influenza strain and subtype. This identification in turn allows authorities to better guess which vaccine should be formulated for the next season of influenza.

Several antiviral drugs, such as amantadine, oseltamivir, rimantidine, and zanamivir, are active against influenza A. These drugs should be started within two days of symptoms to have maximum effectiveness. All but zanamivir are approved for use as chemoprophylaxis (treatment with medicine in an effort to prevent disease) of influenza A. Chemoprophylaxis would be useful, for example, during an influenza A outbreak at a nursing home or health care facility.

Pathogenesis

Of the three types of influenza viruses, only A has subtypes. Subtypes are based on the surface proteins HA (hemagglutinin) and NA (neuraminidase); at present, there are 16 HA and 9 NA subtypes. However, because the virus can mutate, it is possible for new subtypes to evolve. A type A virus is named by combining the first letter of the surface protein with its respective numerical subtype, for example, H1N1, H1N2, and H1N9. Over time, small, continual changes occur in influenza viruses, a process called antigenic drift. Thus, a new vaccine must be formulated every year to keep up with these changes in the virus.

Seasonal flu occurs yearly; pandemic influenza is infrequent, but more deadly. Pandemics occur when there has been a major change in the influenza virus, typically when viruses that infect birds merge their genetic material with influenza viruses that infect humans, creating a new virus to which humans have no immunity. Pandemics require three conditions—a new influenza virus subtype, the capability of this subtype to infect humans, and sustainable transmission. Antigenic shift, a reassortment of genetic material between two viruses creating a hybrid virus, can cause pandemics.

Influenza viruses are passed from person to person and have a particular affinity for cells along the

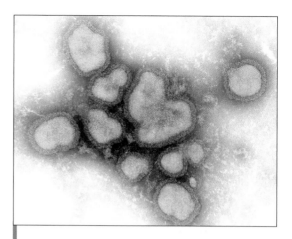

This is a colored electron micrograph of the influenza A virus. Each virus consists of a core of genetic material, surrounded by spikes, which attach to the host cells.

respiratory passages. The virus attaches to respiratory epithelial cells, assisted by neuraminidase present on the virus surface, and invades these human cells. Viral genes enter the cell nucleus, where they make new viral copies; these virus particles exit to continue the same process. When an opportunity presents itself for a bird-flu virus to swap genetic material with a human-flu virus, the resulting hybrid virus can sweep through human populations because there is a lack of immunity to this novel virus.

Prevention

Simple precautions reduce the spread of flu, such as use of surgical masks and covering a cough with a tissue or other such barrier.

The yearly seasonal flu vaccine is recommended for individuals, such as the young or elderly, at high risk of complications should they contract flu, as well as those who can transmit the flu to these at-risk persons—for example, health care workers.

The best time to receive the flu vaccine is in the fall, preferably during October or November (flu season can start as early as October and continue through May). Two types of vaccines are available—a flu shot and a nasal-spray flu vaccine. Once flu vaccine is given, it takes about two weeks to develop antibodies. The vaccines offer protection from influenza, but not from influenza-like illnesses caused by other viruses.

Rita Washko

See also
• Avian influenza • Influenza • Pneumonia

Asperger's disorder

Primarily a social and behavioral disorder, Asperger's disorder shares aspects in common with autism, although Asperger's disorder is a much less severe condition. Affected individuals experience difficulty in complex social behaviors and communication subtleties, particularly in nonverbal interactions with others. Cognitive functioning (related to mental processing) and speech are typically normal. Individuals display compulsive behaviors, stereotypical movement, obsessive interests, and have difficulty forming peer relationships.

One year after Leo Kanner's paper on infantile autism was published in 1943, Austrian psychiatrist Hans Asperger described a group of boys with another disorder, which he referred to as autistic psychopathy. The boys had marked difficulties with social interaction and use of language to communicate; each showed repetitive movement behaviors, possessed narrow, intense interests, and was highly socially isolated. This condition, now called Asperger's disorder, or Asperger's syndrome, is one of the five disorders that comprise the pervasive developmental disorders, or autistic spectrum disorders. Individual symptoms of Asperger's disorder can vary in severity. It is only since the 1980s that American and European doctors have widely recognized Asperger's as a unique personality disorder, and it was not until 1994 that the disorder was officially recognized as being distinct from autism.

Causes

The disorder is considered to be a neurobehavioral syndrome. There is no known prevention or cure of the disorder. Asperger noted that many of the fathers of his patients also showed similar traits, and studies since have supported a genetic basis for the disorder. As with autism, dietary allergies, environmental toxins, vaccines, and neurotoxins used as preservatives for vaccines have all been invoked as contributing to the symptoms. However, scientific studies have consistently failed to prove their definite involvement.

Symptoms

Asperger's disorder is a lifelong condition that may be diagnosed by three years of age. Many children are misdiagnosed as having autism, obsessive-compulsive disorder, or attention-deficit hyperactivity disorder. Affected people have normal intelligence, and thus higher IQs than autistic children; in fact, some researchers refer to Asperger's disorder as high-

KEY FACTS

Description

Member of the autistic spectrum disorders group. Similar to, but milder than, autism; shared features include impaired social interactions and communication, although there is no delay in the development of language.

Causes

Unknown, although the causes are suspected to involve a combination of genetic and environmental factors.

Risk factors

A family history of the disorder.

Symptoms

Problems with social behavior, particularly in nonverbal communication and development of peer relationships. Unable to enjoy activities with others. Repetitive behaviors. Narrow, sometimes obsessive activities and interests.

Diagnosis

Cognitive and behavioral tests for autistic spectrum; autistic symptoms but with age-appropriate language and cognitive development, achievement of self-help skills, and display of curiosity about environment. Absence of other personality disorders.

Treatments

Behavioral therapy. Drugs for the symptoms.

Pathogenesis

Symptoms evident by 3 years of age; the disorder is lifelong.

Prevention

There is no known way of preventing Asperger's disorder.

Epidemiology

Estimated 1 case in 500; 4 times more common in men and boys.

functioning autism. Many people with Asperger's have excellent rote-learning skills and often develop a focused interest in one or two subjects, ranging from cars and dinosaurs to the more unusual, such as train schedules or contents of phone books. However, they may have difficulty with abstract thinking.

Individuals with Asperger's disorder learn many facts about their favorite topic and can talk incessantly about it, even as young children, but with a total lack of regard for their audience. Such focus appears abnormally intense in children. However, for some individuals it evolves into an expertise that supports a successful career in adulthood. Some successful mathematicians, artists, and musicians have Asperger's disorder.

Language skills of children with Asperger's disorder develop at the normal pace, unlike in autism, in which speech is often delayed. Language is grammatically correct, and vocabulary may be quite rich. But the speech tends to sound monotonic and repetitive, and those with Asperger's show a lack of understanding of the context in which language is used. Affected individuals have trouble making eye contact and reading nonverbal cues from the listener's face, and in interpreting another person's tone of voice, which results in great difficulties in carrying on two-way discussions; considered weird or eccentric, they are often teased and bullied at school.

Social isolation is common, but unlike in autism it is not due to an active withdrawal from people, nor from a lack of desire to have friends. Rather, isolation stems from an inability to learn the social rules that would allow affected individuals to respond to the needs of others. Those with Asperger's disorder lack the skills to reciprocate others' emotions and are unable to spontaneously share pleasures or achievements with other people.

Children with Asperger's disorder tend to be clumsy. They sometimes appear to have an odd posture. As with autism, children with Asperger's exhibit repetitive body movements such as spinning or rocking. Asperger himself believed that the primary deficit for these affected individuals was social, and their symptoms were not due to delayed developmental milestones of childhood. Although social impairments are evident before three years of age, the children learn about self-care on a normal schedule, and all exhibit the usual age-appropriate curiosity about their environment.

Diagnosis

Diagnosis is made by a team with expertise in child development, language development, psychiatry,

neuropsychology, and behavior. Personality disorders must be ruled out. The typical age for diagnosis is 11 years, but parents can often trace their worries about the child back to three years of age. Researchers might look at old home videos to try to pick up on symptoms during early life.

Treatments and pathogenesis

There is no one specific treatment for people with Asperger's. Interventions are based on treating the patient's symptoms and behaviors. Available treatments for Asperger's disorder include special education, behavioral training, and sometimes medicines. In milder cases, therapy is primarily aimed at enabling a child to be part of a regular classroom. Sometimes extra help is needed for the individual, and children suffering from the disorder appear to do better if activities are very structured, since adherence to routine is an important part of their condition. For children with more severe symptoms, a special school may be required. Vocational training is an important aspect of the training. The higher the IQ of the child, the better the outcome in terms of adaptation to independent living as an adult.

Behavioral therapy, tailored at an early age to the individual, can improve outcome, as for autistic children. Clinical psychologists can help families cope with problems of behavior, and schools can use methods to help affected children express themselves. Drugs can be given to manage anxiety, compulsive behaviors and obsessive thoughts, and the depression often associated with social isolation but cannot cure Asperger's disorder.

There is some limited evidence to show that music therapy may help some children with communication.

Epidemiology

For a long time, doctors believed that Asperger's disorder affected only boys, but in recent years girls have also been diagnosed. Nevertheless, boys are four times more likely to have the disorder. According to the U.S. National Institute of Child Health and Mental Development, almost 1 in 500 people (or 0.2 percent of the general population) are affected by Asperger's disorder. However, estimates from other sources are two or three times higher.

Sonal Jhaveri

See also
• Autism

Asthma

Asthma is a chronic respiratory condition in which the air passages (bronchial tubes) to the lungs become inflamed, causing the tubes to narrow, which results in intermittent attacks of coughing, shortness of breath, and sometimes wheezing. Each year nearly 500,000 individuals in the United States are hospitalized due to asthma, and more than 4,000 of these cases prove fatal.

Asthma is most commonly found in children; it usually starts before the age of five, although it may begin in adolescence or adulthood. More than 6 percent of children in the United States are asthmatic, and the incidence continues to rise. The reason for this increase has not been established, but the incidence is greatest in urban areas and among Hispanic and African American children. However, with adequate treatment and control of their environment up to half of all asthmatic children outgrow the attacks.

Causes and risk factors

It is not yet understood why some individuals develop asthma when they are exposed to particular substances and circumstances while others do not. No genetic link has been identified, but a child with one asthmatic parent has a 25 percent risk of developing asthma; there is a 50 percent risk if both parents have a history of asthma. Ethnicity is significant because the higher incidence in African American and Hispanic children may be due to the socioeconomic environment in urban areas.

Repeated exposure to inhaled irritants results in chronic inflammation of the lining of the main air passages that transport air to the lungs (bronchial tubes). Large amounts of mucus may be produced, which further compromises the air passages. Exposure, especially for young children, to irritants like dust mites and cockroach droppings is linked to asthma, as is exposure to animal dander (skin, hair, and feathers) and saliva. Molds and pollens from grass and trees may also produce allergic reactions. Other known irritants include cigarette smoke, air pollution, scented products, cold air, and strong paint or cooking odors. Viral infections, stress, anxiety, and even prolonged crying or laughing may precipitate an attack, and physical exercise or weather changes can trigger an episode.

Sulfides used as preservatives in prepared foods and beverages, such as dried fruit, wine, or beer may stimulate an attack, as can tartrazine, an artificial yellow coloring in food and pills. Aspirin and other medications such as beta blockers are known to induce or increase the likelihood of asthmatic symptoms, and chemicals and dusts at work may also cause attacks. Occasionally, especially in children, no cause is identified.

Symptoms and signs

Symptoms vary considerably. Some individuals stay relatively symptom free with occasional episodes of shortness of breath unless a trigger provokes an attack. Others cough and wheeze continually.

Exposure to house dust mites (below) as well as hair, skin, and feathers, is believed to be a risk factor for asthma.

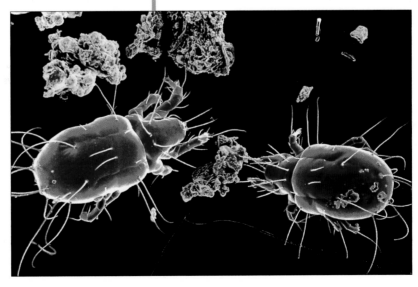

KEY FACTS

Description

Asthma is a chronic respiratory condition in which the air passages (bronchial tubes) to the lungs become inflamed, causing the tubes to narrow and resulting in shortness of breath, coughing, and sometimes wheezing.

Risk factors

Exposure to inhaled irritants and allergens.

Symptoms

Difficulty breathing, a cough, wheezing, and chest tightness.

Diagnosis

Evaluation of personal history with tests and occasionally an X-ray to rule out other causes of the symptoms, such as cystic fibrosis.

Treatment

Medications to reduce inflammation and relax the air passages, along with environmental control and general health maintenance.

Pathogenesis

Exposure to irritants or allergens may cause chronic inflammation of the respiratory air passages in some individuals. More than half of young asthma sufferers outgrow the condition.

Prevention

Avoiding substances and situations that may irritate the respiratory air passages. Timely treatment of common upper respiratory infections to avoid chronic inflammation.

Epidemiology

Asthma affects approximately 18 million people in the United States, and this figure continues to rise. Among children the incidence has increased 75 percent in the past 20 years. Asthma occurs most frequently in urban environments, especially among Hispanic and African American populations.

The classic symptoms are difficulty in breathing accompanied by a high-pitched wheezing sound. Coughing is sometimes the only symptom, and not all wheezing is due to asthma. In severe attacks there may be no wheezing because little air moves into or out of the lungs (see box, page 64).

Diagnosis

The individual, or parents of children, can contribute to the diagnosis by providing details of symptoms and episodes, along with a family medical history of allergies, asthma, or other breathing problems.

A thorough physical examination is carried out and, for patients over the age of five, a pulmonary (lung) function test may be done, in which a device called a spirometer shows how much air can be blown out of the lungs after a deep breath and at what speed. Other tests, such as a bronchial challenge test or exercise tests, may also be done using a spirometer.

A series of allergy tests may reveal if known allergy-causing substances are responsible for the asthma, and other tests can rule out conditions with similar symptoms, such as cystic fibrosis.

Treatment and control

There is no cure for asthma, but the condition can be controlled with various types of drugs. Medications called relievers provide immediate relief for asthma attacks by relaxing (bronchodilation) the walls of the air passages, which widens the passages, allowing air to move freely into and out of the lungs. Long-term treatments called preventers reduce the chronic inflammation of the lining of the air passages, thereby decreasing the likelihood of an attack and relieving day-to-day discomfort.

Relievers, also known as bronchodilators, are most effective when taken as soon as symptoms of coughing, chest tightness, wheezing, or shortness of breath occur. They work within minutes and are effective for four to six hours. The most commonly used bronchodilators are called beta-2 agonists. As these are inhaled they primarily affect the lungs, which means there are fewer side effects. Another type of medication known as anticholinergics may be given after beta-2 agonists in emergencies to further widen the air passages and reduce mucus production.

Some bronchodilators are long-acting medications that last for at least 12 hours and may be used before exercise or before breathing cold air and to prevent symptoms while sleeping. These longer-acting beta-2 agonists are usually used together with inhaled corticosteroids.

One bronchodilator, theophylline, has been prescribed for many years as a long-term control medication for mild to moderate cases of asthma. This is taken daily as a pill, sustained release capsule, or syrup and is particularly effective for reducing symptoms during sleep. Initially it may cause side effects, including rapid and irregular heartbeats (palpitations), restlessness, nervousness, or a headache, but these usually disappear as the body adjusts. To be sure the dose is appropriate, blood levels should be checked periodically. If the level of medication is too low there will be inadequate control of symptoms, while if it is unnecessarily high, serious heart rhythm irregularities or seizures, as well as nausea and vomiting, abdominal pain, or diarrhea may occur. Aminophylline is a more powerful but pharmacologically similar bronchodilator that is only given intravenously in emergencies.

For long-term treatment of severe chronic asthma, corticosteroids, or preventers, are used. Corticosteroids have long been considered the most effective preventer medications because they are anti-inflammatory, and so reduce inflammation in the lining of the air passages. If they are used long-term, however, there is a risk of serious side effects, including cataracts, osteoporosis (loss of bone mass), and decreased resistance to infection, but as corticosteroids usually are inhaled directly into the air passages, rather than taken internally, these effects are lessened. Nevertheless, inhaled corticosteroids may, sometimes temporarily, affect growth in children.

For individuals with moderate asthma, a group of anti-inflammatory medications called leukotriene modifiers may eliminate the need for corticosteroids. They are not used for acute attacks but for protection from attacks. These drugs block substances released during an attack that cause more inflammation in the air passages. For more severe asthma, they may be used together with other medications, including inhaled corticosteroids.

Cromolyn (Nasalcrom) and nedocromil (Tilade) are considered the safest asthma medications currently available for mild or moderate asthma and are frequently prescribed as preventives for use before exercising. For people with mild or moderate asthma, daily long-term use of these medications may prevent attacks by reducing inflammation in the air passages.

For allergic asthma, allergy desensitization injections (immunotherapy) may decrease sensitivity to allergens in substances such as pollen, insect droppings, or molds. When confronted with an allergen, the body's immune system manufactures proteins called antibodies. Immunoglobulin E (IgE) is an antibody frequently associated with respiratory allergies. Based on the idea that an allergic attack may not develop if immunoglobulin E is prevented from attaching to cells that release substances which cause allergic asthma, new injectable treatments are under development.

Management and prognosis

Lifestyle and management of the environment are important in controlling asthma. Identifying and avoiding known causes of attacks are essential, and recognizing early indications of an attack enables action to be taken to prevent serious episodes.

Regular at-home testing to measure lung function using a peak flow meter is a significant aid for control. The handheld device measures how fast air is exhaled forcibly after a deep breath. A single unusual result or a series of changes may warn of a possible attack or

USING A METERED-DOSE INHALER

Many asthma medications are inhaled using metered-dose inhalers. These handheld devices contain pressured gas which, when released, deliver a fine spray directly into the lungs. Each time the inhaler is pressed, a measured dose is released. To be effective an inhaler must be used as instructed or the dose of medication will be wasted.

A dry powder form is easier to use because it requires less coordination with breathing. An attachment called a spacer inserted between the inhaler and the mouthpiece can also help. After using an inhaler it is important to rinse the mouth with water to prevent thrush, an infection of the mouth. The water should not be swallowed to avoid the absorption of medication elsewhere in the body.

For infants, small children, or those unable to use an inhaler, a mask connected to a nebulizer may be used. A nebulizer creates a fine mist of the medication, eliminating the need to coordinate breathing with pressing the inhaler. Nebulizers are increasingly portable, with models available that can be plugged into an automobile cigarette lighter.

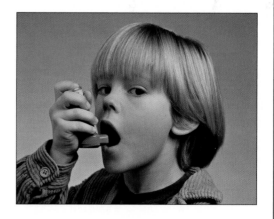

By inhaling a drug that relieves asthma, the person can get faster relief from the symptoms without too many side effects. An anti-inflammatory drug works to relax the muscles around the bronchioles in the lungs and reduce inflammation and swelling in the constricted tubes.

STATUS ASTHMATICUS

Status asthmaticus is the most severe form of asthma and is most likely to occur when asthma has been inadequately treated. Any asthmatic may experience status asthmaticus, and the risk of having repeated attacks increases after the first attack.

During a status asthmaticus attack the air passages are so severely constricted (narrowed) that insufficient air moves into and out of the lungs to provide adequate oxygen. The person may be unable to speak because of the effort it takes to breathe. Wheezing or coughing may not be heard because of the lack of air flow, which leads to a bluish color (cyanosis) of the face, lips, and nails. Untreated, the lack of oxygen and buildup of carbon dioxide may seriously affect many organs, resulting in unconsciousness and death.

Typically, status asthmaticus requires emergency treatment. Any attack that does not respond to inhaled prescribed medication, or lasts for more than 5 to 10 minutes, should be treated as an emergency, and supplemental oxygen should be supplied as quickly as possible. Placing a breathing tube through the mouth into the main air passage (intubation) may be necessary so that a mechanical ventilator can be used. Once the attack has been controlled, the patient will probably be monitored for oxygenation and treated for other effects caused by the attack. Children may be monitored in an intensive care unit.

inadequate medication so that appropriate measures can be taken before symptoms appear. Initially, for several weeks, the test must be done at the same time each day to establish a record and identify the best possible peak flow reading while medication is being adjusted to control symptoms and attacks. The test should then be done every morning and the rate recorded to compare to the known best possible peak flow number. Older children can manage this with a little supervision, which enhances their feeling of being in control of their condition. Education of asthma sufferers and family members is key to developing the safest and least restrictive lifestyle. An action plan

A pall of smog and polluted air is visible above the Hell Gate Bridge over the East River, New York City. Polluted air is one of the risk factors for asthma sufferers.

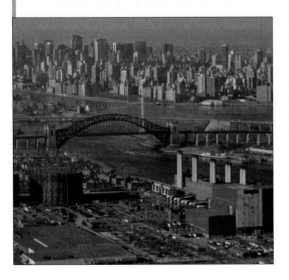

written with the health care provider's direction can detail the appropriate action to take in different circumstances. The plan can describe how to take medication correctly; early signs that indicate a significant change in condition; what medication to take to manage an attack; when to call the health care provider; when emergency treatment is necessary; and what steps to take to provide an optimal personal environment and decrease or avoid known triggers.

Younger children especially require close parental observation, and child care providers should be aware of the child's asthma and her or his prescribed medication, and should understand how to implement the action plan. School nurses should be informed about the child's symptoms and history so that activities can be monitored and appropriate medication be available. Exercise is important to a child's development and general health, so rather than avoiding an activity, a special dose of medication may be prescribed. Some schools allow older children to use inhalers when they are needed.

Like other chronic disorders, such as diabetes, asthma must be continually managed to maintain a normal life. At least 50 percent of children outgrow the condition, although the more serious the symptoms the less likely it is that asthma will be outgrown. With management, asthma need not interfere with otherwise good health and normal activities.

Nance Seiple

See also
• Allergy and sensitivity

Astigmatism

Astigmatism is caused by an irregular curvature of the clear front covering of the eye, the cornea. A perfectly shaped cornea is spherical, like a baseball, allowing all light rays to enter the eye and bringing them to focus on the retina. Astigmatism occurs when the cornea is elongated, much like a football, and causes a vision error or blurring instead of a sharp focus.

Astigmatism results in distorted or blurred vision. It is estimated that 15 percent of adults have some form of astigmatism and 2 percent of adults have significant astigmatism. Astigmatism is considered hereditary, but it may also result from an eye injury that has caused scarring on the cornea, or from keratoconus, a disease that causes a gradual thinning and distortion of the cornea. Some patients experience surgically induced astigmatism after eye surgery. Sutures that are tightly placed can cause a slight wrinkling of the cornea, and the patient will experience astigmatism until the surgical wound is healed.

There are two types of astigmatism: regular and irregular. What is called "within-the-rule," or regular astigmatism, is common. In this case, the eye has more refractive power along the vertical axis, and the patient has difficulty resolving targets with horizontal lines with letters such as E or F. A patient with "against-the-rule" astigmatism has the opposite problem; he or she has difficulty focusing vertically oriented targets. Regular astigmatism of a significant degree is usually corrected with cylinder in eyeglasses, toric soft contact lenses, which supplement the eye's refractive power for the orientation where it is needed, or rigid gas-permeable contact lenses that alter the shape of the cornea.

Irregular astigmatism is present when the different meridians of curvature of the cornea are not 180 degrees apart or the cornea takes on multiple meridians of curvature, which results in a corneal surface that is bumpy in appearance. Irregular astigmatism is diagnosed using corneal topography, also known as videokeratography, which is a noninvasive medical imaging technique that produces a three-dimensional map of the cornea to assist the ophthalmologist in making diagnoses. This type of astigmatism is usually not correctable with glasses or contact lenses. Common causes of irregular astigmatism include dry eyes, corneal scars, pterygium (a raised, wedge-shaped growth of the conjunctiva), contact lens overwear, trauma, and surgery.

Surgical correction of astigmatism allows patients freedom from eyeglasses or contact lenses. Laser surgery is more widely available, with enhanced safety and predictability. For cases of mild (regular) astigmatism, LASIK (Laser Assisted in-Situ Keratomileusis) is a safe and effective technique. LASIK modifies the cornea to allow rays of light to focus on the retina. Topography is an invaluable tool to selectively reshape portions of the cornea. Studies are currently underway to determine if the technique may be expanded to include all types of irregular astigmatism.

Herbert Kaufman and
Josephine Everly

KEY FACTS

Description

An irregular curvature of the cornea of the eye.

Causes

Inheritance; injury to the eye due to keratoconus or surgery; dry eyes; overwear of contact lenses; corneal scarring; pterygium; or trauma.

Risk factors

Genetic predisposition; eye surgery.

Symptoms

Distorted or blurred vision, especially of horizontal or vertical lines.

Diagnosis

Vision test by optometrist; corneal topography, or videokeratography, by an ophthalmologist.

Treatment

Corrective eyeglasses, toric soft lenses, or rigid contact lenses; surgery.

Pathogenesis

Astigmatism is usually hereditary and does not worsen with age.

Prevention

Astigmatism cannot be prevented.

Epidemiology

About 15 percent of adults are astigmatic; about 2 percent of adults have significant astigmatism.

See also
• Macular degeneration • Retinal disorders

Attention-deficit hyperactivity disorder

Attention-deficit hyperactivity disorder, commonly called ADHD, is a brain disorder that manifests as a persistent pattern of inattentiveness, hyperactivity, and impulsive behavior. People who suffer from the disorder may be bright but are unable to focus on tasks at hand, which can result in frustration and a loss of self-esteem.

Attention-deficit hyperactivity disorder (ADHD) is a disorder of the nervous system that presents itself as persistent hyperactivity, inattentiveness, forgetfulness, and impulsive behavior. It occurs worldwide and afflicts 5 to 8 percent of children in the United States. The disorder persists in at least half of these children into adulthood. The symptoms of ADHD may appear as early as toddlerhood; however, they may vary as the child enters adolescence and adulthood. The hyperactivity associated with ADHD is most marked in early to middle childhood but declines significantly with age. By adulthood, feelings of restlessness, subjective hyperactivity (an internal feeling of hyperactivity or restlessness), and the need to be busy or engaged in physical activities are the main symptoms.

Causes and risk factors

The exact cause of ADHD is not known. However, research suggests that a variety of factors, such as a genetic predisposition to the disorder, or an infection, may contribute to the onset of ADHD. Genetics has been found to play a key role in the development of ADHD. Studies show that children who have parents with ADHD are eight times more likely to have the disorder, and a sibling of an affected child is five to seven times more likely to have the disorder. Evidence suggests that an imbalance in neurotransmitters may contribute to ADHD. This imbalance can cause dysfunction of the limbic system. (The limbic system includes various structures in the human brain that are involved in emotion, motivation, and emotional association.) Prenatal exposure to poor nutrition, viral infections, or maternal substance abuse may contribute to the development of ADHD. In early childhood, exposure to lead or other toxins, as well as a brain injury or disorders of the nervous system may produce ADHD symptoms. It appears that boys are five times more likely to develop ADHD than girls.

Symptoms

Hyperactivity, inattentiveness, and impulsive behavior are hallmark symptoms of ADHD. Children with ADHD have difficulty sustaining attention toward activities and respond to distracting events that may draw them away from their task. This situation is further compounded by problems reengaging with the ongoing task after being distracted.

The hyperactivity associated with ADHD often diminishes with age. However, the impulsiveness persists throughout the person's lifetime. It often presents itself verbally by excessive talking, interrupting others, or blurting out the answer before questions are finished. Physically, the impulsiveness manifests itself as doing things on an impulse or as a dare. Those with ADHD suffer two to four times the rate of accidental injuries than their unaffected counterparts because they tend to be more involved in risk-taking activities.

A new subtype of ADHD, called predominantly inattentive type, has been identified. The symptoms of this subtype differ greatly from the classical type, in that they are characterized by hypoactivity (underactivity) rather than hyperactivity. Children with this subtype often appear to be in a daydream, confused, or "spacey."

In adults, ADHD manifests itself as difficulty with time management and organization, careless behavior, and risk taking, such as walking into a street without looking. Affected adults are also easily distracted and behave impulsively. They often lack the ability to structure their lives and plan complex daily tasks. Their greatest problem seems to be an inability to exert self-control, to direct their behavior toward future goals and tasks, and to keep those tasks in mind until completed.

Diagnosis

To confirm a diagnosis of ADHD, a child must have at least six symptoms that fall under the category of inattentiveness or hyperactivity-impulsivity. Also, these symptoms must persist for at least six months and interfere with normal day-to-day activities. Symptoms found in the category of inattentiveness include failure to pay close attention to details, difficulty sustaining attention in work tasks or play activities, inability to listen when spoken to directly, or difficulties engaging in tasks that require sustained mental efforts. Hyperactivity-impulsivity is characterized by constant fidgeting with hands or feet, squirming in a seat, excessive talking, difficulty in waiting one's turn, and interrupting others. The diagnosis also involves a physical examination and a look at family history.

It is of utmost importance that only a trained health care provider makes a diagnosis of ADHD. Proper diagnosis is essential because there is some overlap among symptoms of various disorders. For example, other mental disorders may also have symptoms of inattentiveness, such as depression and anxiety disorders, and distractibility, such as in the manic phase of bipolar illness.

ADHD symptoms are present in many people to a certain extent. However, what defines ADHD as a disorder is the severity and pervasiveness of the symptoms and their ability to significantly impair a person's ability to function within different social settings.

Treatments

Treatment of ADHD usually consists of a combination of drugs, behavior-modification therapy, and educational interventions. First-line drugs for ADHD are stimulants, which activate the areas of the brain responsible for focus, attention, and impulse control. About 70 to 80 percent of people with ADHD treated with stimulant medication experience significant relief from symptoms, at least in the short-term.

Behavior-modification therapy reinforces good behavior and task completion by using a reward system. For example, a child may be rewarded with a sticker for each task he completes or for good behavior. Therapy may also include helping the child to recognize the connection between a negative thinking pattern and poor behavior and providing the tools necessary to change this thinking pattern.

Educational interventions aim to increase the ability of an ADHD child to succeed academically by developing areas of strength and adapting to special needs. Research suggests that children with ADHD tend to fare better in a diverse learning environment, in which teachers use various teaching and communi-

---

KEY FACTS

Description

A neurological and developmental disorder characterized by excessive inattentiveness, hyperactivity, and impulsive behavior.

Cause

The exact cause of ADHD is unknown. Possible causes may be a neurochemical imbalance, a genetic predisposition, a viral or bacterial infection, a brain injury, or a nutritional deficiency.

Risk Factors

Often runs in families.

Symptoms

ADHD is characterized by inattentiveness, hyperactivity, and impulsive behavior. Symptoms may vary with age.

Diagnosis

Based on symptoms, some of which should develop before the age of seven and significantly affect the child's ability to function in two or more settings, such as at home and school, for a period of at least six months.

Treatments

Usually consist of a combination of drugs, most often stimulants, behavior-modification therapy, and educational interventions.

Pathogenesis

The hyperactivity is most noticeable in early to middle childhood; it decreases significantly with age, but impulsivity and inability to stay focused remain.

Prevention

No known scientifically tested prevention.

Epidemiology

Affects 5 to 8 percent of children in the United States. Males appear to be at more at risk.

---

cation techniques, such as role play, music, and the expressive arts. Teachers clearly state directions and use written directions or a pictorial list.

Although anecdotal reports suggest that certain diets or particular teaching and parenting methods may prevent ADHD, none of these methods have been tested scientifically. However, once symptoms have begun and ADHD is diagnosed, various behavioral and learning techniques, as well as drugs, may be provided to improve symptoms.

Sonal Jhaveri

See also
• Autism

Autism

Autism is a severely disabling developmental disorder that occurs in childhood and consists of a range of social, behavioral, and cognitive (mental-processing) defects. The most characteristic symptoms of autism are lack of social skills, including verbal communication; difficulty in relating to others or deriving pleasure from personal interaction; obsessive or compulsive behaviors, including a resistance to change in environment or routine; and repetitive movements. Although there is no cure, behavioral therapy and drugs can relieve symptoms.

The word *autism* is derived from the Greek *autos,* meaning "self." Pediatric psychiatrist Leo Kanner used it in 1943 to describe children exhibiting severely impaired social skills, difficulties with verbal and nonverbal communication, and an inability to cope with change. It is one of five complex brain disorders known as the autism spectrum disorders, or pervasive developmental disorders.

Autism can be diagnosed as early as 18 months of age and its consequences are lifelong. There are wide individual variations—mild to severe—in each symptom associated with the disease. Some parents note that their child is unusual from birth; other children develop normally, then suddenly regress, becoming withdrawn and losing language skills. About 40 percent are nonverbal, whereas others exhibit limited speech or echolalia (repeating others' speech). Autistic people are deficient in their ability to relate socially. As children, they avoid social play, do not make eye contact, and cannot read or use body language, facial gestures, or other social cues—they may not understand the meaning of a laugh, a wink, or a frown and have difficulty seeing the world from another person's point of view. Their voices are singsong or flat and robotic, and they have trouble controlling speech volume. Many reject being cuddled or hugged. They lack empathy and have difficulty developing reciprocal relationships with peers. Many show excessive anxiety and have frequent frustrated outbursts or tantrums. As adults, they are often socially isolated.

Autistic children cannot shift focus easily and have a strong desire for sameness. They may spend hours arranging favorite toys, becoming extremely agitated if this arrangement is altered in the slightest way. They resist change in daily routine—for instance, a child used to a bedtime sequence of brushing teeth followed by reading a book will become exceedingly distressed by a reversal of the order. Sensory perception may also be unusual in autistic individuals—often they are oversensitive to certain sounds, tastes, or smells, yet insensitive to pain and temperature. Frequently, they become intensely fascinated by bright lights and moving parts. They repeatedly perform simple actions with the body, such as rocking, spinning, or flapping

KEY FACTS

Description

Developmental disorder characterized by severe language, cognitive, and behavioral impairments accompanied by lack of normal sociability and an inability to relate to others.

Causes

Unknown. Likely to be due to genetic and environmental factors.

Risk factors

The genetic disorder tuberous sclerosis; fetal exposure to the infection rubella. More likely if a sibling is autistic and also has the disorder fragile X syndrome.

Symptoms

Delayed cognitive, social, language development. Obsessive interests, insistence on routine, repetitive movements, aversion to touch, and difficulty in forming interpersonal relationships.

Diagnosis

Behavioral assessment of symptoms by a psychiatrist.

Treatments

No cure. Early, intense behavioral therapy and drugs relieve some symptoms.

Pathogenesis

Varies widely with individual. Develops from birth or in childhood. Condition is lifelong.

Prevention

Not known. Early intensive intervention reduces severity.

Epidemiology

4 to 40 of every 10,000 people in the United States, depending on the diagnostic criteria used. Between 1987 and 1998, a 273 percent increase recorded in California, in part due to raised awareness and improved diagnosis.

hands but have trouble with complex motor coordination such as kicking a ball or tying shoelaces.

Causes

In the 1940s and 1950s, doctors believed that parental neglect was the cause of autism. In particular, the "refrigerator mother" theory put forward by a number of psychologists claimed that autism was a result of an emotionally cold mother failing to show affection toward her child. This theory has now been clearly dispelled by a number of studies and by findings showing that autistic children have abnormal brains.

Recognizing that autism is not a rare disease, the U.S. Congress passed the Children's Health Act of 2000, commissioning a committee of experts in neurology, mental health, child health, environmental health sciences, birth defects, and other fields to develop a 10-year autism research program. This research has led to new insights about the disease. Scientists now accept autism as a behaviorally defined syndrome with multiple causes. Brain scans reveal that the amygdala (a part of the brain that mediates emotion and social interaction) and the hippocampus (a neural center for learning and memory) are smaller in the brain of autistic individuals. The cerebellum, a large region of the brain involved in motor learning (learning how to make movements smooth and

accurate; responding to changes in the environment), is also abnormal, and there are fewer connections between cell groups that regulate cognitive functions. Eye-tracking studies document that autistic individuals watch the mouth of a person speaking to them rather than the eyes, unlike normal control subjects. A noninvasive imaging technique called fMRI, which indicates brain activity, reveals that when autistic individuals are asked to infer emotion from a set of images, activity in their amygdala is lower than that observed in control subjects.

Although the precise cause of autism is not understood, scientists agree that there are probably multiple triggers. Research with twins suggest that there is a genetic component to the disease, but its exact contribution is unknown. Recent studies of the chromosomes of autistic individuals indicate a possible involvement of perhaps 20 or more genes. If one male child in the family is autistic and also has fragile X syndrome—a form of inherited mental retardation in which part of the X chromosome appears thin, or fragile—there is a higher risk that a sibling will also be

A researcher assesses the social and emotional skills of a boy with autism. This behavioral task analyzes the boy's response to various facial expressions on a computer-generated face.

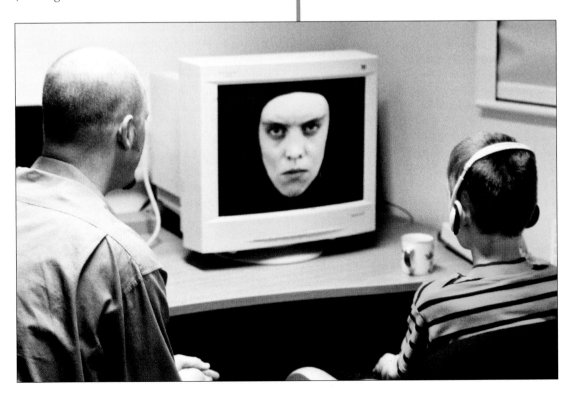

autistic and have the fragile X gene. About 1 to 4 percent of autistic people also have a rare genetic disease called tuberous sclerosis, in which benign tumors grow in a number of organs, including the brain.

Biochemical studies document that the brain of an autistic child has higher-than-normal levels of the hormone neuronal growth factor, suggesting that nerve cell growth may be disordered. This finding could explain why the head of affected children grows disproportionately faster. Recently, researchers have found inflammatory cells in the brains of autistic people of all ages, indicating an ongoing, chronic problem with the immune system. How these and many other findings fit together to solve the puzzle of autism is not yet clear, but the emerging picture is that of a brain that is both structurally and functionally unusual. Whether brain abnormalities are a primary factor in the onset of autism or whether they occur as a result of environmental factors is intensely debated. Autistic children also have abnormal stools, probably as a result of an imbalance between beneficial and nonbeneficial gut bacteria. Repeated antibiotic treatment may lead to high concentrations of yeast in the gut. Researchers are considering the possibility that these disease-causing organisms produce toxins that can have widespread effects in the body.

Other theories have attempted to link the impact of vaccines on the immune system and nutritional deficiencies or allergies with autism. Despite a number of studies, no significant statistical evidence has yet been found to support a link for either of these theories.

Symptoms

Symptoms of autism commonly appear before the age of three. An early indication is the development of language skills, which varies with the type of autism. Some children rarely progress beyond babbling, preferring to sign, type, or use visual aids to communicate. They may also learn songs, jingles, and phrases by rote. At the other end of the autism spectrum are children with a large vocabulary who can talk endlessly about favorite subjects but who rarely share in a normal conversation with another person.

A lack of social interaction with the child's parents and siblings is another early indicator of the condition. Autistic children seem indifferent to others around them and may resist or fail to reciprocate affection. Changes in routine are extremely upsetting to them. Although a few autistic individuals are gifted in specific skills such as music, drawing, rote-learning, or mathematical calculations, two-thirds are mentally

retarded. About 25 percent experience epileptic seizures, especially during adolescence.

Diagnosis and treatments

Because there is no biological marker that can be used to confirm a diagnosis (such as a protein in the blood or urine specific to autism), doctors rely on behavioral assessments. Research has shown that intensive behavioral therapy, initiated early, improves the long-term outcome for autistic children and increases their chance for living more independently as adults.

Diagnosis currently involves a two-step procedure: initial screening, done by the child's pediatrician during routine checkups, and a comprehensive follow-up evaluation. A number of standard tests are available for the first screen. If autism is indicated, the child is referred to a multidisciplinary team that includes a psychologist, neurologist, psychiatrist, and speech pathologist, who use tests that are specifically designed for identifying autism. A future goal is to develop genetic tests or diagnostic biomarkers, such as proteins in the blood or urine, to enable the diagnosis of autistic children to be made soon after birth, thus permitting immediate intervention.

There is no known cure for autism. Drugs can relieve some symptoms, such as seizures, anxiety, depression, and hyperactivity. Early intensive behavioral therapy is effective in helping children learn basic verbal, social, and self-care skills, but it is expensive and emotionally taxing for families.

Epidemiology

According to the Centers for Disease Control, autism is one of the fastest growing childhood disorders in the United States with an estimated 141,000 children, about 1 in 166, classed as autistic. Autism occurs equally across ethnic boundaries but is three times as likely to affect boys and men than girls and women. Autism is less prevalent than mental retardation but more common than childhood cancer and other childhood diseases. California recorded a 273 percent increase in autism from 1987 to 1998, through increased awareness, improved diagnoses, and greater availability of services. Autism remains an urgent threat to public health and poses a heavy financial and emotional burden on affected families.

Sonal Jhaveri

See also
• Asperger's disorder

Avian influenza

In October 2005, researchers digging for clues about the devastating influenza pandemic of 1918 confirmed what many had feared—an avian influenza, or bird flu, had crossed the species barrier, ultimately taking 50 million lives worldwide. In the early years of the twenty-first century, outbreaks of a virulent bird flu in Southeast Asia, called H5N1, stirred fears that another similar pandemic was about to strike.

Avian influenza viruses belong to a group of viruses called type A orthomyxoviruses (there are also types B and C). These pathogens have a history of causing pandemics (worldwide epidemics), resulting in millions of human deaths. Influenza A viruses are carried by migratory birds, which shed the virus in their droppings and secretions. Wild birds seem to suffer no ill effects from the virus. However, domestic birds such as chickens and turkeys are not immune to the viruses. When they contract bird flu from wild birds, domesticated birds usually succumb to the illness.

Although several strains can cause human illness, including H5N1, H7N2, H7N3, H7N7, and H9N2, the strain of most concern is H5N1. This particular strain was identified in Hong Kong in 1997. It is highly pathogenic and is more often associated with pneumonia and death than are other subtypes. H5N1 resurfaced in China and Hong Kong in 2003 and again in other Asian countries in 2004–2005. Although the total number of human deaths has been limited to a few more than 100, health officials view these sporadic cases as a potential public health catastrophe because the virus might mutate, or change its genetic makeup, allowing it to jump from human to human. Such an event could happen if an intermediate host, for example a pig, was infected simultaneously with bird flu and a human influenza strain. Shuffling of genetic material, in a process called reassortment, could then produce a new strain that readily infects humans.

Those who have been affected by avian flu have been mostly very young, old, or have had a chronic (long-term) health problem such as diabetes or lung disease. Because of the avian flu outbreaks in several countries across Asia, avian flu has erroneously been referred to as Asian flu in some reports. True Asian flu outbreaks, however, were caused by the strains H2N2 and H3N2.

Symptoms and signs

After a one-to-five-day incubation period, people infected with bird flu develop fever, cough, sore throat, severe fatigue, and muscle aches. Complications can include pneumonia and other life-threatening problems. In young children, high fevers may be

---

KEY FACTS

Description
Acute viral infection that mainly infects birds. Under certain conditions, humans can become infected.

Causes
Avian influenza viruses, carried by migratory birds and passed on to domesticated birds and other animals, including humans.

Risk factors
Contact with birds infected with the virus or with surfaces that have been contaminated by the body fluids or feces of infected birds.

Symptoms
Fever, cough, sore throat, muscle aches, and severe fatigue. Complications include pneumonia, severe respiratory distress, and death. Milder forms are associated with eye infections and may even go unnoticed.

Diagnosis
Blood tests; tests on infected tissues.

Treatments
Antiviral drugs.

Pathogenesis
So far there is no effective vaccination, and humans have no immunity, so likely progress is severe illness and possibly death.

Prevention
Monitoring health of poultry and culling flocks of sick birds. Avoiding contact with animals at open-air markets and avoiding contact with surfaces potentially contaminated by sick birds.

Epidemiology
More than 100 human cases of avian flu have been identified since 1997, mostly in Southeast Asia. These viruses vary by severity of illness and pathogenicity—the origination and likely progress of the disease. The most virulent bird flu virus is influenza A H5N1, which has a human mortality rate greater than 50 percent.

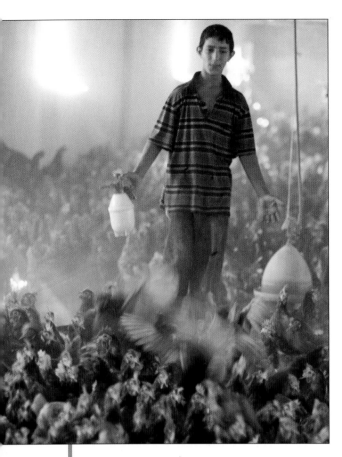

A young man sprays disinfectant on a chicken farm in the Dyala province in Iraq. Governments throughout the world have grown more vigilant about poultry production.

present and can lead to febrile seizures. Other nervous-system and heart complications can also occur. Most of the symptoms last from three to seven days; however, cough and malaise can last two or more weeks.

Diagnosis and treatments

Diagnosis of influenza A can be made using rapid tests, which can be done in a physician's office by staff members without specific laboratory training, or by sending blood or swabs of infected tissue for laboratory tests. Identification of bird flu requires that specimens be sent to state health or Centers for Disease Control and Prevention laboratories.

Several antiviral drugs, including amantadine, oseltamivir, rimantadine, and zanamivir, which are active against influenza A, are available for treatment, but resistance has been reported. To have maximum effectiveness, these drugs should be started within two days of the onset of the symptoms.

Transmission

Only influenza A viruses can infect birds. This type of virus also infects humans, horses, pigs, seals, and whales. If a bird infected with avian flu dies, it can still shed viruses for up to 10 or more days. Those people who come into contact with an infected bird during this period can contract bird flu. Sustained transmission from person to person has not occurred; however, that could easily change through a process called antigenic shift, in which there is a merging of genetic material from subtypes of A viruses. The evolved virus could run rampant in the human population because humans would have no natural immunity to the virus.

Prevention

No vaccine is currently available to prevent bird flu, although research is ongoing to find an effective vaccine. The seasonal flu vaccine is not effective in preventing bird flu infection. Thus prevention rests upon safety measures and changes in behavior.

In general, surgical masks may help prevent transmission of respiratory communicable diseases, especially when used in health care settings. On a more global scale, regions that have experienced or been threatened with bird flu have resorted to destroying sick birds and quarantining farms in an effort to control spread of the virus. In the United States, there is ongoing surveillance of poultry for infection with bird flu, and imports of birds from affected countries have been banned. The U.S. Senate appropriated close to $4 billion in September 2005 for a national emergency response to an outbreak of avian flu.

Travelers to regions where there is transmission of bird flu need to take precautions to avoid contact with animals or contaminated surfaces in open-air markets and should avoid visiting poultry farms. Raw eggs could be contaminated with fecal material from poultry and thus should also be avoided. Because heat destroys avian viruses, thoroughly cooked poultry does not pose a health threat. Finally, even though the seasonal flu vaccine does not prevent bird flu, it should still be considered because simultaneous infection is a possibility.

Rita Washko

See also
• Asian influenza • H1N1 influenza
• Influenza

Backache

Backache, or back pain, is one of the most common conditions for which people seek medical attention. It has been estimated that 80 percent of the population will experience back pain at least once in their lifetime.

The spine is composed of individual vertebrae, each separated by an intervertebral disk (IVD), and can be divided into three regions (cervical, thoracic, and lumbar). Together, the disks and vertebrae function to provide flexibility and shock absorption for everyday activities. Joints exist between each vertebra (facet joints), providing additional flexibility and stability. The lumbar region, often referred to as the lower back, has five vertebrae.

Each IVD is made of fibrous cartilage with a viscous consistency that allows it to absorb stresses while providing flexibility in the spine. In contrast, each vertebra is rigid and provides protection for the spinal cord and its surrounding structures. Nerves originating from the spinal cord exit the spine through bony canals called intervertebral foramina and extend to muscles and other tissues of the back and lower extremities.

The vertebra-IVD complex is held together by ligaments and muscles. The muscles surrounding the spine, abdomen, and pelvis need to be strong for optimal posture and function. The core or deep muscles of the trunk are activated prior to movement to provide stability. The larger spinal muscles are responsible for creating back movement. Proper timing and coordination of these muscles is important to help reduce stresses placed on the lumbar spine during activities. When muscles become weak, instability of the spine may occur, increasing stress on the ligaments and joints, resulting in pain.

Causes and risk factors

Backache can be caused by a combination of factors including poor posture, poor fitness, work or leisure activities that place abnormal stresses on the spine, changes in bony and soft tissues as a result of age, and other coexisting conditions affecting the surrounding structures. For example, sitting with poor posture for prolonged periods of time will overstress the structures that provide protection and stability to the lumbar spine. In the same way, repetitive activities, such as gymnastics, may overwork certain muscles and under-use others. Eventually, this repetition may lead to faulty coordination of muscles and backache.

Symptoms and signs

A person experiencing backache may exhibit a variety of symptoms, including localized ache or pain in the lower spinal region, pain that is central over the spine or more to one side, or pain that originates in the back and travels into the buttock region or leg or both. It might also be felt in just one leg or both legs. Other symptoms include numbness or pins and needles, or both, which may also be felt in the back, buttocks, or legs.

Diagnosis and pathogenesis

Diagnoses of backache are achieved through a variety of methods. Generally, the person with backache will be seen by a health care professional (HP) such as a doctor, physiotherapist, or chiropractor. After conducting a thorough interview, the HP guides the patient through a series of physical tests to determine the

KEY FACTS

Description

Ache, pain, numbness, or tingling in lower back, buttocks, or legs.

Causes

Stress on the spine or degenerative changes.

Risk factors

Poor posture, poor fitness level, family history, types of work, and leisure activities.

Symptoms and signs

Ache, numbness, or tingling in lower back, buttocks, or legs.

Diagnosis

Examination by a health care practitioner.

Treatments

Changing activities; maintaining correct posture; stretching and strengthening muscles; applying heat and cold; taking pain relievers.

Pathogenesis

Dysfunction in one or more tissues.

Prevention

Exercise to ensure strong supple muscles; maintaining good posture.

Epidemiology

80 percent of U.S. population will experience at least one episode of backache.

CURVES OF THE SPINE

The regions of the spine have different functions: The cervical vertebrae support the head, the thoracic vertebrae hold the ribs in place, and the lumbar vertebrae give stability during movement.

brain
medulla oblongata
cervical vertebrae
spinal cord
thoracic vertebrae
cerebrospinal fluid
lumbar vertebrae
filum terminale
sacrum

The spine—vertebrae separated by intervertebral disks—is naturally curved into a shallow S shape.

underlying cause of injury. During this examination the HP attempts to rule out any serious pathology that might be mistaken for a musculoskeletal backache, such as cancerous tumors or serious infections. Diagnostic imaging such as X-rays, magnetic resonance imaging (MRI), and computed tomography (CT) also help the HP determine the cause of pain.

Bony and soft tissues, such as disk, muscle, or nerves, begin to break down and lose function when abnormal stresses are placed on them. In younger people, the disk can migrate beyond its normal barriers. This condition is referred to as disk herniation. Pain can be caused by the disk itself or the pressure that it places on surrounding tissues, such as the joints and nerves. In older people, the disk degenerates and loses its shock-absorbing capabilities. Pain or ache may then result from compression of the nearby joint space.

Bone pain may result from degenerative changes at the joint space. Cartilage lining the joint can break

down through abnormal wear and tear or from trauma. This degeneration can occur at any level of the spine and can result in pain. Pain may be caused by tightness or abnormal tension within the muscles or the fatigue of being tense all the time. In other situations, the muscles may not contract optimally, resulting in abnormal wear and tear of the joint.

Nerve pain is generally caused by compression of the nerves, which will not receive nutrition from the blood supply, resulting in pain. People who experience nerve pain often have symptoms into their buttocks and legs. For most people with backache, anatomical structures are not generally dysfunctional in isolation, but rather in combination. For example, if someone has pain originating from a disk, there is usually also pain from the bones, muscles, and nerves.

Treatments and prevention

Management of backache should help the patient understand that backache need not be a serious problem. Treatments are appropriate exercises, remaining at work or play, maintaining a positive attitude, and avoiding unnecessary medication. Bed rest is not recommended to manage backache. Continuing with usual activities, modifying them if necessary, is critical to recovery. Any postures or activities that increase back pain should be adapted during the most painful period and then reintroduced as symptoms begin to subside.

Proper posture ensures the least amount of stress on the spine, decreasing strain on ligaments, muscles, and joints. During standing, sitting, and lying the spine should be "in line" to maintain the natural S-shape curve. Stretching tight muscles and strengthening weak muscles help to maintain optimal posture and protect the spine. When strengthening muscles it is important to ensure that exercises are specific and functional.

The application of ice or heat to the painful area can act as an analgesic and muscle relaxant. Over-the-counter pain medications can help with pain control.

The primary means of preventing future back pain is exercise and maintaining proper postural alignment. Ensuring optimal body weight and general health will also assist in the prevention of recurring back pain.

Robyn Davies, Euson Yeung, and Sharon Switzer-McIntyre

See also
• Diabetes • Osteoporosis • Sports injury

Bipolar disorder

Also known as manic-depressive illness, bipolar disorder is a mood disorder marked by episodes of significant mood changes, ranging from extremely elevated (mania) to depressed. The disorder usually first appears during the teenage years or early 20s and tends to recur intermittently throughout life. In almost all cases, control of bipolar disorder requires medication.

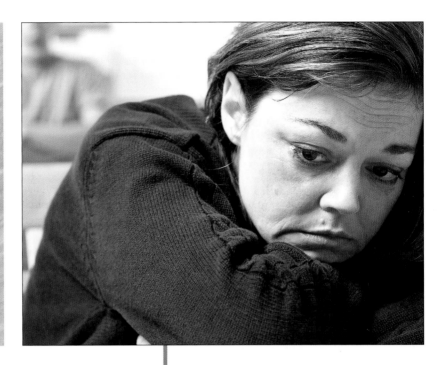

Bipolar disorder is a brain disorder that produces abnormal swings in an individual's mood, energy levels, and ability to function. The mood swings are more severe than the usual highs and lows that people experience and may seriously disrupt a person's life or even result in suicide. The disorder usually first appears during adolescence or in early adulthood and typically persists throughout life, although it can often be controlled effectively with medication. Bipolar disorder affects an estimated 2.6 percent of the adult population of the United States (approximately 5.7 million people).

Causes and risk factors

The immediate cause of bipolar disorder is believed to be an abnormality in the chemistry of the brain. The underlying cause of the abnormal brain chemistry has not been clearly identified, although there are many theories. Most of the theories highlight the importance of risk factors such as a family history of mood disorders or major psychiatric illnesses such as schizophrenia, and environmental factors such as sleep deprivation and major life stressors. Based on current knowledge, the development of bipolar disorder is thought to depend on complex interactions among genetic and environmental factors.

The severity of bipolar disorder varies among individuals but is characterized by severe mood swings from periods of depression, with feelings of hopelessness and a loss of interest in life, to elevated manic episodes.

Symptoms and types

Mania and depression, the two major syndromes of bipolar disorder, each have precise definitions. A manic episode is defined as being a period of at least one week during which an individual experiences a persistently elevated, expansive, or irritable mood. For the mood to be classed as elevated or expansive at least three of the following symptoms must be present: inflated self-esteem or grandiosity, increased goal-directed activity, excessive talkativeness, seemingly random flights of ideas, distractibility, decreased need for sleep, and excessive involvement in pleasurable activities with potentially painful consequences. For the mood to be classed as irritable, at least four of those symptoms must be present.

A depressive episode is defined as being a period of at least two weeks during which time the individual experiences at least four of the following symptoms: a depressed mood, a reduced interest in pleasurable activities, changes in appetite or weight, or both, feelings of guilt, worthlessness, or hopelessness, suicidal thoughts, changes in the individual's sleep pattern, decreased energy levels, and a reduction in the ability to think clearly or concentrate.

Some people experience mixed episodes (also called mixed states), which are defined as being a period of at least one week during which the individual experiences both manic and depressive symptoms simultaneously. In some people with bipolar I and II disorders (see below), manic and depressive episodes alternate frequently. If this phenomenon occurs at least 4 times in a 12-month period, it is known as "rapid cycling." Mania and depression can sometimes follow a seasonal pattern, with a predominance of manic episodes during the summer and depressive episodes during the winter. In addition to mood symptoms, some people with severe bipolar disorder may also have psychotic symptoms, such as delusional beliefs, and auditory or visual hallucinations. People suffering with bipolar disorder are also at an increased risk of attempting suicide, particularly during a depressive or mixed state.

Although bipolar disorder is characterized by fluctuations in mood between mania and depression, there are considerable variations between individuals in the pattern and severity of symptoms. Four subtypes of bipolar disorder have therefore been defined: bipolar I, bipolar II, cyclothymia, and bipolar disorder not otherwise specified (bipolar disorder NOS). In bipolar I disorder, major depressive episodes alternate with severe full manic episodes. In bipolar II disorder, major depressive episodes alternate with hypomanic episodes, which are less severe than full manic episodes. In cyclothymia, hypomanic episodes alternate with less severe depressive episodes. In addition, the cycles tend to be shorter than in bipolar I and II disorders and the mood changes are abrupt and irregular, sometimes occurring within hours of each other. Bipolar disorder NOS is usually diagnosed when an individual has the mood fluctuations of bipolar disorder but the symptoms do not meet the criteria for any of the other subtypes.

Diagnosis

Bipolar disorder is usually diagnosed by a psychiatrist. There are no specific investigative tests or procedures, and the diagnosis is based on a thorough psychiatric interview during which the psychiatrist evaluates the type, severity, and pattern of symptoms. In addition to this report, the individual may be given a thorough medical examination and have a full medical history taken, including information about previous and current medical treatments and lifestyle factors such as

use of over-the-counter medications, herbal remedies, or a history of substance abuse. The medical opinions of other health care professionals may also be sought. All of these measures are necessary to rule out other possible causes of the symptoms.

Treatments

Bipolar disorder is almost always treated with drugs. Mood-stabilizing drugs treat both manic and depressive phases of the illness, and their use between episodes makes future episodes of mania and depression less likely. Depending on the individual case,

KEY FACTS

Description
A mood disorder characterized by mood swings from mania to depression.

Causes
Abnormalities in the brain's chemistry. The underlying cause of the abnormal brain chemistry has not been clearly identified.

Risk factors
Family history of mood disorders, major life stressors, and substance abuse.

Symptoms
Most people with bipolar disorder experience two distinct mood syndromes: mania and depression. The number and severity of mood symptoms vary considerably from individual to individual. Some people experience manic and depressive episodes simultaneously, which are referred to as mixed episodes. The mood disturbances may be complicated by psychotic features such as hallucinations and delusions.

Diagnosis
Evaluation of symptoms by a psychiatrist.

Treatments
Most cases are treated with medications, including mood stabilizers, antipsychotic drugs, anticonvulsants, and antidepressants. Electroconvulsive therapy (ECT) may be used in some cases.

Pathogenesis
The disorder generally emerges between late adolescence and the early 20s and episodes tend to recur throughout life.

Prevention
Compliance with treatment decreases the likelihood of multiple episodes.

Epidemiology
About 5.7 million adults in the United States are affected by bipolar disorder in any given year. It is equally common in men and women.

other drugs may also be used to control specific symptoms. The mood stabilizers most commonly prescribed are valproate, lithium, and carbamazepine.

One of the most commonly prescribed medications for bipolar disorder is valproate. The side effects of this drug include stomach irritation, weight gain, hair loss, and drowsiness, and people taking valproate require regular blood tests to monitor the level of medication. Lithium is the longest-standing drug used to treat bipolar disorder, although it is not recommended for treating mixed states. The side effects include drowsiness, weight gain, gastrointestinal disturbances, thirst, and hand tremors. Long-term use of lithium can affect the kidneys and thyroid gland, and regular blood tests are necessary to monitor the level of medication. Carbamazepine is used mainly for patients who have not responded to lithium or valproate or who are in mixed states. However, it is not commonly prescribed because of its side effects, which include rashes, blurred vision, vertigo, abnormal gait, and drowsiness.

Antidepressants may also be used in the treatment of bipolar disorder, usually during depressive phases. These drugs are typically used on a short-term basis because they can precipitate manic episodes in some patients. The most commonly used antidepressants for bipolar disorder are selective serotonin reuptake inhibitors (SSRIs) such as citalopram, escitalopram, fluoxetine, paroxetine, and sertraline. Monoamine oxidase inhibitor (MAOI) antidepressants are prescribed less commonly because of their side effects. Tricyclic antidepressants are not generally recommended for treating bipolar disorder because they may trigger episodes of rapid cycling.

Depressive episodes may also be treated with the anticonvulsant drug lamotrigine, either by itself or in combination with antidepressants. Side effects of lamotrigine include headaches, nausea, skin rashes, and influenza-like symptoms.

Manic symptoms may be treated with antipsychotic drugs. The newer, second-generation antipsychotics, such as aripiprazole, olanzapine, quetiapine, risperidone, and ziprasidone, may also be used in the long-term management of bipolar disorder, either alone or in combination with mood stabilizers. The side effects of the newer antipsychotic drugs include weight gain, drowsiness, and metabolic abnormalities such as hyperglycemia (high blood glucose). The older antipsychotic drugs such as haloperidol and chlorpromazine are occasionally used, but they are not considered suitable for long-term use because they are poorly tolerated and also carry a high risk of producing movement disorders such as tremors and abnormal face and body movements.

Other drugs that may be used in the management of mania include clozapine and clonazepam. Clozapine is an effective antimanic drug, but again its usefulness is limited by its side effects, which include weight gain, metabolic abnormalities such as hyperglycemia, tachycardia (abnormally rapid heartbeat), constipation, and excessive salivation. Clozapine can also cause agranulocytosis (a severe deficiency of certain white blood cells), which predisposes individuals to potentially fatal infections, and for this reason people taking the drug require weekly blood monitoring tests. Clonazepam, in combination with mood stabilizers and antipsychotics, may be used to rapidly control periods of acute agitation during manic phases. The side effects of clonazepam include drowsiness, slurred speech, impaired memory, and ataxia (shaky movements and unsteady gait).

Electroconvulsive therapy (ECT) remains one of the most effective treatments for bipolar disorder. However, because of the wide range of medications available and the stigma attached to the procedure, ECT tends to be used only when drug treatments have proved ineffective. When it is used, ECT is given under general anesthesia. Its side effects include headaches, muscle soreness, confusion, and temporary loss of memory.

In addition to the above treatments, people with bipolar disorder and their families may be offered psychotherapy. This form of therapy helps patients and their relatives better understand the condition, encourages patients to continue other treatments, and helps decrease the risk of suicide.

Prevention

There is no known way of preventing bipolar disorder, and for most patients the condition is long lasting, with episodes recurring throughout life. Preventive measures are focused primarily on minimizing recurrences. Such measures include reducing life stressors, encouraging people with the disorder to adhere to their treatment regimens, and involving relatives in the ongoing treatment.

Oleg V. Tcheremissine
and Lori M. Lieving

See also
• Mood disorders • Schizophrenia

Birthmarks

Birthmarks are colored areas of skin that are present at birth or soon after birth. Birthmarks come in different shapes, sizes, and colors, including brown, tan, black, blue, pink, white, red, or purple. They may appear on the surface of the skin, raised above the skin, or located under the skin. The two main types of birthmarks are hemangiomas and pigmented birthmarks.

Birthmarks are colored marks on the skin that are present at birth or soon after. No causes are known. Some researchers have correlated premature birth, multiple births, and fertility drugs with birthmarks, although the association with these causes is poor. There are two broad categories of birthmarks: red and pigmented. The medical term for red marks are hemangiomas, from the Greek words *hema*, meaning "blood," and *oma*, meaning "tumor." Because blood vessels are collected together near the skin, hemangiomas are also called vascular birthmarks.

There are four different kinds of hemangiomas. Strawberry birthmarks are pinkish or red. They are most common on the face, scalp, back, or chest; 95 percent of strawberry birthmarks disappear by the time the child is nine years old. Cavernous hemangiomas are similar to strawberry marks but are deep in the skin and may appear as a red-blue spongy mass.

Port-wine stains are flat, maroon hemangiomas consisting of dilated fine blood vessels called capillaries. The face is the most common location of a port-wine stain; of those elsewhere, the size may vary from very small to more than half the body.

Salmon patches or stork bites are small pink, flat spots. They are usually on the forehead, eyelids, or upper lip, between the eyebrows, or on the back of the neck, and they often fade as the infant grows.

The second type of birthmark, pigmented skin markings, includes café-au-lait spots, moles (which can be flat or raised), and Mongolian spots.

Café-au-lait spots are light brown and look like coffee with milk. If these spots are larger than a quarter, they may indicate a genetic disorder that causes abnormal growth of nerve tissue. Moles are small clusters of pigmented skin cells. A Mongolian spot appears bluish or black, resembling a bruise, and is found in dark-skinned people.

KEY FACTS

Description

Colored marks on the skin that may grow, stay the same, or get smaller.

Causes

Unknown. Moles sometimes run in families.

Risk factors

Not known, possibly associated with premature birth, multiple births, or fertility drugs.

Symptoms

They do not hurt and are not the sign of disease. Rarely cause problems, but obvious ones may cause emotional distress.

Diagnosis

A physician needs to check all birthmarks.

Treatments

Most need no treatment; drugs, laser therapy, cryosurgery (freezing), or surgery may remove problematic marks.

Pathogenesis

A birthmark may or may not change; others grow over a period of time. Birthmarks that bleed or grow should always be checked by a physician.

Prevention

No prevention.

Epidemiology

Red birthmarks are common in children, with 10 percent having a birthmark by the age of one. They are seen more often in girls than boys. Port-wine stains occur in 1 percent of newborns but affect boys and girls equally, and salmon patches appear in 30 to 50 percent of newborns but have usually faded by one year.

Treatment

Most birthmarks fade as the child gets older. A birthmark that causes problems with sight, breathing, hearing, speech, or movement may need treatment. Cryosurgery (freezing), surgical removal, or laser surgery may remove marks after the child has reached school age. Port-wine stains on the face can be removed with laser treatment when the child is very young to prevent psychological problems later in life.

Evelyn Kelly

See also
• Cancer, skin

Blood poisoning

Also called septicemia or sepsis, blood poisoning is a potentially fatal illness that occurs when pathogens (infectious agents) flood the bloodstream. The most common causative pathogens are bacteria, but fungi, viruses, parasites, or toxins produced by the pathogens can also cause blood poisoning. The pathogens or toxins, or both, spread rapidly throughout the body, leading to widespread inflammation, organ failure, and death.

Blood poisoning is the common term for the serious illness that results when infectious agents or their toxins enter the bloodstream, spread throughout the body, and cause an exaggerated immune response, which can lead to widespread inflammation, multiple organ failure, and death. The terms *septicemia* and *sepsis* are medical names for the condition. The term *bacteremia* refers specifically to blood poisoning caused by bacteria, which are the most common causative agents.

Causes and risk factors

The initial infection can have various possible sources. For example, it may originate from a burn, ulcer, or other wound that becomes infected, from an unsterilized needle or other equipment, from surgical implantation of a device such as a pacemaker, or through an intravenous line (a tube inserted into a vein). Blood poisoning may also occur as a complication of an existing illness, such as a urinary tract infection, influenza, pneumonia, or a tooth abscess. The most common pathogens that cause blood poisoning are bacteria, often streptococci or staphylococci, but any infectious agent is capable of causing the condition.

In the body the pathogen multiplies too rapidly for the body's defense mechanisms to contain and spreads though the bloodstream to affect organs throughout the body. In addition, the immune system overreacts and produces excessive amounts of immune modulators (substances that combat invading organisms), which inflame the linings of blood vessels, stimulate the blood to clot, and generally produce an exaggerated inflammatory response that causes widespread damage to body systems.

Blood poisoning can affect anybody but certain groups are more vulnerable. Those at increased risk

KEY FACTS

Description
Illness resulting from a pathogen or pathogen-produced toxin spreading through the bloodstream.

Causes
Proliferation of bacteria in the bloodstream; toxins that are released from the bacteria can exacerbate the infection.

Risk factors
Recent illness or hospitalization, an invasive medical procedure or device, a weakened immune system, and intravenous drug use increase the risk of blood poisoning. Babies and older people are also at increased risk.

Symptoms and signs
Symptoms vary according to the source of infection but may include fever and chills, low body temperature, mental changes, low blood pressure, shock, rapid breathing, increased heart rate, and pale skin. The condition may progress to organ and respiratory failure and death.

Diagnosis
Physical examination; laboratory tests of blood, feces, urine, and cerebrospinal fluid; imaging tests to check internal organs; and possibly other tests, depending on the source of infection.

Treatments
Treatment varies according to the type and source of infection. Typically hospitalization is required and intravenous antibiotics or other antimicrobials, intravenous fluids, and oxygen are given. In some cases surgery may be needed to remove the source of infection.

Pathogenesis
Pathogens or their toxins cause an extreme immune response, leading to widespread inflammation, clotting disorders, oxygen-deprivation of the organs, and organ dysfunction or failure.

Prevention
Meticulous hygiene and sterilization measures, prompt treatment of all infections, and avoiding intravenous drug use can reduce the risk.

Epidemiology
In the United States about 750,000 people every year get blood poisoning and about 210,000 of these die. The number of cases is increasing and is predicted to rise to about 1 million by 2010.

include people with weakened immune systems, such as those with diabetes or HIV infection and those who are undergoing chemotherapy or taking immunosuppressant medications; the very old or young, especially premature babies; intravenous drug users; and people with invasive medical devices, such as catheters, intravenous lines, or pacemakers. Anybody who has recently been hospitalized or had a serious illness is also at increased risk.

Symptoms and signs

The initial symptoms and signs vary according to the origin of the blood poisoning. For example, blood poisoning originating from pneumonia may initially cause coughing and shortness of breath, whereas if the origin is a urinary tract infection the first symptom may be frequent, painful urination. In most cases symptoms are initially mild but quickly become severe.

As blood poisoning progresses, typical symptoms and signs include chills, low body temperature, pale skin, increased breathing and heart rates, low blood pressure, reduced urine output, impaired mental functioning, and high fever.

In the later stages, blood poisoning can produce shock, coma, multiple organ failure, respiratory failure, and death.

Diagnosis

Blood poisoning is diagnosed from the symptoms, particularly the presence of high fever, low body temperature, low blood pressure, pale, clammy skin, and reduced responsiveness.

Laboratory tests on samples of blood, urine, feces, and cerebrospinal fluid may be performed to check for infection and to identify the causative pathogen. If there is an infected wound, a skin culture may be done. If the physical examination indicates that internal organs may be affected, imaging tests such as computed tomography (CT) scanning may also be done to check the organs.

Treatments

Blood poisoning can progress rapidly, and early aggressive treatment greatly improves the likelihood of survival. The treatment varies according to the infection involved. Hospitalization is usually necessary, and treatment includes antibiotic or other drugs effective against the specific pathogen responsible, intravenous fluids to normalize blood pressure, and mechanical ventilation with oxygen to stabilize breathing and heart function. If a wound or a particular organ has been identified as the source of infection, surgery may also be needed to remove the source.

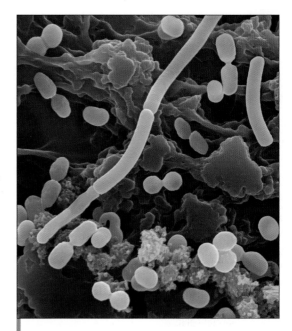

Acinetobacter spp. is a coccobacillus that causes many infections, including blood poisoning. It is found in water, sewage, soil, and on human skin.

Prevention

Blood poisoning will probably never be entirely preventable but there are various measures that reduce the risk of it developing. Because many cases originate in hospitals, meticulous sterilization and other hygiene procedures can reduce the presence and spread of pathogens.

Prompt treatment of even minor infections or wounds can help prevent the development of blood poisoning. Early treatment is particularly important for at-risk groups, such as the young, the old, and those with conditions that compromise the immune system, such as HIV infection and diabetes. Avoiding intravenous drug use also reduces the risk of blood poisoning.

The incidence of blood poisoning is increasing, both in the United States and worldwide, and the development of antibiotic-resistant strains of bacteria makes treatment more problematic in some cases. Efforts are therefore being made to formulate health policies and procedures to control the condition.

Lise Stevens

See also
- Antibiotic-resistant infections
- Food poisoning

Brain tumors

A brain tumor is a mass of diseased brain cells that develops when cells in the nervous system divide in an uncontrolled way. Brain tumors affect nerve cell function by compressing, invading, and damaging healthy tissue. Treatment is surgery, followed by chemotherapy or radiation therapy to eliminate remaining abnormal cells.

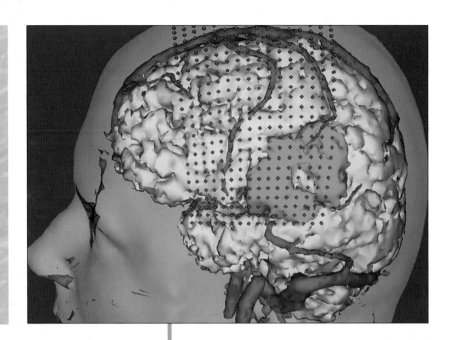

A colored MRI (magnetic resonance imaging) scan of the brain shows a brain tumor (green). Blood vessels are red and a ventricle (cavity) is cyan. Blue dots indicate a map of the motor cortex of the cerebrum; the map will help the surgeon remove the tumor with the least damage to the motor cortex.

Uncontrolled cell division in the brain results in cell masses called brain tumors. If the cell divisions are initially triggered inside the brain, the mass is called a primary tumor; if dividing cells originated from a cancer elsewhere in the body that traveled to the brain and set up a secondary site, the tumor is metastatic. Primary tumors can be benign; they have distinct borders, grow slowly, and do not spread to other parts of the body. Or, they can be malignant; they invade neighboring tissue, grow rapidly, and become life threatening. Metastatic brain tumors are always malignant.

Doctors discuss tumors using a standard terminology. Tumor names are based in part on their cells of origin, following the World Health Organization Classification System. Tumors are also given a grade (I to IV). Grade I describes a tumor that is slow growing, has normal-looking cells, and is the most benign; grade IV describes a tumor that is the most malignant, is rapid growing, and has abnormal cells that infiltrate nearby tissues.

Types of brain tumors

About 120 types of brain tumors have been identified. The most common are acoustic neuromas, astrocytomas, ependymomas, oligodendrogliomas, central nervous system lymphomas, meduloblastomas, meningiomas, metastatic brain tumors, and pituitary tumors.

Acoustic neuromas, also called vestibular schwannomas, develop from Schwann cells, which produce insulating layers of fatty myelin around peripheral nerve fibers. Typically, these tumors form on the sensory nerves that innervate (supply nerves to) the cochlea, which is involved in hearing, and the vestibular apparatus, which is involved in balance. These tumors occur more commonly in women and can be treated surgically.

Astrocytomas originate from astrocytes, which are star-shaped brain glia (cells that support nerve cells). Astrocytomas are slow growing in children and malignant in adults. A malignant grade IV astrocytoma is called a glioblastoma multiforme.

Ependymomas arise in the lining of the ventricles (fluid-filled cavities in the brain and spinal cord). They often block the flow of fluid in these cavities, leading to a buildup of pressure. More common in children, they may be of grade I (papillary ependymomas) through grade IV (ependymoblastomas).

Oligodendrogliomas are tumors formed by oligodendrocytes, which are the myelin-producing cells of the brain. Unregulated growth of oligo-dendrocytes is often accompanied by abnormally multiplying astrocytes, and the tumors therefore contain both cell types. These tumors are called oligoastrocytomas.

Central nervous system lymphomas, often shortened to lymphomas, are tumors of B lymphocytes (a type of white blood cell). They commonly occur in the front part of the brain, but may also be scattered in other regions. Lymphomas may cause personality disorders and symptoms resulting from increased pressure inside the skull. They can be treated with radiation therapy or chemotherapy.

Medulloblastomas are aggressive tumors that comprise more than 25 percent of all childhood tumors and are more frequent in boys. They are usually found in the part of the brain called the cerebellum.

Meningiomas develop from uncontrolled growth of cells that make up the meninges, the membranes that cover the brain and spinal cord. These tumors are benign and rarely invade other tissues. Surgical excision of the tumor is usually successful. However, these tumors have a tendency to recur.

Metastatic brain tumors originate from cancers that develop in other parts of the body and spread to the brain. Cancers of the skin (melanomas), lung, breast, kidney, and colon most often metastasize to the brain.

Pituitary tumors originate in the pituitary gland, which is located deep in the skull cavity and is critical in the production of hormones such as growth hormone, thyroid hormone, and, in women, hormones that regulate milk production and the menstrual cycle. Some pituitary tumors produce too much of a specific hormone, whereas others are nonsecretory. Available drugs are successful in reducing some types of pituitary tumors.

Causes and symptoms

Scientists do not understand what triggers brain-tumor formation. Genetics can be traced in some cases: for example, inherited genes for certain diseases of the nervous system, such as tuberous sclerosis and neurofibromatosis, put a person at increased risk of developing a brain tumor. Other gene mutations can occur spontaneously—that is, they are not inherited. If a tumor-suppressor gene, which normally suppresses unregulated cell division, becomes mutated, cell proliferation may be released from its normal controls. Mutations in proto-oncogenes also contribute to cancer. Some proteins, such as the receptor for a substance called epidermal growth factor (EGF), are

---

KEY FACTS

Description

Mass of abnormally dividing brain cells. May be primary (originates in brain) or metastatic (originates outside brain), benign, or malignant. Many different brain-cell types are affected.

Causes

Unknown. Suspected genetic links.

Risk factors

Radiation or toxin exposure; more likely in those with the disorders tuberous sclerosis or neurofibromatosis; specific gene mutations.

Symptoms

Appear gradually with tumor growth, and are dependent on location. Headaches, nausea, seizures, numbness, altered vision, hearing, speech, memory, and personality change are common.

Diagnosis

Neurological tests of motor function, balance, reflexes, eye movement, speech, and memory. Use of spinal tap, recording of neural activity, MRI or CT scanning, and biopsy.

Treatments

Depends on size or grade of tumor, its location, and age of the patient. Surgery, radiation therapy, chemotherapy, gene therapy, or immunotherapy may help. Medical management of symptoms such as pain.

Pathogenesis

Depends on type of tumor and location. As the tumor grows, pressure affects nearby tissue. Tumor may spread within nervous system, rarely outside. Can be life threatening.

Prevention

Unknown.

Epidemiology

Affect 130 in 10,000 people in the United States. More frequent in children and elderly people. More than 40,000 new cases reported each year. Metastatic tumors are four times more frequent than primary tumors.

---

found at high levels in brain-tumor tissue and are likely to be involved in the development of tumors. Environmental factors such as ionizing radiation and toxins are also suspected risk factors. Much current research is aimed at understanding mechanisms involved in transforming normal cells into cancerous cells and at finding molecules that can be targeted by new therapies.

Many symptoms of brain tumors are similar to those for other growths in the brain, such as aneurysms. Symptoms develop because the growing tumor pushes on normal brain tissue. There may be one or more of many symptoms, including: headaches; nausea; vomiting; loss of vision, hearing, or sensation; slurred speech; motor dysfunction; memory loss; personality disorders; hormonal imbalance; confusion; and seizures. Usually symptoms associated with brain tumors develop gradually, over months or years.

Diagnosis and treatments

If these symptoms are noted, a neurologist performs a basic neurological examination, including tests for normal reflexes, eye movements, pupillary responses to light, and sensory, motor, and memory functions. If a brain tumor is suspected, the neurologist will probably arrange for brain scans. MRI and CT scans are used to locate and visualize the tumor, and angiography (X-rays to investigate the arteries that supply the brain) is used to determine the extent of vascularization (blood-vessel supply) to the tumor, especially prior to surgery. Other types of scans or recordings of electrical activity using electrodes placed in brain tissue are used to map areas involved in critical functions such as speech or memory in order to avoid these regions during surgery. Spinal tap is a diagnostic technique in which the fluid in and around the brain is sampled for proteins that indicate the presence of tumors. Biopsy tissue (small samples of tumor tissue) is collected before or during surgery and is sent to the pathology laboratory, where it is analyzed by a pathologist to identify the type and grade of tumor; results are used to guide treatment options. Once a brain tumor has been detected, the medical team will work with a neuro-oncologist and a neurosurgeon to determine the best treatment options. This decision will depend on the suspected type and grade of tumor, its location, and the age of the affected person.

Surgery is usually the first treatment, in an attempt to remove the tumor tissue completely or at least to reduce its mass. Some tumors cannot be approached surgically because of their position in the brain. In these cases, other options must be used.

Radiation therapy is often used following surgery to eliminate tumor remnants because dividing cells are more vulnerable to radiation than normal ones. However, since many normal brain cells are still dividing in very young children, radiation may not be advisable until a child is older.

Chemotherapy involves using cocktails of drugs that interfere with cell division. The drugs may be given orally or injected. Because these drugs act systemically (throughout the body), chemotherapy is most effective with malignant brain tumors, in which abnormal cells invade tissues in the brain and spinal cord. However, increasingly, drugs may be applied on a wafer and inserted directly into the tumor for easier and more direct access to proliferating cells. Chemotherapy is not commonly used to treat benign tumors. Researchers are testing combinations of these therapies. Formation of new blood vessels, called angiogenesis, which supply the mass of growing cells, is critical for tumors to grow; one therapeutic approach involves inhibiting the growth of new blood vessels in diseased tissue by local application of drugs called angiogenesis inhibitors, which starve the tumor.

Other therapies use tumor-specific toxins or stimulate the body's immune system to kill abnormal cells.

Alternative medicine is increasingly considered by patients as a treatment, in an effort to maintain a good quality of life after a diagnosis of brain cancer. Treatments include homeopathy, yoga, nutritional supplements, and special diets, relaxation techniques, and spirituality. Benefits from these treatments have not been validated by scientific studies, but anecdotal reports of relief from symptoms are widespread. Post-treatment follow-up tests are done periodically to monitor whether or not the treatment worked and to stay vigilant regarding the recurrence of tumors.

Pathogenesis

The progression of the disease depends on many factors: the location of the tumor, its size, and how quickly it is growing. A patient with a slow-growing benign tumor that is removed usually has a better outlook than someone with a malignant tumor.

Epidemiology

About 18,000 new cases of brain tumors arise each year in the United States, but if both primary and malignant tumors are considered, the number is more than 40,000 new cases per year. Statistics show that about 130 in 10,000 people in the United States have brain tumors. Elderly individuals and children are more susceptible. In children, solid tumors (not infiltrating) are the most common, and more than 3,100 cases are diagnosed annually. The five-year survival rate for people with malignant tumors is 32 to 40 percent, and close to 70 percent in children.

Sonal Jhaveri

See also
• Cancer, breast • Cancer, colorectal
• Cancer, lung • Cancer, skin

Bronchitis

Bronchitis, characterized by excessive coughing and sputum production, is caused by inflammation of the large airways in the lungs (bronchi). Bronchitis may be either acute (usually as a result of a viral infection) or chronic; smokers and people with lung disease are most at risk for either type. High atmospheric pollution is also a risk factor.

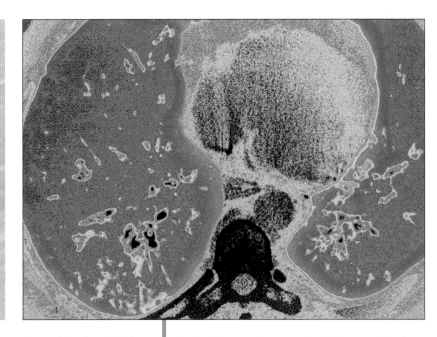

A colored computed tomography (CT) scan of the lungs shows the effects of bronchial inflammation, or bronchitis. The bronchi, or airways, are colored blue; mucus inside the bronchi is colored dark brown.

Bronchitis is an inflammation of the bronchi, the main airways in the lungs. Bronchitis can be acute (short-lived) or chronic (long lasting and recurring). Acute bronchitis is one of the most common reasons for doctor visits in the United States. It is usually caused by a virus, such as the rhinovirus, which causes the common cold, although sometimes it may be caused by bacteria such as chlamydia. Acute bronchitis can last from several days to several weeks. People are more likely to develop acute bronchitis if they have had a recent respiratory illness such as a cold, have other lung diseases like asthma or cystic fibrosis, or are cigarette smokers.

Chronic bronchitis, part of the spectrum of chronic obstructive pulmonary disease (COPD), is the more serious disease. It is defined as a persistent cough with sputum (the liquid secretion that comes up from the lungs when a person coughs) on most days for at least three months and for at least two successive years. It is a slowly progressive type of COPD, limiting airflow in the lungs and causing a chronic cough and difficulty breathing due to shortness of breath. There is no known cure for chronic bronchitis, although smoking cessation and the judicious use of antibiotics can help.

Causes and risk factors

Cigarette smoking is responsible for 85 to 90 percent of chronic bronchitis cases in most developed coun-

tries, including the United States. Toxic gases and particles from cigarette smoke are the main cause of chronic bronchitis, but other pollutants can also be inhaled from pipes, cigars, or other tobacco, and some environmental dusts and chemicals can irritate the lungs. The longer a person smokes or is exposed to smoke, even to secondhand smoke (see box, page 86) the greater the chances of developing chronic bronchitis. Air pollution, repeated lung infections, allergies, and genetic factors may also contribute. Some researchers believe that there are workplace exposures that may cause chronic bronchitis symptoms similar to those caused by cigarette smoking. Suspected workplace exposures include coal, oil mists, cement, silica, silicates, osmium, vanadium, welding fumes, organic dusts, engine exhausts, and fire smoke. Exposure to organic dusts, like cotton, jute, hemp, flax, sisal, wood, and different grains can also cause symptoms of chronic bronchitis.

Symptoms

Symptoms of chronic bronchitis include a cough that produces mucus (liquid secretions produced in the tiny glands lining the airways in the lungs), fatigue, frequent lung infections that worsen symptoms, and shortness of breath.

Diagnosis

Evaluation of patients with suspected chronic bronchitis includes a physical examination and a detailed history for possible environmental exposures. Usually a chest X-ray or a chest computed tomography (CT) scan (or both) are done. Pulmonary function tests can be done in a physician's office to measure how well air flows into and out of the lungs, and how well oxygen travels from the lungs to the blood.

Spirometry uses a handheld device to measure how well a person can quickly and forcefully exhale the air in his or her lungs through the mouth. An arterial blood gas, a blood sample taken from an artery, measures how much oxygen and carbon dioxide are present in a sample of blood and can give information about whether a person's blood is too acidic (called acidosis) or too alkaline (called alkalosis). A laboratory examination of sputum, coughed into a specimen container, may be done to help diagnose bronchitis or other lung diseases, like pneumonia.

Treatments

There is no cure for chronic bronchitis. Quality of life worsens as the disease progresses, limiting even normal physical activity. The goal is to discontinue exposure to environmental irritants, like tobacco; to prevent complications, like pneumonia, emphysema, and heart problems; and to provide relief of symptoms. Some medications can help relax and open up the airways so more oxygen gets into the lungs and may relieve symptoms such as shortness of breath and wheezing (a high-pitched whistling sound produced by breathing through narrowed airways.)

Steroids can be used during flare-ups to decrease lung inflammation. Antibiotics can be used to treat episodes of chronic bronchitis that appear to be related to bacterial infection. Oxygen may be helpful and even life saving in severe cases. Patients with COPD may also benefit from exercise therapy, and rarely, lung transplant in the most severe cases.

Pathogenesis

Chronic bronchitis is a slowly progressive disease with gradual loss of lung function. Through an immune reaction, cells linings the main airways and their mucus-producing glands react to the constant exposure to toxic particles or gases and become inflamed. Inflammation of the airways can be found in otherwise healthy smokers as young as 20 or 30 years old. The damaged glands along the airways produce more mucus than normal. Mucus is a thick, slimy, liquid material produced in the airways, sinuses, and other places in the body. In normal lungs, mucus cleans the airways and is moved along by cilia, the

KEY FACTS

Description
Inflammation of the airways that leads to scarring of airways of the lungs, chronic excess mucus production, and decreased airflow in the lungs that is irreversible.

Causes and risk factors
Toxic particles and gases from cigarette smoke are the main cause. Pipe, cigar, and other types of tobacco, and other environmental pollutants, like dust and chemicals, can contribute.

Symptoms
Chronic cough, increased mucus production in the lungs, wheezing, difficulty breathing, clearing of the throat.

Diagnosis
Medical history, physical examination, chest X-ray or CT scan, pulmonary function tests, spirometry, arterial blood gas.

Treatment
Avoid exposure to environmental irritants like cigarette smoke, smoke from other types of tobacco, and other lung toxins. Some medications and exercise may help.

Pathogenesis
Inflammation from toxins like those in cigarette smoke leaves breathing tubules scarred and narrowed, resulting in permanent damage to the lungs. Airflow in the lungs decreases. An increase in the size and number of glands creates excess mucus. Cilia, the tiny hairlike structures that help clear mucus from the lungs, become damaged.

Prevention
Avoiding smoking is the most important way to prevent or stop progression of the disease. Identify and prevent exposure to other possible lung toxins.

Epidemiology
There are more than 8 million diagnosed cases in the United States, but some estimates put the figure as high as 14 million or more. As more women smoke, the incidence of bronchitis in women is also rising. The incidence of chronic bronchitis is directly related to the number of cigarettes smoked. Occupational exposure may account for as many as 15 percent of cases.

BRONCHITIS AND SMOKING

The inhalation of secondhand smoke, also called environmental tobacco smoke (ETS), is known as passive, or involuntary, smoking. Secondhand smoke is made up of mainstream smoke, the smoky mixture given off by the burning end of cigarettes or other tobacco products, and sidestream smoke, the smoke exhaled by smokers. This kind of smoke contains more than 4,000 known chemicals, depending on the type of tobacco, but there may be more than 100,000 chemicals. Secondhand smoke contains at least 60 carcinogens (substances that cause cancer), including formaldehyde, and can be found in homes, workplaces, and public places like bars and restaurants. It is a risk factor for lung cancer, even in nonsmokers, and is particularly dangerous in the developing lungs of infants and children, for whom it is responsible for an increased risk of sudden infant death syndrome (SIDS), asthma, bronchitis, and pneumonia. More than 8,000 new cases of asthma and more than 150,000 new cases of bronchitis and pneumonia in children each year are caused by secondhand smoke. More than 20 percent of all children younger than age 18 live in a home that is polluted by secondhand smoke.

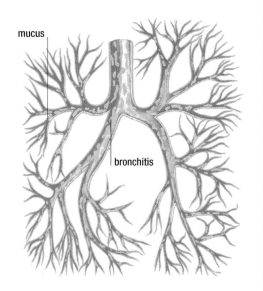

mucus

bronchitis

Bronchitis, which is an inflammation of the bronchi, the airways in the lungs, causes an increased production of mucus, which is shown in the diagram as yellow patches. Bronchitis often follows another respiratory illness.

small beating hairlike structures. Normally, these cilia would move about 17 fluid ounces (500 ml) of mucus per day (a little more than 2 cups) to the lower part of the throat, where it is swallowed and not noticed. However, in chronic bronchitis, the amount of daily mucus is increased by 3 fluid ounces (100 ml) or more. The lining of the airways scar and thicken, the airways narrow, and it is more difficult to cough mucus out to clear the airways. This condition can prevent oxygen from entering some parts of the lungs. The airways can also become a breeding ground for bacteria.

Prevention

Early recognition and treatment, and avoiding irritants like tobacco smoke are the best ways to prevent chronic bronchitis. Lung inflammation is present in every person who smokes tobacco. Some people may be more susceptible to damage in their lungs, but the reason for this susceptibility is not known. Stopping smoking can have a beneficial effect at any age.

Epidemiology

There are more than 8 million people in the United States diagnosed with chronic bronchitis, but the real

figure may be as high as 14 million, since many patients tend to underreport their symptoms. It is estimated that as many as 15 percent of cases are due to occupational exposures, but it may be difficult to identify specific exposures, and many of the workers may also smoke. COPD, which includes chronic bronchitis and emphysema, is the fourth leading cause of death in the United States.

Although chronic bronchitis was previously more common in men, as more women have taken up smoking over the last 50 years, the incidence of chronic bronchitis in women has risen remarkably. In 2004 more than twice as many women than men were diagnosed with chronic bronchitis.

The incidence of chronic bronchitis is related to the number of cigarettes smoked. It affects people of all ages but is more common in people over the age of 45.

Ramona Jenkin

See also
• Asthma • Cold, common • COPD • Cystic fibrosis • Emphysema • Pneumonia

Burns

A burn is an injury to tissue, most commonly the skin, as a result of exposure to heat, chemicals, electricity, or radiation. The majority of burns are relatively minor, and most of the more than 2 million people every year in the United States who sustain burns are treated as outpatients. About 70,000 people have burns that require inpatient treatment, however, and more than 5,000 people die every year from burns.

Burns range from minor skin damage requiring only first aid treatment to catastrophic injuries that need intensive inpatient hospital treatment and have a significant mortality rate. Most burns are caused by heat from a flame, hot liquids or steam (scalds), or by contact with a hot object. However, burns can also be caused by chemicals such as acids and alkalis, electricity, and radiation, both nonionizing radiation such as the ultraviolet radiation in sunlight and ionizing radiation from radioactive sources.

Types, symptoms, and signs

Burns are classified according to their depth. A first-degree burn, such as sunburn, damages only the outer layer of skin (epidermis). The skin is red, inflamed, and painful and becomes dry and flaky as it heals. The skin usually heals in about five days and does not scar. A second-degree burn damages the epidermis and extends into the dermis (the layer beneath the epidermis). Such a burn produces fluid-filled blisters and is very painful. Healing is slower than with first-degree burns and may take up to about 14 days. In addition, healing often produces scar tissue, which may contract and interfere with normal functioning. A third-degree burn destroys the entire thickness of the skin. The appearance of the burned area may vary from white and waxy to black, charred, and leathery. Third-degree burns are generally not painful because the nerves in the skin are destroyed. Such burns can only heal by migration of tissue from the wound's edges, which is a slow process for all but small wounds and carries an increased risk of infection and the chance of severe scarring. Rare burns in which the damage penetrates the skin to body tissues such as muscles and bones may be referred to as fourth-degree burns and are usually the result of contact with a very hot flame or electricity.

COMMON TYPES OF BURNS

Burns are classified according to the depth of penetration in the skin layers. First-degree (superficial) burns damage the outer layer of skin. The skin usually recovers in a few days because the basic structure, which is necessary for the growth of new skin, remains. In second-degree (partial thickness) burns, healing is much slower; all but the deepest glands and hair follicles are destroyed. In third-degree (full thickness) burns, no basic cellular structure remains from which new skin can start to reform. These burns are not painful, apart from areas where some nerves still remain. Fourth-degree (subdermal) burns penetrate to muscles and bones.

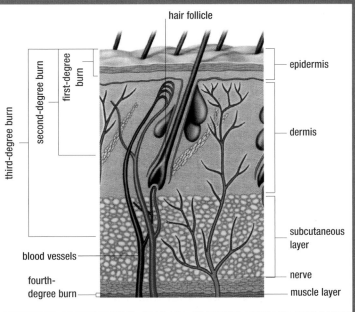

87

Description and causes

Tissue injury caused by exposure to heat, chemicals, electricity, or radiation.

Risk factors

Certain occupations (such as electricians and chemical workers), some activities (such as cooking), and unsupervised children have a higher risk of burns.

Symptoms and signs

First-degree burns produce redness, swelling, and pain. Second-degree burns produce blistering and pain. Third-degree burns cause the skin to become white and waxy or charred; such burns often do not initially cause pain because nerves in the skin are destroyed. Rare types of burns that penetrate the skin to muscle and bone are called fourth-degree burns.

Diagnosis

Diagnosis is usually obvious from the skin injury and circumstances. Blood tests and bronchoscopy may be done to aid diagnosis of inhalation injury. Cardiac monitoring may be done to check for heart problems with electrical burns.

Treatments

Immediate first-aid treatment is aimed at stopping the burning process and protecting the burned area. Subsequent treatment centers on controlling pain, preventing infection, and aiding healing. Intravenous fluids may be necessary in some cases, and assistance with breathing may be given if smoke has been inhaled. People with severe burns may also require skin grafts or reconstructive surgery, or both; physical therapy; and psychological support.

Pathogenesis

The external agent causes cellular death in the affected tissue. The severity of the burn depends on duration of contact and, with heat burns, on the temperature. Further damage may occur as a result of chemicals that are released from the damaged tissue.

Prevention

Educational programs and safety measures in the home and workplace can help reduce likelihood of burns. Specific home preventive measures include reducing the water-heater temperature, installing smoke detectors, and having fire-resistant furnishings and clothing.

Epidemiology

In the United States more than 2 million people a year sustain burns, and about 70,000 of these require hospitalization. About 5,000 people a year die as a result of burns. Serious burns are most common in adult males between ages 20 and 29 and in children younger than 9. Fire is the most common cause, followed by scalds.

As well as determining the depth of tissue damage, burns are also assessed according to the percentage of the body area affected. For this assessment physicians use the "rule of nines," by which the body surface is divided into areas that are multiples of 9 percent. The head and neck make up 9 percent; each arm is 9 percent; each leg is 18 percent (2 x 9 percent); the front of the trunk is 18 percent; and the back of the trunk is 18 percent. Children, who have a different surface area ratio, are assessed by other methods.

If a burn is due to fire there is a risk of inhalation injury, which can cause difficulty in breathing, hoarseness, soot in the airways, and redness of the back of the throat. Chemical burns may produce inhalation injury if chemical vapors are inhaled. There may be symptoms of toxicity, depending on the chemical involved. With both types of burns, the combination of inhalation injury and a large burn area significantly increases the probability of death.

Electrical burns cause injuries to the skin and may disrupt the normal functioning of internal organs. Symptoms depend on the route taken by the current through the body, the size of the current, and its duration. Other symptoms include confusion, rapid breathing, and unconsciousness. If the current passes through the heart there may be cardiac damage or even cardiac arrest. With any burn most of the tissue damage is a direct result of the causative agent, but additional tissue damage may occur as a result of harmful chemicals released from the damaged tissue and the associated inflammatory response. With large burns released chemicals can impair the functioning of other organs.

Diagnosis

The initial medical assessment is focused on evaluating the overall condition of the patient, including evaluating the extent and severity of the burns and checking for associated problems, such as inhalation injury, damage to the heart from electrical injury, or toxic effects of chemicals. A definitive diagnosis of inhalation injury may require blood tests of the levels of oxygen and carboxyhemoglobin and direct examination of the airways with a bronchoscope. Cardiac monitoring may be carried out if heart damage is suspected from an electrical injury.

Treatments

First aid treatment of burns involves stopping the burning process, then protecting the burned area. Any burn except the most minor should also receive professional medical help. The patient's vital signs,

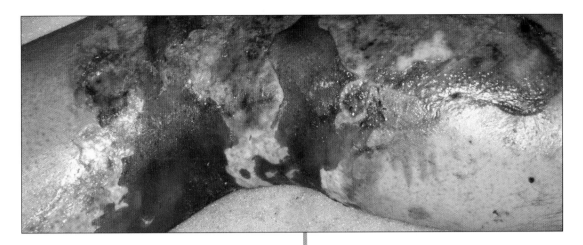

including breathing, heartbeat and circulation, and consciousness, should be monitored until help arrives.

The first step is to remove the source of burning. Clothing can usually be extinguished by the "stop, drop, and roll" maneuver. Dry chemicals should be brushed off the skin. Wet chemicals and hot liquids should be immediately washed off with large amounts of cool, clean water. Specific chemical neutralizing agents should not be used. With electrical burns the electricity supply should be turned off or the victim removed from contact with it. With radiation burns the victim should be removed from the radiation source. However, the rescuer should never endanger him- or herself to help the victim; instead, emergency services should deal with the problem. When the source of burning has been removed, the injured area should be cooled using large amounts of clean water. The injured area should then be covered with a cool, damp, clean cloth. Home remedies, such as butter or other salves, should not be put on the burn.

After initial first aid, treatment consists of controlling pain, preventing infection, and facilitating healing. If the victim is also suffering from inhalation injury, she or he may require breathing assistance with a mechanical ventilator. Any other associated problems, such as heartbeat irregularities from electrical injury, toxic effects of chemicals, or effects of radiation exposure may also require treatment. For first-degree burns and small second-degree burns, the wound may be treated with a topical cream, such as an antibiotic or silver sulfadiazine, and then covered with a dressing; or a medicated dressing may be used. Extensive second-degree burns and third-degree burns require hospital treatment. If an extensive area of the body is burned, the victim may lose large amounts of fluid. In such cases intravenous fluids are necessary to ensure that the victim remains ade-

A third-degree burn has damaged the entire thickness of the skin of this leg and penetrated to the nerves that lie beneath the dermis. The appearance of the skin is charred and waxy.

quately hydrated and to maintain blood pressure and blood flow through the body's organs. With the loss of the epidermis, nerve endings are exposed, which usually causes severe pain that requires strong analgesics to control. Open burn wounds are vulnerable to infection, and patients are usually given antibiotics as a preventive measure. Nutritional support is also important, to encourage wound healing and help the patient resist infection.

The main treatment of third-degree burns is skin grafting. When possible, skin is removed from an uninjured area of the body and transplanted over the injured areas, but with extensive third-degree burns there may not be sufficient uninjured skin available. In such cases tissue culturing may be used to grow skin for later transplantation. If a burn site takes more than about three weeks to heal, there is a significant risk of scarring, which may not only affect appearance but also impair function, particularly if there is scarring on the hands or across joints. In such cases, plastic or reconstructive surgery may be recommended; physical and occupational therapy may also be helpful.

Recovery from major burns can be slow, painful, and traumatic, and some patients suffer post-traumatic stress disorder. Psychiatrists, psychologists, and social workers can help provide support for both the patients and their families.

David Wainwright

See also
• Radiation sickness • Sunburn and sunstroke

Cancer, bladder

A cancer of the bladder lining can spread throughout the body. The most common cause of bladder cancer is cigarette smoking. For reasons that are not clear, men are at much higher risk than women.

Industrialized countries such as the United States may have a higher standard of living, but industrialization also increases the risk of bladder cancer. In Asia and South America there are much lower rates of this cancer. For reasons no one understands, bladder cancer is much more common in men than in women.

Causes and risk factors

For both men and women, the number one cause of bladder cancer is cigarette smoking. The carcinogens inhaled in smoke can enter the bloodstream and reach the urine. Exposure to these chemicals in the environment can also increase the risk of bladder cancer. Genetic factors determine how well the body can prevent these chemicals from damaging genes. Ultimately, it is a genetic change that turns healthy cells into cancerous cells. Other risk factors include a family history of the disease, recurrent bladder infections, diet, and increasing age.

Symptoms and diagnosis

The most striking symptom of bladder cancer is blood in the urine. However, many noncancerous conditions also produce this symptom. Therefore a physical examination is essential. A doctor uses an endoscope called a cytoscope to look inside the bladder. If bladder cancer is suspected, a biopsy, or small sample of bladder tissue, is removed. The tissue is examined to confirm the diagnosis. If the cells are cancerous, further tests may be done to determine if the cancer has invaded the muscular bladder wall or spread to other parts of the body.

Treatments and prevention

Radiation therapy and chemotherapy are standard treatments for bladder cancer following surgery. Superficial tumors can be removed, leaving the bladder intact. With invasive tumors, the entire bladder will be removed, as well as nearby lymph nodes and organs. When caught in its earliest stage, the five-year survival rate is 85 percent. However, only 5 percent of those diagnosed with invasive bladder cancer survive more than two years. Novel therapies are being developed to improve the survival rate. Immunotherapy uses special vaccines to stimulate the immune system into fighting the spread or recurrence of bladder cancer.

The best preventive measure is not to smoke. Drinking plenty of fluids and eating a low-fat diet can also reduce the risk. According to one study, men who regularly ate broccoli and cabbage also had a lower risk.

Chris Curran

KEY FACTS

Description

A cancer of the bladder lining and wall.

Causes

Both genetic and environmental factors contribute to bladder cancer.

Risk factors

The biggest risk factor is cigarette smoking. Increasing age, a high-fat diet, and a family history of the disease are also risk factors.

Symptoms

There may be no symptoms in the early stages. Blood in the urine is a warning sign but does not always indicate cancer. Other symptoms mimic those of the bladder infection cystitis.

Diagnosis

Cystoscopy and a biopsy of bladder tissue.

Treatment

Surgery, radiation therapy, chemotherapy, and immunotherapy.

Pathogenesis

Cells in the bladder lining divide abnormally. Invasive bladder cancer can spread into the muscular bladder wall and elsewhere in the body.

Prevention

Quitting smoking; eating a low-fat diet; drinking lots of water.

Epidemiology

The highest rates are in industrialized countries, with 50,000 new cases in the United States each year. Men are two to three times more likely to develop bladder cancer than women.

See also
• Cystitis

Cancer, breast

Breast cancer is the most common cancer of women in the United States after skin cancer. Early diagnosis is important because treatment given at the onset of the disease can increase the chance of recovery. Screening programs based on mammograms are widely available to help detect the disease when it is in its early stages.

In the United States one in eight women will be diagnosed with breast cancer during her lifetime, and about one in thirty will die from the disease. It is the second most common cause of death of women in the United States, after lung cancer. Seventy-five percent of diagnosed cases are in women aged 50 or older. Some cases of breast cancer are called in-situ cancers, meaning that the cancer typically does not spread beyond the local tissue where it begins. Most in-situ breast cancers can be cured. The majority of breast cancers, however, are invasive, meaning that the cancer is able to spread within and beyond the breast, and these cancers are more serious.

In 2005, according to the National Cancer Institute and the American Cancer Society, there were 211,000 new cases of invasive breast cancer in women, more than 58,000 new cases of in-situ breast cancer, and more than 40,000 breast cancer deaths. Breast cancer also occurs in men, but the numbers are small, about 1,700 cases each year.

Causes and risk factors

The cause of most breast cancer is unknown, but there are several risk factors associated with the disease. Increasing age is the most important risk factor in the United States. The following factors can also increase risk: a previous personal history of breast cancer or other breast abnormalities, including in-situ breast cancer; family history (a mother, a sister, or a daughter, or all three, with breast cancer, especially if diagnosed before age 50); reproductive history (the older a women is when she has a first child, the higher her risk); early menstruation (before age 12); late menopause (after age 55); dense breast tissue, with more glands and ligaments and less fatty tissue; radiation therapy to the chest before age 30 for any type of cancer; a personal history of other cancers, such as ovarian, colorectal, or uterine cancer; race (white women are at higher risk);

increased body weight after menopause; moderate alcohol intake (risk may increase with increased alcohol consumption); and long-term hormone replacement therapy. Mutations in certain known genes such as *BRCA1* and *BRCA2*, which are also a risk factor for ovarian cancer, account for less than 10 percent of breast cancers.

Symptoms and pathogenesis

Symptoms of breast cancer include changes in the way the breast or nipple feels, or a lump or thickening in or near the breast, or in the underarm area. The breast may change in size; the skin or the area around the

---

KEY FACTS

Description

Cancer originating in the milk-secreting tissues of the breast.

Causes and risk factors

Causes mostly unknown. Several risk factors, of which increasing age is most important. Genetic mutations account for less than 10 percent of cases.

Symptoms and signs

Change in how a nipple or breast looks and feels; swollen lymph nodes under arm; fluid discharge from nipple. Many women have no symptoms.

Diagnosis

Mammography (breast X-ray) is the most important technique.

Pathogenesis

Cancer may be in situ (nonspreading and less dangerous) or invasive (spreading). Invasive forms are more common and can spread beyond the breast to other parts of the body, including bones, lungs, liver, and brain.

Prevention

Complete prevention not generally possible, though some high-risk groups can choose preventive surgery or other treatment.

Treatments

Depends on the individual case, but usually a combination of surgery, radiation, chemotherapy, and sometimes hormone therapy.

Epidemiology

The most commonly diagnosed cancer in women in the United States after skin cancer. Seventy-five percent of all diagnosed cases are in women age 50 or older.

nipple may turn inward or become flaky, red, or swollen; or fluid may leak from the nipple. Many women with breast cancer, however, have no obvious signs or symptoms until the disease is advanced.

Breast cancer arises in the milk-producing tissues of the breast, which consist of lobes and ducts surrounded by fatty tissue. Each breast has about 20 lobes; each lobe is made up of smaller sections called lobules, which in turn contain dozens of tiny milk-secreting bulbs. Narrow ducts convey the milk from the bulbs and lobules to the nipple. Breast cancer most commonly starts in the ducts and less commonly in the lobes and lobules.

Breast cancer is one of the broad group of cancers classed as carcinomas. Most breast cancer can be classified as either in situ (localized) or invasive (also called infiltrating) carcinoma. Ductal (of the ducts) carcinoma in situ is a noninvasive condition. Eighty percent of such carcinomas can be detected by a mammogram, and it is almost always curable. Lobular (of the lobes) carcinoma in situ is also non-invasive, but it identifies women at increased risk of developing invasive breast cancer later.

Invasive ductal carcinoma starts in a milk duct but breaks through the duct wall and invades the breast's fatty tissue. It makes up 80 percent of the cases of invasive breast cancer. Invasive lobular carcinoma is less common, making up about 10 percent of invasive breast cancer. Both of these cancers can spread to the breast's lymphatic system , and thence to other parts of the body. The lymphatic system, found in all tissues of the body, filters and drains fluid from tissues, and also helps fight infection and disease, but it is also a route by which cancers can spread. The lymphatic system consists of narrow vessels plus small bean-shaped structures called lymph nodes. Groups of lymph nodes are found near the breast, under the arms and collarbone, and in the chest. When cancer spreads outside the breast, to bones, liver, lungs, or other parts of the body, it is called metastatic, and the new cancer colonies are called metastases.

Other types of breast cancers include inflammatory breast cancer, an uncommon but very serious form usually found in younger women. It is almost always in an advanced stage by the time it is diagnosed. In inflammatory breast cancer, the cancer cells block the lymph vessels. The breast becomes swollen, very red, and hot, and the breast skin is ridged or pitted, giving an appearance called *peau d'orange* (orange-peel skin). Inflammatory breast cancer can arise from invasive ductal, lobular, or other breast cancer. Sometimes it is misdiagnosed as an infection.

ANATOMY OF THE BREAST

The breasts of women are the mammary glands; their function is to produce milk for a baby. Breasts are also important as part of normal sexual development. The breasts are composed of largely fatty tissue with lactating glands and ducts that conduct milk to about 15 to 20 openings in the nipples. The pigmented area around the nipples is called the areola, which contains nerves, sweat glands, and hair follicles. Although the breasts do not have any muscles, they are supported by bands of ligaments. Surrounding each breast is a network of lymph vessels, which connect to lymph nodes in the armpit.

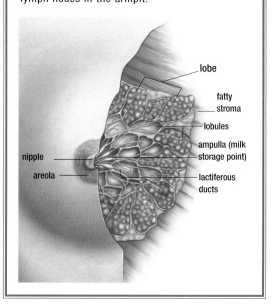

lobe
fatty stroma
lobules
ampulla (milk storage point)
nipple
areola
lactiferous ducts

Diagnosis

A mammogram (an X-ray of the breast) is the most important method of detecting breast cancer early. Mammograms can detect some tumors up to four years before they would be found through a clinical breast examination. They can also detect tiny deposits of calcium in the breast that can be a clue that breast cancer is present. Not all breast lumps turn out to be cancer. Most are benign (noncancerous) lumps or growths.

Mammograms can miss up to 20 percent of cancers that are actually present. Such failures in detection are called false negatives and occur more commonly in younger women because their breasts are denser, so there is less contrast between a cancer and normal tissue. As women age, their breasts have more fatty tissue, so cancers are easier to spot on mammograms. False positives happen when mammogram results are read as abnormal when they are actually normal. False positives are more common in women who are younger, have already had breast biopsies, or have a family history of breast cancer, and in women taking the hormone estrogen. There are various recommendations about how often mammograms should be carried out. If a mammogram detects an abnormality, further tests are then initiated.

United States health agencies also recommend that women aged 20 to 39 years should have a clinical breast examination by a health expert at least every three years, and every year after age 40. Experts now believe that the benefits of a women examining her own breasts (breast self-examination, or BSE) may be limited, however. Any breast examination should include checking how the breasts look and feel, looking for lumps, skin irritation, discharge from or changes in the nipple, or redness or scaly skin.

Ultrasound testing bounces high-frequency sound waves off breast tissue and produces a picture called a sonogram. Ultrasound can help decide whether a breast lump is a solid mass or a fluid-filled cyst, help examine lumps that are hard to see on a mammogram,

A woman having a mammogram, during which the breasts, which are examined separately, are pressed firmly between two plates. The tissue is then exposed to X-rays at a low dosage. The mammogram is then examined by a doctor.

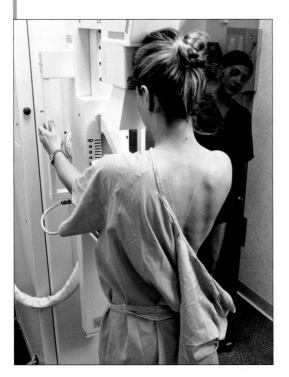

or help guide a doctor performing a breast biopsy. Ultrasound alone is not usually used as a test to find early breast cancer because it does not always detect the tiny deposits of calcium that are an important diagnostic clue.

A biopsy is a procedure in which material is removed from a suspicious region of tissue for laboratory examination. There are several biopsy techniques, including removing all or part of a breast lump, or taking samples of cells or fluid from the breast, so they can be examined under a microscope and checked for signs of cancer.

Treatments

Breast cancer is usually treated with various combinations of surgery, radiation therapy, chemotherapy, and hormone therapy (for general descriptions of these treatments, see CANCER). Treatment and prognosis, or chance of recovery, depend on the type of cancer and also the stage that it has reached. Other factors that influence prognosis include the presence of receptors for the hormones estrogen and progesterone in the cancer tissue, as well as age, general health, and menopause status; postmenopausal women may have a slightly better prognosis then premenopausal women with this cancer.

Surgery is performed in most patients with breast cancer to remove the main cancerous tissue and to see whether the cancer has spread to lymph nodes close to the breast. Most women have the choice between breast-conserving surgery and total mastectomy, the complete surgical removal of a breast. Long-term survival rates are similar for both options for most types of early breast cancers, although neither guarantees that the cancer will not return.

Breast-conserving surgery includes lumpectomy (removal of the tumor and some normal tissue around it) and partial or segmental mastectomy (removal of the part of the breast that includes the cancer). When the whole breast is removed the options include: total mastectomy, or simple mastectomy, which is the removal of the whole breast and some lymph nodes under the arm; modified radical mastectomy, which is removal of the whole breast, some lymph nodes under the arm, and parts of the chest wall muscles; and radical or Halsted mastectomy, the removal of the breast, parts of the chest wall muscles, and all lymph nodes under the arm. Radical mastectomy was the standard operation for many years, but is now used only when the cancer has spread to chest muscles. After mastectomy some women choose to have breast reconstruc-

MAMMOGRAM TO SCREEN FOR BREAST CANCER

Regular screening with mammograms along with timely treatment have been shown to lower the death rate from breast cancer in women aged 40 to 69 years (for age 70 and older it is not clear whether mammograms are helpful). A mammogram can find many cancers too small to feel on manual breast examination. In the United States a mammogram usually costs between $100 and $150. Most states have laws requiring health insurance companies to cover all or part of the cost, and some state and local health programs provide mammograms at low cost or free of charge. Experts disagree about the frequency of mammograms beginning at age 40, some recommending them every year (American Cancer Society), others every one to two years (National Cancer Institute and Centers for Disease Control and Prevention). Women at higher risk, even if under age 40, are recommended to talk to their doctors to decide when they should start and how often they should have mammograms. The number of women in the United States over 40 who have had a mammogram in the past two years increased

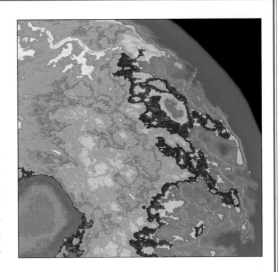

A color-enhanced mammogram shows a cancerous tumor. The tumor has a pink core surrounded by a darker red.

from about 30 percent of all women in 1986 to about 70 percent in 2003.

tion, using implants and stretching muscles to restore the shape of the breast.

Radiation therapy, or radiotherapy, uses high-energy X-rays or other types of radiation to kill cancer cells or keep them from growing. External radiation directs radiation to the breast cancer cells not removed by surgery. Internal radiation uses radioactive substances that are placed into or near the cancer cells. Women who have lumpectomies or partial mastectomies almost always have radiation therapy.

Chemotherapy is sometimes used to shrink the cancer before surgery and to lower the chances that the cancer will recur after surgery. Chemotherapy may help control the cancer if it has spread beyond the breast. The treatment is usually given in cycles—daily, weekly, or monthly—depending on the type and stage of breast cancer.

Some female hormones such as estrogen can cause certain breast cancer cells to grow. A laboratory test, called the estrogen and progesterone receptor test, can be carried out to find out the extent to which a particular cancer is affected by body hormone levels. If the cancer is stimulated by estrogen, then tamoxifen, an anti-estrogen drug, can be given as a pill to block the growth or recurrence of the cancer.

Prevention

While early diagnosis can help detect and eliminate existing breast cancer, total prevention is not generally possible, since the causes are still mainly unknown. Sometimes, changes to breast tissue that may later become cancerous can be detected by biopsy. Risk factors may be modified, but not all can be avoided. Women who are at a high risk of developing hormone-responsive breast cancers sometimes take tamoxifen as a preventive measure. The hormone estrogen, targeted by tamoxifen, is primarily produced in the ovaries, so in some cases, as in those women with mutations in the *BRCA1* or *BRCA2* genes that make breast cancer more likely, the surgical removal of the ovaries may reduce risk of both breast and ovarian cancer. Some high-risk women with a family history of breast cancer may consider prophylactic (preventive) mastectomies before cancer develops. Preventive surgery is carried out only after very careful consideration.

Ramona Jenkin

See also
• Cancer, colorectal • Cancer, ovarian
• Cancer, uterine

Cancer, cervical

A cancer that develops on the surface or lining of the cervix is the second-most common malignancy among women worldwide and the leading cause of cancer-related deaths in developing countries. With the help of regular screening, such as Pap smear tests, cervical cancer can often be detected and cured during its early stages.

Cervical cancer is the second most common malignancy in women throughout the world and it remains the number one cause of cancer-related deaths among women in the majority of developing countries. Each year, cervical cancer strikes more than 10,000 American women, and more than 3,000 women die of the disease in the United States.

The cervix is the lower part of the uterus and is connected to the vagina. Cervical cancer develops either on the surface of the cervix or in its lining. The cancer generally develops over time, and sometimes it takes normal cervical cells a few years to develop precancerous changes that eventually turn into cancer. The early stages of cervical cancer generally do not produce symptoms. For some women precancerous cells can remain unchanged and eventually disappear without any treatment. With cervical cancer screening such as the Pap smear test, almost all the abnormal changes in cervical cells can be observed, and most cases of cervical cancer can be cured at an early stage.

Causes and risk factors

The exact cause of cervical cancer is as yet unknown, but studies have shown a direct relationship between cervical cancer and sexual activities. Major risk factors for cervical cancer include human papillomavirus (HPV) infection, starting to have sex at a young age, having multiple sex partners, a history of sexually transmitted disease, lack of regular Pap smear tests, a weakened immune system, contraceptive pills, and an unhealthy lifestyle, such as smoking.

Evidence of HPV infection has been found in more than 80 percent of cervical carcinomas, and HPV is therefore believed to be a major contributing factor to cervical cancer. Because HPV is sexually transmitted, certain sexual activities, such as having multiple sex partners and starting sexual relations at an early age, can increase the risk of cervical cancer by increasing the likelihood of exposure to HPV.

Infection with the human immunodeficiency virus (HIV) weakens the immune system and therefore also increases the likelihood that precancerous cells develop into cancer. Like most cancers, smoking increases the chances of contracting cervical cancer. For those who do not have access to medical care or regular cervical screening, the rate of developing cervical cancer is significantly increased.

Prevention

Not all women with HPV infection will develop cervical cancer; regular Pap smear screening ensures that most abnormal cell changes in the cervix can be observed at an early stage. With proper treatment, abnormal cells can be removed and the progression of the disease can be halted. Avoiding known risk factors lessens the chances of developing cervical cancer.

Along with reducing possible exposure to HPV, regular Pap smear tests are the most common way to prevent cervical cancer. Due to the widespread use of the Pap smear test, the incidence of cervical cancer and mortality rates have declined significantly during the past few decades. The purpose of conducting a Pap smear test is to detect early changes in the cells that might develop into cancer. In a Pap smear test some loose cells on the surface of the cervix are gently scraped off and put on a glass slide to examine any changes or abnormalities under a microscope. For women who are older than 18 or who become sexually active before the age of 18, a Pap smear test is recommended every year. A woman may receive the test less frequently if she has had negative Pap smear results three years in a row or is not sexually active. There is no suggested upper age limit for the test.

Treatments

According to the National Cancer Institute in the United States, women with cervical cancer may be treated with surgery, radiation therapy, chemotherapy, or a combination of two or more of these methods. Most women with the early stages of cervical cancer have local surgery to remove the cervix and uterus (hysterectomy). However, at a very early stage, a total hysterectomy may not be needed. For a small number of women who cannot have surgery because of medical reasons, radiation therapy may be suggested

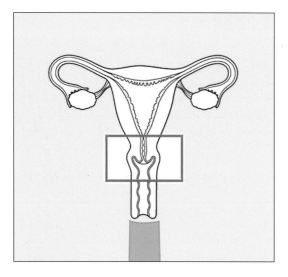

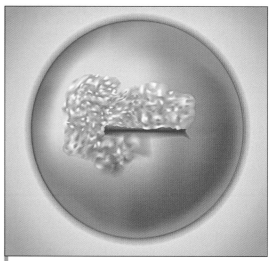

The area in the red box (above left) shows the location of the cervix. A colposcopic view (above) shows cancer of the cervix, which must be treated promptly.

KEY FACTS

Description
A cancer occurring on the surface of the cervix.

Causes
Unknown, but human papillomavirus (HPV) infection is thought to be directly associated with cervical cancer.

Risk factors
HPV infections, lack of access to medical care and Pap smear screening, smoking, unhealthy diet.

Symptoms and signs
No symptoms in early stages. Signs that may relate to cervical cancer include abnormal vaginal bleeding, abnormal vaginal discharge, low back pain, painful sexual intercourse, painful urination.

Diagnosis
Pap smear examination and biopsy.

Treatments
Local surgery, radiation therapy, and chemotherapy.

Pathogenesis
HPV infection is considered a major factor in the development of cervical cancer.

Prevention
Limiting exposure to HPV; regular Pap smears.

Epidemiology
Each year in the United States more than 10,000 women are diagnosed with cervical cancer and more than 3,000 women die of the disease. In the majority of developing countries, cervical cancer is the number one cause of cancer-related deaths among women. Younger women, especially those in their 20s, are more likely to contract cervical cancer than older women. In the United States, cervical cancer rates are highest in African Americans, Hispanics, and Native Americans.

instead. Two types of radiation therapies, external and internal radiation, are often used. External radiation is conducted in the hospital or a clinic five days a week for several weeks, and patients generally do not have to stay in the hospital. But women who receive internal radiation may have to stay in the hospital during this time and may not be able to have visitors, who could be affected by the radiation. Internal radiation may be given from a few hours up to a couple of days and may be repeated two or more times over several weeks.

Chemotherapy is generally combined with radiation therapy, but if cancer has spread to other organs chemotherapy alone may be used. Women usually receive the treatment in an outpatient part of the hospital, at a doctor's office, or at home. A woman rarely needs to stay in the hospital during the treatment.

A vaccine to protect women from cervical cancer by blocking HPV infection has now been approved for use by the Food and Drug Administration. Trials of the vaccine, called Gardasil, have shown it to be extremely effective. This vaccine could help to save thousands of lives each year.

Yanni Wang

See also
• Cancer, breast • Cancer, ovarian
• Cancer, uterine • HPV infection

Cancer, colorectal

In most cases, colorectal cancer (a malignant tumor in either the colon or the rectum) develops from polyps (growths) in the large intestine that become cancerous—growing uncontrollably and invading neighboring tissues. Colorectal cancer is one of the most common cancers in Western countries; a high-fat, low-fiber diet is thought to contribute to its occurrence.

About 130,000 people in the United States are diagnosed each year with cancer of the colon or rectum (colorectal cancer), and about 56,000 people in the United States die each year of the disease. Colorectal cancer affects men, women, and most racial and ethnic groups in relatively equal numbers. However, exceptions include African Americans and Ashkenazi Jews, two groups that have a higher incidence of this cancer.

Colorectal cancer is slow growing and usually remains undetected for many years before it is diagnosed. Prior to becoming invasive, colorectal cancer usually appears as a growth of tissue, called a polyp or adenoma, on the inside of the large intestine.

Colorectal cancer—like many other types of cancers—is further classified by the type of body cell that becomes cancerous. More than 95 percent of cases of colorectal cancers are adenocarcinomas. These are cancers of the glandular cells in the epithelium—the lining of the inside of the colon and rectum. Lymphomas—cancers of lymphoid tissue—can affect either the colon or rectum. This form of colorectal cancer is rare, accounting for about 0.5 percent of all colorectal cancer cases. Other uncommon types of colorectal cancer include gastrointestinal stromal tumors, which can form anywhere in the stomach or intestines, and carcinoid tumors, which develop from hormone-producing cells in the intestine.

Causes and risk factors

The underlying cause of all types of cancers is changes in certain genes in a cell that lead to uncontrollable growth. These genetic changes may be inherited or acquired during the course of a person's life, usually for unknown reasons. An uncommon form of colorectal cancer called hereditary nonpolyposis colorectal cancer (HNPCC) is due to inheriting a faulty gene. Another condition called familial adenomatous polyposis (FAP) increases the risk of colorectal cancer. In FAP, the colon is lined with polyps, and there is a high chance that some of the polyps will eventually become cancerous. In most cases, the faulty gene is inherited from a parent, but in about a quarter of cases of FAP the faulty gene appears spontaneously.

In addition to the presence of benign polyps in the intestine, there are various other risk factors for colorectal cancer. These factors include: increasing age; having a close blood relative who has had colorectal cancer; having inflammatory bowel disease (IBD); and lifestyle factors.

Increasing age is a risk factor for colorectal cancer. Most diagnoses are made in people over the age of 50. The risk of most types of cancers increases with age due to general wear and tear in the body. Having a close relative who has had colorectal cancer, especially at a young age (less than 45 years), also increases a person's risk of developing the disease. For someone who has already had colorectal cancer, there is a high risk that it will recur. There is an increased risk of colorectal cancer in women with ovarian, uterine, or breast cancer and also in those with diabetes mellitus.

People with a long-term IBD, such as Crohn's disease or ulcerative colitis, are at higher risk of developing colorectal cancer. The increased risk is thought to be due to the constant repairing of the damaged intestinal lining, increasing the chances that new cells will become dysplasic, a change in cell structure that sometimes leads to cancer.

Lifestyle factors that increase the risk of colorectal cancer include cigarette smoking, excessive alcohol consumption, obesity, and a sedentary lifestyle. Diet is also thought to be a key factor: the Western high-fat, low-fiber diet seems to increase the risk of this cancer. In developing countries, where the diet generally contains less meat and saturated fat and more fruits, cereals, and vegetables, the incidence of colorectal cancer is much lower.

Symptoms and signs

Polyps generally do not cause any symptoms while they are small. When polyps become large, regardless of whether or not they have become cancerous, they can bleed, which leads to rectal bleeding. Polyps that grow large enough or turn cancerous can cause partial obstruction of the colon or rectum, leading to discomfort ranging from a feeling of bloating to severe abdominal pain, and they can even cause vomiting.

Abdominal pain, changes in bowel habits (constipation or diarrhea), and rectal bleeding are generally the first symptoms of colorectal cancer. However, these are also the symptoms of many other gastrointestinal disorders—such as inflammatory bowel disease (IBS), diverticulitis, and short-term gastrointestinal distress caused by infectious agents such as viruses, bacteria, or parasites. These symptoms should always be checked by a clinician (a doctor, nurse practitioner, or physician assistant), but someone who develops these symptoms should not become overly frightened that these symptoms signal cancer.

Diagnosis

Whether someone has symptoms of gastrointestinal distress or requires routine colorectal-cancer screening, a number of tests can be performed. A digital rectal exam should be conducted in any routine physical for any adult. In this test, a clinician inserts a lubricated, gloved finger into the anus to check for any abnormalities in the rectum. During this examination, the clinician takes a small smear of stool to perform a fecal occult blood test (FOBT) to look for blood. Even if an individual does not see blood after a bowel movement, there may be small amounts of hidden, or occult, blood in the stool.

The presence of blood signals the need for further examination. One of three tests can be performed next. Sigmoidoscopy involves the insertion of a short fiberoptic tube into the anus to examine the rectum and sigmoid colon (the last six inches or so of the colon). Sigmoidoscopy can be performed with or without sedation. Any polyps that are found can be removed by instruments inserted through the sigmoidoscope, and sent to a laboratory for pathological testing to determine if cancer cells are present.

A double-contrast barium enema involves taking X-rays of the colon and rectum after the individual is administered an enema containing a solution of barium. Air is also pumped into the colon to fill it. Polyps can often be detected in the colon using this test, but they cannot be removed. Sedation is not required for a barium enema.

Most polyps are detected through a test called a colonoscopy, in which a thin fiberoptic tube with a

camera is inserted through the anus into the large intestine while an individual is sedated. The doctor performing the colonoscopy, usually a gastroenterologist (a doctor who specializes in diseases of the digestive system), can remove small polyps or portions of large polyps through the colonoscope. These tissue samples are sent to a pathology laboratory and examined under a microscope to determine if any cancerous cells are present.

KEY FACTS

Description
Noncommunicable, invasive cancer of the inside wall of the large intestine that, if untreated, can metastasize (spread) to the lungs, liver, and other organs.

Causes
Faulty genes causing uncontrolled spread of cancerous (malignant) cells in the wall of the large intestine.

Risk factors
Age (over 50); colorectal polyps; inflammatory bowel disease; diet; smoking; diabetes; obesity; personal history of colorectal, ovarian, uterine, or breast cancer; family history of colorectal cancer; the inherited disorders FAP and HNPCC.

Symptoms
Evidence of colorectal polyps, rectal bleeding, change in bowel habits, and abdominal pain.

Diagnosis
Digital rectal examination; fecal occult blood test; sigmoidoscopy; double-contrast barium enema; colonoscopy.

Treatments
Surgery, either alone or in combination with radiation therapy and chemotherapy.

Pathogenesis
Left untreated, early-stage colorectal cancer grows through the outer walls of the large intestine, invades the lymph system, and metastasizes in the liver and lungs.

Prevention
Regular screening beginning at age 50 or earlier for those at increased risk; changes in diet may decrease the risk.

Epidemiology
About 130,000 new cases in the United States each year and 56,000 deaths. Estimates are that better screening and detection could reduce the death rate by up to 30,000 annually. Colorectal cancer affects an equal number of men and women. Incidence of colorectal cancer is higher among African Americans and Ashkenazi Jews than other groups.

STAGING COLORECTAL CANCER

There are three competing systems for staging (assessing the spread of) colorectal cancer. The Dukes and Astler-Coller systems classify colorectal cancer as stage A, B, or C (there is a stage D in Astler-Coller but not in Dukes). The American Joint Committee on Cancer (AJCC) uses a system that describes the extent of the tumor (T), whether cancer cells are present in lymph nodes (N) close to the tumor, and whether any cancer cells have metastasized (M), or traveled, to distant organs, especially the liver or lungs.

The AJCC system classifies colorectal tumors as Stage 0, I, II, III, or IV. Stage 0 and I cancers have a five-year survival rate of over 90 percent, whereas some Stage III cancers, in which there is invasion of the local lymph nodes but without distant metastasis, have a five-year survival rate of about 44 percent. Stage IV, in which there is metastasis, has a five-year survival rate of only 8 percent.

For Stage 0 or I colorectal cancers, surgical removal of the cancerous polyp or tumor that has invaded only the inside mucosal layer of the colon is all that is necessary. For Stage II colon cancer, radiation therapy is often given after surgery. For Stage III colon cancer, chemotherapy and some-times radiation therapy is given after surgery. For

Stage IV colon cancer, any surgery performed is only to relieve blockage of the colon by the tumor, not for any hope of curing the cancer. If only a few metastases are present in the liver, surgery may be performed to remove them. Chemotherapy or radiation may be performed to relieve symptoms or prevent the recurrence of tumors.

If someone with Stage 0 or I rectal cancer is too old or too ill due to other disorders to withstand surgery, radiation is used to try to shrink the tumor. Some minimally invasive rectal cancers can be removed through the anus, but most tumors require an incision in the lower abdomen and removal of the rectal tissue. Many rectal surgeries require a colostomy (a rerouting of the bowel through an opening in the abdomen) for future waste removal, because the rectal muscle is damaged and bowel control is lost.

In stage 0 (left) a cancerous polyp attaches itself to the mucosal membrane lining the colon. In stage I (middle) the polyp starts to invade the colon wall but is still contained within it. At stage II (right) the cancer has penetrated the wall and begun to spread into surrounding tissue. By stage III the cancer has spread to the lymph nodes, and in stage IV has reached distant organs such as the liver and lungs.

Stage 0	Stage I	Stage II
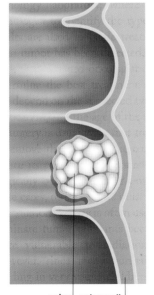	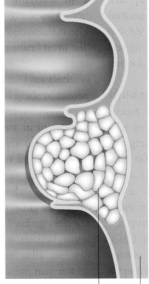	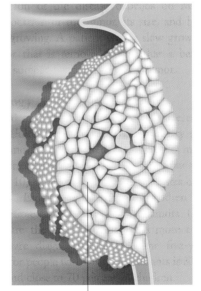
polyp colon wall	Polyp has invaded colon wall. surrounding tissue	Polyp is causing bleeding into the colon and has spread to surrounding tissue.

Screening

The National Cancer Institute considers colonoscopy the "gold standard" for colorectal cancer detection, and suggests that everyone in the United States have their first colonoscopy for the purpose of cancer screening at or around the age of 50 years. A plan for routine cancer screening every two to five years can then be developed, assuming the results of the colonoscopy are negative.

People with a family history of colorectal cancer and women with a history of cancers of the uterus, ovary, or breast are often urged to begin colorectal-cancer screening earlier. Individuals at higher risk of developing colorectal cancer because of inflammatory bowel disease (IBD), such as Crohn's disease or ulcerative colitis, are generally screened every two years beginning 10 to 15 years after their IBD is diagnosed.

Treatments

Most cases of colorectal cancer are treated with surgery, either alone or in combination with radiation therapy and possibly chemotherapy. The particular treatment regimen is determined by whether or not the tumor is in the colon or the rectum, and the "stage," or extent, of the disease (see box, page 99). Sometimes it is possible to determine the stage of colorectal cancer by using minimally invasive diagnostic tests, such as blood tests, colonoscopy, ultrasound, CT scanning, and chest X-ray. Other times the stage cannot be determined until after surgery is performed to remove the tumor.

New drugs are being developed to combat colorectal cancer. One type is designed to counteract tumor growth factors, naturally occurring substances in the body that promote cell growth. Epidermal growth factor (EGF) and vascular endothelial growth factor (VEGF) have been shown to promote the development of colorectal cancer. Scientists are working on anti-BGF and anti-VEGF compounds. Scientists are also experimenting with various forms of immunotherapy to bolster the immune system in an effort to get the immune system to seek out and destroy colorectal cancer cells.

Pathogenesis

If early-stage colorectal cancer is left untreated, the cancer grows through the outer walls of the large intestine, invades the bloodstream and lymph system, from where cancerous cells can travel to and invade other organs—a process called metastasis—in particular, the liver and lungs.

Prevention

In addition to screening, specialists in colorectal cancer believe it is possible for people to reduce their risk of developing the disease. Changing diet by decreasing intake of meat and saturated fats and increasing the amount of natural fiber from fruits, vegetables, cereals, and legumes is related to a lower incidence of colorectal cancer. Recent research has shown that people who take a daily multivitamin that includes the B vitamin folic acid have a lower incidence of colorectal cancer. Quitting smoking and cutting down alcoholic-drink intake may also help prevent colorectal as well as other types of cancers.

Epidemiology

Less than half of all Americans older than 50 have had an initial screening for colorectal cancer. In the African American community, the incidence of screening is lower than for the population at large, yet African Americans are diagnosed with colorectal cancer at a higher rate than other racial or ethnic groups in America. To date, no one has found a genetic link that suggests African Americans should be any more susceptible to colorectal cancer than any other population subset; the higher incidence of diagnosis is thought to be a direct result of less screening and detection of noncancerous or precancerous polyps.

The incidence of colorectal cancer is also higher in people of Ashkenazi Jewish descent. Up to 1 in 10 of this ethnic group—whose ancestors were from Eastern Europe—have a faulty gene called *I1307K*, which possibly may predispose them to this type of cancer.

Researchers believe that up to 30,000 deaths annually from colorectal cancer in the United States could be prevented with proper early detection and effective treatment. The National Cancer Institute puts the five-year survival rate for colorectal cancer discovered in its earliest stage at about 93 percent; whereas for colorectal cancers not discovered until they have reached later stages, the five-year survival rate is less than 50 percent.

Jon Zonderman and
Laurel Shader

See also
- Alcohol-related disorders • Cancer, liver
- Cancer, lung • Colitis, ulcerative
- Crohn's disease • Diabetes • Diverticulitis

Cancer, kidney

In kidney cancer, a tumor usually starts in the kidney but can occur in the cells lining the renal pelvis. Renal cell carcinoma is the most common kidney cancer, in which cancer cells grow in the kidney's lining. Rarely, it spreads to the kidney from another organ in the body.

There are three types of kidney cancers: renal cell carcinoma; Wilm's tumor, a fast-growing tumor that affects children under the age of five; and transitional cell carcinoma, which occurs in the urine-collecting region of the kidney. Very little is known about the exact cause of kidney cancer, but it has been shown that smokers are twice as likely to contract this disease than nonsmokers. In addition, certain materials used in industries, such as cadmium, asbestos, and lead used in paints, are linked to kidney cancer. Certain medical conditions, such as diabetes, obesity, chronic kidney failure, or high blood pressure, and overuse of painkillers may also increase the risk of developing kidney cancer. Since certain genetic mutations are believed to account for the tendency to develop kidney cancer, this form can run in families.

Prevention and treatments

If the disease is diagnosed and treated at an early stage, kidney cancer can often be cured. Surgery is the most common treatment for kidney cancer. Depending on the stages of the disease and the overall health situation of a patient, several surgical options can be applied. When the tumor is small and confined to a certain portion of the kidney, only part of the kidney may be removed, but sometimes the entire kidney and the adrenal gland, or even the surrounding tissue, may have to be removed if the cancer has spread over a large area. In some cases, hormonal treatment or biological treatment can be used either after surgery or when a cancer cannot be removed surgically. Occasionally radiation therapy is used. In rare cases, kidney cancer spontaneously improves without any treatment.

Although it is not possible to prevent kidney cancer, quitting smoking, eating healthy food, staying physically active, maintaining a healthy weight, reducing high blood pressure, and avoiding exposure to environmental toxins can all help reduce the risk of developing kidney cancer.

Yanni Wang

KEY FACTS

Description

A disease in which cancer cells develop in the kidney and may spread to other organs.

Causes

The exact causes are unknown, but certain genetic changes in the kidney are accountable for the development of the cancer.

Risk factors

Smoking; misusing pain medications (ibuprofen, acetaminophen, aspirin) for a long time; obesity; high blood pressure; environmental toxins such as cadmium and organic solvents; dialysis; radiation; family history of kidney diseases.

Symptoms

Blood in urine, blood clots in bladder, lump in kidney area, dull ache in back or side, or persistent high temperature and weight loss.

Diagnosis

Blood and urine tests, intravenous pyelogram (IVP), ultrasound scan, computed tomography (CT) scan, CT-guided biopsy, magnetic resonance imaging (MRI) scan.

Treatments

Surgery is the standard treatment for kidney cancer; radiation therapy, chemotherapy, and biologic therapies may also be used, depending on the health of the patient.

Pathogenesis

Cancerous cells develop in the kidney and eventually grow into cancer.

Prevention

Quit smoking, eat healthy food, including a large portion of fruits and vegetables, stay physically active, maintain a healthy weight, reduce high blood pressure, and avoid exposure to environmental toxins.

Epidemiology

Renal cell cancer is the most common; in 2005 there were 21,300 new cases in the United States, with around 8,800 deaths from the disease. Men are more than twice as likely to develop kidney cancer than women. African American men have a slightly higher risk of the disease. Most people who develop kidney cancer are more than 50 years old.

See also
• Adrenal disorders

Cancer, liver

Two types of primary liver tumors occur: hepatomas, which develop in liver cells; and cholangiocarcinomas, in the cells lining the bile ducts. Cancer of the liver can be primary (arising in the liver) or much more commonly, secondary (spread from another organ).

The liver is the largest internal organ in the human body. Since it consists of different types of cells, several types of tumors can form in the liver. Depending on where the cancer starts to develop, liver cancer is divided into primary liver cancer and metastatic (secondary) liver cancer. In primary liver cancer, the cancerous cells develop in the liver. In metastatic liver cancer, the cancerous cells begin in other parts of the body and spread to the liver.

The prognosis of liver cancer is very poor. Without proper treatment, patients usually die in three to four months. Treated patients may live 6 to 18 months if they respond to therapies. Men are twice as likely to develop liver cancer as are women. In the United States, Asian Americans have the highest incidence of liver cancer due to high rates of hepatitis B infection.

Causes and risks

The exact cause of liver cancer is not known. It may start with genetic damage in liver cells. Possible risk factors for primary liver cancer include having hepatitis B or hepatitis C (or both), having a close relative with both hepatitis and liver cancer, and having cirrhosis. Excessive alcohol consumption can lead to liver damage and increase the risk. Smoking is also a risk factor.

Treatments and prevention

Surgery is currently the best and the most common treatment for localized liver cancer. In some cases, the affected area of the liver is removed. Radiation therapy can be used following surgical removal of the tumor and may be used alone to destroy cancerous cells. Chemotherapy, using drugs to kill cancer cells, is another option to treat liver cancer. Chemotherapy may cause side effects, such as nausea and vomiting.

It is not always possible to prevent liver cancer, but the risk of developing it can be reduced. The hepatitis B vaccine is the most effective way to prevent primary liver cancer. The protection can last years or be lifelong.

A vaccine for hepatitis C is not yet available, but practicing safe sex and not sharing needles can reduce the risk of hepatitis C infection and liver cancer.

Quitting smoking can reduce the risk of developing lung and stomach cancer and is an effective way to reduce the risk of metastatic liver cancer. A healthy diet and a low intake of alcohol can also reduce the risk of developing liver cancer.

Yanni Wang

KEY FACTS

Description
A cancer in the liver.

Causes
The exact cause is unknown. It is possibly related to genetic damage in liver cells.

Risk factors
Common risk factors include chronic infection, diabetes, excessive alcohol consumption, and smoking.

Signs and symptoms
Possible signs related to liver cancer include a hard lump below the right side of the rib cage, discomfort in the upper abdomen on the right side, pain around the right shoulder blade, unexplained weight loss, yellow skin, unusual tiredness, nausea, and loss of appetite.

Diagnosis
Physical exam; serum tumor marker test; complete blood count (CBC); laparoscopy; biopsy; CT scan; magnetic resonance imagining (MRI); ultrasound.

Treatments
Surgery; radiation therapy; chemotherapy; alcohol injection; radio frequency ablation or cryotherapy to destroy cancerous cells; liver transplantation.

Pathogenesis
Liver cancer is strongly associated with chronic hepatitis B infection.

Epidemiology
Liver cancer occurs more frequently in men than women. This type of cancer is rare in the United States but is a common cancer in parts of Asia and Africa.

See also
- Cancer, colorectal • Cancer, pancreatic
- Cancer, stomach • Cirrhosis of the liver
- Hepatitis infections

Cancer, lung

Lung cancer is the uncontrolled growth of abnormal cells lining air passages in one or both of the lungs. These abnormal cells form lumps or tumors that disturb normal lung function. The principal function of the lungs is to exchange gases such as carbon dioxide and oxygen. Normally, carbon dioxide exits from the bloodstream with each exhalation, and oxygen enters the bloodstream with each inhalation. With each breath, air is carried into and out of the lungs through the airways, comprising the trachea, bronchi, bronchioles, and alveoli. The trachea divides into the bronchi, which in turn branch into progressively smaller airways called bronchioles that end in alveoli, where gas exchange occurs. When there are tumors in any part of the airways, gas exchange is impaired and lung function is restricted.

There are two major types of lung cancers: small cell lung cancer (SCLC) and non–small cell lung cancer (NSCLC). Sometimes a lung cancer may have characteristics of both types, which is known as mixed small cell–large cell carcinoma. Non–small cell lung cancer is the most common type of lung cancer; it accounts for 80 percent of all lung cancer cases. This type of cancer usually spreads or metastasizes to different parts of the body more slowly than SCLC. There are three main types of non–small cell lung cancers. They are named for the type of cells in which the cancer develops: squamous cell carcinoma, adenocarcinoma, and large cell carcinoma. Small cell lung cancer, also called oat cell cancer, accounts for the remaining 20 percent of all lung cancers. This type of lung cancer grows more quickly and is more likely to spread to other organs in the body.

Symptoms

Some of the symptoms of lung cancer may be confused with other illnesses, but should not be ignored. Signs and symptoms to cause concern are having a cough most of the time, a change in a cough that one has had for a long time, being short of breath, coughing up phlegm (sputum) with blood in it, an

A computed tomography (CT) scan shows lung cancer. The blue areas are the spine, heart, and other organs; the cancer is the yellow area on the right of the scan, toward the bottom of the lobe.

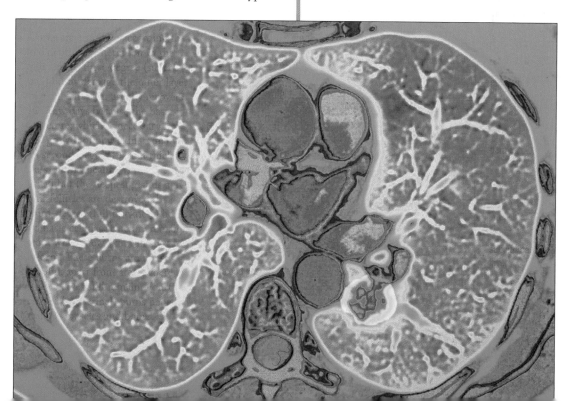

ache or pain when breathing or coughing, loss of appetite, fatigue, and losing weight. If the cancer has invaded surrounding tissues, it may cause paralysis of the vocal cords, leading to hoarseness, or shoulder pain that travels down the outside of the arm; this condition is called Pancoast's syndrome and is a result of nerve invasion. Difficulty swallowing (dysphagia) might be a symptom that indicates that the lung cancer has metastasized to the esophagus. If one of the airways is obstructed, a portion of the lung may collapse and cause infections, such as abscesses or pneumonia in the obstructed area. Although pneumonia can occur independently, recurring pneumonia should be evaluated for cancer.

Causes and risk factors

The most common cause of both types of lung cancer is cigarette smoking. It is estimated that 87 percent of lung cancer cases are caused by smoking. Even those who smoked cigarettes and quit are at risk for developing lung cancer, but the risk falls with every year that a smoker has stopped smoking. After 10 years of not smoking, a person who has quit will have reduced the risk of developing lung cancer from 50 percent to 30 percent. Nonsmokers who breathe in smoke from others' cigarettes (secondhand smoke) are also at increased risk of lung cancer. Nonsmoking spouses of smokers have a 30 percent greater risk of developing lung cancer than do spouses of nonsmokers. Also, workers exposed to tobacco smoke at work are more likely to develop lung cancer. Lung cancer may be considered one of the most tragic forms of cancers because in most cases it is preventable. Although cigarette smoking is the largest risk factor, marijuana smoke is also known to increase the risk of developing lung cancer.

It is estimated that radon gas is the second leading cause of lung cancer. Radon is a colorless, odorless radioactive gas formed by the radioactive decay of radium, which is dispersed naturally throughout Earth's crust. Thus, radon leaking into buildings and homes can be a serious problem.

The number of deaths from lung cancer caused by radon exposure is approximated to be between 15,000 and 21,000 in the United States annually. Researchers report that even at concentrations far below official guideline levels, residential radon may lead to a 2.5-fold rise in the risk of lung cancer.

Lung cancer can also be caused by exposure in the work environment to asbestos, uranium, or coke, which is an important fuel in the manufacture of iron

KEY FACTS

Description
Malignant growth of cells in the lungs. There are two major types of lung cancer: non–small cell lung cancer (NSCLC) and small cell lung cancer (SCLC).

Causes
Changes in a cell's genes that alter its ability to control growth. The most common cause of lung cancer is cigarette smoke.

Risk factors
Exposure to tobacco or marijuana smoke, asbestos, air pollution, radon; personal history of recurring lung infections; a combination of any or all of these risks; family history of cancer.

Symptoms
Chronic cough, hoarseness, coughing blood, weight loss, shortness of breath, wheezing, repeated bouts of bronchitis or pneumonia, and chest pain.

Diagnosis
Examination of sputum (mucus from lungs) and imaging scans.

Treatments
Surgery, radiation, or chemotherapy, or a combination of all three treatments.

Pathogenesis
Develops from a localized tumor to widespread cancer if not treated in early stages.

Prevention
Reduce exposure to tobacco or marijuana smoke, asbestos, air pollution, and radon.

Epidemiology
Lung cancer is the leading cancer killer in both men and women in the United States.

in smelters, blast furnaces, and foundries. In one study, researchers found that long-term exposure to fine particles in air pollution was associated with approximately an 8 percent increased risk of death as a result of lung cancer.

The role of diet in lung cancer risk and prevention is debatable. While there is substantial data to support that a diet rich in soy products, grains, carrots, spinach, broccoli, and other fruits and vegetables has a protective effect against cancer in general, it is not known if this applies to lung cancer specifically.

Those at highest risk include men and women who have had previous lung tumors or chronic obstructive pulmonary disease, or who are 60 years of age and currently smoke or have a history of smoking.

Diagnosis and treatment

All cancer patients benefit from early detection and treatment. The chances of curing lung cancer are greatest when the tumor has not spread to other parts of the body. Lung cancer poses a particular problem because there may be very few symptoms in the early stages. Without signs such as coughing, pain, or shortness of breath, the cancer may have metastasized by the time it is discovered. In fact, only 15 percent of lung cancer cases are found before they have spread.

Diagnosis involves a doctor taking a patient's medical and lifestyle history, including exposure to hazardous substances at either work or home. During the physical exam, a doctor checks for swollen lymph nodes in the neck or collarbone area and listens to the lungs with a stethoscope to hear any abnormal breathing sounds or patterns. If a patient's cough produces sputum (mucus), it may be examined for cancerous cells. Imaging technologies applied to the chest such as X-rays, computed tomography (CT), positron emission tomography (PET) scan, and magnetic resonance imaging (MRI) allow visualization of tumors and indicate how far they may have spread. Bronchoscopy involves viewing the lungs through a hollow, flexible tube (bronchoscope) that is passed through the nose and throat into the main airway of the lungs. If abnormal areas or tumors are seen, biopsies (a piece of tissue) can be taken through the bronchoscope for laboratory examination.

Based on the results of these tests, a doctor is able to determine the type of cancer, the stage of the cancer, and prognosis (outlook) for the patient. Staging is the process of finding out how much cancer there is in the body and where it is located. For SCLC, there are two stages: the limited stage in which a tumor is found in one lung and in nearby lymph nodes, or the extensive stage in which the tumor has spread beyond one lung or to other organs. In NSCLC, the stages are more detailed. Stage I a/b is used to denote that a tumor of any size is found in the lung only. In stage II a/b, the tumor has metastasized to the lymph nodes that are associated with the lung. In stage III a, the tumor has spread to the lymph nodes in the tracheal area and other parts of the chest, and in stage III b, the tumor has metastasized to the lymph nodes on the opposite lung or in the neck. The last stage is stage IV, in which the tumor has spread beyond the chest. Once a stage is determined, a prognosis and treatment plan specific to that type and stage of cancer is developed.

Standard treatments include surgery, radiation, chemotherapy, or a combination of approaches. Lung cancers found early in development can be treated by surgery or radiation alone because these are localized treatments, that is, they can be used specifically at the site of the cancer. If there is a chance that the cancer has metastasized, chemotherapy, which affects the entire body, may be used. In chemotherapy, toxic chemicals used to kill cancer cells also kill healthy ones, so there are serious side effects.

Novel approaches such as biological therapies are less invasive than standard treatments. Biological therapy (also called immunotherapy, biotherapy, or biological response modifier therapy) uses the body's immune system, either directly or indirectly, to fight cancer or to decrease the side effects that may be caused by standard cancer treatments.

An approved biological therapy available to those who suffer from NSCLC is Tarceva, a drug treatment in which cancer cells displaying a protein called HER1/EGFR are specifically targeted for treatment. Tarceva binds to the protein and blocks cell growth of NSCLC. In some patients, Tarceva can be effective in both improving survival and slowing or stopping the growth of cancer. At the current time, Tarceva treatment is

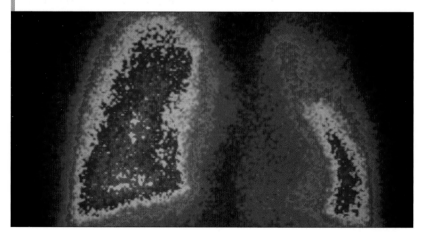

A nuclear medicine scan called a scintigram shows cancer in the left lung (at the right of the picture). Lung cancer is one of the leading killers of men and women in the United States. Tumors may spread to the lungs from other areas.

LUNG CANCER

Lung cancer is one of the most common of all cancers. Cancerous tumors in the lungs can spread to other areas of the body, particulary the brain, liver, and bones.

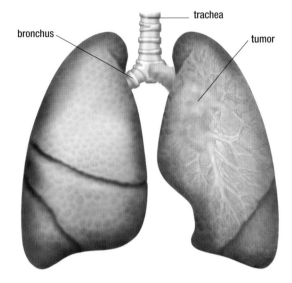

trachea

bronchus

tumor

A cancer is shown in the left lung and bronchus. A bronchoscopy is usually carried out by a physician to confirm the diagnosis

reserved for those who have not responded to chemotherapy.

Other therapies that are being developed for lung cancer treatment and prevention include substances that repair some of the genetic damage done by smoking, vaccines that can alter tumor cells, gene therapy using tumor suppressor genes, and new combinations of chemotherapy drugs.

Prevention

Lung cancer can be largely prevented or slowed down by limiting exposure to cigarette smoke, radon gas, asbestos, and air pollution. If exposure is unavoidable, an important factor in prevention is protection and routine screening. Although currently there is no approved screening test for lung cancer that has proven to improve survival or detect localized disease, such as colonoscopy for colon cancer, a personalized screening plan can be performed by a physician. For example, if someone works in a building with known asbestos exposure, then that person should protect him- or herself by wearing a mask and making regular visits to the doctor to have chest X-rays or sputum examinations.

Similarly, if smokers cannot stop smoking, they should be screened for lung cancer.

For individuals who are at the greatest risk, chemoprevention may also be used. These methods, including the use of chemotherapy, vitamins, diet, and hormone therapy, are being tested to not only reduce the risk of cancer, but also to reduce the chance that the cancer will come back.

Epidemiology

Lung cancer is the leading cancer killer in both men and women in the United States. In 2006, it was estimated that 31 percent of men and 26 percent of women suffering from cancer would have lung cancer. About 6 out of 10 people with lung cancer die within a year of being diagnosed with the disease. Lung cancer is predominantly a disease of the elderly. From 1998–2002, the median age at diagnosis was 70 years of age.

Men have higher rates of lung cancer than women. In 2002, 77.8 per 100,000 men compared to 50.8 per 100,000 women were diagnosed with lung cancer in the United States. However, since the 1970s, the lung cancer incidence rate has decreased in males and increased in females.

Although lung cancer occurs in Americans of all racial and ethnic groups, the rate of occurrence varies from group to group; for example, African Americans are more likely to develop and die from lung cancer than persons of any other racial or ethnic group. The lung cancer incidence rate among African American men is more than 50 percent higher than for Caucasian American men, even though their overall exposure to cigarette smoke is lower. Similarly, the lung cancer incidence rate for African American women is equal to that of Caucasian American women, despite the fact that they smoke less.

Lung cancer is the leading cause of cancer death in the United States, and in most cases it can be prevented.

Rashmi Nemade

See also
• Cancer, mouth and throat • Pneumonia

Cancer, mouth and throat

Mouth and throat (oropharyngeal) cancer is the uncontrolled growth of cells in either the mouth or throat. Oral cancer includes abnormal growth in the lips, mouth, tongue, gums, and salivary glands. Throat cancer involves malignant growth in the part of the throat just behind the mouth.

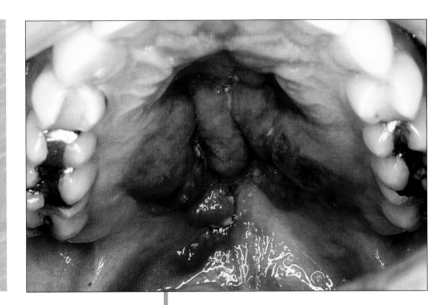

This Kaposi's sarcoma lesion of the soft palate is an oral cancer, which is often a complication of AIDS. This cancer is at an advanced stage.

Almost all oral and throat cancers are of the squamous cell type. Squamous cells are firm and flat, and they form the lining of the oral cavity and upper throat as well as the surface of the skin. Squamous cell cancer begins with abnormal cells located only on the surface. As it progresses, malignant cells invade deeper layers of the oral cavity and upper throat and may spread, or metastasize, to lymph nodes as well as to other parts of the body.

Signs and symptoms

An early indication of oral and throat cancer is one or more changes in the way the soft tissues of the mouth look or feel. Signs and symptoms may include: a sore in the mouth that doesn't heal or a sore that increases in size; persistent pain in the mouth; lumps or white, red, or dark patches inside the mouth; thickening of the cheek; difficulty chewing or swallowing or moving the tongue; swelling, pain, or difficulty moving the jaw; soreness of the throat or a feeling that something is caught in the throat; pain around the teeth or loosening of teeth; numbness of the tongue or elsewhere in the mouth; changes in the voice; a lump in the neck; or severe pain in one ear with a normal eardrum. Many oral cancers occur inside the cheeks, on the gums, or on the roof of the mouth; however, most arise on the tongue or on the floor of the mouth.

Causes and risk factors

The leading cause of mouth and throat cancer is tobacco use, excessive alcohol consumption, or both. About 90 percent of people who develop these cancers use some form of tobacco. Those who use smokeless or chewing tobacco are at even higher risk of cancers of the cheek and inner surface of the lips. In addition, about 75 to 80 percent of people with oral and upper throat cancers frequently drink alcohol. The combination of numerous carcinogens (cancer-causing agents) in chewing tobacco and the irritation of excessive drinking causes a much higher risk of oral and throat cancer. Other risk factors include chewing lips and cheeks, excessive exposure of the lips to ultraviolet light, and wearing loose-fitting dentures. Many oral and throat cancers are not detected until they are far advanced. When detected early, squamous cell cancer can almost always be successfully treated.

Diagnosis and treatments

To determine if mouth or throat cancer is present, a small tissue sample (biopsy) from the area in question is taken for laboratory analysis. If the biopsy results

107

show cancerous cells, endoscopy or imaging procedures may be used to determine how far the cancer may have spread. Endoscopy is the use of a thin, lighted tube called an endoscope to examine areas inside the body. In the case of mouth and throat cancer, a laryngoscope is inserted through the mouth to view the larynx, an esophagoscope is inserted through the mouth to examine the esophagus, and a nasopharyngoscope is inserted through the nose to inspect the nasal cavity and nasopharynx.

Imaging procedures such as X-rays, computed tomography (CT), magnetic resonance imaging (MRI), or ultrasound help establish the size and location of a tumor and possible metastases. Two-dimensional images produced by X-rays of the head, neck, and chest reveal if any masses are visible. Three-dimensional images of slices through the affected area created by CT scanning and MRI allow a doctor to see not only if a tumor is present but approximately how deep it is in the body. Ultrasound uses reflected high-frequency sound waves to visualize moving images on a computer screen. Ultrasound is especially good for providing information about the shape, texture, and makeup of tumors.

Doctors use surgery, radiation therapy, and chemotherapy either alone or in some combination to treat oral and throat cancer. Choice of treatment depends on the location of tumors, the stage of the cancer, and prognosis. If surgical treatment involves removing vital parts of the mouth and throat, reconstructive surgery and rehabilitation may be included in the treatment plan.

The goal of reconstructive surgery is to improve the appearance and to help patients adjust to difficulties with chewing, swallowing, speaking, or breathing. Sometimes grafts of skin or tissue from other parts of the body are used to rebuild areas in the mouth, throat, or jaw. A dental prosthesis may be implanted to replace a part of the jaw that was removed during surgery. Extensive surgery of the neck may require the creation of a hole in the neck (tracheostomy) to help breathing. If muscles involved in swallowing have been removed, there is usually another surgery (gastromy) to create a hole in the abdomen to receive food directly into the stomach through a feeding tube.

After surgery, speech therapy can help with problems of speech and swallowing, and a dietitian can help choose foods that match the ability to swallow or chew for particular patients. Physical and occupational therapists may help make adjustments to personal and work life.

KEY FACTS

Description

Malignant growth of cells in the lips, mouth, tongue, gums, salivary glands, and throat just behind the mouth.

Causes

Any substance that damages the genes of cells inside the mouth and throat. Using tobacco or excessive alcohol consumption, or both, can damage these tissues.

Risk factors

The combination of smoking or chewing tobacco and excessive drinking creates a much higher risk of developing these cancers.

Symptoms

Lumps in mouth or throat; white, red, or dark patches inside the mouth; difficulty chewing or swallowing; changes in voice; pain and swelling in jaw.

Diagnosis

Oral biopsy.

Treatments

Surgical removal of the tumor followed by radiation therapy or chemotherapy, or both.

Pathogenesis

Develops from localized tumor in the mouth or throat to widespread cancer if not treated in early stages.

Prevention

Reduce exposure to tobacco or alcohol, or both.

Epidemiology

An estimated 8,000 Americans die of these cancers annually. They are twice as common in men as in women.

Prevention and epidemiology

Mouth and throat cancer can be largely prevented or slowed down by limiting the use of tobacco and alcohol.

In addition, not chewing on the tissues of the inner cheek, limiting exposure to the sun by using sunscreen lip balm and hats, using well-fitting dentures, routine self-exams, and check-ups with a doctor or dentist can considerably reduce the risk of developing mouth and throat cancer.

Around 30,000 people in the United States are diagnosed yearly with oral cancers, and 8,000 die.

Rashmi Nemade

See also
• AIDS • Alcohol-related disorders

Cancer, ovarian

Ovarian cancer is not one of the most common cancers in women, but it is one of the most deadly forms of cancer to strike women because most women are not diagnosed until the cancer has spread to other parts of the body. Despite some progress in research, and because the disease remains difficult to detect, death rates from ovarian cancer have not changed much in the last 50 years.

This cancer is one of the deadliest in women, being the fifth leading cause of cancer deaths in women. It often begins with relatively benign symptoms, but these mild symptoms make the disease difficult to diagnose in its earliest stages when it is most treatable. As a result, thousands of women die each year.

Causes and risk factors

The discovery of the *BRCA1* and *BRCA2* genes made headlines several years ago when mutations of these genes were found to increase a woman's risk of breast cancer. These same mutations also increase a woman's risk of ovarian cancer. However, only 5 to 10 percent of ovarian cancers have a clear hereditary link. The environmental factors responsible are largely unknown, although exposure to gene-damaging agents such as radiation can increase a woman's risk. There are three types of ovarian cancers, but the most common (ovarian epithelial cancer) is also the deadliest. The other forms arise from different cell types in the ovaries and are rare.

Symptoms, diagnosis, and pathogenesis

Early symptoms include abdominal pain, fatigue, bloating, and gastrointestinal or urinary problems. These symptoms are so common that it makes ovarian cancer difficult to diagnose, but the persistence of symptoms after any treatment should be a warning sign. About 80 percent of women with ovarian cancer will not be diagnosed until the disease has spread.

Regular pelvic examinations and a blood test for a molecule associated with ovarian cancer (CA-125) can help doctors, but neither test is particularly good at finding ovarian cancer before it spreads. Ultrasound and biopsies are needed to confirm a diagnosis of ovarian cancer.

Prevention and treatment

Women with a family history of breast or ovarian cancer can have a genetic test to see if they are carrying mutations in the *BRCA1* or *BRCA2* gene. If they have the disease gene, they can have their ovaries and uterus removed or have more frequent medical examinations.

Women with ovarian cancer undergo surgery to remove cancerous tissue, followed by chemotherapy and occasionally radiation therapy. New studies show that intravenous chemotherapy injected into the abdomen can increase survival rate in ovarian cancer patients.

Chris Curran

KEY FACTS

Description
A malignant tumor in one or both ovaries.

Cause
A combination of genetic and environmental factors.

Risk factors
Family history, gender, age, and living in an industrialized country.

Symptoms
Persistent abdominal pain, gastrointestinal or urinary problems, and fatigue.

Diagnosis
Blood tests, ultrasound, CT scans, or X-rays are usually followed by a confirmatory biopsy.

Treatments
Surgery, followed by chemotherapy or radiation therapy, or both.

Pathogenesis
Most women are not diagnosed until the late stages of the disease, so ovarian cancer generally reaches the metastatic or invasive stage, which is typically fatal.

Prevention
Genetic screening and regular gynecological exams. In extreme cases, removal of the ovaries in women with a positive test for genes linked to the disease.

Epidemiology
Approximately 22,000 women will be diagnosed with ovarian cancer in the United States each year. More than 15,000 will die of the disease.

See also
- Cancer, breast • Cancer, cervical
- Cancer, uterine

Cancer, pancreatic

Pancreatic cancer, also called cancer of the pancreas, is a malignant tumor that occurs in the tissues of the pancreas. Early stages of the disease do not show noticeable symptoms. It is one of the most serious types of cancer and is the fourth leading cause of cancer-related deaths in the United States.

Pancreatic cancer develops in the tissues of the pancreas. Due to the difficulties of diagnosis, the aggressive nature of the disease, and limited treatment options, the survival rate is extremely low. Very few patients who are diagnosed with pancreatic cancer can survive for five years afterward.

Causes and risk factors

The exact causes of pancreatic cancer are still unknown. It is believed that many cases are caused by environmental factors or an unhealthy lifestyle. Among all the possible risk factors, smoking is probably the leading cause of pancreatic cancer. A diet high in animal fat and low in fruits and vegetables may also increase the risk of the disease. People who are overweight and physically inactive also have a higher rate of contracting pancreatic cancer. It has also been shown that people who work with petroleum compounds, including gasoline and other chemicals, have a higher incidence of pancreatic cancer than people who are not exposed to these chemicals. The risk of pancreatic cancer gets higher as people become older. Most of the patients are older than 50 years of age. Rarely, pancreatic cancer may run in families. About 3 percent of cases are related to genetic disorders.

Treatments and prevention

Pancreatic cancer is extremely difficult to cure, and surgical removal of the cancer is currently the only option. Whipple procedure, a surgical resection of most of the pancreatic cancers, is the most advanced surgical treatment for the disease. At Johns Hopkins hospital, 25 percent of patients who have undergone the Whipple procedure have survived five years. When a tumor cannot be removed surgically, chemotherapy and radiation therapy are offered.

Although it is not always possible to prevent pancreatic cancer, certain healthy lifestyle measures can reduce risks of the disease. Not smoking, maintaining a healthy weight, exercising regularly, and eating a diet containing high amounts of fruits and vegetables, but low in animal fat, can reduce the risk of pancreatic cancer. The American Cancer Society recommends that people eat five servings of fruits and vegetables daily.

Yanni Wang

KEY FACTS

Description

A disease in which malignant cells grow in the tissues of pancreas.

Causes

Exact causes are unknown, but certain genetic changes in the cells of the pancreas might be responsible for the development of the cancer.

Risk factors

Age, smoking, diabetes, family history, gender, ethnicity, environment.

Symptoms

No symptoms at the early ages; as the cancer grows, symptoms may include pain in the upper abdomen or upper back, yellow skin and eyes, dark urine, weakness, loss of appetite, nausea and vomiting, and weight loss.

Diagnosis

Physical exam, lab tests, computed tomography (CT), ultrasonography, endoscopic retrograde cholangiopancreatography (ERCP), percutaneous transhepatic cholangiography (PTC), biopsy.

Treatments

Currently only surgery can cure the disease if it is found at an early stage.

Pathogenesis

Symptoms do not appear until the cancer has spread, so progression can be rapid.

Prevention

Not smoking, limiting fat, especially animal-fat intake, increasing intake of fruits and vegetables, exercise, regular tests.

Epidemiology

The risk of pancreatic cancer is higher in men and especially African American men. U.S. mortality rate for pancreatic cancer is 97 percent.

See also
• Cancer, liver

Cancer, prostate

Prostate cancer, a disease in which cells of the prostate gland divide uncontrollably, is one of the most common types of cancers in men, especially in older men. However, the survival rate from the disease, if diagnosed and treated at an early stage, is high.

Only men have a prostate gland, which forms part of the male reproductive system, secreting some of the seminal fluid that carries sperm during ejaculation. The gland lies in front of the rectum and below the bladder and is about the size of a walnut. It also surrounds part of the urethra, the tube that carries urine out of a man's body from the bladder through his penis. When a group of abnormal cells in the prostate grow out of control, prostate cancer occurs.

Most prostate cancers grow very slowly but, as with other cancers, the cancer cells may spread and form colonies in other parts of the body if the disease is left untreated. However, overall survival rates are good. According to the American Cancer Society (ACS), 99 percent of men diagnosed with prostate cancer will survive at least five years, 92 percent will survive 10 years, and 61 percent will survive 15 years.

Causes and risk factors

The exact causes of prostate cancer are still unknown. Scientists still cannot explain why some men develop prostate cancer while others do not. However, researchers have identified some risk factors that are, or may be, associated with the disease, and studies are currently underway to learn more about these factors.

Age is the most significant risk factor for prostate cancer, which is rare among men under the age of 40. According to the National Cancer Institute (NCI) in the United States, the average age of prostate cancer patients when they are diagnosed with the disease is 70.

Ethnicity is a second major risk factor. It has been shown that African American men have the highest risk of developing prostate cancer in the world, and the lowest survival rate. In the United States, prostate cancer mortality rate among African Americans is twice as high as that among white men, although the reasons for this are still unknown.

A family history of prostate cancer is also an important risk factor. A man's risk of developing prostate cancer is much higher if his direct family members

have had the disease than if they have not. Studies suggest that heredity may play an important role in the early onset of prostate cancer. The mortality rate of hereditary prostate cancer is much higher; it is diagnosed at younger ages, and as a result of its early onset, more men with hereditary cancer die of the disease.

It is possible that diet plays a role in developing prostate cancer. There are suggestions that a diet high in animal fat may increase the risk, whereas a diet high in fruits and vegetables may decrease risk. Obesity, as well as certain lifestyle patterns, including lack of exercise, smoking, and risky sexual activity, may also increase the risk of developing prostate cancer, although the evidence is not conclusive.

Studies found that higher concentration of insulin-like growth factor (IGF-1) were associated with an increased risk of prostate cancer, because IGF-1 can

KEY FACTS

Description
A disease in which cancerous tissue forms in the prostate gland in men.

Causes
Not known.

Risk factors
Age, race, relatives with prostate cancer, and perhaps diet.

Symptoms
Usually symptomless in early stages. First symptom may be difficulty or pain on urination, although other diseases can also cause this.

Diagnosis
Digital rectal examination and blood test, followed up by a biopsy.

Treatments
Various treatments possible, alone or in combination, including "watchful waiting," surgery, radiation therapy, hormone therapy, chemotherapy, and high-intensity ultrasound.

Pathogenesis
Gland cells within the prostate become cancerous and may eventually spread elsewhere in the body.

Epidemiology
More than 75 percent of all prostate cancers are found in men above the age of 65, and the disease rarely affects men younger than age 40. African American men are at greater risk, as are men with a family history of prostate cancer.

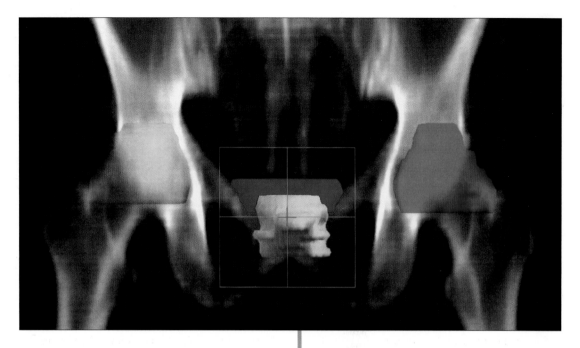

stimulate the division of prostate epithelial (lining) cells. Further studies on the relationship between IGF-1 levels and prostate cancer are needed.

This computed tomography scan of the pelvis shows the mapping of radiation therapy for prostate cancer. Inside the frame, the prostate is orange. X-rays focus on the cancerous area; nearby structures are not affected.

Symptoms and pathogenesis

Early stage prostate cancer usually develops unnoticed, and the first symptom a man is likely to experience is difficulty or pain when urinating. The prostate gland surrounds the urinary duct (urethra), and growth of cancerous tissue may press against the urethra and partly block the tube. Pain in the lower back or elsewhere can be a symptom of primary prostate cancer or metastatic prostate cancer. However, such symptoms can be caused by other diseases, including noncancerous enlargement of the prostate gland. Whether or not cancer is involved can be revealed by a biopsy.

Although the prostate contains several types of cells, including muscle cells, more than 99 percent of prostate cancers develop from gland cells that secrete the seminal fluid. As with other cancers, the spread of prostate cancer is commonly described in terms of four successive stages. At stage I, the cancer is localized in the prostate and cannot be detected during a digital rectal examination. The cancer is usually only found by chance when surgery is done for other reasons. Stage II is more severe than stage I but is still localized in the prostate. At stage III, the cancer has spread outside the prostate, but it has not spread to the lymph nodes. (The body's lymphatic system is a common route by which cancers can spread.) At stage IV, the cancer may

have already spread to the lymph nodes, as well as to other parts of the body. Sometimes the disease seems to disappear, then it returns in the same location or it spreads to other parts of the body. Prostate cancer showing this type of pattern is called recurrent cancer. Recurrent prostate cancer may be found in or near the prostate. It may also recur anywhere in the body, especially in the bones.

According to the ACS, most prostate cancers grow slowly, and autopsy studies have shown that many older men who died of other diseases also had prostate cancer that never affected them. Even with the latest methods, it is difficult to predict which type of prostate cancer will grow slowly and which will grow quickly.

Diagnosis and screening

If a man's symptoms suggest that he may have prostate cancer, various diagnostic tests can be carried out. One simple procedure is the digital rectal examination, in which the physician's gloved finger is inserted into the rectum. The physician can feel the back surface of the prostate through the wall of the rectum and can detect any swelling or lumps. A blood test can detect the levels of a substance produced only by the prostate gland, called prostate specific antigen (PSA). Often a raised blood PSA level is associated with prostate cancer, but there is not always a connection, and a PSA test cannot prove prostate cancer on its own.

The only way to prove that prostate cancer exists, and not some other disorder, is to carry out a biopsy. In this procedure a small amount of prostate tissue is removed and examined under a microscope. Based on how different the tissue looks from normal tissue, the physician detects whether cancer is present at all, and also assigns the cancer a number from 2 to 10 on a standard scale called the Gleason score. The higher the Gleason score, the more dangerous the prostate cancer is likely to be. The extent and spread of any cancer can also be checked by imaging methods such as ultrasound.

Screening for prostate cancer aims to detect the disease before a man reports any symptoms. Currently, there is no standard screening procedure, although a combination of digital rectal examination and a PSA test may be used. Biopsies are not used for initial screening because they may cause side effects, such as bleeding and infection. There is some controversy about prostate screening programs, because most prostate cancer grows slowly and may never become a problem, whereas screening may lead to many more biopsies and other procedures that can cause problems themselves.

Treatments

The overall survival rate has been improved dramatically during the past years. According to the ACS, current five-year survival rate is nearly 100 percent if the cancer is still confined within the prostate when diagnosed.

Common treatments include surgery and radiation therapy, which may be used alone or in combination. Each type of treatment has its own advantages and disadvantages. The treatments a patient is given will depend on his age, the stage of his cancer, and which risks and side effects he is prepared to accept. If the cancer has spread in the body and a complete cure is not possible, palliative treatments, which help relieve symptoms and suffering, can still be important.

If prostate cancer is detected at an early stage and is growing slowly, a so-called "watchful waiting" policy may be adopted. During this time, the patient is monitored with regular checkups, including frequent PSA and digital rectal examination tests. If the cancer gets worse or symptoms become more acute, or both, treatments like surgery or radiation will be considered. Watchful waiting may also be recommended to men who are older and have other serious medical problems.

The main goal of surgery is to remove cancer cells before they spread to other parts of the body. Unlike breast cancer, which starts from a single tumor, prostate cancer consists of a number of small tumors scattered throughout the prostate. To get rid of all the cancer cells, the entire prostate, as well as some surrounding tissues, must be removed. Surgery is a common treatment for patients who are younger than 70 years old and have early stage prostate cancer. The

A patient is treated for prostate cancer with a form of radiation therapy. Surgeons are implanting radioactive sticks around the tumor. Sometimes radioactive pellets are placed in the prostate gland.

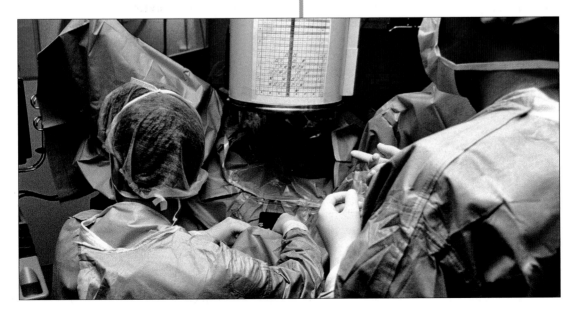

most common surgical procedure is called radical prostatectomy. This surgery removes the whole prostate gland and nearby lymph nodes. After surgery, as a temporary measure, a narrow rubber tube is inserted through the penis and connecting to the bladder, to carry urine out of the body. Major side effects of radical prostatectomy for prostate cancer include involuntary urination and erectile dysfunction. Involuntary urination usually lasts for a few days or weeks, but more serious cases can often be corrected with minor surgery. The chance of impotence can decrease if it is possible for a surgeon to avoid cutting the nerves on either side of the prostate that control erectile functions. However, it may not be possible to avoid cutting the nerves if the tumor is large and the erectile dysfunction will be permanent.

In cases where surgery is not appropriate (when the disease has spread to other parts of the body, or the patient is too old or weak to endure surgery), other therapies such as radiation therapy and hormone therapies may be used instead. Radiation therapy uses various methods that deliver high-energy X-rays to kill cancer cells. Radiation may also be recommended after surgery to destroy any cancer cells that may remain in the area. In some cases, radiation is used in combination with hormone therapy. Both surgery and radiation therapies have shown promising outcomes as curative treatments, with more than 90 percent cure rates for men who have cancer that has not yet spread beyond the prostate.

The goal of hormone therapy is to lower the levels of male hormones in the body. Male hormones such as testosterone stimulate the growth of normal and cancerous prostate cells. Androgens are male hormones, and hormone therapy is also called androgen deprivation therapy (ADT) or androgen suppression therapy (AST). Studies have shown that hormone therapy can usually shrink larger tumors and hence make it easier to remove or kill them using surgery or radiation therapy. Hormone therapy using drugs or surgery can also be used after these other treatments to prevent the cancer from recurring, as well as for cases when prostate cancer has spread to other parts of the body. The therapy reduces the production of the male hormone testosterone, which is needed for prostate cancer cells to grow. Possible side effects of hormonal therapy include impotence, loss of sexual desire, and thinning of bones. Hormone therapy also often causes hot flashes; the exact causes are currently not clear.

Chemotherapy uses drugs to kill cancer cells by interfering with how the cells divide. Chemotherapy often has unpleasant side effects. In prostate cancer, it is generally reserved for very advanced cases that no longer respond to hormone therapy. Often a combination of different drugs is used. Like hormone therapy, chemotherapy is unlikely to kill all the cancer cells, but it can slow the cancer growth and reduce symptoms.

Other new or still-experimental types of treatment include cryosurgery, vaccine therapy, and high-intensity focused ultrasound. The goal of cryosurgery for prostate cancer is to freeze and eventually kill the cancer cells using very cold liquid nitrogen. In this procedure, an instrument known as a cryoprobe is inserted through the penis to directly interact with and freeze the cancer cells in the prostate.

Cryosurgery is only effective in small areas. It can be used to treat men with early stage prostate cancer, in which the cancer is still confined to the prostate gland, but cryosurgery is not designed to treat prostate cancer that has spread to other parts of the body. Cryosurgery is an option for patients who want to avoid the customary surgical procedures. There is minimal pain and discomfort, and patients can return to their routine after a few days. Another advantage is that the procedure can be repeated.

Scientists are currently trying to develop vaccines that would stimulate the body's immune system to attack prostate cancer cells. The ultimate goal of vaccine therapy is to stimulate the patient's immune system to attack specific targets in the cancer cells.

High-intensity focused ultrasound targets a specific area with high-frequency sound waves. Absorption of the ultrasound energy results in an increase in temperature, which can destroy the tissues in that area. High-intensity focused ultrasound can be used for early stage prostate cancer.

Prevention

In general, prostate cancer cannot be prevented. However, lifestyle can be altered to modify some possible risk factors, such as those relating to diet. Studies are underway to assess whether taking food supplements that include substances such as vitamins D and E, selenium, and lycopenes (antioxidants that are found naturally in some fruits) have any potential benefits in preventing prostate cancer.

Yanni Wang

See also
- Cancer, bladder • Cancer, colorectal
- Prostate disorders

Cancer, skin

Uncontrolled growth of skin cells—skin cancer—is the most common cancer, accounting for almost half of all cancer cases. The majority of these, 80 percent, are either basal cell carcinoma (BCC) or squamous cell carcinoma (SCC), which account for 16 percent. The remainder are malignant melanomas.

The risk of developing a skin cancer is directly proportional to the amount of exposure to ultraviolet (UV) radiation over someone's lifetime, including exposure by tanning beds. It is more common in some families, people at advanced ages, and in those with fair skin and blond or red hair. Certain chemicals (arsenic) and exposure to X-ray radiation can also lead to its development. BCC is most common on sun-exposed areas such as the face, neck, arms, and hands, but SCC can also develop in other areas and is most common on the palms and soles in people with dark complexions.

Symptoms, diagnosis, and treatments

Although there are some differences in the appearance of BCC and SCC, they should be suspected whenever a new skin growth develops or there is a change in a preexisting lesion, such as enlargement, elevation, scaliness, or an open sore that does not heal. Regular self-examination can identify suspicious lesions early.

BCC can take many forms but usually develops as a raised, red, waxy nodule with visible blood vessels that eventually develops a central open sore. It can be very slow growing and spreads only locally. SCC generally begins as a small scaly, red patch on the skin that progresses to an open, crusted sore that fails to heal. It can enlarge and spread locally. However, SCC also has the ability to metastasize, or spread, to distant tissues.

Once a skin cancer is suspected, a skin biopsy should be taken and examined under a microscope to confirm the diagnosis. If small, the lesion can be completely excised and the skin closed. Other methods include destroying the cancer by freezing, radiation, chemicals, or electrodesiccation (burning). More than 95 percent of these skin cancers can be cured by these methods.

Prevention and epidemiology

Prevention includes reducing exposure to dangerous UV radiation by limiting exposure during the peak sun hours (10 A.M. to 4 P.M.) and by using protective clothing and broad-spectrum sunblocks that have a sun protection factor (SPF) of 15 or greater.

Skin cancers are most commonly seen in geographic locations with yearlong high-intensity sunlight such as Australia and Florida. More than 1 million new cases develop in the United States each year, and this number is increasing as the amount of leisure time is greater and a tanned body is considered attractive.

David Wainwright

KEY FACTS

Description

Squamous cell carcinoma and basal cell carcinoma are the most common skin cancers.

Causes and risk factors

By far the most common cause of skin cancers is long exposure to ultraviolet radiation. Other causes include chemicals and radiation, and it is seen more frequently in some families and people with lighter skin and hair color.

Symptoms, signs, and diagnosis

The diagnosis should be suspected when a new, enlarging skin lesion is found or there are changes in the appearance of a preexisting skin lesion; it is confirmed with examination of a skin sample under the microscope.

Treatment

Both BCC and SCC can be successfully removed or destroyed by surgical excision, freezing, chemicals, radiation, or electrodesiccation.

Pathogenesis

Ultraviolet radiation damages the cellular genes, and if the cell is unable to repair itself, uncontrolled cell multiplication and growth will occur.

Prevention

Limiting harmful sun exposure with avoidance, adequate protective clothing, and sunblock are the primary methods of preventing skin cancers.

Epidemiology

More than 1 million cases develop in the United States each year and are more common where the average yearly sun intensity is high. Malignant melanoma causes 75 percent of all deaths from skin cancer.

See also
- Melanoma

Cancer, stomach

Although it is rare in Caucasian people, stomach cancer, also known as gastric cancer, is very common among Asian people and Pacific islanders. Diet and lifestyle appear to be significant risk factors.

Like other types of cancers, the causes of stomach cancer are still unknown, but researchers have identified risk factors linked to this cancer.

Long-term infection of the stomach with the bacterium *Helicobacter pylori*, which may cause inflammation and damage to the inner layer of the stomach, is a major risk factor of stomach cancer. However, the majority of people who carry this bacterium in their stomach will never develop stomach cancer.

A diet high in smoked, salted, and pickled foods is suggested as another major risk factor for stomach cancer. Other risk factors include age, gender, lifestyle, and history of stomach diseases. Men more than 60, smokers, and people who have had stomach surgery have a much higher risk of developing stomach cancer.

Treatment and prevention

Surgery is the most common treatment for stomach cancer. Depending on the stage of the cancer, a doctor can choose between two different types of surgery. Partial gastrectomy is recommended when the cancer is still localized. Parts of the stomach are removed, and part of the esophagus or the small intestine and nearby tissues may also be removed. The entire stomach is removed in total gastrectomy. During surgery, a feeding tube is connected to a patient's small intestine.

Chemotherapy drugs are injected into the bloodstream; these chemicals kill cancer cells. Chemotherapy is often used after surgery to prevent the cancer from recurring. The side effects of chemotherapy vary, but the most common side effects include tiredness, losing hair, lack of appetite, nausea and vomiting, diarrhea, and mouth and lip sores.

Radiation therapy, using high-energy X-rays to kill the cancer cells, targets only the area where cancer grows. External radiation, in which the radiation is from a machine outside the body, is normally performed in the hospital or clinic. Radiation therapy may cause stomach or intestinal pain. Patients may suffer from nausea, diarrhea, and tiredness, as well as skin discomfort in the treated area.

KEY FACTS

Description
Malignant tumor in the stomach.

Causes
Exact causes are unknown.

Risk factors
Age, sex, ethnicity, diet, *Helicobacter pylori* infection, smoking, history of stomach diseases, family history of stomach cancer.

Symptoms
No symptoms in early stage stomach cancer. As cancer grows, the most common symptoms include discomfort in the stomach area, constantly feeling full, nausea or vomiting, weight loss.

Diagnosis
Physical exam, X-ray, endoscopy, biopsy.

Treatments
Surgery, chemotherapy, and radiation therapy.

Pathogenesis
A disease in which a malignant tumor develops in the stomach. Without treatment, it can spread.

Prevention
A diet high in fresh fruits and vegetables; low intake of smoked, salted, and pickled foods; quitting smoking.

Epidemiology
Normally occurs in older people. More than twice as common in men as it is in women. The American Cancer Society estimated that in 2005 around 20,000 people were diagnosed with the disease; half died.

A nutritious diet will help recovery. Due to the side effects of the treatments, it is difficult for a patient to eat well. Weight loss after surgery for stomach cancer is common. Receiving nutrition by a feeding tube or by injection can help a patient deal with the problem.

To prevent recurrence, follow-up care is recommended. Checkups include a physical exam, lab tests, X-rays, CT scans, and endoscopy. Reducing salt intake and having a healthy diet can reduce the risk of stomach cancer. Screening can help find any abnormal changes or diagnose stomach cancer at an early stage.

Yanni Wang

See also
• Cancer, mouth and throat

Cancer, thyroid

Thyroid cancer is the most common cancer of the endocrine system, and the number of cases continues to increase in the United States. Almost three times as many women will be diagnosed as men; however, the fatality rates are highest in men.

The number of thyroid cancers more than doubled from 1973 to 2002 in the United States. Many health professionals are unconcerned, however, because the death rate has not increased. Many doctors believe better screening methods are simply detecting more tiny tumors that pose little risk to the patient.

Causes and risk factors

The most important risk factor for thyroid cancer is early exposure to radiation. The radiation source can be X-rays or radioactive fallout. For example, the thyroid cancer rates in children exposed following the Chernobyl nuclear reactor accident in 1986 were ten times higher than expected. Radiation can damage genes, leading to mutations that allow cancer to develop and spread. Family history and gender are also important. Rates of thyroid cancer in women are almost three times higher than those seen in men.

Symptoms and diagnosis

The first symptoms of thyroid cancer are lumps in the neck. The thyroid gland is a butterfly-shaped organ located on the front of the neck underneath the larynx (voice box). As the tumor grows, a person might have difficulty speaking, swallowing, or breathing. The lumps are often detected during a routine physical exam. Fine needle aspiration is the most common test to confirm the presence of cancer. The needle pulls out a small group of cells for diagnosis. Other diagnostic tests include imaging using radioactive iodine, X-rays, MRI, and ultrasound scanning.

Pathogenesis, epidemiology, and treatments

There are four distinct categories of thyroid cancers, depending on the type of cell where the cancer begins. The vast majority of cancers are follicular or papillary. Both types, as well as medullary thyroid cancer, are easily treated with surgery and follow-up therapy. Anaplastic thyroid cancer is rare but spreads easily

throughout the body and is usually fatal. It occurs in about 1 to 2 percent of all patients with thyroid cancer.

Most thyroid cancer patients will have surgery to remove most or all of the thyroid gland. Because the thyroid produces important hormones, these patients will need thyroid hormone replacement therapy for the rest of their lives. Other follow-up treatments include radioactive iodine to destroy the remaining cancerous cells or other types of chemotherapy and radiation therapy.

Chris Curran

KEY FACTS

Description
A cancer of the thyroid gland.

Causes
Genetic mutations and radiation, including X-rays.

Risk factors
Family history, gender, age, insufficient iodine in the diet, and exposure to radiation.

Symptoms and signs
A lump in the neck, difficulty swallowing, hoarseness, and difficulty breathing.

Diagnosis
Biopsies, ultrasound, X-rays, MRI, or imaging using radioactive iodine.

Treatment
Surgery, followed by hormones, radioactive iodine, chemotherapy, or radiation therapy.

Pathogenesis
There are four different types of thyroid cancers. Most are treatable, but the rarest form is aggressive and usually fatal.

Prevention
Frequent checkups for those with a family history of thyroid cancer; avoiding radiation exposure, especially early in life.

Epidemiology
In the United States, Caucasians are at higher risk than African Americans. Women are at higher risk than men. Most cases are diagnosed after the age of 40. About 30,000 new cases will be diagnosed each year, and about 1,500 people will die from the disease in the United States.

See also
• Thyroid disorders

Cancer, uterine

Uterine cancer affects either the lining of the uterus or, more commonly, the cervix, which is the lower part, or neck, of the uterus. Failure to ovulate and taking estrogen hormones and certain drugs are risk factors.

According to the National Cancer Institute, uterine cancer is the most common cancer of the female reproductive system in the United States. The risk of developing endometrial (lining of the uterus) cancer is much higher in Caucasian women. African American women have a higher risk of developing uterine sarcoma (cancer of connective tissue).

Causes and risk factors

The exact causes of uterine cancer are still not clear. However, researchers have identified a number of risk factors associated with uterine cancer. High levels of estrogen are believed to increase the risk of uterine cancer. It has been shown that the risk of developing uterine cancer is at least 10 times higher in women who take estrogen replacement therapy (ERT) alone for more than 5 years. Certain ovarian diseases such as granulose-theca cell tumors may increase the risk of uterine cancer via increasing estrogen levels and decreasing progesterone levels. Tamoxifen, an anti-estrogen drug used to treat breast cancer, may also increase the risk of uterine cancer. For women who take this drug to treat breast cancer, regular gynecological exams are recommended.

It is also suggested that starting menstruation before the age of 12 or experiencing menopause at a late age can increase the risk of developing uterine cancer. Women who have never been pregnant have a higher risk of developing uterine cancer than those who have had children. Obesity and other medical conditions, such as hereditary nonpolyposis colorectal cancer (HNPCC), a genetic abnormality, can also increase the risk of developing uterine cancer.

Treatments and prevention

The choice of treatment generally depends on the stage of the disease. Most women choose surgery to remove the uterus. Sometimes, fallopian tubes and ovaries as well as nearby lymph nodes must be removed. After treatment, most women can return to their normal activity within four to eight weeks.

Radiation therapy, including external radiation and internal radiation, is a common treatment for uterine cancer. It is often used after surgery to kill remaining cancerous cells or prevent recurrence. It is often used before surgery to shrink the tumor. Side effects of radiation therapy include tiredness, reddened skin in the treated area, diarrhea, and discomfort urinating.

For those unable to have surgery or receive radiation therapy, hormonal therapy may be used. Unlike surgery and radiation therapy, hormonal therapy affects cancer cells throughout the body. For women with uterine cancer that has spread to other parts of the body, hormonal therapy is often used. The therapy may increase appetite and result in weight gain.

Yanni Wang

KEY FACTS

Description
Malignant cancer of the uterus.

Causes
Exact causes are unknown.

Risk factors
Age, endometrial hyperplasia, hormone replacement therapy, ethnicity, tamoxifen, obesity.

Symptoms
Abnormal vaginal bleeding, painful urination, painful intercourse, pain in the pelvic area.

Diagnosis
Pelvic exam, transvaginal ultrasound, biopsy.

Treatments
Surgery, radiation therapy, hormonal therapy.

Pathogenesis
Malignant tumor develops in the lining of uterus and spreads to other parts of the body.

Prevention
Healthy diet, breastfeeding, adding progestin therapy to HRT, use of oral contraceptives.

Epidemiology
About 40,000 new cases in the United States in 2006; the American Cancer Society suggests that around 7,400 of those will die. Caucasian women are at a higher risk of endometrial cancer. Women with uterine cancer are normally older than 50.

See also
- Cancer, ovarian

Cataract

A cataract is a painless clouding of the eye's lens that diminishes the passage of light to the retina, resulting in blurred vision. As the eye ages, proteins in the lens are degraded and begin to aggregate, clouding a small area of the lens. As the cataract progresses, the clouding becomes denser and more expansive, resulting in reduced visual acuity. Although the exact cause is unknown, age appears to be the most significant risk factor, as an estimated 70 percent of Americans over the age of 75 have cataracts that interfere with their vision.

Everyone is at risk of developing a cataract because problems with vision are a by-product of the aging process. Most people develop some lens clouding after the age of 60 years, and about 50 percent of people in the United States between the ages of 65 to 74 have cataracts. Why the composition of the lens changes with age still remains elusive.

Causes

Damage caused by unstable molecules known as free radicals as well as the general wear and tear on the lens over the years may contribute to protein degradation and aggregation. However, not all cataracts are age-related. Some children are born with a cataract, and others may develop a cataract during childhood. Such cataracts may be the result of rubella during pregnancy or may be caused by certain metabolic disorders. Congenital cataracts do not always affect vision, but if they do, they can usually be surgically removed soon after detection.

In addition to age, a family history of cataracts, smoking, diabetes, a previous eye injury or surgery, and prolonged use of corticosteroids are all predisposing factors for developing cataracts. Environmental factors such as the exposure to sunlight and ioninizing radiation may also contribute to their onset.

Symptoms and signs

A cataract usually develops gradually without any detectable symptoms at its onset. However, as it progresses and less light is able to reach the retina, vision becomes impaired. A more advanced cataract is often associated with sensitivity to sunlight and oncoming headlights. In addition, a person may experience blurred or double vision, a fading or yellowing of colors, poor night vision, and frequent changes in eyeglasses prescription.

Diagnosis

An ophthalmologist utilizes an array of comprehensive eye examinations to detect a cataract. The first examination given is a typical visual acuity examination. This examination uses an eye chart and measures the eyesight at various distances. Other eye examinations

KEY FACTS

Description
A painless clouding of the eye's lens that prohibits light from reaching the retina.

Causes
Although the exact cause is unknown, damage by free radicals may contribute to cataracts.

Risk Factors
Age is the single greatest risk factor. Additional risk factors include smoking, excessive exposure to sunlight, or a previous eye injury.

Symptoms and signs
Gradual blurring of vision, poor night vision, double vision, and the perception of excessive glare from headlights or sunlight.

Diagnosis
A medical history, a physical examination, and a battery of eye exams are all necessary to confirm a diagnosis of cataracts.

Treatments
Surgical removal of the clouded lens is the only effective method of treating cataracts.

Pathogenesis
If a cataract is left untreated, the person will experience a loss of vision.

Prevention
Because age is a key risk factor, not much can be done to prevent cataracts, but some doctors think that having regular eye tests, not smoking, and eating a healthy diet may be helpful.

Epidemiology
Around 20.5 million people in the United States who are older than 40 years have a cataract in either eye. More than two-thirds of people who are affected are over 60 years old. Women in the United States generally develop cataracts at an older age than men.

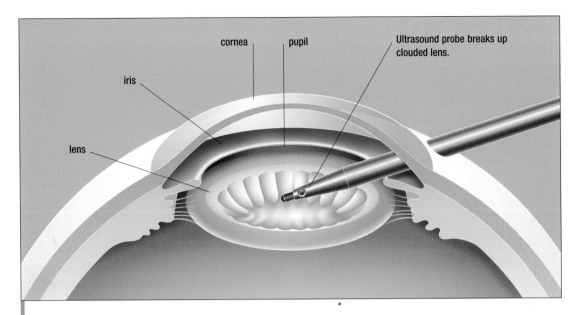

cornea   pupil   Ultrasound probe breaks up clouded lens.

iris

lens

Cataract removal is usually performed as a day-patient operation. A local anesthetic is administered to numb the eyeball, and drops are applied to widen the pupil so that the surgeon can see the lens. A small incision is made through the eye into the lens. An ultrasound probe is inserted, which produces sound waves that shatter the lens material. The pieces of lens are then sucked out. A new lens made from plastic or silicone is inserted. The original incision is so small that it does not need to be stitched.

may include a slit lamp and retinal examination, as well as tonometry. A slit lamp is a microscope that uses an intense line of light to illuminate and magnify the various structures of the eye, allowing the doctor to detect any small abnormalities. For a retinal examination, the pupil is dilated with eyedrops, and a special magnifying lens is used to examine the retina and the optic nerve for signs of damage. In addition, tonometry, which measures the pressure inside the eye, may also be used to detect a cataract.

Treatments

An early cataract may be remedied with new eyeglasses, brighter lighting, anti-glare sunglasses, or magnifying lenses. However, once the cataract progresses to the point where it interferes with vision, surgery is the only effective treatment. Surgery involves removing the cloudy lens and replacing it with an artificial lens. Removal of a cataract is one of the safest and most effective types of surgery. About 90 percent of people who have this surgery experience improved vision afterward.

Pathogenesis

Cataracts are painless but do cause visual problems. The vision becomes blurred and distorted, and color perception may alter. At night, a person with cataracts may experience a scattering of light from any bright lights.

The appearance of the pupil of the eye may look cloudy as a result of the cataract. The cataract keeps growing until the whole lens becomes white.

Prevention

Because age is the most significant risk factor for developing a cataract, the condition may be unavoidable. However, regular eye examinations are key to early detection. Furthermore, some simple lifestyle modifications, such as not smoking, protection from the sun, and eating a balanced diet, may also help prevent the development of cataracts.

Epidemiology

About 17 percent of people in the United States over 40 years of age, or an estimated 20.5 million people, have cataracts. The National Eye Institute predicts that this figure will rise to over 30 million by 2020, as the proportion of older people in the population of the United States increases.

Sonia Gulati

See also
• Diabetes • Macular degeneration • Retinal disorders • Sunburn and sunstroke

Celiac disease

Also known as celiac sprue, celiac disease is an inherited autoimmune disorder in which an intolerance to the protein gluten (found in wheat and rye) causes intestinal damage that impairs the absorption of nutrients from food and may lead to malnutrition.

A digestive and autoimmune (caused by an over-active immune system) disorder, celiac disease causes damage to the small intestine and interferes with the absorption of nutrients from food. People with the disease are allergic to a protein called gluten, which is found in wheat, rye, and barley as well as products such as vitamins, medications, and stamp and envelope adhesive. Celiac disease is estimated to affect about 2 million people in the United States, about 1 in 133 of the population. It affects more women than men and is most common in Caucasians and people of European ancestry.

Causes and risk factors

The underlying cause of celiac disease is a genetic defect that causes the body's immune system to produce antibodies, which, in the presence of gluten, attack the lining of the small intestine. As a result, the tiny, fingerlike protrusions (villi) that line the small intestine become damaged and can no longer absorb nutrients properly. Impaired nutrient absorption in turn causes the person to become malnourished, irrespective of the amount of food eaten.

Because celiac disease is a genetic disorder, people with family members who have the disease are at an increased risk of developing it themselves. A genetic predisposition to celiac disease combined with various trigger factors, including surgery, pregnancy, childbirth, viral infection, and severe emotional stress, may lead to the onset of the disease.

Symptoms and signs

The symptoms associated with celiac disease vary greatly among individuals, sometimes affecting different areas of the body and varying in severity. One person may have severe physical symptoms, such as diarrhea, constipation, or abdominal pain, whereas another may experience emotional symptoms, including irritability or depression. Irritability is one of the most common symptoms found among children with celiac disease. Other symptoms of the disease include gas, recurring abdominal bloating and pain, weight loss, fatigue, bone or joint pain, seizures, muscle cramps, tooth discoloration or loss of enamel, and itchy skin rashes such as dermatitis. Some people with celiac disease have no symptoms, although they are still at risk of developing complications.

Because celiac disease impairs the absorption of nutrients, people with the disease are at risk of developing complications such as malnutrition and anemia. Malnutrition is especially serious for children because

KEY FACTS

Description
An autoimmune disorder that causes damage to the small intestine and interferes with the absorption of food.

Cause
Inherited intolerance to the protein gluten. Exposure to gluten causes the immune system to attack the lining of the small intestine, impairing the absorption of nutrients.

Risk factors
Those who have a family member with the disease are at increased risk.

Symptoms and signs
A wide variety of symptoms and signs, ranging from physical symptoms such as chronic diarrhea or constipation to emotional symptoms such as depression and irritability. There may also be malnutrition. Some people with the disease have no symptoms.

Diagnosis
Laboratory blood tests for specific autoantibodies that indicate the presence of celiac disease.

Treatments
Following a strict gluten-free diet. In some cases nutritional deficiencies may require supplements.

Pathogenesis
The disease may appear at any age. Sometimes it is triggered by surgery, pregnancy, childbirth, viral infection, or severe emotional stress.

Prevention
The only preventive measure is to follow a strict gluten-free diet.

Epidemiology
An estimated 2 million people in the United States have celiac disease. It is most common in Caucasians and those of European ancestry, and occurs more often in women than in men.

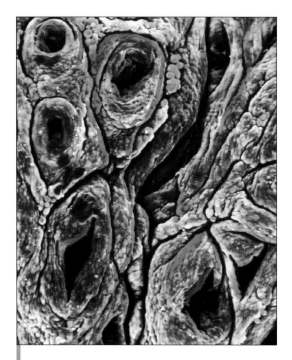

This detailed scan of the small intestine clearly demonstrates the effects of celiac disease. The intestine wall has atrophied and flattened due to the loss of villi, fingerlike projections that facilitate the absorption of food from the intestine.

they need adequate nutrition for proper growth and development. Poor absorption of calcium may increase the risk of osteoporosis in later life, a condition in which the bones become brittle, weak, and prone to breaking. In pregnant women with celiac disease, an impaired absorption of nutrients increases the risk of miscarriage and of congenital malformations. People with celiac disease have a greater tendency to suffer from other autoimmune disorders, including thyroid disease, systemic lupus erythematosus (SLE), type 1 diabetes mellitus, liver disease, collagen vascular diseases, and rheumatoid arthritis. Celiac disease also increases the risk of developing intestinal cancers.

Diagnosis

Celiac disease can be difficult to diagnose because its symptoms are so varied and resemble those of other disorders. For example, disorders that may be confused with celiac disease include irritable bowel syndrome, iron-deficiency anemia, Crohn's disease, diverticulitis, intestinal infections, and chronic fatigue syndrome.

Sufferers of celiac disease have higher than normal levels of substances called autoantibodies in their blood. Whereas antibodies are proteins produced by

the immune system as a protective mechanism when foreign substances enter the body, autoantibodies are proteins that react against the body's own molecules or tissues. Tests therefore can be carried out to measure the blood levels of these specific autoantibodies and in turn diagnose celiac disease. However, screening for the disease is not carried out routinely.

Treatments and prevention

The treatment for celiac disease is to eat a gluten-free diet. This is also the only known means of preventing symptoms from occurring because the underlying genetic cause cannot be treated or prevented. With the help of a dietitian, patients can learn to read ingredient lists when making food choices to identify foods that contain gluten. The foods to avoid are wheat, rye, and barley, as well as all food products made from these grains. To stay healthy the patient must follow this gluten-free diet for the rest of his or her life because eating even a small amount of gluten can lead to damage of the small intestine. Many grocery stores now carry a variety of gluten-free bread and pasta products, and thus people with celiac disease can enjoy a well-balanced diet with a wide variety of foods. In some patients additional complications may develop as a result of the celiac disease, in which case further treatment may be required. For example, if a patient develops malnutrition, then he or she will require treatment with nutritional supplements.

For most patients a gluten-free diet stops the symptoms, allows the intestine to heal, and prevents further intestinal damage. In children the intestine usually heals in three to six months; in adults healing may take up to two years. When the small intestine has healed, the intestinal villi can then resume absorbing nutrients from food into the bloodstream. In some patients a gluten-free diet seems to be ineffective, resulting in a condition known as unresponsive celiac disease. However, it is often found in such cases that trace amounts of gluten are still present in the patient's diet. A dietitian may be needed to identify the source of the gluten because gluten is sometimes hidden in foods. Hidden sources of gluten include additives such as modified food starch, preservatives, stabilizers, thickeners, and texture modifiers.

Julie McDowell

See also
• Anemia • Diarrhea and dysentery
• Osteoporosis

Chicken pox and shingles

Chicken pox is a highly contagious viral infection that is common in children who are not vaccinated. It is caused by the varicella-zoster virus, a member of the herpes family of viruses (its cousins include the viruses that cause cold sores and genital herpes). Shingles, or herpes zoster infection, is caused by the chicken pox virus reactivating in later life, after remaining dormant in nerve cells.

Prior to 1995, when routine vaccination against chicken pox began in the United States (the vaccine has been used since the 1970s in Japan and some other industrialized countries), chicken pox was a common childhood disease. Through the 1970s, the majority of American children who developed chicken pox did so during their early school years (ages six to nine years). From the 1970s and until immunization became common, the age that children contracted chicken pox became lower as an increasing number of children attended preschool and day-care programs. In 1995 the most common age to acquire chicken pox was from two to five years.

Symptoms

Chicken pox moves rapidly through communities of children because an individual becomes contagious one to two days before the rash appears, and the incubation period is generally 10 to 21 days; outside limits are as few as 7 and as many as 28 days.

The rash—generally described as a "tear drop on a rose petal"—usually appears first on the scalp or face, or both, and spreads rapidly to the trunk; within two or three days the body may be covered with as many as 250 to 500 small, red, itchy, and often fluid-filled blisters. People who have chronic skin conditions like eczema or who have a compromised immune system may have as many as 1,500 blisters.

While symptoms, including headache, fatigue, lethargy, and sometimes fever, often begin before the rash appears in adults and some children, in other children the rash is the first symptom, and many children continue to go to school or to other activities for a day or two while they are contagious. An individual is contagious from two days before the rash

KEY FACTS

Description

An infectious, highly contagious disease in which the person develops dozens to hundreds of small, itchy, fluid-filled blisters, accompanied by fever, headache, and fatigue.

Causes

Varicella-zoster virus, a member of the herpes virus family.

Risk factors

No risk factors for becoming ill with chicken pox, although skin problems such as eczema or a compromised immune system are risk factors for more severe disease and complications.

Symptoms

Fever, headache, fatigue for one to two days, followed by a classic rash that typically begins on the scalp or face and trunk, or both, before spreading to the rest of the body.

Diagnosis

By exam of rash (red, fluid-filled blisters) and fever.

Treatments

Mostly palliative; acetaminophen or ibuprofen to reduce fever (not aspirin), soothing lotions, and oatmeal or baking soda baths. Antiviral medications can be used to reduce symptoms and speed recovery.

Pathogenesis

In uncomplicated cases, the blisters continue to appear for a few days, and within 10 days of the first blisters appearing, all have begun to crust over; they heal completely over time with no scarring, unless individual blisters have become infected. In complicated cases, blisters and tissues around blisters can become infected, and viral pneumonia or viral encephalitis can occur.

Prevention

As of 1995, a chickenpox vaccine has been in use in the United States and is currently one of the components of routine vaccination for preschool children.

Epidemiology

Chicken pox appears throughout the world and has long been thought of as a rite of passage of childhood. In countries where vaccine is used, incidences have been greatly reduced, although in countries without vaccine, it is still one of the most common childhood illnesses. Chicken pox is less often seen in children in tropical climates, although the incidence is higher among adults in these areas.

appears to five days after the last blister appears—usually a total of about 10 days.

The chicken pox virus is highly contagious and can be transmitted not only through direct contact but through airborne droplet (coughing or sneezing), or by sharing food or drink, or by touching objects such as utensils or toys. It is possible to contract chicken pox from someone in the same room who does not know he or she is sick. Two children exposed to the same contagious child can develop chicken pox up to two weeks apart, and each will, in turn, be contagious to all other children before the rash appears.

In most cases, chicken pox is not a serious illness. However, complications can arise, especially in people with severe skin conditions, teenagers and adults who were not infected as children and therefore have no immunity, women in their third trimester of pregnancy, infants, and individuals who are immunocompromised because of disease or immunosuppressed because of medications (for example, chemotherapy treatments and corticosteroids) or radiation treatment.

Maternal chicken pox in the first 20 weeks of gestation has been associated with a constellation of birth abnormalities collectively known as congenital varicella syndrome. These abnormalities include low birth weight, as well as abnormalities of the extremities, heart, and brain. The incidence is very low, less than 2 percent. Maternal chicken pox after 20 weeks of gestation has been associated with a higher incidence of infants who develop chicken pox. Maternal chicken pox between five days before and two days after giving birth can cause fetal exposure to varicella without the development of any maternal immunity, and may result in a baby born with chicken pox. Although this occurs rarely, the infant mortality in such cases is 30 percent.

Rare complications

There is a risk of complications, including pneumonia (especially in adults), skin infection, blood infection, or brain infection. If a fever persists or there are signs of infection such as warmth, redness, or swelling of the skin, medical opinion should be sought.

Treatments

Treatment of uncomplicated cases of chicken pox generally involves making sure the person is comfortable. Fever can be reduced by acetaminophen (Tylenol) or ibuprofen (Advil, Motrin). Aspirin should not be used; use of aspirin by someone with chicken pox has been associated with the development of Reye's syndrome.

Reye's syndrome is a rare but serious complication of chicken pox and other viral infections such as influenza. It is believed to be associated with use of aspirin during a viral illness. Symptoms of Reye's syndrome include nausea and vomiting, lethargy, liver enlargement, and changes in mental status that may lead to coma and even death. Most children recover from Reye's syndrome after therapy in the hospital.

Lotions such as calamine and oatmeal or baking soda baths in warm water can reduce the itching, and fingernails should be kept very short to prevent skin infections. Antiviral drugs such as acyclovir, which works specifically against herpes viruses, can be used. To be effective, antiviral treatment must be started within 24 hours of the rash becoming apparent. Because most cases of chicken pox in children are uncomplicated, many physicians and other health care providers do not believe antiviral treatment is worth the cost, unless the child is at risk for complications. Adults or teens who have the disease are routinely treated with antiviral medication if the symptoms are noticed early, since they are more prone to severe complications than younger children.

SHINGLES

Shingles, also known as herpes zoster infection, appears as a small strip or cluster of painful blisters that usually occurs along a nerve path on one side of the trunk, scalp, or face, but can appear anywhere.

The outbreak is usually preceded by two to three days of severe pain in the area where the rash will appear. Sometimes a nerve supplying the eye may be affected; this can cause corneal inflammation. Occasionally a facial nerve is affected and can cause paralysis.

Antiviral medication may be used for shingles and can be helpful if it is started soon after the outbreak of the rash. Acetaminophen or ibuprofen can be used for pain relief, and lotions or soaks can be used to soothe the rash.

Shingles usually resolves within a week to 10 days after onset. However, it can often be a recurrent problem, since one attack does not provide immunity, and in people who are over 50 years old, the pain may continue for several months after the rash has cleared up. Pain that continues to affect people in this way is called postherpetic neuralgia; the condition can sometimes be relieved with anticonvulsants such as carbamazepine.

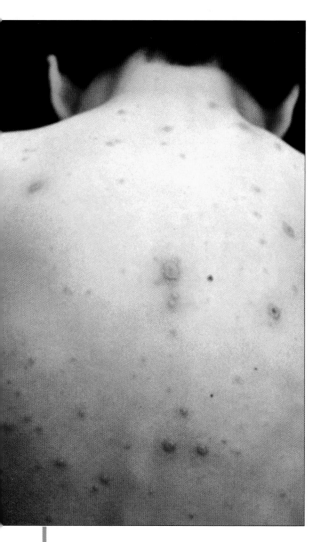

A chicken pox rash typically consists of many small fluid-filled blisters that are intensely itchy. Once the blisters are formed, they usually dry out and form scabs. The spots appear in crops for one to six days.

Prevention

Varicella-zoster immune globulin (VZIG) can be given to any high-risk person who has knowingly come into contact with a person with chicken pox in the contagious phase, even if they have been ill with chicken pox as a child. While it is rare that a person who has had chicken pox will catch it a second time, it is not unheard of. VZIG must be given within 96 hours of exposure to be effective. People who should call their physician and receive VZIG treatment if they have been exposed to chicken pox include women who are pregnant; individuals with immunodeficiencies caused by such diseases as HIV/AIDS or some autoimmune diseases such as rheumatoid arthritis, lupus, or inflammatory bowel disease; people who are receiving drugs that suppress the immune system, such as chemotherapy or corticosteroids; children with leukemia or lymphoma who have not been vaccinated; and newborns whose mothers develop chicken pox between five days prior to and two days after delivery.

Another common complication of chicken pox is shingles (varicella-zoster). After an outbreak of chicken pox has cleared, a little bit of the virus remains in the body for life, sitting dormant on a nerve root. Later in life (typically after age 50 but frequently earlier in people with autoimmune diseases) the virus is reactivated and sets off an episode of shingles. The trigger for reactivation may be the use of immunosuppressant drugs, a flare-up of an underlying autoimmune disease, or simply stress.

Vaccination

Today, throughout the industrialized world, chicken pox vaccine has become part of the routine vaccination program for children. The vaccine has been shown to be about 85 percent effective against all cases of chicken pox and essentially 100 percent effective against severe cases. Over its first decade of routine use, chicken pox vaccine has been responsible for greatly reducing the number of hospitalizations and deaths due to chicken pox. In 2007, the Centers for Disease Control recommended a second dose for lifetime protection.

Epidemiology

Prior to 1995, in a typical year, approximately 4 million Americans became ill with chicken pox, and approximately 11,000 people had to be hospitalized, according to the Centers for Disease Control and Prevention; 2 to 3 children in 100,000 needed hospitalization, as opposed to 8 in 100,000 teens and adults.

The death rate was approximately 1 in 100,000 for children aged 1 to 14 years, 2.7 in 100,000 for teens 15 to 19, and 25.2 in 100,000 for adults. Routine vaccination has cut the death rate to nearly zero.

Jon Zonderman
and Laurel Shader

See also
• AIDS • Herpes infections • Lupus

Chlamydial infections

Infections caused by *Chlamydia* bacteria are among the most common diseases worldwide. There are three main species of *Chlamydia* that cause diseases in humans. *Chlamydia trachomatis* causes the sexually transmitted disease commonly known as chlamydia; this species also causes the eye disease trachoma. *Chlamydia pneumoniae* causes the respiratory diseases bronchitis and pneumonia. *Chlamydia psittaci* causes the influenza-like illness psittacosis.

Chlamydial diseases are a major threat to human health. Of the three main species of *Chlamydia* that cause diseases in humans, *Chlamydia pneumoniae* is particularly common in children of school age. An estimated 10 percent of all cases of pneumonia each year are caused by this species of *Chlamydia*, and there is preliminary evidence that it may also be associated with cardiovascular disease. The species *Chlamydia psittaci* is carried by many birds, including parakeets and parrots. Humans can become infected by contact with bird feathers and droppings and also through being bitten by an infected bird. In humans the bacteria can cause psittacosis, a potentially serious disease that produces fever, cough, and a severe form of pneumonia. The species *Chlamydia trachomatis* can cause the eye disease trachoma, which may lead to blindness

An electron micrograph shows two Chlamydia trachomatis *bacteria. These parasitic bacteria survive by invading human cells and multiplying. Infection can cause both a serious eye disease and the STD commonly referred to as chlamydia.*

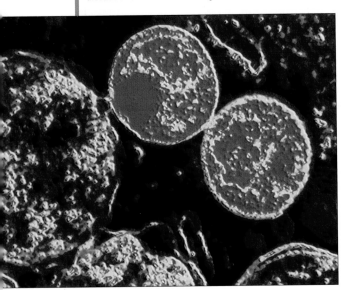

if it is not treated. However, more importantly, this species is the cause of the sexually transmitted disease (STD) generally known simply as chlamydia, which is the most common STD in the world, affecting millions more people than HIV, genital herpes, and gonorrhea combined.

Causes and risk factors for chlamydia

Chlamydia are unusual infectious agents. The bacteria behave more like viruses, invading target cells and multiplying inside them. For *Chlamydia trachomatis* the target cells are often those of the mucous membranes lining the genital tract, the mouth, and the rectum, which become infected during sexual intercourse. Untreated the infection can spread to other structures, such as the fallopian tubes in women or the prostate gland in men.

Chlamydia (the STD) is spread between adults by intimate sexual contact, and those at highest risk are people with multiple sex partners, especially if they have unprotected sex, whether vaginal, oral, or anal. Also at high risk are people with other STDs, such as gonorrhea. Babies of infected mothers are at risk of being infected during vaginal births. Chlamydial infection is not spread by casual contact such as sitting on a toilet or using someone else's towel.

Symptoms and complications for chlamydia

About 75 percent of women with chlamydia do not have any symptoms; in men, about 50 percent are symptom free. When symptoms do occur they usually appear one to three weeks after infection. The symptoms in both sexes include itching in the genital area and a burning sensation or pain while urinating. Men may also have a discharge from the penis.

Women have a higher risk of developing complications than do men. In women the infection may spread and cause pain in the lower abdomen, fever, and vaginal bleeding between menstrual periods. If the

KEY FACTS: CHLAMYDIA

Description

A sexually transmitted disease (STD).

Cause

Infection with the bacterium *Chlamydia trachomatis*.

Risk factors

Unprotected sexual intercourse (vaginal, oral, or anal) with an infected partner. An infected mother who gives birth vaginally may infect her baby.

Symptoms

Most women have no symptoms, but if the infection spreads it may cause pain in the lower abdomen, fever, and bleeding from the vagina. Men may have no symptoms or they may have a discharge from the penis and burning or itching during urination.

Diagnosis

Laboratory tests on genital secretions or urine.

Treatments

Antibiotics. All sexual partners must be treated to avoid repeat infections.

Pathogenesis

The bacteria invade the mucous membranes lining the genital tract, mouth, and rectum and reproduce inside the lining's cells. Untreated infections can spread, leading to pelvic inflammatory disease (PID) and infertility in women, or epididymitis and prostatitis in men.

Prevention

Sexual abstinence is the only certain method of prevention. For sexually active individuals, using latex condoms and regular health screenings.

Epidemiology

More than 900,000 cases are reported in the United States each year, but the actual number is probably closer to 3 million per year. Worldwide an estimated 90 million people are infected with *Chlamydia trachomatis* each year.

infection is not treated, pelvic inflammatory disease (PID) may develop. The infection may spread to the fallopian tubes (the tubes leading from the ovaries to the uterus), where it can cause scarring and obstruction. A fertilized ovum (egg) may then be trapped in the damaged tubes, causing a potentially life-threatening ectopic pregnancy. The blockage in the fallopian tubes may be so severe that the woman becomes infertile.

In men, the spread of infection may lead to epididymitis (inflammation of the epididymides, the coiled structures behind the testes in which sperm mature before ejaculation) or prostatitis (inflammation of the prostate gland).

Newborns infected by their mothers face two major risks. The bacteria may infect the eyes, which can cause conjunctivitis or even blindness if the infection is not treated. In areas of the world where medical treatment is not readily available, chlamydia is a leading cause of blindness. Babies are also at risk of pneumonia from untreated chlamydia.

Diagnosis, treatment, and prevention

The symptoms of chlamydia and gonorrhea are so similar that a medical examination by itself does not enable a physician to make a definite diagnosis. Furthermore, *Chlamydia trachomatis* does not grow in culture. Diagnosis may be made by taking a swab from the genital region or a urine sample and examining them under a microscope for the *Chlamydia* bacteria. Alternatively, a urine sample may be tested for the presence of chlamydial DNA (genetic material).

Treatment of chlamydia is with antibiotics, both for adults and newborns. In many cases medications are prescribed for chlamydia and gonorrhea because the two infections often occur simultaneously. Infected people should refrain from sexual intercourse until the treatment is finished to prevent infecting or reinfecting others. The sexual partners of those infected should also be tested for chlamydia and treated if necessary. A pregnant woman at risk of contracting an STD, that is, a woman who has multiple sex partners or who has had sex with someone who has multiple sex partners, should be tested for chlamydia before she gives birth.

Abstinence from sexual activity is the only certain way of preventing chlamydia, although the risk of infection is greatly reduced for partners in a monogamous relationship. Latex condoms are effective when used properly and consistently. Spermicides and douching are not effective and, in fact, they can increase a woman's risk of contracting chlamydia because they irritate the vaginal lining. Regular screening of sexually active people at risk of an STD can help limit the spread of the infection.

Chris Curran

See also
• Bronchitis • Pelvic inflammatory disease
• Pneumonia

Cholera

An acute, potentially fatal diarrheal disease caused by infection with the bacterium *Vibrio cholerae*, cholera is usually contracted by consuming food or water contaminated with infected feces. Cholera is rare in developed countries but still occurs in developing countries with poor sanitation and unclean drinking water.

Cholera has been largely eradicated in developed countries, mainly because of public health measures such as water purification and modern sewage systems. In developing countries, however, where clean water and sanitation measures may be lacking, the disease is still prevalent. In 2004 more than 100,000 cholera cases and at least 2,000 associated deaths were reported to the World Health Organization (WHO). However, there were only five cases in the United States that year, and all occurred in people who had contracted the disease elsewhere; none of those cases was fatal.

From time to time, major outbreaks of cholera occur, usually in parts of Africa, Asia, or South America, and during such outbreaks the fatality rate may be as high as 41 percent.

Causes and risk factors

Cholera is caused by infection with comma-shaped bacteria called *Vibrio cholerae*. Typically the bacteria are ingested in food or water that has been contaminated with infected feces. However, cholera bacteria also live naturally in some warm coastal seawater and can contaminate local fish and shellfish. Human infection can then occur through eating raw contaminated seafood. Direct person-to-person transmission of cholera is extremely rare.

In developed countries the risk of contracting cholera is almost nonexistent. Travelers to areas where a cholera outbreak is occurring are at a slight risk of infection, which can be minimized by following simple precautions when eating and drinking. People with conditions in which stomach acid production is reduced may be at increased risk of contracting cholera. Similarly, those who take acid-reducing medications, such as antacids, histamine receptor blockers, and proton pump inhibitors, are also at increased risk. People who live in areas without clean water or sanitation are at the greatest risk, and young children are particularly vulnerable. Refugee camps are common sites for cholera outbreaks.

Symptoms and signs

Some people infected with cholera bacteria have no symptoms, although these people are still a potential source of infection because the bacteria pass out of the body in their feces. When symptoms do occur they may appear anywhere between six hours and five days after the initial infection with the bacteria. The most common symptom of cholera is mild diarrhea, and in about 10 percent of cases the symptoms are severe, with profuse watery diarrhea and vomiting. In such cases fluid loss may be substantial, as much as a quart (about a liter) of fluid per hour, which can lead to rapid dehydration. The dehydration itself causes additional symptoms and signs, including a dry mouth and mucous membranes, thirst, lethargy, rapid heart rate, and leg cramps. If not treated, severe dehydration can be fatal within hours.

Diagnosis

Cholera can be diagnosed by culturing the bacteria from a sample of feces or from a rectal swab. Sometimes a blood sample is taken to test for the presence of antibodies against the cholera toxin. However, cholera is no longer routinely tested for in the United States.

Treatments

The most important treatment is the prompt replacement of fluid lost through diarrhea and vomiting. For mild or moderate dehydration, fluid replacement may be done by oral rehydration therapy. However, severe dehydration is a medical emergency that requires intravenous rehydration (infusing fluid directly into the bloodstream). Oral rehydration therapy simply involves drinking a solution consisting of a balanced mix of glucose (a type of sugar), salts (also sometimes known as electrolytes), and water. When diarrhea is severe, this solution is more effective than water alone, which passes through the intestine too quickly to be absorbed by the body tissues. The WHO glucose-based oral rehydration salts are premixed so that they can be easily prepared with water. The rehydration solution contains sodium, glucose, chloride, potassium, and citrate. For each quart (liter) of water, there are about eight teaspoons (40 ml) of sugar and one teaspoon (5 ml) of table salt. Sports drinks should not be used as rehydration solutions because they contain too much sugar in relation to salts.

The amount of oral rehydration solution that should be given depends on the degree of dehydration in the patient. For mildly or moderately dehydrated patients,

caregivers should initially give small amounts of rehydration solution (about one teaspoon) and then gradually increase the amount to about 1–2 fluid ounces per pound of body weight (50–100 ml/kg body weight) over a period of two to four hours. Small amounts of fluid are more easily given using a teaspoon, syringe, or medicine dropper. Travelers should consider including oral rehydration salts in their medical kits, because they can be used to treat dehydration from any cause, not just cholera.

In severe cases of cholera, antibiotics may also be given to reduce the amount and duration of diarrhea. Because antibiotics destroy the cholera bacteria, the drugs also prevent the infection from being passed on to others. Tetracycline is the antibiotic of choice, but the cholera bacteria have become resistant to it in some areas, and other antibiotics may be used instead. Alternatives include ciprofloxacin and erythromycin, although ciprofloxacin resistance is also beginning to emerge in some regions.

Pathogenesis

Typically, infection occurs when cholera bacteria are ingested with contaminated food or water. Ingesting as few as 100 individual bacteria can cause the disease. In most cases the bacteria are destroyed by the acid in the stomach. The bacteria that do survive, however, pass into the small intestine, where they adhere to the intestinal lining and produce a toxin called enterotoxin. This toxin disturbs the biochemical balance of the intestinal cells, causing them to leak profuse amounts of fluid and salts into the intestine, which results in diarrhea. The fluid loss from the diarrhea may lead to dehydration, which can be fatal if not treated quickly. Cholera bacteria pass out of the body in the watery feces and, if the feces comes into contact with food or drinking water, the bacteria may infect other people. The bacteria continue to be passed out in the feces for one to two weeks after infection, regardless of the severity of the disease.

Prevention

Public health measures, notably providing adequate sanitation and clean water that has not been contaminated by sewage, are the most important ways of preventing cholera. In areas of the world where there are no modern sewage or water treatment systems, then following simple recommended precautions when eating and drinking can help prevent cholera and other diarrheal diseases. When traveling to areas where cholera is present, the advice given by the

---

KEY FACTS

Description

An acute bacterial infection of the intestine, spread by water and food contaminated with infected feces.

Cause

Infection with the bacterium *Vibrio cholerae*.

Risk factors

Lack of clean water; lack of hygienic disposal of feces. Low stomach acidity.

Symptoms and signs

Mild to severe watery diarrhea; vomiting. Profuse diarrhea may lead to severe dehydration, which may be rapidly fatal. Some people infected with cholera bacteria have no symptoms.

Diagnosis

Culture of fecal or rectal swab samples; blood test for cholera toxin.

Treatments

Oral rehydration therapy or intravenous rehydration for dehydration. Antibiotics can reduce the amount and duration of diarrhea and can destroy the causative bacteria.

Pathogenesis

Bacteria adhere to cells that line the small intestine, where they secrete a toxin called enterotoxin. The enterotoxin causes an influx of fluid into the intestine, resulting in diarrhea.

Prevention

Public health measures such as providing safe water and adequate sanitation; avoiding contaminated food and water in high-risk areas. Vaccines against cholera are available in some countries but they are not recommended by the U.S. Centers for Disease Control.

Epidemiology

In 2004 there were just five cases of cholera in the United States, all contracted in other countries; worldwide there were more than 100,000 cases during the same year. Epidemics of cholera occur in some countries where there is poor sanitation or a lack of clean water.

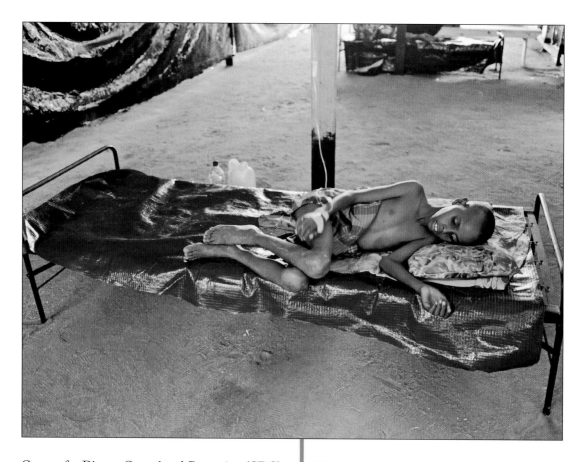

Centers for Disease Control and Prevention (CDC) states: "Boil it, cook it, peel it, or forget it." Food and water that may be contaminated, including raw vegetables and fruits that have been washed with untreated water, should not be eaten. Fruits with peels are generally safe to eat as long as they are hygienically peeled. Raw fish or shellfish such as oysters, clams, crabs, or mussels that originate from coastal waters where the cholera bacteria live should be avoided. If visiting or living in an area where cholera is endemic, only drink water that has been boiled or treated. Other safe beverages include tea and coffee made with boiled water and bottled drinks. The cholera bacteria can survive freezing, and therefore ice is safe only if it has been made from boiled or treated water. Temperatures above 160°F (about 70°C) kill the bacteria, and it is generally considered safe to eat freshly prepared food that has been thoroughly cooked. Foods and beverages that are bought from street vendors are best avoided altogether, but commercially prepared food from cholera-affected countries is generally considered safe. In areas where cholera is endemic, breastfeeding infants is recommended as breast milk can help protect them from severe diseases.

This boy is on an intravenous drip in an attempt to replace water and salts lost through diarrhea and vomiting brought on by cholera. Cholera is a common disease in developing countries, especially where the water is contaminated. It is also prevalent in refugee camps and disaster areas.

Although there are several vaccines against cholera, none is licensed for use in the United States, and the CDC does not recommend cholera vaccination for international travelers. Additionally, no country requires proof of cholera vaccination as a condition of entry or exit. The vaccines available in some countries include an old, injectable one and three newer oral vaccines. The old, injectable vaccine has only limited effectiveness; however, the oral vaccines are both effective and safe and are considered to be an additional public health measure. The World Health Organization is beginning to use the oral vaccines in some developing countries and refugee settlements.

Mary Quirk

See also
• Diarrhea and dysentery

Chronic fatigue syndrome

This condition is characterized by severe, long-standing fatigue. Other symptoms include sore throat, muscle and joint pain, tender lymph nodes, and headaches. There is no obvious cause for the syndrome; sometimes it develops after a stressful episode or a viral illness.

Chronic fatigue syndrome (CFS) is a disorder that causes many symptoms, including extreme and persistent fatigue, pain, headache, and sore throat. Estimates of the prevalence of CFS in populations have been highly variable, with some estimates being as high as 3 percent or more. Most CFS cases are initiated by a short-term stressor or trigger event, with viral or bacterial infection being the most common. Instead of recovering from such infections, some people become afflicted by CFS, an illness that is often life-long. Recovery from CFS occurs in only about 10 percent of cases, although partial recoveries are more frequent. Some experts have called CFS chronic fatigue and immune dysfunction syndrome (CFIDS); in the United Kingdom, CFS, or a similar condition, has been called myalgic encephalomyelitis (ME). The symptoms of CFS are more complex than just chronic fatigue, leading many to query the accuracy of its name.

Causes

Other short-term stressors are suspected to cause some cases of CFS, including toxoplasmosis, physical trauma, severe psychological stress, and exposure to toxins such as carbon monoxide, organophosphorus pesticides, and ciguatoxin. In other cases, no initiating short-term stressor has been identified. The eight stressors described here are all known to, or reported to, increase levels of nitric oxide in the body, so they may all act biochemically through a common mechanism even though the stressors are very diverse.

CFS often occurs with other illnesses or diseases, or both, including fibromyalgia, multiple chemical sensitivity, and post-traumatic stress disorder. Gulf War syndrome sufferers are reported to be afflicted to various extents by all four of these. Diseases that often occur with CFS and these other illnesses include asthma, intestinal hyperpermeability, tinnitus, irritable bowel syndrome, migraine headache, tinnitus, and such autoimmune diseases as lupus and rheumatoid arthritis. The occurrence of these disorders together, or comorbidity, suggests that they may share some or all of the same causes.

Risk factors

Being female is the best documented risk factor for CFS, with at least two-thirds of cases occurring in women. There is fairly extensive evidence for a genet-

---

KEY FACTS

Description

A complex illness causing profound chronic fatigue, multiorgan pain, cognitive dysfunction, post-exertional malaise, and unrefreshing sleep. Symptoms and signs of illness are variable.

Causes

It is important to distinguish between initial causes and the ongoing causes of chronic illness. Initial causes include various viral and bacterial infections and a variety of other short-term stressors. There is no consensus on the cause or causes of the chronic illness. Attempts to show that CFS is caused by a chronic infection or by an autoimmune disease have been unsuccessful, although chronic opportunistic infections do occur.

Risk Factors

Being female and certain genes are both important in increasing susceptibility.

Diagnosis

Diagnosis is currently based on the pattern of symptoms. There is no established specific biomarker for CFS.

Treatments

Treatments have ranged from those aimed at symptomatic relief to those aimed at lowering the presumed basic cause. Certain nutritional supplements as well as some conventional pharmaceuticals may both have considerable promise. Complex treatment protocols are perhaps the most promising.

Epidemiology

Estimates of prevalence in populations have been highly variable, with some estimates being as high as 3 percent or more of the population.

ic role in determining susceptibility, with certain specific genes being implicated. Cases can be initiated in various age ranges, but cases starting before puberty are relatively few. It used to be claimed that CFS mainly struck white, middle-class people, but that has been shown not to be the case. Prevalence is reported to be somewhat higher in some other racial groups and in individuals from lower socioeconomic classes.

Symptoms and signs

The symptoms and signs of illness are highly variable from one case to another. Some researchers have proposed that there may be several subsets of CFS with distinct causes (etiology) but thus far have been unable to clearly define what those distinct subsets may be or how they may differ etiologically. An alternative view is that the variability may be due to a vicious biochemical cycle that may be localized to different tissues in different cases, leading to this high variability.

Diagnosis

Diagnosis has been based on symptoms, often using the 1994 U.S. Centers for Disease Control (CDC) definition. This requires at least 6 months of unexplained profound fatigue accompanied by at least 4 of the following 8 symptoms: impaired memory or concentration; sore throat; tender lymph nodes; muscle pain; multijoint pain; headaches; unrefreshing sleep; and post-exertional malaise. Cognitive dysfunction, including learning and memory dysfunction and confusion, is common. Anxiety and depression are common symptoms. The more recent Canadian diagnostic criteria have considered a wide range of symptoms but have focused on post-exertional malaise as possibly the most characteristic symptom of CFS. Patients are said to have post-exertional malaise if when they exercise to excess (and excess may be very little in the more severe cases) the patients suffer from exacerbation of their whole range of symptoms for at least 24 hours.

Studies have shown that people with CFS have certain abnormal, or aberrant, biochemical pathways in the body, such as the pathways involved in oxidative stress (damage to cells and tissues caused by free radicals and other reactive chemicals) and energy production by mitochondria in body cells. People with CFS often have neuroendocrine dysfunction—problems with the interaction of nerve cells and hormones—particularly what is called hypothalamic-pituitary-adrenal (HPA) axis dysfunction. They often have immune dysfunction, particularly low natural killer (NK) cell function, and circulatory system dysfunction,

when the blood pressure is not controlled properly. Gastrointestinal problems are common in CFS, such as irritable bowel syndrome and intestinal permeability, with the latter often leading to food allergies.

A number of inflammatory markers have been reported to be elevated in comparisons of groups of CFS cases. Controls include levels of some inflammatory cytokines, C-reactive protein, neopterin, and nitric oxide. SPECT (single-photon emission computed tomography) brain scan studies are reported to often show aberrations. However, these markers are highly variable and often within normal ranges in individual CFS patients. They provide at best limited help in developing objective tests for diagnosis and are nonspecific, as they are also elevated in other diseases. However, they provide clear evidence for a physiological cause or set of causes for CFS. A specific biomarker for CFS is needed to aid diagnosis.

Treatments and prevention

Much of CFS treatment has focused on improving sleep patterns or using cognitive behavioral therapy. Four physicians have independently developed complex treatment protocols that are aimed at lowering etiologic mechanisms. These have focused on antioxidant therapy to lower oxidative stress, on restoring mitochondrial function, and in some cases, on restoring hormone balance or improving brain function by lowering excitotoxicity (excessive stimulation of certain receptors in the central nervous system). These protocols have used both numerous nutritional supplements as well as conventional pharmaceuticals. One treatment that has been used for more than three decades in many countries involves intramuscular injections of vitamin B_{12}, especially the hydroxocobalamin form of vitamin B_{12}, which is a potent nitric oxide scavenger. This treatment may act primarily by lowering nitric oxide levels. Two of the complex treatment protocols and the hydroxocobalamin injections have been tested in clinical trials and have shown significant efficacy. Other agents, such as magnesium and L-carnitine or acetyl-L-carnitine have been reported to be efficacious. In most cases, if agents produce improvement—and this is often contentious—it is only modest improvement.

No established prevention measures exist. Avoidance of stressors is expected to lower the incidence of CFS.

Martin L. Pall

See also
- Asthma • Irritable bowel syndrome • Lupus
- Migraine • Post-traumatic stress disorder

Cirrhosis of the liver

In cirrhosis, normal liver cells are damaged and replaced by scar tissue. The condition, which is irreversible, prevents the liver from functioning normally and can lead to serious problems in other parts of the body. Although there are many causes of cirrhosis, the two most common in the United States are chronic alcoholism and infection with the hepatitis C virus.

More than 25,000 people in the United States die each year from cirrhosis of the liver, according to the National Institutes of Health, and half of these deaths are caused by chronic alcoholism. Cirrhosis often develops over a prolonged period without causing symptoms and may not be detected until the condition is advanced enough to cause complications. The liver plays a vital role in a large number of body processes, and if this organ ceases to function a person cannot survive.

The term "cirrhosis" comes from the Greek word *kirrhosis*, meaning yellow—the color of the eyes and skin seen in advanced stages of the disease.

Causes and risk factors

Chronic excessive alcohol use is a major risk factor for cirrhosis. Heavy drinkers have the greatest chance of dying from the disease. Not all people who drink will develop cirrhosis, and some moderate drinkers can also develop the condition. It can take 10 or more years of heavy drinking for cirrhosis to develop, and many people are not aware that they have liver damage. About a third of all cases of cirrhosis are discovered only on autopsy.

Viral causes of cirrhosis are hepatitis types B, C, and D, which cause chronic inflammation of the liver. It may take as long as 20 to 30 years for cirrhosis to develop from hepatitis C. Heavy drinking in combination with hepatitis infection increases the risk of cirrhosis more than alcoholism alone. Some inherited diseases, like Wilson's disease (in which copper accumulates in the body), and hemochromatosis (excess absorption of iron from the diet), can also lead to cirrhosis. Nonalcoholic fatty liver disease (also called nonalcoholic steatohepatitis) is another cause of cirrhosis. One rare type of cirrhosis, called primary biliary cirrhosis, which destroys the small bile ducts in the liver, is a progressive autoimmune disease that is more likely to affect women; the causes of this disorder are unknown.

Symptoms and signs

The symptoms of cirrhosis vary according to the progression of the disease and can range from none to life threatening. In some people, the only signs of cirrhosis are abnormalities in blood tests called liver function tests, which can detect enzymes leaking from damaged liver cells. At an early stage of cirrhosis the liver may swell, but later scarring may cause it to shrink. Common symptoms are fatigue, loss of appetite, and weight loss. The palms of the hands may become red (called palmar erythema) from increased blood flow. The liver can lose its ability to make albumin, a protein that helps regulate the body's water balance, causing swelling of the legs (edema) and of the abdomen (ascites). The liver may no longer make key proteins needed for blood clotting, resulting in bruising and bleeding. The eyes and skin may be stained

KEY FACTS

Description

Replacement of healthy liver cells with scar tissue, damaging liver structure and function.

Causes and risk factors

In the United States the most common causes are chronic alcoholism and hepatitis C infection.

Symptoms and signs

Sometimes none; can include fatigue, weakness, loss of appetite, swelling of abdomen and legs, nausea, weight loss, bleeding, jaundice, coma.

Diagnosis

Physical exam, liver function (blood) tests, liver biopsy, CT scan, MRI scan, ultrasound, liver and spleen scans.

Treatments

Treatment of underlying disease. In severe cases, liver transplant.

Pathogenesis

Scarred liver cells interfere with normal liver and other body functions.

Prevention

Avoid alcohol and high-risk activities associated with hepatitis. Treat underlying diseases.

Epidemiology

More than 25,000 deaths in the United States each year.

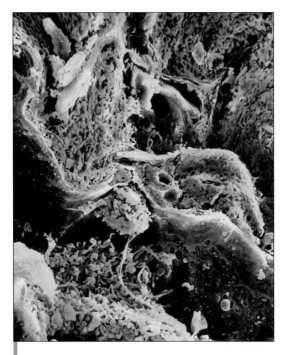

The liver cell (called a hepatocyte) seen in this electron micrograph shows damage caused by cirrhosis. Scar tissue, which appears as pale brown bands at the top left and center of the image, has developed, impairing liver function.

yellow as bilirubin, a yellow pigment usually broken down in the liver, accumulates in the blood.

Cirrhosis can affect the production of bile, a digestive fluid secreted by the liver. Bile salts can accumulate in the skin and whites of the eye, causing itching, and gallstones, which are largely made of bile pigments, can form in the gallbladder. Some people with cirrhosis develop insulin resistance, which is associated with type 2 diabetes. The destruction of normal liver function can lead to toxins collecting in the blood or brain, causing encephalopathy, a state of confusion that can progress to coma. Blood flow to the liver from the digestive tract can be slowed, and blood can back up in veins in the esophagus and stomach, increasing pressure in the portal vein, which carries blood to the liver. This pressure, called portal hypertension, causes enlarged blood vessels (varices), which become fragile and can burst, with life-threatening bleeding.

Diagnosis

Together with any obvious symptoms and a physical exam, cirrhosis may be diagnosed by liver function tests, as well as a CT (computed tomography) scan or MRI (magnetic resonance imaging). A liver scan using a radioactive substance that collects in the liver, or ultrasound, may also be helpful. A liver biopsy (tissue sample) confirms the diagnosis.

Prevention and treatment

Although cirrhosis is not reversible, most deaths from the disease are preventable. Treatment is used to halt the progression of liver tissue damage and avoid the complications that develop in the later stages of cirrhosis. When alcohol-related cirrhosis is treated by halting consumption of alcohol, survival rates increase. A vaccine for hepatitis B is 95 percent effective in preventing chronic infection from developing, but there is no vaccine for hepatitis C. People who already have viral hepatitis may be given drug treatment. A special diet can minimize toxins from the digestive tract and reduce swelling in the legs and abdomen. Drugs to reduce blood pressure may help control portal hypertension. Special injections may help stop bleeding from swollen blood vessels. In severe cases of cirrhosis, a liver transplant may be considered.

Pathogenesis

Damage to liver cells in cirrhosis can be caused by direct injury, such as occurs in hepatitis, or by indirect injury, when there is obstruction or inflammation of the bile ducts. Scarred liver tissue can block the flow of blood through the liver from the stomach, intestines, and spleen, causing portal hypertension. Waste materials normally processed by the liver, including those from food breakdown, can cause ammonia and other toxins to build up in the blood or brain. About 5 percent of people with cirrhosis develop hepatocellular carcinoma, which is primary cancer of the liver.

Epidemiology

In the United States, cirrhosis is the seventh most common cause of death from disease. The death rates are almost twice as high in men as in women. With a decrease in alcohol consumption in the general population, death rates from cirrhosis have fallen. However, an increase in hepatitis C infections, predicted to peak by 2015, may affect these death rates, even if alcohol consumption remains at its present level or decreases.

Ramona Jenkin

See also
- Alcohol-related disorders • Cancer, liver
- Diabetes • Gallstone • Hemochromatosis
- Hepatitis infections

Cold, common

The common cold is the world's most widespread infectious disease, accounting for more than 1 billion cases per year in the United States alone. There is no specific treatment for the common cold, nor is there a vaccine. Nevertheless, about 25 million Americans seek medical attention annually for treatment of symptoms caused by this viral illness.

The common cold is a disease of the membranes lining the nasopharynx, the air passages leading from the nose to the back of the throat. Although not in itself a serious illness—it usually cures itself in a week or less—it has a huge impact on productivity. It is estimated that in the United States 23 million days are lost from work every year due to colds, which account for about 40 percent of lost time from work overall. Among U.S. children, colds account for more than 20 million days of lost school days.

More than 200 different viruses cause symptoms of the common cold, and there is generally little point in testing for a particular virus. A diagnosis is made by noting the symptoms, including the absence of certain symptoms such as a high fever, which might indicate influenza instead of a cold.

Causes, risk factors, and epidemiology

A cold happens when viruses attack the cells lining the nose and upper throat. The viruses find their target cells by identifying specific molecules on the cells' surface. Of the many viruses that cause the common cold, the most important are the rhinoviruses (from the ancient Greek *rhinos*, which means "nose"). There are at least 100 different types of rhinoviruses; among them they cause about 40 percent of colds.

Colds follow a seasonal pattern. They usually occur in the fall and winter, although the belief that a cold climate increases the risk of contracting the common cold has never been validated. There is also no proof that going outdoors with wet hair or getting chilled leads to the common cold. However, the humidity of the air may be a factor: most common cold-producing viruses survive better in low humidity, which is more common in the winter months. Low humidity also has a drying effect on the nasal passages, making infection more likely.

Common cold viruses spread very easily. Infection occurs through direct contact with mucous secretions, by breathing in water droplets containing the virus, or from contaminated surfaces. Viruses remains infectious for two hours on human skin and for several hours on inanimate objects. Children are especially susceptible since they have had less time to develop immunity to cold viruses. Also, typical child behaviors such as sharing toys and touching objects with hands contaminated by mucous secretions make transmission more likely. In the United States, preschool children have as many as seven episodes per year, while adults have two to three episodes per year.

Symptoms

Symptoms of a common cold start to appear within 24 to 72 hours of infection and include a runny or stuffy nose, sneezing, and often a mildly irritated throat. Sore throat is followed by cough, while some people may complain of a mild headache. Fever in adults, if

When someone with a cold sneezes, he or she sprays out tiny droplets containing the virus. Other people can catch the cold by breathing in the infected droplets.

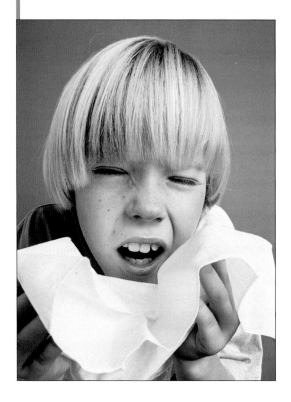

present, is usually low-grade, with temperatures of less than 102°F (39°C). The coughing and sneezing of a cold helps spread the cold viruses to new hosts.

Pathogenesis

Viruses enter via the nose, eyes (spreading down the tear ducts), or mouth before invading the cells of the nasopharynx. As viruses begin to reproduce in their target cells, the body's immune response is triggered. White blood cells and other agents of the body's immune system congregate at the infected sites. This response is largely responsible for symptoms such as swollen nasal passages and discharge of mucus. The body also starts producing specific antibodies against the invading virus, and recovery is usually quick if there are no complications.

Colds tend to be more serious where individuals live in crowded conditions, are malnourished, or have underlying chronic health conditions such as emphysema, diabetes, or heart disease. Younger individuals and premature and low birth weight babies are also at higher risk.

Sometimes a common cold leads to complications such as bacterial sinusitis, pneumonia, or middle ear infections in children. Worsening of asthma may also occur. If cold symptoms last longer than one week, and especially if they are accompanied by a new fever, it is likely that a complication has developed. Contrary to a common belief, a discharge of colored mucus from the nose does not generally mean a bacterial infection.

Treatments

At present there is no cure for the common cold, although antiviral drugs are under development that may be able to shorten its duration in the future. Antibiotics are only of use against secondary bacterial infections, not the cold itself. Most treatments therefore concentrate on relieving symptoms. Rest is important, and inhaling humidified air may also help. Drugs commonly used include mild analgesics (painkillers) such as acetaminophen or aspirin, antihistamines, cough suppressants, decongestants, and medications called expectorants that make mucus easier to cough up. The evidence in favor of popular remedies such as zinc, vitamin C, and echinacea is not conclusive, and zinc may also have undesired side effects.

Most of the above treatments are not appropriate for treating children, because of potential side effects. Aspirin and over-the-counter remedies containing

KEY FACTS

Description
A short-lived viral infection of the upper respiratory system.

Cause
Infection with any of a variety of viruses.

Risk factors
Children are more likely to catch colds and to have them for longer. Poor health makes complications more likely.

Symptoms
Stuffy or runny nose, sneezing, coughing, sore throat.

Diagnosis
By observation of the symptoms.

Treatments
Rest; drugs to alleviate symptoms and to treat complications.

Pathogenesis
Viruses invade via the nose, eyes, or mouth, and attack the cells lining the nasal passages (nasopharynx).

Prevention
Avoiding contact with sufferers; covering coughs and sneezes; washing hands; avoiding touching eyes, nose, and mouth.

Epidemiology
Easily transmitted: around 1 billion cases in the United States per year.

aspirin are now treated with caution because of links with a disorder in children called Reye's syndrome, which affects the brain and the liver.

Prevention

A vaccine against the common cold is not possible because it is caused by so many different viruses. Prevention relies upon frequent hand washing, avoiding the touching of one's mouth, nose, and eyes, and avoiding the sharing of drinking glasses and eating utensils. If possible, it is wise to avoid being around someone who is ill with the common cold. Those already infected should cover their sneezes and coughs to reduce the number of infectious airborne particles and should also wash their hands frequently.

Rita Washko

See also
• Allergy and sensitivity • Croup • Influenza
• Sinusitis

Colitis, ulcerative

Ulcerative colitis is one of two types of inflammatory bowel diseases and occurs most frequently in industrialized countries. It can be the cause of much pain and suffering for affected patients, in part related to reticence in discussing digestive diseases. The cause of ulcerative colitis remains unknown, but there have been several recent advances in treatments.

The precise cause of ulcerative colitis is not yet known, but it is believed to have a genetic component. The most widely accepted theory holds that susceptible individuals have a defect in the immune system that causes them to mount an inappropriate response to normal gut bacteria (that unaffected individuals find innocuous). This response results in the recruitment of inflammatory cells and the release of substances (called cytokines) that injure the cells that line the colon, causing ulceration. The resulting damage to the barrier between the colon and its contents allows additional bacterial products to access the immune system, further perpetuating inflammation.

Symptoms and diagnosis

Ulcerative colitis is a chronic disease usually marked by periods in which the disease is silent, interspersed with acute attacks that can last from weeks to months. Almost all patients experience diarrhea, which can be bloody. Other frequent symptoms include abdominal pain, weight loss, and in severe cases, fever. The primary diagnostic tool is colonoscopy with biopsy of the colonic lining. There is a sharp demarcation between involved and uninvolved segments of the colon. The lining becomes reddened and swollen, and ulcers are seen both through the endoscope and under the microscope. The tissue also becomes filled with many inflammatory cell types. It is important to distinguish between ulcerative colitis and colonic inflammation caused by an infectious organism, as well as Crohn's disease, the other form of inflammatory bowel disease.

Treatments

Anti-inflammatory drugs are used to control the disease but may have side effects. Newer biological agents block the inflammatory effects of cytokines. Antidiarrheal drugs and analgesics may also be helpful. In some patients, the colon may ultimately be removed (colectomy). This surgery is curative, and a pouch may be constructed from a portion of the small intestine to allow the patient to regain continence and avoid the use of an ostomy device. Colectomy also frees sufferers from an increased risk of colon cancer.

Kim Barrett

KEY FACTS

Description
A chronic inflammation of the large intestine that results in ulceration of the intestinal lining.

Causes
Unknown but is thought to involve an inappropriate interaction between the patient's immune system and bacteria that reside normally in the colon.

Risk factors
A family history of the disease is the best known risk factor. Nonsmokers and those who have quit have an increased risk of developing ulcerative colitis.

Symptoms
Abdominal pain, weight loss, and diarrhea. Children with the disease may have delayed development. Ulcerative colitis is also associated with an increased risk of colon cancer.

Diagnosis
Colonoscopy and a biopsy of the tissue lining the colon. Imaging and blood tests may also be used.

Treatments
Anti-inflammatory drugs and symptomatic therapies are the mainstay of treatment. For severe disease, surgical removal of the colon is curative.

Pathogenesis
Immune and inflammatory cells inappropriately damage the body's own tissue, injuring the lining of the intestine and setting up a vicious cycle in which more damage can occur.

Prevention
No known prevention, although many patients resolve their symptoms spontaneously at least for certain periods of time.

Epidemiology
The highest rates occur in industrialized, Western countries, with the peak onset of disease between ages 15 and 25. Some ethnic groups (for example, Jewish origin) have increased incidence.

See also
• Cancer, colorectal • Crohn's disease • Diarrhea and dysentery

137

Color blindness

Also known as color vision deficiency, color blindness is a group of disorders in which individuals cannot perceive or have difficulty distinguishing specific colors. Red-green color blindness is the most common type; complete color blindness is rare. Color blindness is usually inherited but may also result from diseases that affect the retina or from exposure to chemicals. Impaired color vision may sometimes be associated with aging.

The human eye perceives light using two different types of specialized cells (rods and cones) in the retina at the back of the eye. Rods distinguish black and white and provide low-light vision. The less prevalent cones are responsible for color vision. Human color vision is trichromatic: we can detect the three colors red, green, and blue. There are three varieties of cone cells, each variety containing a pigment that is sensitive to one of the three colors. The pigments in turn contain proteins called opsins, with one type of opsin for each of the three colors. If an opsin is defective or missing, the result is a color vision deficiency, commonly called color blindness.

Types, causes, and risk factors

Most cases of color blindness are inherited and result from a defective gene. The most common forms of color blindness involve the red and green opsins. Red color blindness (called protanopia) and green color blindness (deuteranopia) both result from defective opsin genes on the X chromosome (female sex chromosome) and are called sex-linked recessive genetic disorders, found more commonly in males. A man may inherit a defective opsin gene from a color-blind mother or from a mother with normal color vision but who carries a defective gene. A woman must inherit a defective gene from each parent to be color blind.

Individuals with blue color blindness (called tritanopia) have difficulty distinguishing blue from yellow and sometimes blue from green. This form of color blindness is rare, affecting fewer than 1 in 500 people in the United States. It is caused by a defective opsin gene on chromosome seven and can be inherited from either parent, who must also have the condition. It is equally common in men and women.

The inability to perceive any color is called achromatopsia, or rod monochromatism. This condition is rare in the United States, affecting about 1 in 30,000 people. In a few isolated populations, however, such as on the island of Pingelap in the Pacific Ocean, the incidence is as high as 1 in 10 of the population. The high rate is the result of unusual circumstances. In the 18th century most of the population was wiped out by

KEY FACTS

Description

Inability to perceive colors correctly because of problems with cones (color-sensing cells) in the retina (light-sensitive layer of the eye). There are several forms of the condition, depending on the types of cones affected.

Causes

Inheritance of a defective gene, a disease that affects the retina, certain toxins, or medications.

Risk factors

For inherited forms, a family history of color blindness. Factors for acquired forms include various diseases, such as glaucoma and diabetes mellitus, exposure to toxins, taking certain medications, and aging.

Symptoms

Inability to perceive or distinguish specific colors or a complete lack of color vision.

Diagnosis

Color-vision test carried out by a physician or optometrist.

Treatments

There is no treatment for color blindness.

Pathogenesis

Inherited forms affect both eyes, are present at birth, and do not change over time. Acquired forms may affect only one eye and may change in severity over time.

Prevention

Inherited color blindness cannot be prevented. Acquired forms may be prevented by limiting the severity of the associated disease or exposure to the associated substance.

Epidemiology

In the United States about 3.8 million people (1.3 percent of the population) have a form of color blindness. In those of northern European descent, an estimated 8 percent of males and less than 1 percent of females are affected; the rate is lower in other ethnic groups. About 1 in 33,000 individuals has complete loss of color vision.

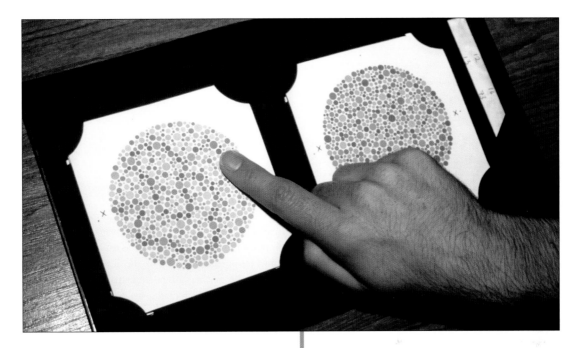

Color blindness is diagnosed by means of a simple test often carried out during childhood. Here, a pattern of green dots is concealed within a random group of colored dots. A person with defective color vision is unable to distinguish the pattern.

a typhoon. Several of the survivors are thought to have been carriers of the defective gene that causes achromatopsia, and this gene became more common as the survivors repopulated the island. In addition to complete color blindness, achromatopsia also causes extreme sensitivity to light. The condition is inherited through recessive genes, so a person must inherit two copies of the gene, one from each parent, to be affected.

In addition to being inherited, color blindness may also be acquired. Some eye diseases, such as glaucoma (raised pressure inside the eye) and macular degeneration (progressive degeneration of the macula, the most sensitive area of the retina) can cause the condition. However, diseases that can cause color blindness are not restricted to those of the eye. Liver diseases, diabetes mellitus, multiple sclerosis, nervous system disorders, Alzheimer's disease, and leukemia may also produce color blindness. Exposure to toxic chemicals, such as lead-based compounds, carbon monoxide, and some substances used industrially, can produce color blindness, especially after long-term exposure. In some cases of substance-induced color blindness, normal vision may eventually return after exposure to the causative substance has stopped. Certain medications are also associated with color blindness. Normal aging may result in an impaired ability to distinguish certain colors and therefore may be considered to cause color blindness. Unlike inherited forms of the condition, acquired color blindness may affect only the vision of one eye and can change in severity over time.

Diagnosis, treatment, and prevention

The condition is diagnosed with color vision tests called pseudoisochromatic tests. The most common forms of these tests are the Ishihara test and the American Optical/Hardy, Rand, and Ritter (AO/H.R.R.) test. Each test utilizes a series of pictures that consist of a background of colored dots, usually red, green, yellow, or blue, and a central area with a pattern of colored dots that resemble a number. A person with normal vision is able to see the number among the background dots, whereas somebody with a color vision deficiency cannot see the number. The tests are usually carried out by a physician or optometrist and may be done at any age but are often done in childhood if color blindness is suspected.

Color blindness cannot be treated, and inherited forms cannot be prevented. Substance-induced color blindness may be prevented by limiting exposure, and color blindness associated with an underlying disease may be prevented by treating the disease.

Michael Windelspecht

See also
• Glaucoma • Macular degeneration

Coma

A coma is a state of deep unconsciousness resulting from injury or other damage to the brain. Unlike a sleeping person, someone in a coma is totally unresponsive and cannot be roused by noise or a physical stimulus. The length of time a coma lasts, and whether there is full recovery afterward, varies enormously depending on what caused the coma and how the sufferer is managed.

Many circumstances can lead to a person going into a coma, from head injuries to the effects of toxins. The common factor is that there is some kind of damage to or interference with the deeper parts of the brain that control wakefulness and alertness. Coma therefore differs from the so-called vegetative state, in which the brain still shows the basic cycle of sleeping and waking even though the patient is not conscious because of damage elsewhere in the brain. Coma also differs from brain death, when all electrical activity of the nerve cells in the brain has stopped permanently.

Causes

Causes of coma are numerous and include severe head injuries, strokes, epileptic seizures, cancer, infections of the brain, drug overdoses, poisoning, and some forms of heart disease. Causes that involve an imbalance of the body's metabolism include a malfunctioning thyroid gland and liver and kidney disorders, leading to accumulations of toxins in the body, and side effects of diabetes.

Pathogenesis

The brain is very sensitive to small changes in its own environment. Direct physical injury to the head can cause bleeding, which increases pressure on the brain. Lack of oxygen, low blood sugar or hypoglycemia, and low sodium in the blood are all examples of metabolic changes that can cause coma. Awareness, or being conscious, is linked with different regions in the brain, so damage to one or more of these areas can cause varying levels of consciousness, including coma.

A person with injuries can continue to heal while in a coma, and the coma may even act as a phase of recovery after a severe brain injury. Comas tend not to persist indefinitely. Many coma patients who survive begin a gradual recovery within one to two weeks.

Others may evolve to a vegetative state, which is described as persistent if it lasts longer than one month. If the vegetative state still exists 12 months after a physical injury, or three months after a nonphysical injury such as poisoning, it is considered to be permanent and irreversible. When the injury is very severe, the coma may end in death.

Diagnosis

A person admitted to hospital in a coma is typically a medical emergency, and urgent tests may be needed to pinpoint the cause of the coma as quickly as possible. Information about a person's medical history, such as whether he or she suffers from diabetes or epilepsy, can be vital to a quick diagnosis. A neurologist (physician specializing in the nervous system) will usually check whether the body's natural reflexes are working properly or not, which helps assess how much the brain has been damaged. Blood tests may be carried

---

KEY FACTS

Description

A state of deep unconsciousness from which a person cannot be wakened.

Causes and risk factors

Many causes, including head injury, stroke, epilepsy, heart failure, diabetes, drug overdoses and poisoning, and infections.

Symptoms and signs

Cannot be awakened, even with a painful stimulus or loud commands.

Diagnosis

Various tests and examinations to determine the underlying cause. Depth of coma is usually assessed using the Glasgow Coma Scale (GCS).

Treatments

Coma is a medical emergency. The underlying cause needs to be treated, and the patient provided with supportive care.

Pathogenesis

Disruption of brain pathways responsible for wakefulness, without which consciousness is not possible.

Prevention

Depends on cause. For example, many physical injuries to the brain can be prevented by measures such as wearing a seat belt, using child safety seats, and wearing appropriate helmets during athletic activities.

out to check for the presence of toxins, or of disturbances to the body's natural metabolism. Sometimes the basic cause of coma is obvious, such as when a person has suffered head injuries in an accident, but for a detailed picture of the damage the brain has suffered, imaging techniques such as CT scans and MRI may be used.

For assessing and describing the depth of the coma itself, various scoring systems are used, based on how the patient is responding. By far the most common scoring system used worldwide is the Glasgow Coma Scale (see box, below). Scoring systems can help health professionals communicate the medical condition of a patient easily and consistently. The scoring can be done every day, or more often, so that the progress of a person in a coma can also be assessed.

Treatment

As with diagnosis, treatment is usually a matter of urgency, especially at first. Some states of coma may interfere with basic reflexes and motor functions such as breathing, so the patient may need to be put on a ventilator. The patient requires a full evaluation to determine and treat the underlying cause: quick action can save lives as well as help prevent permanent disabilities afterward. Coma patients need ongoing supportive care, including nutrition, water, and constant bed care.

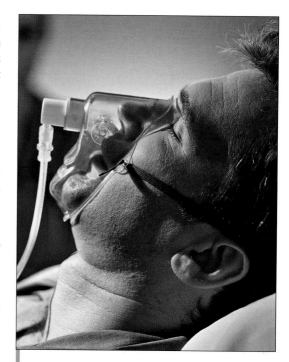

A coma patient has a ventilator to assist breathing because his breathing is faulty. Sometimes people in deep comas maintain their ability to breathe and perform reflex actions such as blinking.

GLASGOW COMA SCALE

The Glasgow Coma Scale (GCS) provides a common language for describing states of coma and decreased consciousness. It was developed in the early 1970s by physicians Graham Teasdale and Bryan Jennett of Glasgow, Scotland, as a simple and easy way to evaluate how deeply impaired a patient's level of consciousness is during and after a brain injury. The GCS is based on three categories: eye opening, verbal response, and responses involving movement, and whether these responses happen spontaneously or from painful or other stimuli. Each of the three categories is scored separately using a points sytem, and the three totals are added up to give an overall score ranging from 3 to 15.

Patients are classified as follows: mild, GSC 13–15; moderate, GSC 9–12; and severe, GCS 3–8. In severe GCS, or coma, there is no eye opening, no ability to follow commands by movement, and an inability to utter any words.

Epidemiology and prevention

Coma and related types of brain damage account for more than 73,000 hospital admissions in the United States each year. Preventing the underlying causes of coma, like accidents that result in brain injury, or uncontrolled diabetes or thyroid disease, stroke, infections or poisonings, is critical.

One cause of coma is traumatic brain injury (TBI). There are 1.4 million TBIs of varying severity (only a portion result in coma) in the United States each year. Many TBIs could be prevented by wearing seat belts and using child safety seats in motor vehicles, and by fitting window guards in homes to prevent young children from falling out.

Males are about twice as likely to suffer from a TBI, and the two age groups most at risk are between 0 to 4 and 15 to 19 years.

Ramona Jenkin

See also
- Diabetes • Epilepsy • Head injury
- Stroke and related disorders
- Thyroid disorders

Conjunctivitis

In this condition the conjunctiva, a transparent membrane in the eye, is inflamed and red. There is discharge from the eye and swelling of the eyelid.

Also known as pink eye, conjunctivitis is an infection of the conjunctiva, the membrane that lines the inside of the eyelids and covers the white of the eye. Conjunctivitis is a common condition and usually causes no threat to vision. *Chlamydia trachomatis* infection, however, causes a form of conjunctivitis that is the most significant cause of preventable vision loss in the world, especially in the Middle East, including northern Africa.

Causes

The most common types of conjunctivitis are viral, allergic, and bacterial. Viral conjunctivitis is usually associated with an upper respiratory infection, common cold, or sore throat spread by coughs and sneezes or by contact with contagious viruses. Allergic conjunctivitis occurs more often among children, adults with hay fever, and people with intolerance to cosmetics, perfume, deposits on contact lenses, or drugs. Irritant conjunctivitis is caused by chemicals such as those in chlorine, soap, air pollutants, or natural toxins, such as ricin.

Symptoms and diagnosis

Viral conjunctivitis causes a watery discharge, a gritty sensation, redness, sensitivity to bright lights, or infection in one eye, which may spread to the other eye. Allergic conjunctivitis usually affects both eyes, causing itching, tearing, a ropey thin discharge, and swollen eyelids. Bacterial conjunctivitis involves a heavy discharge, sticking together of the eyelids, swelling of conjunctiva, redness, tearing, irritation, and foreign body sensation. The incubation period is 5 to 12 days before symptoms begin. Irritant conjunctivitis is painful; there is redness, but no discharge and itching.

Diagnosis is by a routine eye exam using a slit lamp microscope and taking cultures to determine the type of bacteria causing the infection.

Risk factors and prevention

Viral conjunctivitis is highly contagious and is spread by droplet and hand-to-eye inoculation. To avoid cross-contamination of the noninfected eye, hand washing is essential after contact with the infected eye. No sharing of shaving utensils, washcloths, towels, pillowcases, or eye cosmetics should be done with a suspected or confirmed contagious person.

Treatments

Viral conjunctivitis lasts one week in mild cases and up to three weeks in severe cases. Although there is no cure for viral conjunctivitis, cool compresses and artificial tears may give symptomatic relief. Bacterial conjunctivitis requires treatment with topical antibiotics for seven to ten days. Chlamydia infection may require oral antibiotics and topical medication for 10 to 14 days. The use of cool compresses and artificial tears relieves discomfort in mild cases of allergic conjunctivitis. Conjunctivitis due to burns, toxins, and chemicals require washout with saline beneath both eyelids and may also require topical steroids.

Isaac Grate

KEY FACTS

Description

An infection of the membrane of the eye.

Causes

Viral or bacterial infection, allergic reaction, irritants.

Symptoms

Viral infections cause watery discharge, redness, irritation, sensitivity to light. Allergic irritations affect both eyes, with intensive itching, tearing, discharge, and swollen eyelids. Bacterial infections in one eye initially, heavy discharge, redness, tearing, irritation, eyelids sticking together.

Diagnosis

Eye examination with a slit lamp microscope.

Risk factors

Spread by cough droplets, hand-to-eye inoculation, and cross contamination, such as sharing towels, cosmetics.

Treatments

Cool compresses and artificial tears for viral infections. Topical antibiotics for 7–10 days for bacterial conjunctivitis. For allergic conjunctivitis, compresses, artificial tears, and antihistamine drops.

See also
• Allergy and sensitivity

COPD

Chronic obstructive pulmonary disease, or COPD, is really two related diseases: chronic (long-term) bronchitis and emphysema. Both of these diseases cause airflow obstruction and progressive lung damage, and both are usually related to smoking. COPD results in irreversible structural change in the lungs, which blocks the airflow and makes breathing more difficult. Frequently, chronic bronchitis and emphysema coexist in the same person and either one may be dominant. There is no cure for COPD, but its symptoms can be alleviated.

It is estimated by the National Institutes of Health that as many as 24 million people in the United States have COPD, although as many as half of these cases may be undiagnosed. COPD is the fourth leading cause of death in the United States, after cardiovascular disease, cancer, and stroke. The condition causes 120,000 deaths a year. About 85 percent of cases result from smoking tobacco. Cigarette smokers are 10 times more likely to contract and die from COPD than people who have never smoked. Over a 20-year period (1980–2000) the death rate from COPD in the United States grew faster in women because of an increasing number of women who had taken up smoking. According to the Centers for Disease Control and Prevention there has also been a decrease in mild and moderate cases of COPD in 25- to 54-year-olds because of the overall decrease in smokers in the United States since the 1960s. Most people with COPD are at least 40 years old when symptoms begin to develop, and the disease is most commonly found in those over 65 years of age. However, COPD can develop in younger people.

COPD limits normal daily activities in more than half the people it affects, and the total annual health care costs for COPD are greater than $32 billion.

Causes and risk factors

Cigarette smoking is overwhelmingly the main cause of COPD. Other risk factors for the disease include smoking a pipe, cigars, or other tobaccos, air pollution, secondhand smoke, genetic factors, and frequent respiratory infections during childhood, although this last risk is less of a problem during the age of antibiotics. Occupational exposure to dusts and chemicals is thought to account for as much as 15 percent of COPD cases. Industries with a higher risk for COPD include rubber, plastics, textile mills, agriculture, and construction. In developing countries indoor air quality may be a more significant risk factor for COPD than in the United States. In a small number of cases emphysema is caused by a rare genetic disorder called alpha-1-antitrypsin deficiency, in which there is a mutation of a gene called P1. In people who carry the alpha1-antitrypsin deficiency gene and who also smoke, emphysema progresses at a quicker rate.

143

Symptoms

In the early stages of COPD there may be no symptoms. As the disease progresses, patients experience difficulty breathing and fatigue. This may be mild at first, and only with exertion; later in the disease, they may be short of breath during simple daily activities, like showering or dressing. Later in the disease, patients have difficulty breathing even at rest. If chronic bronchitis is present, cough and sputum will also be prominent symptoms.

Diagnosis

A thorough history, including symptoms (difficulty breathing and cough), history of smoking, and information about allergies and exposure at work and at home is important. Physical examination, chest X-rays, and arterial blood gases, in which blood extracted from an artery is tested for levels of oxygen and carbon dioxide, are other tests useful in diagnosing and treating patients with COPD. Pulmonary function tests (PFTs), which measure the pattern and degree of lung dysfunction, confirm the diagnosis. The history, physical exam, X-ray, and PFTs help distinguish COPD from other causes of cough and shortness of breath, including asthma, pneumonia, and heart disease.

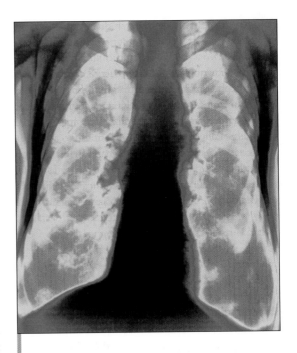

This X-ray shows the effects of COPD on the lungs. The yellow areas indicate fibrosis, where the lungs have become scarred by inflammation. The red areas show where emphysema has destroyed the alveoli, reducing gas exchange.

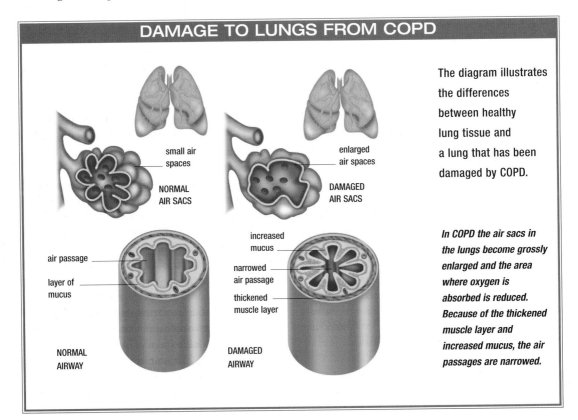

DAMAGE TO LUNGS FROM COPD

small air spaces

NORMAL AIR SACS

enlarged air spaces

DAMAGED AIR SACS

air passage

layer of mucus

NORMAL AIRWAY

increased mucus

narrowed air passage

thickened muscle layer

DAMAGED AIRWAY

The diagram illustrates the differences between healthy lung tissue and a lung that has been damaged by COPD.

In COPD the air sacs in the lungs become grossly enlarged and the area where oxygen is absorbed is reduced. Because of the thickened muscle layer and increased mucus, the air passages are narrowed.

SPIROMETER

During the 1840s, the English physician John Hutchinson (1811–1861) devised the first spirometer—a pneumatic device used to measure flow of air in and out of the lungs. About the size of an adult male, Hutchinson's spirometer was a calibrated bell that was inverted in water and captured exhaled air from the lungs. Hutchinson collected data from more than 1,100 men of various occupations, including sailors, policemen, royal horse guards, gentlemen, craftsmen, and paupers. He determined the lung capacity of each man—how much air could be voluntarily expelled from the man's chest. From his observations, Hutchinson concluded that disease in the chest limited the lung's normal capacity, as did abnormal curvature of the spine.

Modern spirometers—based on the principles of Hutchinson's invention—are small, handheld devices that are used for the diagnosis and monitoring of the progression and response to the treatments of various lung diseases such as COPD and asthma. Spirometers also record the rate at which air is inhaled and exhaled, as well as the total volume.

PFTs include several tests of lung function. One of these, spirometry, involves having the patient breathe into a machine that measures the depth of breathing and how quickly air can be inhaled and exhaled. Spirometry can detect COPD early, before symptoms arise, and can distinguish COPD from other lung diseases. PFTs can also be used to monitor the effectiveness of medicines used in treating COPD.

Pathogenesis

COPD is caused by inflammatory processes inside the lungs that damage the airways (chronic bronchitis), the air sacs (emphysema), or both. New research has shown that components of cigarette smoke not only cause inflammation, but also poison cells that protect the lung against inflammation. In chronic bronchitis, inflammation and scarring narrow the bronchial airways, making it harder to breathe. The number and size of mucus-producing cells increase, and there is progressive trouble clearing mucus from the airways, which causes a chronic cough.

The airways end in small sacs called alveoli, which are like tiny balloons that inflate and deflate with each breath. Tiny capillaries filled with blood run along these air sacs, and the exchange of oxygen and carbon dioxide takes place there. In emphysema these sacs become enlarged, thin, and fragile. They lose their delicate elasticity, and walls between air sacs break, forming larger air sacs called bullae. If normal healthy airways were opened up, their total surface area would be the size of a football field. When larger bullae form there is less surface area for gas exchange, resulting in difficulty breathing, shortness of breath, and other symptoms of COPD.

The loss of healthy elastic lung tissue has other effects. Because the lung tissue becomes thin and flabby, the lungs no longer easily return to normal size after a breath. Patients must use extra effort to exhale, which adds to the sensation of difficulty in breathing. As a result, patients breathe at high lung volumes, which is very uncomfortable.

Treatments and prevention

There is no cure for COPD, but eliminating exposure to possible causes, most importantly cigarette smoke, can help prevent progression of the disease. In some cases medications called bronchodilators may be inhaled to relax muscles in the airways, which helps air flow and breathing. Other drugs called corticosteroids can be inhaled to decrease airway inflammation. In severe cases the patient's blood oxygen decreases and supplemental oxygen is needed. Antibiotics may be used to treat bacterial lung infections. Since influenza can cause serious problems in COPD sufferers, a flu vaccine should be considered as a preventive measure, and the pneumoccocal vaccine is recommended to prevent common pneumonia. A special program of exercise, nutrition, and education can help a person with COPD manage the disease. In severe COPD, surgery called bullectomy—removal of part of a lung with bullae—may improve symptoms, as the bullae may be compressing healthy lung tissue. In very severe cases, and particularly in younger patients, a lung transplant may be done.

Avoiding risk factors such as smoking and pollution are the best preventive measures. Carrriers of the alpha1-antitrypsin deficiency gene may not be able to prevent emphysema, but avoiding known risk factors such as smoking may slow the progress of COPD.

Ramona Jenkin

See also
• Asthma • Bronchitis • Emphysema
• Influenza • Pneumonia

Coronary artery disease

Coronary artery disease (CAD) is a progressive narrowing of one or more coronary arteries, which restricts the blood supply to the heart. It is caused by atherosclerosis, a buildup of fatty material and plaque on the inner lining of the blood vessels. CAD can lead to chest pain (angina), heart attacks (myocardial infarction), heart failure, abnormal heart rhythms (arrhythmias), and sudden cardiac death.

Coronary artery disease is the most common form of heart disease and is a leading cause of death in the Western world. It is a chronic condition affecting one or more coronary arteries, which are the blood vessels that supply the heart with oxygen-rich blood. CAD occurs when these arteries become narrowed and the blood supply to the heart is restricted. Without sufficient oxygen and nutrients, the heart muscle cannot function properly, leading to a range of problems. CAD is also known as coronary heart disease (CHD), ischemic heart disease (IHD), and atherosclerotic heart disease.

Causes and risk factors

CAD is caused by atherosclerosis, a common disorder characterized by thickening and hardening of the arteries. As atherosclerosis develops, fatty substances, calcium, cellular debris, and other substances are deposited on the inner lining of the arteries to form "plaques." Large plaques can cause the artery to narrow, restricting the flow of blood and oxygen. In addition, plaques may rupture and release their contents into the bloodstream, triggering the formation of blood clots that can completely block the artery.

In an individual with CAD, atherosclerosis develops in the coronary arteries. Restricting the blood flow to the heart can have a range of consequences, from chest pain (angina) and abnormal heart rhythms (arrhythmias) to heart attacks (myocardial infarction), heart failure, and sudden cardiac death (death of the heart muscle).

Many factors are known to increase the likelihood of developing CAD, and they are usually grouped according to whether or not they can be changed or controlled. An important nonmodifiable risk factor for CAD is older age. Atherosclerosis develops over many

KEY FACTS

Description

Narrowing of coronary arteries, which restricts the supply of oxygen-rich blood to the heart.

Causes

Atherosclerosis, a buildup of fatty substances, calcium, cellular debris, and other particles to form plaques.

Risk factors

Older age, a family history of early CAD, cigarette smoking, high blood pressure, high blood cholesterol levels, overweight and obesity, physical inactivity, diabetes mellitus, low consumption of fruit and vegetables, and excessive alcohol intake. Other risk factors include C-reactive protein, homocysteine, fibrinogen, and lipoprotein(a).

Symptoms

The most common symptom is chest pain (angina); other symptoms include shortness of breath, swollen feet and ankles, and pain in the shoulder, arm, jaw, or back.

Diagnosis

Patients undergo a variety of investigations and tests such as an electrocardiogram, echocardiogram, and coronary angiography.

Treatments

Many different treatments are available. All patients should make healthy lifestyle changes such as eating a low-fat, low-salt diet, maintaining a healthy weight, stopping smoking, and getting regular exercise. Medications can help control risk factors (such as high blood pressure, high blood cholesterol, and diabetes) and keep the heart and arteries healthy. In more severe cases, a minimally invasive procedure called balloon angioplasty may be used to widen the coronary arteries, and a stent is implanted. Coronary artery bypass surgery may also be done.

Pathogenesis

CAD can become more severe as the coronary arteries become narrower and the heart's blood supply is more restricted. Left untreated, CAD can lead to serious complications, including heart attack and sudden cardiac death.

Prevention

It is possible to reduce the chance of developing CAD by controlling risk factors through healthy lifestyle changes and, in some cases, medication.

Epidemiology

The risk of developing CAD after 40 is 49 percent for men and 32 percent for women.

BLOCKAGE IN CORONARY ARTERY LEADING TO HEART ATTACK

The coronary arteries can become narrowed by atherosclerosis, a condition in which plaque, consisting of substances such as fatty deposits and cholesterol, can build up. The plaque develops a fibrous layer that can rupture, causing a roughened area that platelets and blood cells can adhere to. This buildup can form a clot, which may block the artery and cause a myocardial infarction (heart attack), because fresh oxygenated blood cannot reach the heart muscle, which may lead to death of the heart muscle. Often there are no warning symptoms; the first sign may be chest pain or angina, or a heart attack.

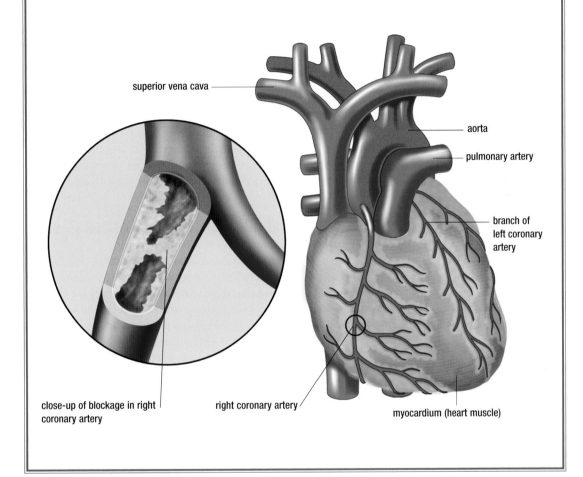

superior vena cava

aorta

pulmonary artery

branch of left coronary artery

close-up of blockage in right coronary artery

right coronary artery

myocardium (heart muscle)

years and may even begin in childhood, but it typically starts causing problems after the age of 45 years in men and 55 years in women.

The second nonmodifiable risk factor is an inherited predisposition to the disease. Although the genetic mutations involved in CAD are not understood, people with a family history of early heart disease (occurring before the age of 55 in a father or brother or before the age of 65 in a mother or sister) are at increased risk of developing CAD themselves.

Many other risk factors for CAD have been identified and can be modified through lifestyle changes, medications, or both. The most important modifiable risk factors are cigarette smoking, high blood pressure, raised blood cholesterol levels, overweight and obesity, physical inactivity, diabetes mellitus, low consumption of fruit and vegetables, and excessive alcohol intake.

The risk factors listed above are often referred to as "traditional" CAD risk factors. However, CAD can also affect people without any of these factors, an observation that has prompted the search for new factors. Many of these "novel" or "emerging" risk factors for CAD are substances that are present in the bloodstream, such as C-reactive protein

(CRP), homocysteine, fibrinogen, and lipoprotein(a). Their precise role in contributing to CAD is currently unclear.

Symptoms and signs

The signs and symptoms of CAD vary. In some people the condition produces no symptoms whatsoever until it causes a heart attack or sudden death. But the most common symptom of CAD is chest pain (angina). Less common symptoms include shortness of breath and swollen feet and ankles.

Angina occurs when the blood supply to the heart is insufficient to meet the heart's demand for oxygen. Typically, angina feels like a pain behind the breastbone and is characterized by a heavy or squeezing feeling. Other forms of angina may radiate up the left arm or neck and can even be felt in the shoulder, elbows, jaw, or back.

The characteristic symptoms of angina often arise when the heart's demand for oxygen cannot be met by the blood supply, such as during exercise. However, in more severe cases, angina can also occur during normal everyday activities or at rest. Angina may be mild and intermittent, or pronounced and steady. The symptoms tend to become more severe as the disease progresses and the coronary arteries become narrower.

Over time, CAD can gradually weaken the heart muscle. This weakening can give rise to other forms of heart disease, such as heart failure and abnormal heart rhythms.

Diagnosis

CAD is diagnosed on the basis of medical and family history, a physical exam, and one or more tests or investigations. The latter are important to determine if CAD is present, to assess the extent and severity of the disease, and also to rule out other possible causes of the symptoms.

An electrocardiogram (ECG or EKG) is commonly used to measure the rate and regularity of the heartbeat. Small electrodes are attached to the patient at various points on the body, and electrical activity of the heart produces signals that are recorded as a trace on the ECG machine. The test takes several minutes and is painless for the patient. It may be performed in a medical facility, or the patient may be given a portable ECG device, also called a Holter monitor, to wear at home. Another test, called an echocardiogram, uses ultrasound waves to create a detailed image of the heart. Both ECG and echocardiogram may be performed while the patient exercises (for example on a

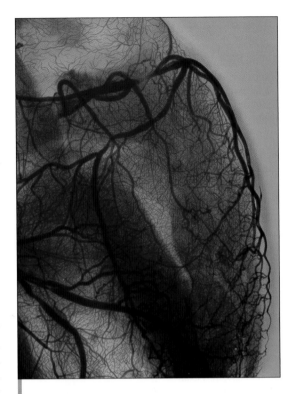

This color-enhanced angiogram of the heart shows stenosis (obstruction) in a major coronary artery, one of the arteries that supplies the heart with blood. The stenosed section of the artery is shown as the break in the dark red vessel at the center top of the picture. Arteries become obstructed by the buildup of atheroma (a fatty plaque that occurs on the inner arterial wall), resulting in coronary artery disease, which causes a reduction in the blood supply to the heart, chest pains, and in the worst case, death of the heart muscle.

treadmill or exercise bike) to see how well the heart copes with an increased demand for oxygen. This procedure is often called a stress or exercise test.

Another test for CAD is coronary angiography (or arteriography), also known as cardiac catheterization. This is a minimally invasive procedure; the patient is awake throughout but receives mild sedation and a local anesthetic. A long, thin tube (catheter) is inserted into an artery in the arm or leg and guided to the coronary arteries. A special dye is then injected through the catheter, allowing the arteries to be seen on an X-ray machine and revealing the presence of any narrowing or blockage.

Other investigations used to diagnose CAD include electron-beam computed tomography, myocardial nuclear perfusion scan, and magnetic resonance angiography.

Treatments and prevention

The aims of treating CAD are to relieve symptoms, prevent worsening of atherosclerosis, reduce the risk of blood clots, and improve blood flow to the heart. These steps will reduce the likelihood of complications such as myocardial infarction, heart failure, and sudden death.

There are many different treatments for CAD; the right one (or combination of treatments) for a particular patient will depend on the severity of symptoms and how far the disease has progressed. Nevertheless, all patients with CAD should make lifestyle changes such as eating a low-fat, low-salt diet, maintaining a healthy weight, stopping smoking, and getting regular exercise. Many patients are also prescribed medications aimed at modifying the risk factors for CAD (if present) and improving the blood flow to the heart. Medications used in patients with CAD include: cholesterol-lowering drugs; antiplatelet and anticoagulant drugs; glycoprotein IIb/IIIa inhibitors; beta-blockers; nitrates; calcium-channel blockers; angiotensin-converting enzyme (ACE) inhibitors; angiotensin receptor blockers; and diuretics.

If the symptoms of CAD persist despite drug therapy and lifestyle changes, more aggressive treatments may be needed. Sometimes these are performed on an emergency basis, such as during a heart attack.

Angioplasty (or percutaneous coronary revascularization) is a minimally invasive procedure. It is often performed in patients who have just undergone coronary angiography and have been found to have a narrowing or blockage in a coronary artery. A catheter with a balloon at the tip is guided to the blockage, where the balloon is inflated to widen the artery. In most cases, a tiny metal tube (stent) is then placed inside the vessel to help hold the artery open. Some stents release medications that help keep the blood flowing freely and prevent the artery from becoming blocked again.

Another treatment for CAD (and for angina that is difficult to control), is coronary artery bypass surgery (CABG), also known as a heart bypass. This is a surgical procedure in which a vessel is taken from another part of the body and used as a bypass to re-route the blood supply around a blockage, thereby restoring adequate blood flow to the heart.

Bypass surgery is a major surgical procedure performed under general anesthetic, during which the patient may be connected to a heart-lung machine. A vein or artery from another part of the body (usually the arm, leg, or chest) is removed and reattached to the coronary artery, allowing blood to flow around the blockage. If more than one artery is blocked, more blood vessels will be used to bypass them (double, triple, or quadruple bypass surgery).

Other procedures used to open coronary arteries include atherectomy, laser revascularization, coronary brachytherapy, catheter-based thrombolysis, and mechanical thrombectomy.

Not all cases of CAD can be prevented. However, the likelihood of developing CAD can be minimized by controlling risk factors through lifestyle changes and, in some cases, medications. Important ways of preventing CAD include not smoking, eating a low-fat diet, getting regular exercise, maintaining a healthy weight, and controlling blood pressure, blood cholesterol, or blood glucose levels.

Pathogenesis

As the coronary arteries become progressively narrower, CAD becomes more severe and the blood supply to the heart is more and more restricted. The disease may begin to weaken heart tissue so that other disorders start to occur, such as heart failure and arrhythmias (abnormal and irregular heart rhythms). If CAD is not treated, eventually there will be serious complications such as heart attack, or even sudden cardiac death.

Epidemiology

CAD is the most common form of heart disease and accounts for more than half of all cases of cardiovascular disease. The lifetime risk of developing CAD after the age of 40 years is 49 percent for men and 32 percent for women. In the United States, CAD causes one in five deaths, making it the single largest killer of men and women. The death rate from CAD fell substantially between 1993 and 2003. The incidence of angina has fallen in the United States and in Europe over the last three decades, mainly owing to a healthier lifestyle and better treatments. The estimated direct and indirect costs of CAD in the United States in 2006 were around $142.5 billion. In many other parts of the world, the incidence of CAD is rising; it is believed that this may be a result of changing lifestyles, such as diet, obesity, and lack of exercise.

Joanna Lyford

See also
- Alcohol-related disorders • Diabetes
- Heart attack

Creutzfeldt-Jakob disease

A degenerative disorder of the brain in which the brain's neurons (nerve cells) are progressively destroyed, causing the brain to become spongelike, Creutzfeldt-Jakob disease leads to progressive dementia, a decline in physical abilities, and is ultimately fatal.

Creutzfeldt-Jakob disease (CJD) is a progressively debilitating and fatal degenerative disorder of the brain that affects about 200 people a year in the United States and about one person per million every year worldwide. It belongs to a group of diseases called transmissible spongiform encephalopathies (TSEs). These diseases are characterized by the development of numerous holes in the brain, with the result that the brain tissue eventually resembles a sponge when it is examined under the microscope. The predominant characteristic symptom of CJD is rapidly progressive dementia, although initially the most obvious features of the disease are those of memory problems, lack of coordination, impaired vision, and behavioral changes. As the disease progresses, mental dysfunction becomes more pronounced and is sometimes accompanied by blindness and jerking movements (myoclonus). The disease is fatal, and death usually occurs within about a year of the appearance of symptoms.

Types and causes

There are four known forms of CJD. The most common form is called sporadic or classical CJD, which accounts for about 85 percent of all diagnosed cases. It affects primarily those over the age of 50 and is associated with dementia and impaired balance and coordination. The course of sporadic CJD is often short, and the underlying cause of the illness is not known. The second form, familial CJD, accounts for between 5 and 15 percent of all cases and is caused by an inherited mutation in a specific gene (known as the *PrP* gene). This mutation is inherited in an autosomal dominant pattern (only one parent has the abnormal gene); therefore either parent may pass on the gene to a child, who then may develop CJD later on in life. With familial CJD, symptoms typically appear at a

KEY FACTS

Description

A degenerative and fatal brain disorder.

Causes

Aggregation in the brain of infectious prion proteins that produce brain damage. The underlying cause is not known in most cases. In a minority of cases, the cause may be genetic or the prions may be acquired during medical procedures or by eating contaminated cattle.

Risk factors

Eating nerve tissue of cattle with bovine spongiform encephalopathy (BSE), commonly called mad cow disease, or infection with the causative prions during medical procedures.

Symptoms and signs

Initial symptoms include changes in sleep patterns and appetite, personality changes, poor coordination, impaired memory and vision, and mild dementia. Dementia worsens rapidly, and there may be muscle spasms and involuntary jerking movements (myoclonus). Ultimately the condition is fatal.

Diagnosis

Neurological investigations including electroencephalography (EEG) and magnetic resonance imaging (MRI) or computed tomography (CT) scans; spinal fluid analysis may be done. Definitive diagnosis is by brain biopsy.

Treatments

There is no cure and no known treatment that may slow progression of CJD; symptoms may be relieved by medication.

Pathogenesis

An aberrant form of prion protein aggregates in the brain, leading to progressive loss of brain tissue, increasingly severe mental and physical symptoms, and resulting in death.

Prevention

There is no known way of preventing sporadic CJD or familial CJD. Other forms of CJD may be prevented by better screening for infected tissue, by using sterilization techniques that inactivate prions, and by avoiding eating the high-risk parts (brain, spinal cord, offal) of cattle.

Epidemiology

In the United States there are about 200 cases a year. Worldwide about one person in a million is infected per year.

younger age than they do with sporadic CJD, and the pattern of symptoms tends to vary according to the particular mutation the *PrP* gene has undergone. The course of this type of CJD is typically longer than that of sporadic CJD. The third form of the disease is known as iatrogenic CJD, and this form is thought to be caused by contamination with infectious prions during medical procedures, such as organ transplantation, brain surgery, or the administration of human-derived pituitary growth hormones. Iatrogenic CJD is more commonly associated with impaired balance and coordination than with dementia. During the mid-1990s a fourth form of CJD, called variant CJD (vCJD), was identified. This form of the disease is believed to be caused by eating contaminated beef from cattle with bovine spongiform encephalopathy (BSE), which is commonly called mad cow disease. In variant CJD, symptoms typically first appear at a young age (most commonly between the ages of 10 and 20), and the duration of the disease is longer than in sporadic CJD. The initial symptoms of variant CJD are usually psychiatric abnormalities.

In all forms of CJD the common immediate cause of the disease is the presence in the brain of infectious forms of proteins called prions. Normal prions occur naturally in the brain, and these are harmless. However, the structure of prions can become distorted, which causes them to become infectious. When an infectious prion comes into contact with other normal prions, it transforms them into infectious forms, which can then in turn transform other normal prions. As a result of this pattern, infectious prions build up and form clumps, which leads to the loss of neurons and brain damage and eventually results in holes in the brain tissue that give the brain a spongelike appearance when viewed under the microscope.

Symptoms and signs

The initial symptoms of CJD include weakness, changes in sleep patterns, depression, loss of appetite, weight loss, loss of sexual drive, difficulty in balancing, and a deterioration in coordination; in these early stages there may also be mild dementia. As the illness progresses, the most characteristic symptom of CJD is rapidly progressive dementia. Dementia is characterized by an array of cognitive impairments, including loss of memory, poor judgment, decreased attention span, disorientation, and psychosis (a loss of contact with reality, with features such as delusions, hallucinations, depression, manic behavior, disordered thinking, and emotional disturbances). In the later stages of the

disease, dementia and mental impairment become increasingly severe and individuals also often develop involuntary muscle jerks (myoclonus) and may go blind. They eventually lose the ability to move or speak and enter into a coma. Pneumonia and other infections often occur in these patients and are usually the cause of death.

Diagnosis

There is as yet no single diagnostic test for CJD and therefore diagnosis is based on the patient's medical history, a physical examination, and neurological investigations. Electroencephalography (EEG) is often used; if the patient has CJD the EEG readout shows a characteristic pattern. Magnetic resonance imaging (MRI) or computed tomography (CT) scans may also be carried out. These scans typically show atrophy (degeneration) or loss of brain tissue in patients with CJD. In addition, the spinal fluid may be tested for a protein that is released from damaged nerve cells and is present in more than 90 percent of patients with sporadic CJD.

None of these neurological investigations by itself is sufficient to give a diagnosis of CJD, but if at least two out of the three tests are positive, a CJD diagnosis is virtually certain. The only conclusive test for CJD is an examination of a sample of brain tissue (removed by biopsy) under the microscope. However, a brain biopsy can be dangerous and for that reason is rarely performed.

Treatment and prevention

There is at present no cure for CJD nor any treatment that can slow the progression of the disease. Treatments are therefore aimed at relieving symptoms. For example, opioid drugs may be given to relieve any pain, and anticonvulsant drugs such as clonazepam and sodium valproate may help relieve myoclonus. Similarly, antidepressant drugs may be used to help deal with the symptoms of depression.

There is no known way of preventing sporadic CJD or familial CJD. Iatrogenic and variant CJD may be prevented by improved screening for infected tissue, by using sterilization techniques during surgery that inactivate prions, and by avoiding eating high-risk parts, such as beef on the bone and organ meats, of cattle.

Sonia Gulati

See also
• Dementia

Crohn's disease

A chronic inflammatory disease of the intestines, Crohn's disease usually begins between the ages of 15 to 25. It primarily causes ulcerations of the small and large intestines, but it can affect the gut anywhere from the mouth to the anus. It is named after New York physician Burrill B. Crohn, who described the disease in 1932.

Crohn's disease is a long-term inflammatory disorder that affects the digestive tract. The disorder commonly begins in early adulthood and usually continues to cause ill health throughout the life of the person affected.

Causes and pathogenesis

The cause of Crohn's disease is unknown. Crohn's disease is not contagious. Although diet may affect the symptoms in patients with Crohn's disease, it is unlikely that diet is responsible for the disease. Since Crohn's disease is often found in families of patients with Crohn's disease and ulcerative colitis, it is possible that it has a genetic component. It is more prevalent in white people of Jewish origin.

It is difficult to predict the likely progression of Crohn's disease. Treatment to control rectal bleeding, abdominal pain, and inflammation may reduce recurrences of the disease, but there is no cure. Some people have long remissions when they are symptom free; but about three-quarters of sufferers will need surgery. Poor digestion causes nutritional deficiencies, and intestinal blockages are common in this disease.

Symptoms

The symptoms of Crohn's disease include abdominal pain, diarrhea, and weight loss. Less common symptoms may include poor appetite, fever, night sweats, rectal pain, and bleeding. Symptoms are dependent on the location, the extent, and the severity of the inflammation. Fatigue, prolonged diarrhea with abdominal pain, weight loss, and fever with and without gross bleeding are the hallmarks of Crohn's disease. However, 10 percent of patients do not have diarrhea.

Subtypes

Crohn's colitis is inflammation confined to the colon (large bowel). Abdominal pain and bloody diarrhea are common symptoms. Anal fistula (opening near the anus) and perirectal abscesses also can occur. Approximately 20 percent of patients with Crohn's have this form of the disease, which can be difficult to distinguish from ulcerative colitis.

Crohn's enteritis is inflammation confined to the jejunum (second portion of the small intestine) and the ileum (third portion of the small intestine). Disease restricted to the ileum alone is referred to as Crohn's ileitis. Abdominal pain and diarrhea are common. Obstruction of the small intestine can occur. Around 30 percent of Crohn's patients have the enteric form of the condition.

KEY FACTS

Description
Chronic inflammatory disease of the intestines causing ulceration of the small and large bowels from mouth to anus.

Causes
Unknown; possibly multiple causes (genetic, environmental, immune).

Pathogenesis
The gut wall becomes unable to regulate its immune response, resulting in inflammation.

Symptoms
Abdominal pain, loss of appetite, diarrhea, weight loss, fever, rectal pain, and bleeding occurs in up to 80 percent of cases.

Diagnosis
Endoscopy to examine the intestine, including a biopsy of intestinal tissue. Definitive diagnosis is made by X-ray. Blood tests may be done for anemia, and fecal tests for occult (hidden) blood.

Treatments
Dependent on the severity of the disease. The goal is to control the amount of inflammation occurring in the gut with restoration of normal hydration and nutrition. No cure is known.

Prevention
None known at this time.

Epidemiology
It is estimated that 1 million people in the United States have Crohn's disease. Peak incidence is between 15 to 30 years. It is four times more common among Jewish people. There is a 3.5-fold risk of developing Crohn's disease in a relative of someone with the disease. CDC has launched research to gather statistics about the disease.

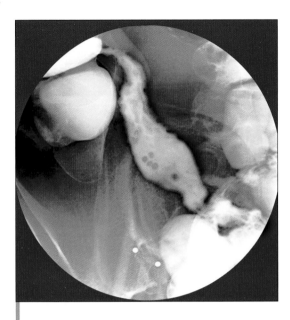

A colored abdominal X-ray shows the terminal part of the ileum (center of picture) inflamed by Crohn's disease.

Crohn's disease affecting the very last part of the small intestine is called terminal ileitis. Abdominal pain and diarrhea are common. The majority of patients have terminal ileitis. Crohn's enterocolitis describes inflammation of both the small intestine and the colon. Bloody diarrhea and abdominal pain are common. About 50 percent of patients with Crohn's disease are affected. Perianal (around the anus) disease occurs in one-third of patients with Crohn's disease and is characterized by abdominal abscess, painless fissure, and fistula (a channel connection between the intestine and other adjacent organs).

Around 8 to 40 percent of patients with Crohn's disease have bowel obstruction and perforation of the small intestine, abscesses, fistulae formation, and intestinal bleeding. Massive bowel distention (megacolon) and perforation of the intestine are potentially life threatening, and generally require surgery. Perianal disease affects 25 to 50 percent of patients. Other complications may involve the skin, joints, spine, liver, eyes, and bile ducts. They include shallow ulcers of the mouth, painful nodes on the lower legs, and ulcers on the ankles. There may be visual difficulties. These manifestations are reported in over one-third of the patients hospitalized with Crohn's disease.

Diagnosis

The diagnosis is usually established with endoscopic findings in a patient with compatible clinical history.

The physical examination can be normal or show non-specific signs, such as pallor and weight loss suggestive of Crohn's disease. Endoscopic features show focal ulcerations next to areas of normal mucosa and polypoid mucosa changes, which give a cobblestone appearance. Typically there are segments clear of inflammation where the bowel appears normal, interrupted by large areas of obvious disease. An intestinal biopsy usually confirms the diagnosis. There is no blood test to confirm the disease, but a complete blood cell (CBC) count may show anemia secondary to chronic or acute blood loss. Stool examination may show hidden blood and fecal white blood cells (indicative of infection).

Treatments

To date, no cure is known for Crohn's disease. The symptoms and severity of Crohn's disease vary among patients. For initial stabilization, intravenous fluids for volume replacement are necessary if the patient is dehydrated or in the early stages of shock. A blood transfusion is required if significant blood loss has occurred. Suctioning by a nose to stomach tube is used if obstruction or toxic megacolon is suspected. Treatment depends on the location and severity of the disease and may include drugs, nutrition therapy, or surgery, or all three. Drugs commonly used are anti-inflammatory drugs, such as 5-ASA agents, corticosteroids, immune system suppressors, antibiotics, anti-diarrheals and fluid replacements. When there is bowel wall perforation, intestinal or gut obstruction (or both) massive blood loss, toxic megacolon, and perforation with abscess formation, surgery may be needed.

Epidemiology

The onset of Crohn's disease is usually between 15 to 30 years or between 50 to 70 years old. Since many of the symptoms of Crohn's disease and ulcerative colitis are similar, diagnosis is arduous, time-consuming, and invasive. About one-third of the patients have a history of perianal disease, which may be the most prominent or initial complaint. Approximately 70 percent of Crohn's disease patients will ultimately require surgery. Estimates suggest that up to 1 million people in the United States have the disease. The incidence and prevalence of the disease is rising. There is no preventive measure known at this time.

Isaac Grate

See also
• Colitis, ulcerative • Diarrhea and dysentery

Croup

A common disease of the upper respiratory tract, croup usually affects young children. Although its characteristic barking cough can be alarming, the disease usually clears up in a few days. In a few cases, breathing difficulties may require emergency attention.

Croup is any infection of the upper respiratory tract that results in a distinctive barking cough. This cough is often likened to the sound of a seal. Most cases of croup are caused by viruses called parainfluenza viruses, although other infectious agents such as the influenza virus can also cause croup. It is most common in children aged three years and under. Croup-causing viruses usually spread through water droplets in the air that result from coughing or sneezing.

The different kinds of parainfluenza viruses are more common at different times of the year. For example, type 1 tends to cause croup infections in the fall, whereas type 3 causes outbreaks during the spring and summer. After a croup infection, the body develops immunity to the particular virus that caused the attack, but this immunity does not extend to croup caused by other viruses, so repeated attacks of croup may occur.

Pathogenesis and symptoms

The alternative medical term for croup is laryngotracheobronchitis. The term refers to the areas of the respiratory tract that get attacked by the virus: the larynx, trachea, and bronchi; -itis means "inflammation." Like many viral infections, croup-causing viruses trigger inflammation of the mucus-producing lining of the throat and air tubes, causing hoarseness, wheezing on breathing in, and the barking cough, as well as some fever.

Croup can come on suddenly, often in the middle of the night. In the small breathing tubes of young children, the swelling may be enough to make breathing difficult, especially if the infant is also crying. In some cases, the breathing difficulty can become dangerous.

Treatments and prevention

Bringing a child into a warm, steamy bathroom can help ease the symptoms of croup and make breathing easier. Running a cold-water humidifier at night, or allowing the child to inhale cool, moist night air, can also help. If breathing becomes a serious struggle, medical emergency services should be called.

Because croup infections are caused by viruses and not bacteria, antibiotics do not work against them. In severe cases, where the airways are partly obstructed by swelling, physicians may prescribe a steroid medication to reduce inflammation and swelling in the throat. These anti-inflammatory drugs may shorten the illness. In rare cases, hospitalization for oxygen treatment or to treat an obstructed airway is necessary.

As with many viruses, frequent hand washing and not sharing eating utensils help prevent the spread of infection. Scientists are currently seeking to develop vaccines against the parainfluenza viruses that cause most croup, but these are not yet available.

Mary Quirk

KEY FACTS

Description
An upper respiratory tract infection of childhood leading to a characteristic barking cough.

Causes
Various viruses, especially parainfluenza viruses.

Risk factors
Contact with infected people.

Symptoms
Hoarseness, cough, breathing difficulties, fever.

Diagnosis
Barking cough. Laboratory tests to detect which virus is responsible.

Treatments
Breathing moist warm or cool air. In serious cases, emergency treatment for breathing difficulties and treatment with steroid drugs.

Pathogenesis
Infection spreads in water droplets produced by coughing and sneezing. Viruses infect surface cells of breathing tubes, causing inflammation.

Prevention
Avoiding infected people.

Epidemiology
Outbreaks tend to be seasonal, in spring and fall.

See also
- Bronchitis • Cold, common • Influenza
- Whooping cough

Cystic fibrosis

Cystic fibrosis (CF) is a genetic disorder that can be treated but not cured. Many people think of CF as a disease that only affects the lungs, because most patients experience respiratory problems first. However, the genetic change that causes the disease has devastating effects on many different parts of the body.

Cystic fibrosis (CF) hit the cover of *Sports Illustrated* in 1993 when NFL quarterback Boomer Esiason's young son Gunnar was diagnosed with the disease. Gunnar is one of about 30,000 people with CF in the United States. Although the disease is often fatal, newer and more effective treatments now allow many patients to lead active lives and survive into adulthood. Gunnar, for example, has been able to play soccer, lacrosse, and ice hockey while attending high school in New York. However, despite all this progress, there is still no cure for this deadly genetic disorder.

Cystic fibrosis was first described in 1938 by Dorothy Andersen, who wrote about its devastating effects on both the digestive system and the respiratory tract while working at the New York Babies Hospital. Her report focused on the damage to the pancreas. She called the disease cystic fibrosis (CF); less commonly, it is called mucoviscidosis. This name comes from the primary pathology: the production of excessively thick and sticky mucus in the lungs and digestive tract. Although the hereditary nature of the disease was recognized in the 1940s by Andersen and her colleagues, the gene responsible for the disease was not found until 1989. The disease's gene, cystic fibrosis transmembrane conductance regulator (CFTR), changes the way chloride, a key component of salt, is moved across cell membranes. As a result, there is a high level of salt in secreted mucus and sweat. Finding the CF gene raised hopes for a quick cure or more effective treatments, but those hopes were soon dashed. More than 1,000 mutations have been found in the CFTR gene since its initial discovery. This variation makes treating and identifying carriers and patients more complex.

Cause and risk factors

In classic cystic fibrosis, the child inherits one abnormal gene from each parent. Each child has a 25 percent chance of getting the disease. The risk is equal for boys and girls. This pattern of inheritance is called autosomal (not a sex chromosome) recessive. It is called recessive because unless there are two faulty copies of the gene, there will be no abnormality.

Some studies suggest that males are more likely to develop problems with infertility and reduced lung function. Fertility problems result from abnormal transport of developing sperm, but it is unclear why males are at higher risk of declining lung function.

KEY FACTS

Description
A genetic disorder primarily affecting the lungs and digestive system.

Cause
A gene mutation resulting in abnormal chloride transport across cell membranes.

Risk factors
People of northern European descent are at highest risk.

Symptoms
Frequent coughing, wheezing, and respiratory infections. Infants may show delayed growth, unusual or delayed bowel movements, or salty-tasting skin.

Diagnosis
A sweat test shows whether the amount of salt secreted is abnormally high.

Treatments
Dietary supplements and digestive enzymes improve nutritional status. Antibiotics prevent lung infections, and special medicines reduce the thick mucus that clogs the lungs. Gene therapy remains experimental.

Pathogenesis
Patients' lungs become damaged over time from frequent infections and excessive mucus. The mucus also disrupts the transport of digestive enzymes and absorption of nutrients from the gut. Most CF patients die from respiratory failure.

Prevention
Genetic testing can identify parents at risk. Newborn screening can identify patients early.

Epidemiology
Each parent carrying one copy of the mutant gene.

Cultural background is very important in determining a person's risk for having a child with cystic fibrosis. The CF gene is much more common in northern European populations than in Asian, Hispanic, and African populations. The risk of having a child with cystic fibrosis ranges from 1 in 377 live births in England to 1 in 90,000 births in Hawaii's Asian population. With increased immigration and an increase in intercultural marriages, it will become more difficult to predict an individual's actual risk.

Risk also depends on which CF mutation is inherited. Not all of the mutations have the same effect on patients. There is also some evidence that other genes or environmental factors might play a role in the development of cystic fibrosis. Research is continuing to identify these factors.

Symptoms and diagnosis

The most common test to diagnose cystic fibrosis is the sweat test, which has been used since the 1950s. Doctors analyze the amount of salt in sweat to determine if it is in the normal range. Parents may notice this high level of salt when cuddling or kissing their babies, so a salty taste to the skin may be the first symptom of the disease. It is more likely that children will be diagnosed because they do not grow as rapidly as healthy children. Some patients show signs of serious illness in their very first days of life. It may take 24 to 48 hours before a newborn's first bowel movement, and the stools may be unusually foul smelling or appear to be greasy. This is an indication that CF has already affected the digestive system. Two-thirds of CF patients will be diagnosed by their first birthday, because they fail to thrive or they develop frequent respiratory infections.

If two sweat tests show abnormal salt levels, genetic tests can be used to confirm the diagnosis. At least two mutations in the CFTR gene should be present. Other common tests include an analysis of the fat content in stools. High fat content is indicative of cystic fibrosis. Other tests assess the level of the digestive enzyme trypsin in infant stools. If the levels are low, that indicates that the pancreas is not functioning normally. However, enzyme tests must be combined with other tests before a final diagnosis can be made.

Treatments

As CF patients grow older, they are likely to face frequent and repeated lung infections. Bacteria that are especially common and dangerous for CF patients are *Pseudomonas aueruginosa*, *Burkholderia cepacia*, and *Staphylococcus aureus*. These infections can be extremely difficult to treat, although early diagnosis is helpful in avoiding chronic infections.

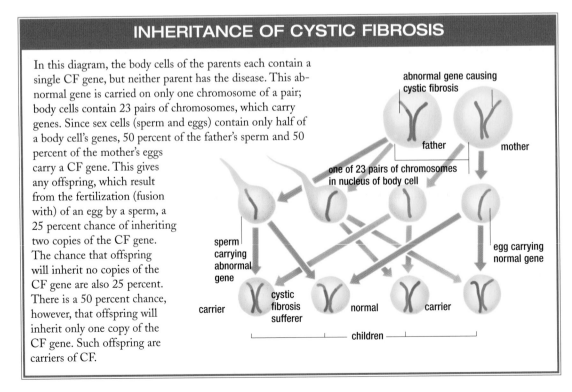

INHERITANCE OF CYSTIC FIBROSIS

In this diagram, the body cells of the parents each contain a single CF gene, but neither parent has the disease. This abnormal gene is carried on only one chromosome of a pair; body cells contain 23 pairs of chromosomes, which carry genes. Since sex cells (sperm and eggs) contain only half of a body cell's genes, 50 percent of the father's sperm and 50 percent of the mother's eggs carry a CF gene. This gives any offspring, which result from the fertilization (fusion with) of an egg by a sperm, a 25 percent chance of inheriting two copies of the CF gene. The chance that offspring will inherit no copies of the CF gene are also 25 percent. There is a 50 percent chance, however, that offspring will inherit only one copy of the CF gene. Such offspring are carriers of CF.

abnormal gene causing cystic fibrosis

father

mother

one of 23 pairs of chromosomes in nucleus of body cell

sperm carrying abnormal gene

egg carrying normal gene

carrier

cystic fibrosis sufferer

normal

carrier

children

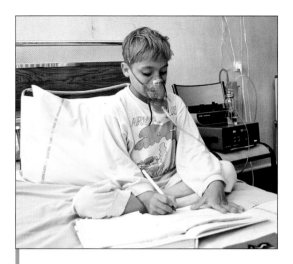

A young boy breathes through a nebulizer in hospital. The nebulizer breaks up the thick mucus that builds up in the lungs by passing a fine mist into the airways. This treatment eases breathing difficulties.

Antibiotics have been used to help treat and prevent lung infections in cystic fibrosis patients. The downside of these treatments is the development of resistant strains of bacteria. When a person is infected with an antibiotic-resistant strain, the infection takes longer to cure, and others can be infected as well. Treating patients with ibuprofen as well as antibiotics helps prevent inflammation, which can further damage the lungs.

Nutritional therapy is important in helping CF patients grow at a normal rate. Special diets have been used to increase the amount of calories and vitamins absorbed by the digestive tract. Patients also receive enzyme therapy, so they can break down more of the food they eat. A standard treatment might include as many as 25 pills each day. Without treatment, much food, especially fats, cannot be digested properly.

There are several treatments used to keep the lung passages from being clogged with thick mucus. A drug called dornase alfa helps thin the mucus so it can be cleared more easily from the lungs. Parents and therapists can also use a drumming or percussive pounding on the back to help patients cough up the mucus. These treatments are done once or twice a day for about 30 minutes each time. The treatments are beneficial in reducing the frequency of respiratory infections and improving respiratory function.

Lung transplants are an option for patients with severe symptoms and extensive lung damage. They are not performed on patients with mild symptoms.

About 10 percent of all lung transplants in the United States are performed on CF patients. Nearly half of CF patients receiving lung transplants are alive five years after the operation, but the lack of donor organs means this option is not available to all CF patients.

Prevention

There is no way to prevent cystic fibrosis without the use of genetic testing. Genetic testing can identify individuals who are carriers for the disease. This testing can be done before a pregnancy occurs or after a woman becomes pregnant. Current tests cannot identify all carriers because there are so many different mutations in the CFTR gene. Only the most common mutations are included in the screening tests.

Embryos and fetuses can also be tested to determine if they carry two copies of the disease gene. Pre-implantation diagnosis requires expensive in vitro fertilization and genetic tests on a cell taken from an early embryo. Fetal diagnosis is done through chorionic villus sampling or amniocentesis, which uses cells from the fetus for genetic analysis. Both pre-implantation and fetal diagnoses raise social and ethical issues; not all parents can afford the tests, and the results can be used to justify destroying embryos or choosing an elective abortion. These tests are not 100 percent accurate because there are so many mutations of the CF gene.

Gene therapy is a technique being developed to deliver copies of a healthy CF gene into a patient's cells, so they can begin to produce the normal protein. Viruses carry healthy CFTR genes into a patient's respiratory tract, and the gene becomes part of the cell's genetic makeup. The first CF gene therapy trial began in 1993, when a modified cold virus was used. There was some evidence that the genes were taken into patient cells and normal proteins produced. However, there are many issues surrounding the use of gene therapy. Viruses can sometimes provoke an immune response, and repeated dosing might be required. The cells in the body's lining often turn over, with new cells replacing older cells over time. Unless these new cells also carry the healthy gene, they will be unable to produce normal proteins and transport chloride normally. Protein therapy is being tried as an alternative. In this case, researchers aim to activate or repair the actual CFTR protein.

Chris Curran

See also
• Pneumonia

Cystitis

A bacterial infection of the urinary bladder, cystitis is more common in women than men, because the urethra that empties the female bladder is shorter. The disease is not considered a serious health threat unless the infection spreads into the kidneys.

A woman who has a frequent urge to urinate should consider whether she is suffering from a bladder infection such as cystitis. This common bacterial infection will strike the majority of women at some point in their life, but in general cystitis is not a significant health threat.

Causes and risk factors

The primary cause of bladder infections is *Escherichia coli*, the bacteria that normally live inside our digestive tract. If these bacteria come in contact with the urethra, where urine leaves the body, they can move upward into the bladder and cause infection. Women are at highest risk, because the urethra is only about 1½ inches (4 cm) long, compared with about 8 inches (20 cm) in men. Sexually active women and women who use tampons may experience more bladder infections. After menopause the vaginal lining changes, making it easier for infection-causing bacteria to grow. Congenital defects can restrict the flow of urine in some people and leave them at higher risk.

People with cystitis have a frequent urge to urinate. They may wake up several times during the night to use the bathroom. They may also experience pain and a burning sensation and notice a foul odor to the urine. Children may have bed-wetting accidents and a low-grade fever. Interstitial cystitis can cause many of the same symptoms, but it is not caused by a bacterial infection and is considered a separate disorder.

The infection is normally short-lived unless it spreads to the kidneys. A kidney infection is a serious complication and needs rapid attention. Urine can be cultured to determine what type of bacteria is causing the infection, or a special diagnostic dipstick provides an instant diagnosis in the physician's office.

Treatment and prevention

Standard antibiotic drugs are effective against most bladder infections. They are needed to stop bacteria from traveling upward to the kidneys. Patients may also drink a solution to change the pH of the bladder. Drinking lots of water and cranberry juice are recommended to help prevent cystitis. Liquids flush out the bladder and change the acidity of the bladder lining, making it difficult for bacteria to grow. It also helps to avoid irritants such as soaps and deodorants in the genital area, and to choose showers over baths.

Chris Curran

KEY FACTS

Description
An inflammation of the urinary bladder.

Cause
Bacterial infection, most commonly *Escherichia coli* (E. coli).

Risk factors
Women are at greater risk than men, especially when sexually active or after menopause.

Symptoms
Lower abdominal pain, a frequent urge to urinate, cloudy or bad-smelling urine, and burning during urination.

Diagnosis
Lab tests on urine samples.

Treatments
Antibiotics are normally used, but drinking large amounts of water is also helpful in clearing many infections.

Pathogenesis
Bacteria move up the urethra into the bladder, where they multiply and cause an inflammation of the bladder lining.

Prevention
Drinking a large amount of fluid regularly—particularly water or cranberry juice—can help prevent cystitis. In the bathroom, wiping from front to back avoids spreading fecal bacteria near the urethral opening.

Epidemiology
Millions of women suffer at least one case of cystitis each year. The disease affects men and children less often.

See also
• Menopausal disorders

Dementia

A loss of mental skills and intellectual functioning that can become so severe as to affect daily life, dementia is not a specific disease but a symptom of a number of different conditions that affect the brain. People with dementia have trouble remembering, thinking clearly, and planning ahead, and over time will not be able to care for themselves. The word *dementia* means "deprived of mind."

Dementia is not a disease but a descriptive term for a collection of symptoms found in a number of conditions. The one common factor in people suffering with dementia is impaired intellectual functioning that interferes with normal daily activities and relationships.

Dementia is classified under five different categories depending on which part of the brain is affected and how the disease progresses. These five divisions are: cortical dementia, which is located in the brain's outer layer, or cortex, and affects memory, language, and social behavior; subcortical dementia, which targets parts of the brain below the cortex and causes changes in emotions and movement in addition to memory; progressive dementia, which worsens over time; primary dementia, which does not result from injury or another disease; and secondary dementia, which results from a physical injury. Many conditions such as Alzheimer's disease (AD) are categorized as both cortical and progressive dementias.

Some kinds of dementia can be reversed once the underlying condition causing the dementia has been treated. For example, hypothyroidism, caused by an underactive thyroid gland, vitamin B_{12} deficiency, heavy metal poisoning, late-stage syphilis, and alcoholism can all cause dementia but can all be treated and therefore the symptoms reversed.

Types and causes of dementia

Alzheimer's disease, the most common dementia in the United States, causes the individual to lose nearly all brain functions, including movement, judgment, behavior, and abstract thinking. Some people can live for up to 20 years after being diagnosed but eventually are reduced to a state of lying in bed in a fetal position. Two abnormalities are found in the brains of AD victims: neurofibrillary tangles, which consist of abnormal twisted protein within neurons (nerve cells), and clumped proteins (groups of amino acids) called amyloid plaques found between neurons. Trapped in these plaque deposits is a substance called "tau," which in normal brains helps neurons communicate. AD

KEY FACTS

Description

Loss of mental functioning that affects daily life.

Causes

Difficult to determine, but damage or changes in the brain always occur.

Risk factors

Age, genetics, and family history, smoking and alcohol use, atherosclerosis (hardening of the arteries), plasma homocysteine (a protein), cholesterol, diabetes, Down syndrome.

Symptoms

Memory loss, having trouble understanding words, becoming lost in familiar places, having trouble doing simple tasks like balancing a checkbook or grocery shopping, depression, irritability, or acting in irrational ways.

Diagnosis

A medical history, a physical exam, and mental status exam test by health professionals. In the mental exam the person does simple tasks, such as identifying the day, month, or year, or repeating a series of words. Magnetic resonance imaging (MRI) and computed tomography (CT) scans are used.

Treatments

Medications slow the progress of the condition but cannot cure dementia.

Pathogenesis

A progressive condition that worsens over time.

Prevention

Avoidance or control of the risk factors: lowering cholesterol, blood pressure, and homocysteine (protein) levels. Exercise and keeping engaged in social and mental activities. Some studies recommend controlling inflammation and use of nonsteroidial anti-inflammatory drugs (NSAIDS).

Epidemiology

Prevalence increases with age and doubles every five years after age 60. Dementia affects only 1 percent of those aged 60 to 64 but 30 percent of those over 85. The U.S. Congress of Technology Assessment estimates that as many as 6.8 million people in the United States have dementia.

patients often die not from their condition but from pneumonia because of impaired swallowing. As a result, bits of fluid and food are breathed into the lungs and cause infection.

Vascular dementia, the second most common cause of dementia, results from brain damage incurred as a result of a heart attack or from other cardiovascular problems such as a stroke. Patients usually have a history of high blood pressure, vascular diseases, or previous strokes or heart attacks. Damage usually begins in the midbrain but may progress to other parts of the brain. People with vascular dementia often maintain their personality until the later stages of the disease.

Frontotemporal dementia describes a group of diseases in which an abnormal form of the protein tau accumulates in the neurofibrillary tangles, and nerve cells in the frontal and temporal lobes of the brain disintegrate. This type of dementia occurs in about 2 to 10 percent of all cases and appears to have a strong genetic factor. Because the frontal and temporal lobes are related to judgment, individuals may steal or exhibit other inappropriate social behavior. One type of frontotemporal dementia is called Pick's disease, in which abnormal brain cells swell before they die.

Lewy body dementia (LBD) is a common type of dementia that can occur in people with no known family history of the condition. In this type of dementia, cells in the brain's outer cortex die and in the midbrain abnormal structures called Lewy bodies appear. The person may have visual hallucinations, a shuffling gait, and flexed posture. Patients with LBD live an average of seven years after diagnosis.

Other causes of dementia are HIV/AIDS, Huntington's disease (a genetic disease), boxer's dementia caused by repeated blows to the head, and Creutzfeldt-Jakob disease, a rare degenerative disorder similar to mad cow disease.

Diagnosis

A diagnosis is made after taking a medical history, a physical examination, and a mental status test in which the individual is given simple mental tasks such as identifying the day, month, or year, or asked to repeat word patterns. Magnetic resonance imaging (MRI) or computed tomography (CT) scans may be carried out to identify areas of impaired brain activity.

Treatments and prevention

Although no treatments reverse or halt the progress of most dementias (apart from those caused by treatable conditions), medications may relieve symptoms, and

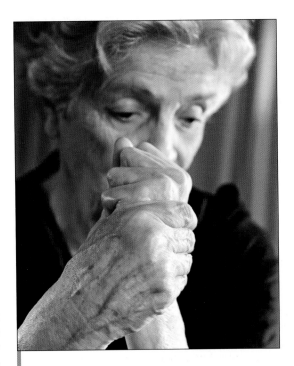

The symptoms of dementia develop gradually over a period of months or even years. In the early stages there may be anxiety and depression; as the disease progresses there can be a loss of intellect and personal neglect.

behavior modification training can sometimes help. Alzheimer's disease is the target of extensive drug testing. A group of pharmaceuticals called cholinesterase inhibitors improve or slow mental decline in AD, and a drug called memantidine has recently been approved to treat AD. Vascular dementia has no standard treatment, but some drugs relieve symptoms.

A number of factors may prevent or delay the onset of dementia. People who have stable blood glucose levels appear to maintain cognitive functions longer. Lowering cholesterol levels and blood pressure reduces the risk of heart attacks, which can sometimes cause dementia.

Above all else, individuals should keep themselves in good shape by exercising, eating a healthy, balanced diet, and avoiding smoking. Keeping both body and mind active helps maintain mental agility.

Evelyn Kelly

See also
- AIDS • Alcohol-related disorders
- Alzheimer's disease • Creutzfeldt-Jakob disease • Huntington's disease • Syphilis
- Thyroid disorders

Dengue fever

Dengue fever is caused by a virus carried by an infected mosquito. There is no treatment; prevention by protection against mosquitoes is the best measure.

Dengue fever and its potentially fatal complication, dengue hemorrhagic fever, are a rapidly growing threat to human health throughout the world. The disease was uncommon prior to World War II (1939–1945) but has become more common since then because the geographic distributions of dengue viruses and their mosquito carriers have grown larger.

The most common form of dengue may make the patient miserable but is rarely fatal. Dengue hemorrhagic fever, however, can kill as many as 20 percent of its victims unless medical treatment is available.

Causes and risk factors

The viruses are spread from human to human via the bite of an infected female mosquito. *Aedes aegypti* is a common carrier because of its preference for urban habitats. It is a threat throughout the increasingly urbanized countries in the tropics and subtropics. Another species, *Aedes albopictus*, recently spread from its native Asia to Africa, the Americas, and Europe; this species' penchant for riding in shipments of used tires has contributed to its spread. Any exposure to dengue-carrying mosquitoes increases risk of infection. Patients acquire immunity only to strains they have been infected with. Subsequent infections by other strains increase the risk of developing dengue hemorrhagic fever, however.

Symptoms and signs

Symptoms for dengue fever vary, ranging from mild fever and rash to severe fever, headache, and muscle and joint pains. Dengue fever often begins with sudden onset of high fever (up to 105°F or 41°C); bruising, bleeding from mucous membranes of the nose and mouth, enlarged liver, damage to and leakage from blood and lymph vessels, shock, and convulsions. Symptoms usually subside after the fever breaks, but patients can go into severe shock and die in a day or so.

Treatment and prevention

No drugs exist to combat dengue and dengue hemorrhagic fevers. The primary treatment is to manage pain and fever for the milder forms, and to maintain fluid volume and blood pressure in patients with severe forms. Researchers are developing a vaccine, but the effort is complicated by multiple viral strains.

David Lawrence

KEY FACTS

Description

A flulike viral disease with potentially fatal complications.

Causes

Infection by one of four strains of closely related Flavivirus.

Risk factors

Bites by infected mosquitoes, mainly *Aedes aegypti*.

Symptoms and signs

For dengue fever, symptoms include high fever, severe headache, severe joint and muscle pain, nausea, vomiting and rash; for dengue hemorrhagic fever, symptoms include those already mentioned, along with marked damage to blood and lymph vessels, bruising, and bleeding from mucous membranes in the nose and mouth.

Diagnosis

Examination by experienced medical personnel; blood tests for antibodies to virus.

Treatments

All that can be done is to manage the symptoms with bed rest, fluids, and drugs to moderate fever.

Pathogenesis

Mosquitoes transmit the viruses as they bite humans; recovery from infection by one strain of dengue viruses provides immunity only to that strain; sequential infections by other strains may increase the risk of dengue hemorrhagic fever.

Prevention

Controlling the mosquito population with insecticides; habitat management such as draining potential breeding sites and properly disposing of refuse; or using repellants, clothing, or barriers such as closed windows or mosquito netting to prevent contact with mosquitoes.

Epidemiology

As many as 50 million people may be infected every year; 40 percent of the world's population is at risk, mostly in Africa, North and South America, the eastern Mediterranean, southeastern Asia, and the western Pacific.

See also
• Ebola fever • Malaria

Depressive disorders

Depressive disorders are characterized by severe and persistent sad moods as well as disruptions in thinking and daily body cycles, such as eating and sleeping. Severe depression typically results in poor performance at work or school and strains in relationships with family and friends.

Mood disorders include disorders that have a disturbance in mood as the predominant feature. Depressive disorders and bipolar disorders are the two most common types of mood disorder. The three types of depressive disorders are major depressive disorder, dysthymic disorder, and depressive disorder not otherwise specified. Historically, depressive disorders were called melancholia, but more currently are referred to as depression, clinical depression, or unipolar depression. The focus here is on major depressive disorder and, to a lesser extent, dysthymic disorder.

Causes and risk factors

No specific cause for depression has been identified. A combination of genetic, psychological, and environmental factors contribute to depressive disorders. Causal theories for depression are evolving over time as new research findings emerge. Life stressors are associated with the onset of depression. A serious loss, difficult relationship, financial problems, or any stressful (unwelcome or even desired) change in life patterns can trigger a depressive episode for some. Other risk factors include a history of trauma or abuse and being raised in a family with severe strife. Current views about the causes of depression also emphasize that a biological vulnerability for depressive disorder can be inherited. Indeed, some types of depression run in families. Major depression is 1.5 to 3 times more common in people who have parents, siblings, or children with depression as compared to the general population, and families may have depression occurring generation after generation. Depression can also occur in people who have no family history of depression.

Whether directly inherited or not, depression is often associated with changes in brain functioning and associated regulatory systems in the body. Sleep abnormalities are common. Sleep studies reveal abnormalities that include difficulty getting to sleep, staying asleep, and abnormal patterns of rapid eye movement (REM) sleep as well as non-REM periods.

Abnormalities in how the mind and body react to stress are often associated with severe depression. That

is, a number of immediate and more prolonged changes ensue when the body responds to stress, including engagement of the hypothalamic-pituitary-adrenal axis (for example, producing hormones like cortisol). Problems with regulating this stress response are commonly associated with severe forms of depression.

A number of abnormalities in neurotransmitters, including serotonin, noradrenaline, and GABA, have been found to be associated with depression. Because these neurotransmitters are used to allow the electrical signals to move from one nerve to another, a shortage of these chemicals or their receptors may interfere with efficient processing in the brain. Also, the two hemispheres (or sides) of the brain may process different types of emotion, and accordingly the brain's activation patterns have been found to be differently associated with depression. Brain activation patterns in the right frontal lobe are associated with withdrawal and negative emotions, and underactivation of the left frontal lobe is associated with depression.

Symptoms

Depression in adulthood has been recognized as a disorder for as long as psychology has existed as a formal discipline. However, the same cannot be said for depression in childhood. Although accounts in the 1940s observed depressive-like symptoms in institutionalized infants, even up until the 1980s there was considerable debate about the existence of depression in children. Currently, clinicians use near identical evaluation procedures to diagnose depression in children, adolescents, and adults.

The most common types of depressive disorders are major depressive disorder and dysthymic disorder. Depression is episodic, meaning there are periods when these symptoms cause problems and periods of recovery or at least more moderate problems.

Symptoms of major depressive disorder include disruptions in mood, thinking, and in the body's regulatory system. Mood changes include a severe and persistent (nearly every day) depressed mood or irritability, or both. Many people with depression experience a loss of interest or pleasure in hobbies and activities that were once enjoyed, including a diminished interest in sex. Changes exhibited in the body may include a loss of appetite or overeating, having difficulty sleeping or sleeping a lot, and feelings of restlessness or moving very slowly. Tiredness or feeling low in energy are additional symptoms of depression. Changes in thinking patterns may include difficulty in thinking clearly, making decisions, or concentrating. Excessive feelings of guilt, self-blame, worthlessness, or hopelessness, or all of these feelings, may also be experienced. At times, people suffering with depression may have recurrent thoughts of death or suicide.

Dysthymic disorder (dysthymia) is a more persistent but less severe form of depression that lasts for several years (at least 2 years for adults and 1 year for children). Dysthymic disorder and major depression share very similar symptoms. They include depressed mood (for more days than not) coupled with other symptoms such as appetite, sleep, or energy disturbances and cognitive disturbances (for example, low self-concept, poor concentration, difficulty making decisions, feelings of hopelessness). Often people with major depressive disorder also have dysthymia, a condition referred to as "double depression."

Depression is often accompanied by other psychological problems, including severe anxiety and substance abuse. More than half of the people who have depressive disorders may also have an anxiety disorder, and some have suggested that anxiety often precedes depression. Also, it has long been debated whether substance abuse is a risk factor for depression or if people who experience depression use drugs as a method of self-medicating their symptoms.

Depression is associated with a number of medical conditions, including metabolic syndrome, diabetes, heart disease, and a number of autoimmune disorders. Furthermore, several medical conditions or medication or drug reactions may mimic depression. These alternative disease processes should be examined to plan an effective treatment.

Diagnosis

Most people diagnosed with depression can be helped with treatment, which typically includes psychotherapy (counseling) or medication, or a combination of both of these treatments. Depression is often left untreated because people fail to recognize the symptoms and believe their depression is just normal sadness, a sign of weakness, or that they should "just pull themselves together."

The first step in getting treatment for depression is an examination by a physician. Certain medications as well as some medical conditions such as a viral infection can cause the same symptoms as depression, and the physician should rule out these possibilities through examination, interview, and lab tests. If a physical cause for the depression is ruled out, a diagnostic evaluation should be completed by a physician, psychiatrist, or psychologist.

KEY FACTS

Description
Depression is characterized by a severe and persistent sad mood. It affects the way a person thinks and also impacts daily patterns like eating and sleeping. When untreated, depression can linger, affecting almost every aspect of life.

Causes
A combination of genetic, psychological, and environmental factors are involved in the onset of a depressive disorder.

Risk factors
Life stressors, history of abuse.

Symptoms
Disruptions in mood; disruptions in thinking; recurrent thoughts of death or suicide, or both; disturbances to the body's regulatory system.

Diagnosis
A diagnostic interview completed by a physician or a mental health professional is used to assess depression.

Treatments
Most people diagnosed with depression can be helped with treatment. This treatment typically includes psychotherapy or counseling, or medication, or all of them.

Pathogenesis
Depression is a recurrent disorder. The length of the episodes is variable (lasting from two weeks to several years). People may have one episode of depression, a few episodes, or many episodes.

Prevention
Although there are approaches that can help reduce the risk of depression and suicide, there are no known ways to completely prevent depression and suicide.

Epidemiology
About 16 percent of the U.S. population will experience depression sometime in their life. Depression is rare in young children, but it is more common in adolescence and adulthood. Depression is two to three times more common in women than it is in men.

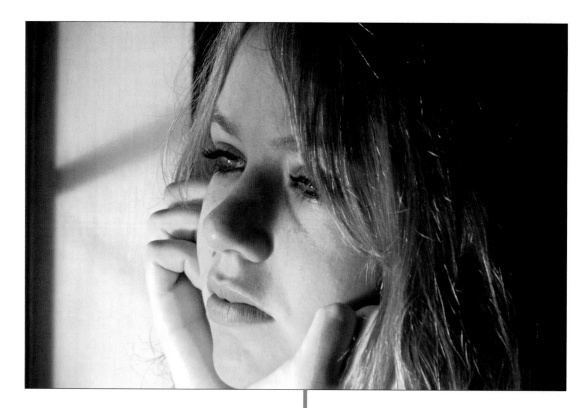

Adolescents are vulnerable to depressive disorders, and there is a rise in the incidence of depression from adolescence to adulthood. Women are two to three times more likely to suffer depression than are men.

A diagnostic interview is used to assess depression. Ideally, during the evaluation, the clinician will ask about which aspects of depression are currently being experienced and a history of symptoms (that is, when they started, whether the symptoms were treated, and whether there is a family history of depression). The evaluator will also ask questions about how the person is coping with these feelings of distress, including if the person has thoughts about suicide and if the person uses alcohol or drugs. The clinician typically asks about how these symptoms affect other areas of life functioning, including school or work performance and relationships with others. The prescribed treatment will depend on the outcome of the evaluation. Depressive disorders may be mild, moderate, or severe with or without psychotic features, such as delusions (having thoughts that are not based in reality) and hallucinations (seeing or hearing things that are not there). Currently, no laboratory tests are available to accurately diagnose depression.

Treatments

The prescribed treatment depends on the outcome of the evaluation. There are a variety of psychotherapies and antidepressant medications that can be used to treat depressive disorders. The diversity of both biological and social factors associated with depression supports a multimodal treatment plan. Some people with milder forms of depression may do well with psychotherapy alone. People with moderate to severe depression most often benefit from antidepressant medications in addition to psychotherapy. Given the high rate of relapse and recurrence of depression and the mortality risk associated with suicide, monitoring after the termination of therapy is recommended.

A trained mental health professional provides psychotherapy, also referred to as counseling or talk therapy. Psychiatrists, psychologists, social workers, or psychiatric nurses conduct individual or group psychotherapy sessions. There are many forms of psychotherapy. One type of psychotherapy that research has shown helpful for depression is cognitive behavioral therapy (CBT). CBT theories assume that cognitive and emotional processes mediate the disease process, and accordingly, CBT therapies effect a change in symptoms through changes in thinking patterns. In CBT, the therapist helps the depressed person learn to recognize and change faulty and nonproductive thinking patterns, behavior, and emotional responses. This approach is highly structured and involves collaboration between the client and the therapist to identify problems, set goals and use problem-solving strategies that will provide alternative methods of coping. Other forms of psychotherapy (for example, psychodynamic therapy and family therapy) may be useful, but there is little research support available. For example, in psychodynamic therapy, therapies help the depressed person gain insight into the cause of the problems and to resolve problems through talking with the therapist. In family therapy, altering family patterns is the focus of intervention.

There are several types of antidepressant medications used to treat depressive disorders. These include newer medications, chiefly the selective serotonin reuptake inhibitors (SSRIs) and more established medications, such as the tricyclics and monoamine oxidase inhibitors (MAOIs). The SSRIs affect neurotransmitters such as dopamine or norepinephrine and are commonly prescribed, in part because they have fewer side effects than tricyclics and MAOIs. Alternative medicines such as herbal remedies (for example, St. John's wort) and dietary supplements have also been used, but research is lacking as to their benefit.

When depression is particularly severe, or life threatening, or when it does not respond to psychotherapy and antidepressant medication, alternative methods of treatment, including electroconvulsive therapy (ECT), have been shown to be effective. ECT uses short bursts of a controlled electrical current into the brain to induce a brief seizure when the patient is under anesthesia. Additional techniques that are under investigation involve stimulation to selective brain structures. These approaches include magnetic stimulation, repetitive transcranial magnetic stimulation, and surgical insertion of electrodes (vagus nerve stimulation). Although these more invasive approaches remain controversial, they may provide a more marked and immediate relief of symptoms than do other forms of psychotherapy or medication.

Pathogenesis

Depression is a recurrent disorder. Although the length of the episodes is variable (lasting from 2 weeks to several years), an untreated depressive episode usually lasts 6 months. People who suffer from depression may have one, several, or many episodes of depression throughout their lifetime. People who first become depressed in childhood or adolescence typically experience more episodes of depression than do those with

an adult onset. Initial episodes are usually associated with severe life stressors. Later episodes may be brought on when the person is experiencing only a mild stressor or no obvious stressor.

Depression is the leading cause of disability in the United States, as well as in other countries, and according to the World Health Organization is expected to become the leading cause of disability worldwide by 2020. Even more tragic is the rise in suicide, because suicide is now one of the most common preventable deaths.

Prevention

There are no known ways to prevent depression and suicide. However, there are approaches that aid in reducing the risk of these problems. Currently, there are many efforts in place to educate the public about the signs of depression and options for treatment, including public service announcements and high school health class curricula. Preventionists may also direct their efforts in changing systems, such as altering how the media reports on suicide, attempting to restrict lethal means, such as handguns, and providing training about useful responses to those who are likely to come in contact with a depressed or suicidal person.

Another focus is to provide more in-depth preventive interventions to people who are at high risk for depression or for those who are already experiencing some problems associated with depression. For example, because depression runs in families, there are some preventive programs that provide guidance and support to children who have a depressed parent.

Epidemiology

The estimates of depression vary widely. Some estimates indicate that about 16 percent of the U.S. population experience depression sometime in their lives. In young children depression is rare, and there are no gender differences in depression in childhood. There is a rise in the incidence of depression from childhood to adolescence and into adulthood. Gender differences emerge in adolescence and persist in elderly people.

Depression is two to three times more common in women than in men. Several factors may contribute to the increased rate of depression in women. Hormonal factors appear to increase the risk of depression, including menstrual cycle changes, pregnancy, miscarriage, the postpartum period, and menopause. Many women also face additional stresses, such as responsibilities both at work and home, single parenthood, and caring for children and aging parents.

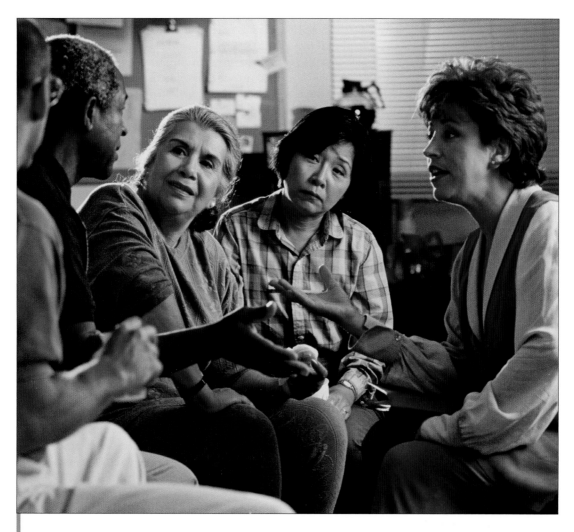

Some people find that the informality of a group therapy session enables them to express themselves more easily than in one-to-one therapy. Because a facilitator or therapist is always present, vulnerable people are protected.

When depression occurs in women within 2 years of childbirth, it is referred to as postpartum depression. It is common for women to experience some crying or sadness during the initial weeks after giving birth, referred to as the "baby blues." It is less common for women to experience a depressive disorder during this period. It is extremely rare for women to experience psychotic depression (delusions—having thoughts that are not based in reality; hallucinations—seeing or hearing things that are not there). Untreated psychotic postpartum depression at times results in severe lapses in the mother's judgment and may put her child's safety at risk. Although men are less likely to suffer from depression than women, it is still a signifi-

cant problem. Men may experience depressive symptoms differently, they are less likely to seek help when depressed, and they are four times more likely than women to commit suicide.

The rate of occurrence in depression increased in the later part of the twentieth century, manifesting at younger ages of onset for mild and moderate depression. The documented rate of suicide also rose considerably over this period. The rates and symptoms of depression may differ around the world. Westernized cultures have higher rates of depression than do non-Westernized cultures.

Bonnie Klimes-Dougan

See also
• Anxiety disorders • Menopausal disorders
• Menstrual disorders • Mood disorders
• Sleep disorders

Dermatitis

Dermatitis is an inflammation of the skin. The term is derived from the Greek words *dermat,* meaning "skin," and *itis,* meaning "inflammation." Dermatitis covers a wide range of conditions that result in red, dry, itchy skin. There are many causes of this noninfectious condition, but treatment and prevention are similar for most types. The term "eczema" can also be used to describe the condition.

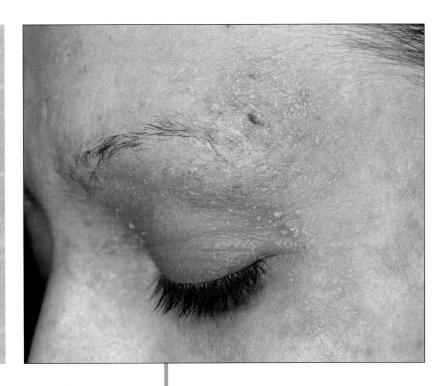

Seborrheic dermatitis commonly affects the skin on the face and scalp. Characterized by a red, scaly rash, the condition is thought to be linked to a growth of yeast on the skin and can be triggered by stress or illness.

The skin is the largest organ in the body, covering about 21 square feet (2 m²). The role of the skin is to act as a protective barrier to the inner organs of the body. As a large exposed area, the skin is constantly bombarded by outside elements, some of which can prove harmful and result in irritation. Dermatitis is the skin's reaction to such irritants. There are several categories of dermatitis, each with specific symptoms, but all types produce redness, swelling, and blisters.

Types of dermatitis

The different types of dermatitis are: contact, atopic, seborrheic, nummular, stasis, neurodermatitis, generalized exfoliative, and perioral dermatitis.

Contact dermatitis

Contact dermatitis consists of two forms: irritant and allergic dermatitis. Irritant contact dermatitis occurs when a harmful substance directly damages the skin. Such irritants include detergents, nail-polish remover, antiperspirants, formaldehyde (found in permanent press fabrics), unwashed new clothes, and strong soaps. Allergic contact dermatitis occurs when the body's immune system reacts to a substance contacting the skin. Usually the sensitivity develops slowly over a period of time, although occasionally just one exposure to a substance will cause the skin to be sensitized. Thousands of things can cause an allergic reaction, the most common culprits being plants, perfumes, and jewelry. About 10 percent of women are allergic to nickel, a common component of jewelry. About 50 to 70 percent of people are sensitive to urushiol, the oil in poison ivy, oak, and sumac. The oils are quickly absorbed in the skin but may remain active on clothing and pet fur for a long time. Smoke from burning poison plants can irritate the eyes and skin of susceptible people, and some people may even react to the creams and lotions that treat dermatitis.

Regardless of the cause, the symptoms of contact dermatitis are swelling, rash, and sometimes itching. The rash may have tiny blisters that appear first in sensitive skin areas. Chronic forms appear as thickened, inflamed skin, and in babies, as diaper rash. Breaking the blisters does not cause the rash to spread.

Atopic dermatitis

Atopic dermatitis is a chronic (long-lasting), severely itchy skin condition that often develops in people who suffer from hay fever or asthma. The condition frequently runs in families, usually beginning during infancy, varying in severity throughout childhood and adolescence, and then tending to subside during adulthood. The suspected cause is a combination of dry skin and the malfunction of the cytokines, chemicals produced by the immune system, which cause the skin to overreact to certain substances. Excessive bathing, hand washing, or swimming may trigger symptoms, along with contact with irritants such as detergents. Excessive or prolonged heat, such as hot showers or electric blankets, can trigger a flare-up. Emotional stress, low room humidity, bacterial skin infections, and irritating materials, such as wool, can all worsen the condition. The problem is aggravated by uncontrollable scratching, which can break the skin surface and introduce bacterial infections.

Seborrheic dermatitis

Seborrheic dermatitis consists of a red rash and greasy, yellowish scales. In infants it occurs on the scalp and is commonly known as cradle cap. In adults the rash occurs on the hairy areas, such as the scalp, face, and genitals, in skin creases under the nose, breasts, and the armpits, and on the ankles. The condition is common in people with oily hair or skin and may vary with the seasons. In adolescents and adults it is caused by an overgrowth of a yeast that inhabits the skin. This type of dermatitis can recur, and illness or periods of stress can trigger a flare-up.

Nummular dermatitis

Nummular dermatitis consists of distinctive coin-shaped red patches on the skin that have tiny blisters, scabs, and scales. It is commonly seen on the legs, hands, arms, and torso. The dry, round spots start as itchy patches of pimples and then form blisters that ooze and form crusts. It is much more common in men than women, and the peak ages of onset are between 55 and 65 years. People who live in very dry climates or take very hot showers may develop this condition. The cause is unknown.

Stasis dermatitis

Stasis dermatitis is caused by poor circulation from varicose veins and congestive heart failure. In these conditions, veins in the lower legs do not return the blood to the heart, and pooled blood causes fluid to accumulate in the lower legs, resulting in irritation around the legs and ankles. At first, the skin becomes red and scaly, and within a number of weeks turns brown. The skin may break down and form open sores that become infected with bacteria. Stasis dermatitis is not usually painful, but the ulcers may become a serious problem.

Neurodermatitis

Neurodermatitis develops in areas where tight garments rub the skin or anywhere that someone picks or rubs. The person scratches that area constantly and may continue after the initial cause has gone. Anxiety and stress can make the itching worse. More women than men have this condition, and it is common among Asians and Native Americans.

KEY FACTS

Description
Itchy, red, inflamed skin; also called eczema.

Causes
Allergies, genetic factors, physical factors, mental stress, and irritants.

Risk factors
Contact with irritants, winter conditions when air is dry. Scratching can expose underlying skin to infection.

Symptoms
Redness, swelling, itching, and blisters.

Diagnosis
Observation of skin; confirmation made by a patch test.

Treatments
Corticosteroid creams relieve inflammation and itching.

Pathogenesis
Left untreated, any open sores may become infected with bacteria.

Prevention
Avoiding harsh soaps or plants such as poison ivy. Self-care is important in managing and preventing dermatitis.

Epidemiology
Prevalence of atopic dermatitis in the United States is 12 percent, around 15 million people; almost 66 percent of people with atopic eczema develop it before six months of age and 90 percent by five years of age. Seborrheic dermatitis occurs mostly in infants, usually within the first three months of life, and then between the ages of 30 and 70 years. Women are more susceptible to dermatitis than men.

Generalized exfoliative dermatitis

Generalized exfoliative dermatitis affects the entire surface of the skin. Certain drugs, especially penicillin and sulfonamides, may cause the disease, and in some cases it is a complication of contact dermatitis or infection. The condition starts slowly with red, shiny patches that gradually become covered with scales. Over time hair and nails may even fall out. Many people have an accompanying fever, although they may feel chilled and lose considerable fluid through damaged skin. The symptoms are similar to those of many skin infections where there is swelling and discomfort. Early diagnosis and treatment are important to stop the skin from becoming infected.

Perioral dermatitis

Perioral dermatitis is a disorder of unknown cause that produces a red, bumpy rash around the mouth and on the chin that resembles acne. It most commonly affects women between the ages of 40 and 60. The use of strong corticosteroid creams to clear the condition is not advised as the dermatitis often returns after treatment is stopped. Oral tetracyclines or other antibiotics are the recommended treatment. Physicians may also advise against using sunscreens, moisturizers, makeup, and dental products that may aggravate the condition.

Diagnosis, treatment, and prevention

Physicians can reach a diagnosis of dermatitis after reviewing the patient's symptoms and carefully looking at the skin. They may scrape a small amount of skin to be sent for microscopic examination. If allergic contact dermatitis is suspected, the physician may order a patch test that involves placing tiny amounts of potential allergens onto small disks, which are then attached to a piece of tape and in turn stuck on the wide surface of the back. The disks and tape are left in place for a couple of days and then removed; the skin is then examined for any sign of a reaction, which will appear as a red patch on the skin. Treatment varies according to the cause or condition of the dermatitis. If a cause is identified, then the affected person should avoid the source as much as possible.

Because many types of dermatitis have the same initial symptoms, the physician may recommend a bath taken at room temperature followed by fragrance-free moisturizer and a corticosteroid cream. For some conditions, there are specific treatments. For example, seborrheic dermatitis usually responds to shampoos with a coal-tar base, zinc pyrithione, or sulfur. People with nummular dermatitis or acute contact dermatitis may soak the area to dry the oozing before applying a corticosteroid cream. Antihistamines are sometimes prescribed for contact dermatitis to relieve itching.

For stasis dermatitis, the treatment is first to correct the condition that causes fluid to accumulate in the legs and ankles. This may involve wearing elastic support stockings or having surgery to treat varicose veins. A zinc paste may be given to treat the ulcers or sores of stasis dermatitis.

For a patient with neurodermatitis the most important thing is to stop scratching. Sometimes a surgical tape saturated with a corticosteroid cream is used to cover the affected area, thus protecting the skin from damaging fingernails.

Generalized dermatitis is a serious condition, and early diagnosis and treatment are important to keep the skin from infection and avoid fluid and protein loss; people with severe generalized dermatitis often need to be hospitalized.

Although dermatitis is not normally serious, it can affect a person's quality of life, and prevention and management are key. Affected people must learn to avoid irritants, such as household substances, deodorants, or certain kinds of soaps, which cause the problems. Taking a daily bath or shower may be recommended as long as it is followed by the rapid application of a moisturizer, ideally to skin that has been only slightly patted dry before application. Thorough drying should be avoided. The bath should be limited to 5 to 10 minutes. A good preventive strategy is to use mild soaps, which clean without removing natural oils, on the face, underarms, genitals, hands, and feet, with clear water elsewhere. Children should be given sponge baths.

Other self-care tips include avoiding scratching the skin whenever possible, dressing with layers to avoid sweating, and wearing smooth-textured cotton clothing that will not irritate the skin. Clothes should be washed in mild laundry soap and rinsed well. To prevent exacerbating dermatitis, affected people must be vigilant in avoiding possible irritants. People with contact dermatitis should wear a thin pair of cotton gloves inside rubber gloves for all wet work. With care, most forms of dermatitis are preventable.

Evelyn Kelly

See also
- Allergy and sensitivity • Asthma
- Hay fever

Diabetes

A serious and potentially fatal disease, diabetes is a metabolic disorder. It is characterized by inadequate secretion or use of insulin, which results in high levels of sugar in the blood. Uncontrolled, diabetes can lead to fatal stroke, heart attack, kidney failure, nerve and blood vessel damage, blindness, and the amputation of body extremities affected by the disease.

Diabetes results from abnormal insulin production. Insulin is a hormone produced in the pancreas by cells called beta cells. It enables body cells to take in glucose (a sugar) from the blood to provide energy.

When food is eaten and digested, it is broken down into glucose, which fuels body cells. Normally, the pancreas produces the appropriate amount of insulin to transport glucose from the blood into the cells. In people with diabetes, either the pancreas produces little or no insulin or the cells respond improperly to insulin produced; glucose accumulates in the blood and is eventually excreted in the urine without being properly absorbed by the cells in the body. As a result, the main fuel source for cells and energy is greatly depleted. There is no cure for diabetes, but there are treatments available that can keep a person with diabetes healthy.

There are several types of diabetes, and all types can be managed, but not cured, with a careful program of monitoring glucose levels, sensible diet, exercise, and (in some cases) medication.

Type 1 diabetes

Previously known as insulin-dependent diabetes mellitus or juvenile-onset diabetes, type 1 diabetes accounts for 5 to 10 percent of all diabetes cases. It usually occurs in children or adolescents, but can occur at any time in life. Symptoms such as dry mouth, frequent urination, and excessive thirst develop quickly, although the underlying disease may have been present for years. Type 1 diabetes is an autoimmune disease, meaning that the body's own immune system, which normally serves to fight infection, malfunctions and sabotages processes that keep the body functioning normally. In people with type 1 diabetes, the immune system attacks the insulin-producing beta cells in the pancreas and destroys them. Researchers

have not yet determined what causes the immune system to turn on itself, although several factors (genetics, environment, and viruses) are under study. People with type 1 diabetes have to take synthetic insulin injections every day to regulate glucose levels. Without insulin, people with diabetes lapse into a life-threatening coma, a condition in which ketones (organic acids that can build up in the blood) cause ketoacidosis through incomplete breakdown of fats. Ketones become toxic when the body is starved of insulin. Usually ketone accumulation is gradual, but in some cases it develops suddenly.

It is important that people with type 1 diabetes are able to recognize ketoacidosis and seek medical assistance. Symptoms include nausea, vomiting, abdominal pain, thirst or dry mouth, dry or flushed skin, confusion, and disorientation.

Type 2 diabetes

Also known as insulin-resistant diabetes, this type of diabetes is the most common form. It accounts for 90 to 95 percent of cases, and was once more usual in older people. However, type 2 diabetes is becoming more common in children and young adults.

Type 2 diabetes develops more gradually than type 1, and people with a family history of diabetes, a history of obesity, and no or low physical activity, or a history of gestational diabetes, are at greater risk. Also Native Americans, African Americans, and Hispanic people are more likely to acquire type 2 diabetes.

In type 2 diabetes, the pancreas produces enough insulin, but for unexplained reasons, the body does not use the insulin efficiently, and over time, insulin production drops. The result is the same as in type 1 diabetes—glucose builds up in the blood and is excreted in the urine. Symptoms include abnormal thirst, weight loss or weight gain, nausea, blurred vision, and slow healing of wounds.

Gestational diabetes

This type of diabetes develops in pregnant women who were free from diabetes before becoming pregnant. During pregnancy all women become insulin resistant, so the body has to make extra insulin to compensate. Most women are able to compensate and maintain normal blood glucose levels, while those with gestational diabetes become hyperglycemic. These women are at risk for type 2 diabetes later in life. Gestational diabetes must be treated aggressively to keep the baby healthy.

Prediabetes

This fairly new category has been added to the diabetes family of diseases. It is a condition that shows risk based on sugar levels and other tests. Prediabetes develops over time.

There are two indicators of pre-type 2 diabetes: impaired fasting glucose, in which blood glucose levels are elevated but not yet at a level indicative of diabetes, and impaired glucose tolerance, in which glucose is elevated on oral glucose tolerance tests but not yet at the level of diabetes. In the United States, about 35 million people of ages 40 to 74 have impaired fasting glucose and 16 million have impaired glucose tolerance; this is of concern, because without taking steps to reverse the condition, many people will develop type 2 diabetes. In people with prediabetes, developing diabetes is not a certainty; with improvements in diet and exercise patterns, prediabetes can be delayed or even reversed.

Pre-type 1 diabetes is characterized by antibodies in the blood that show that the pancreas is being attacked by the immune system.

Diabetic retinopathy

Diabetes mellitus can affect blood vessels anywhere in the body. When the blood vessels in the retina are affected, it is called diabetic retinopathy, and the condition affects the vision of both eyes. It is one of the most common causes of blindness.

THE ROLE OF INSULIN

The pancreas produces the hormone insulin, which enables glucose to be stored in the liver. Glucose is essential for the production of energy in body cells. When the body requires more energy, it needs glucose to make that energy. The glucose will then be released from the liver into the body's cells. Insulin from the pancreas enables the cells to utilize the glucose in the production of energy. Without sufficient insulin, glucose cannot be stored or used and is lost in the urine.

The hormone insulin (green spots) is produced by the pancreas. Insulin is essential for glucose (red spots) to be absorbed by body cells, where glucose is converted into energy, and for the liver to store excess glucose.

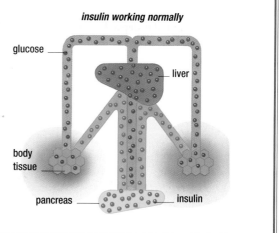

insulin working normally

glucose

liver

body tissue

pancreas

insulin

Causes and risk factors

Type 1 diabetes seems to have very different causes from other types of diabetes. Since researchers believe it is a disease of the immune system, there is no easy way to prevent it. The immune system is made up of a complex network of organs, including the appendix, lymph nodes, spleen, and thymus. White blood cells and proteins called antibodies combat foreign agents such as bacteria or viruses that enter the body. In type 1 diabetes, an autoimmune reaction occurs. The immune system makes a mistake and launches an inappropriate attack on certain targets, and destroys or alters healthy, normal cells in the body. In type 1 diabetes, researchers believe the body turns on the insulin-producing beta cells in the pancreas, eliminating or reducing their ability to produce insulin. Researchers are not exactly sure why that happens, but it is known that genetics plays a part, since people (especially Caucasians) are more likely to develop type 1 diabetes if their relatives have the disease.

Environmental factors play a role as well because type 1 diabetes develops more often during cold weather and more frequently in people who live in cold climates. Viruses may also trigger it, although this is still under investigation. Diet could also be a factor; people who were breast-fed (rather than bottle fed baby formula) and who began eating solid foods at a later age get diabetes less often.

Type 2 diabetes has an even greater link to genetic background, yet it also depends greatly on environmental factors in people who live in the Western Hemisphere. So, although people who have a family history of diabetes have a high risk of developing type 2 diabetes, lifestyle factors play an even stronger role. The combination of a diet high in fat and low in carbohydrates and fiber and the low level of exercise prevalent in the West place Americans and Europeans at greater risk than people in non-Westernized countries, where diabetes is much more unusual, even among people whose relatives have diabetes. In the United States, African Americans, Mexican Americans, and Pima Indians have the highest risk of all. There are other behavioral risk factors for type 2 diabetes besides a poor diet. Heavy alcohol use can lead to type 2 diabetes because it causes inflammation of the pancreas, called pancreatitis, which can affect its ability to secrete insulin. Smoking is a risk factor because it increases blood sugar levels and decreases the body's ability to use insulin; chemicals in tobacco damage blood vessels, muscles, and other organs besides the pancreas. Carrying excess weight, especially around the

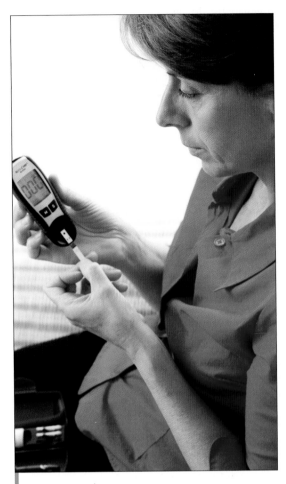

A woman with diabetes monitors her blood sugar (glucose). A drop of blood is placed on a test stick and analyzed in a glucometer, which measures the levels of glucose present.

abdomen, also increases risk. Risk factors that are not controllable include being over 30 years old, a low birth weight, ethnicity (Native American, African American, and Hispanic) and, rarely, deficiency of chromium. The risk factors for prediabetes are the same as for diabetes.

To date, the causes behind gestational diabetes are still not well understood, although women who get diabetes while pregnant are more likely to have a family history of diabetes, to smoke, to be older, and tend to be overweight.

For diabetic retinopathy, risk factors include having diabetes mellitus, which may not be well controlled, and lifestyle factors such as smoking.

Symptoms and associated disorders

Prediabetes often has no symptoms at all until it develops into diabetes. Usually there are no symptoms in gestational diabetes, but some women experience excessive thirst and increased urination.

Symptoms of type 1 diabetes often follow a flulike illness and develop quickly over a few weeks. People may have all or some of the following symptoms: Increased thirst or frequent urinating, or both, may occur because the excess glucose that builds up in the blood is excreted in the urine, causing body water to be excreted with it, which leads to dehydration and thirst. Excessive hunger is also typical because there is not enough fuel provided to muscles and organs, so a hunger response is triggered. Although eating fills the stomach, the glucose that should be absorbed from carbohydrates does not reach the necessary tissues. Weight loss is also typical because since the body's tissues, muscles, and organs are not receiving the correct amount of fuel, they shrink. Blurred vision is also typical because the lens of the eye loses fluid, decreasing its ability to focus. Fatigue is common because the glucose-deprived cells do not have enough energy, making the body feel tired.

Type 2 diabetes shares some of the same symptoms as type 1 diabetes, but it develops much more slowly. Again, people may have all or just some symptoms. Increased thirst and frequent urination are common, because the excess glucose draws water from the body, causing constant thirst, then urination to excrete extra fluid intake. Sometimes type 2 diabetes may be mistaken for influenza, because flulike symptoms such as fatigue and weakness may develop due to the lack of energy provided to the body. Weight loss may occur, as in type 1 diabetes, due to tissues shrinking from a lack of fuel. Some people gain weight; because fuel is not reaching tissues and organs efficiently, the body may crave more food than is normal, leading to overeating and weight gain. The difference between this and type 1 diabetes is that there is enough insulin present to allow weight gain even though the body is not using the fuel efficiently. Blurred vision is also common because less fluid is able to reach the eye, which affects the ability of the eye's lens to focus. If blood sugar levels are reduced, vision improves. Diabetic retinopathy may lack symptoms at first, but if left untreated, irreversible visual loss occurs.

Complications

Complications occur when diabetes is not managed properly and hyperglycemia is present for many years. They are avoidable with careful control of blood sugar levels. Diabetes affects the body's ability to heal quickly and fight infections, which makes the body vulner-

able to bladder infection and to common ailments such as the cold and the flu, which a healthy person can fight off; also, cuts and other wounds heal more slowly because the immune system is not working properly. In extreme cases, wounds on the hands and feet can become so infected that they cannot be treated, and amputation of the affected limb becomes necessary to avoid the spread of infection to the entire body. Skin infections and resulting sores are also common. Boils, carbuncles, and fungal infections typically affect diabetics but can be treated with antibiotics and antifungal creams. Some people also suffer blistering on the backs of the hands and feet and sometimes on the legs or forearms. The blisters are not painful and heal after sugar levels have been brought under control. One particular skin condition that may occur in people with diabetes is acanthosis nigricans, in which the skin can grow thick and dark in body folds and creases such as the armpits, groin, and neck. It is not an infection or health threat, but the condition affects a person's appearance.

Nerve damage, called neuropathy, is common because high levels of glucose in the blood damage the small blood vessels, which are numerous in the hands and feet. Neuropathy causes tingling, loss of feeling, and burning in the hands and feet, and sometimes in the legs and arms. Autonomic neuropathy can cause digestive problems, vomiting and diarrhea, and reduced or increased sweating; it can also affect the eye's ability to react to light and dark and may make the patient less aware of the warning signs of low blood sugar. Nerve damage can also affect the sex organs in men and affect the ability to have or maintain an erection. Careful control of blood sugar and regular care of the feet can reduce the impact of these problems.

Tooth and gum disorders may trouble people with diabetes. Because high glucose increases the risk of infection, it affects oral health, resulting in gum infections that may cause the gum to pull away from the tooth, making teeth loose. Sores or pockets of infection may appear on the gums, and the teeth may actually become so loose that they fall out.

Diabetic hyperosmolar syndrome may develop when people with type 2 diabetes do not control their glucose levels; blood sugar is too high and the body tries to remove excess sugar by excretion in the urine. This leads to dehydration, a lack of adequate fluid in the body that, left untreated, can cause seizures, coma, and death.

Circulation disorders are common in people with type 2 diabetes. Atherosclerois may occur; this is the hardening of the blood vessels that carry oxygen and nutrients from the heart to the entire body. Such stiffness in the walls of the arteries can restrict blood flow to organs and tissues. The effect on arteries that serve the heart can lead to a stroke or heart attack. Blood vessel problems may also lead to high blood pressure and peripheral arterial disease (PAD) in which arteries that supply the limbs becomes blocked.

Kidney disease is also a complication of poorly treated diabetes. A transplant or dialysis may be necessary if the kidneys fail.

Treatments

For type 1 diabetes, insulin is the only treatment. People with type 1 diabetes cannot help getting the disease since it is not a result of being overweight, lack of exercise, smoking, or the other factors that can lead to type 2 diabetes. There is no vaccine or medication that prevents type 1 diabetes from developing, and once it is diagnosed, people who have it must take insulin through daily injections or an insulin pump for the rest of their lives to stay alive. To determine the amount of insulin needed, the diabetic person must prick his or her finger and test the blood glucose level, then inject the appropriate amount of insulin to create a normal level in the blood. There are many types of insulin available, and a doctor will prescribe what is suitable for each individual patient.

People with type 1 diabetes can also manage the disease by paying close attention to their eating habits. Since glucose rises when the body takes in food, the amount of insulin required will vary based on food intake and energy expended on a daily basis. Usually type 1 diabetics can eat a completely normal diet, as long as they correctly balance their food and insulin. Also, reactions of insulin with other medications taken concurrently are a consideration. Alcohol intake must also be carefully monitored, since alcohol can cause blood sugar levels to drop.

Many people with type 2 diabetes can control their condition (at least for a while) by making lifestyle changes. Maintaining a weight proportional to height and body type, exercising regularly, quitting smoking, restricting alcohol intake, and eating a healthful diet that is low in fat and sugar and high in fiber can reduce glucose in the blood.

Oral medications may also be recommended for type 2 diabetes. There are several available. Some drugs stimulate the pancreas to release insulin. Other drugs make the body more sensitive to the effects of insulin. These drugs may be used in combination or singly. Lifestyle changes will enhance their effect in improving diabetic symptoms.

Frequent monitoring of blood sugar levels can help the patient make decisions about appropriate diet, physical activity, and medications.

Type 2 diabetes is a progressive disease, and people with this condition usually require more aggressive therapy over time. If their disease is not controlled by lifestyle changes, medications, or both, they may have to take insulin as the disease progresses.

People with type 1 or 2 diabetes who face kidney or liver failure because the disease has progressed uncontrollably may have to undergo a kidney transplantation. However, shortages in donor organs, organ rejection, infection, and other complications make an organ transplant a difficult option.

For diabetic retinopathy, laser surgery removes damaged vessels and, if carried out early enough, may prevent further loss of sight.

New therapies are under development. Researchers have recently transplanted cells into the pancreas to enable it to produce insulin normally. Early results have been promising, and more research is underway.

Women with gestational diabetes can often control their blood sugar with diet and exercise during their pregnancy, but some may require insulin injections to lower their blood sugar. Women who control their glucose levels during pregnancy have fewer problems during childbirth.

Losing weight, quitting smoking, and eating a healthful diet can delay or prevent the progression to type 2 diabetes.

Prevention

Because diabetes may arise from a number of factors—genetic predisposition, lifestyle choices, or pregnancy—there is no way to eradicate it. In face of the growing number of obese and sedentary people worldwide, rates of obesity may grow over the coming decades. However, there are measures that can be taken to either prevent or manage diabetes.

Eating a diet low in sugar and fat and high in fiber, keeping off extra weight, getting regular physical activity, and quitting smoking can have a tremendous effect on reducing or preventing glucose intolerance.

Lise Stevens

See also
- Macular degeneration • Obesity
- Retinal disorders

Diarrhea and dysentery

Diarrheal illnesses have plagued mankind since time immemorial. Although these illnesses are most often simply an inconvenience in industrialized countries, they cause much discomfort and are associated with an economic impact stretching into billions of dollars each year. In developing countries, however, diarrheal diseases are the second leading cause of infant mortality. In some cases, however, diarrhea can be considered a protective response that rids the body of infections or toxins, albeit at the risk of pain and dehydration.

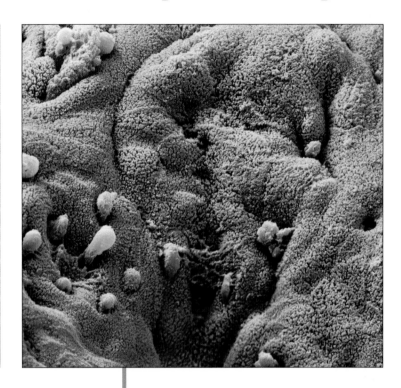

This colored scanning micrograph (SEM) shows Entamoeba histolytica *protozoa (blue) invading the lining of the large intestine. These parasites are a common cause of dysentery in hot regions of the world with poor sanitation.*

Diarrhea is a multifaceted condition that can arise from a variety of causes. It is often helpful to distinguish between acute diarrhea, lasting at most a few weeks, and chronic diarrhea, which lasts for more than six weeks in duration, because this distinction aids in diagnosis. Acute diarrhea is mostly caused by infectious agents, such as bacteria, viruses, or parasites, or is drug-induced. Dysentery is defined as a severe form of diarrhea in which the stools are bloody and contain mucus, and it is most often caused by infection, particularly when acute. Infectious diarrhea is transmitted among people by way of the fecal-oral route, and those living in circumstances with inadequate sanitation and thus a lack of clean food and water are especially at risk. Infectious diarrhea is also seen frequently in travelers.

Common infections causing diarrhea include salmonella, shigellosis, cholera, rotaviruses, giardiasis, and various types of *E. coli*. Other important causes of acute diarrhea include the use of broad-spectrum antibiotics, which are believed to cause diarrhea by disrupting the normal community of bacteria resident within the intestine such that harmful species, such as *Clostridium difficile*, predominate. Patients receiving chemotherapy for cancer also frequently develop diarrhea because the drugs used are harmful to the epithelial cells lining the intestine that normally control the movement of water into and out of the intestinal contents.

On the other hand, chronic diarrhea is often indicative of an underlying systemic disease, such as celiac disease, inflammatory bowel disease, food allergies, irritable bowel syndrome, or rarely an endocrine tumor. It is important to recognize, however, that in many cases of either acute or chronic diarrhea, an underlying cause is either not sought nor ever identified, and in a significant proportion of people with chronic diarrhea, the symptoms are actually due to the intentional abuse of laxatives (drugs to treat constipation).

With respect to the mechanisms that underlie diarrhea, the symptoms can be caused primarily in one of two ways, or a combination of these. In "osmotic" diarrhea, water is retained within the intestine because the intestinal contents contain a substance or substances that cannot be digested or absorbed, or both.

175

In "secretory" diarrhea, the epithelial cells that line the intestine are stimulated to secrete salt into the intestinal contents, which in turn drives the secretion of water in amounts too large to be reabsorbed into the body before they are lost to the stool. A classic example of secretory diarrhea is cholera, which is caused by a bacterium *Vibrio cholerae*. This bacterium reproduces in the small intestine and secretes a toxin that promotes salt and thus water secretion and also inhibits water absorption. In diseases such as cholera, fluid losses to the stool may exceed 25.4 pints (12 liters) per day compared with a normal stool volume of less than 6.7 fluid ounces (200 ml). Inflammation or injury to the intestine may both decrease its ability to digest and absorb nutrients and may result in the release of inflammatory substances that directly stimulate salt and water secretion. Thus, inflammatory diarrheas may include both osmotic and secretory components. No matter what the underlying mechanism of a particular diarrheal illness, the increased volume of intestinal contents can distend the bowel and trigger it to contract and propel the contents along its length more rapidly, further worsening the symptoms because there is less time for fluid to be absorbed.

Symptoms and signs and diagnosis

Patients with diarrhea exhibit increased daily stool volumes, often associated with an increased frequency of defecation and increased urgency to defecate. The stools may be watery (particularly in secretory diarrhea) or bulky with evidence of maldigested nutrients. Nocturnal bowel movements point to a secretory cause. The presence of excess fat in the stool, referred to as steatorrhea, is often the first sign of a generalized problem with digestion or absorption (that is, osmotic diarrhea). Patients may also complain of abdominal pain and cramping, and there may be blood in the stool, which reflects injury to the bowel. In severe cases, patients may have a fever or symptoms consistent with dehydration. If severe diarrhea is left untreated, death can result.

Acute diarrhea is often mild and self-limited, and a specific cause is not sought. However, if the disease is more severe or lasts longer than a few days, stools can be cultured for the presence of specific microorganisms (although this is time-consuming, and positive results are not assured even if an infection is present). Diagnosing the cause of chronic diarrheal diseases rests initially on a detailed history and physical examination of the patient. The stool can again be cultured for the presence of infectious agents, particularly

KEY FACTS

Description

Diarrhea is a sign of a variety of intestinal diseases and is defined as increased stool weight, with or without an associated increase in stool frequency. Dysentery refers to bloody diarrhea with fever.

Causes

A variety of causes, including malabsorption, infections, adverse effects of drugs (especially antibiotics and chemotherapy), inflammation, and abuse of laxatives.

Risk factors

Poor sanitation and the use of broad-spectrum antibiotics are significant risk factors. Children, elderly people, those with a weakened immune system, and those housed in institutions and hospitals are also at increased risk.

Symptoms and signs

The primary symptoms are an increase in stool volume and urgency, which may be accompanied by abdominal pain and fever. In severe cases, dehydration with accompanying problems with other body systems can result.

Diagnosis

The patient's history and physical examination are useful in identifying possible causes. Stool cultures and evaluation for malabsorbed substances (especially fat) may be helpful. Tests for antibodies can diagnose celiac disease. Endoscopy and biopsy may be important to evaluate chronic diarrhea.

Treatments

Relieving symptoms and replacing lost fluids are the mainstays of treatment. Antibiotics are used where appropriate. Celiac disease is treated by eliminating gluten from the diet.

Pathogenesis

Water is drawn into the bowel contents, beyond the amount that can be reabsorbed before being lost to the stool. This occurs either in response to malabsorbed substances or secondary to the active secretion of salts by epithelial cells lining the intestine, or both.

Prevention

Avoidance of contaminated food and water is critical. Probiotic microorganisms may improve illness in patients taking broad-spectrum antibiotics.

Epidemiology

The highest rates are recorded in developing countries, where diarrheal illness kills millions, especially young children, every year. Even in industrialized countries, individuals may report one to two episodes of diarrheal illness each year.

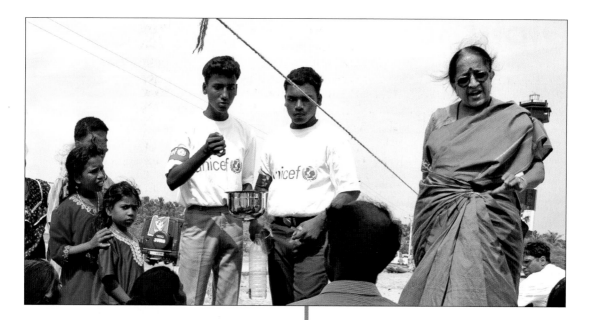

Workers from UNICEF demonstrate how to make oral rehydration solution (ORS) to people made homeless after a tsunami struck the coast of India on December 26, 2004, killing 10,000 people. ORS treats severe diarrhea, thus avoiding further deaths, especially of children.

parasites, and blood tests are used to provide evidence of malabsorption, the presence of antibodies consistent with celiac disease, or elevated levels of hormones that might reflect the presence of an endocrine tumor.

Osmotic diarrheas also frequently respond to fasting, and a comparison of the salt composition of the stool with that of plasma may reveal the presence of a nonabsorbed osmotically active substance that is causing excess fluid loss (such as fat or carbohydrate). Screening for ingested laxatives is often also conducted. Finally, endoscopic examination with biopsies may reveal specific inflammatory diseases or celiac disease. However, many cases of chronic diarrhea will defy a specific diagnosis, even with extensive testing.

Treatments

Diarrhea can be treated symptomatically with antidiarrheal drugs that act predominantly by slowing the movement of intestinal contents along the length of the bowel, allowing more time for water to be reabsorbed. Fluid replacement is also critical in moderate to severe disease, either intravenously or in the form of oral rehydration solutions. The latter contain both salt and sugars and revolutionized the treatment of diarrhea in developing countries where the ability to deliver sterile intravenous solutions may be severely limited or even absent. If a specific infectious cause can be identified, appropriate antibiotics can also be administered, although often the symptoms subside before the infection is identified. However, if the pa-

tient has weakened immunity or suffers concurrently from other serious conditions, such as heart disease, antibiotic treatment with ciprofloxacin may be considered, although this is controversial because some infectious diarrheal illnesses and their consequences—for example, those caused by the strain of *E. coli* called the "hamburger" bacterium—can be worsened considerably by the use of antibiotics. Similarly, if the stool is bloody, antidiarrheal drugs should most likely be avoided.

In chronic diarrhea, treatment centers on the underlying cause, assuming it can be identified. Celiac disease can be treated by witholding gluten-containing products, such as bread and pasta, from the diet. Inflammatory bowel diseases such as ulcerative colitis and Crohn's disease are treated with anti-inflammatory drugs. Some endocrine tumors can be removed surgically, and those who surreptitiously ingest laxatives can often be helped by psychological counseling.

Kim Barrett

See also
- Allergy and sensitivity • Celiac disease
- Cholera • Colitis, ulcerative • Food poisoning • Giardiasis • Irritable bowel syndrome

Diphtheria

Diphtheria is an infection of the throat, nose, and sometimes skin caused by the bacterium *Corynebacterium diphtheriae*. Once a leading cause of death in developed countries, diphtheria is now a rare disease due to a comprehensive immunization program.

Since 1980 there have been less than five cases of diphtheria annually in the United States, according to the Centers for Disease Control and Prevention. During the 1990s in Russia, however, more than 150,000 people contracted the disease and 5,000 died as a result of a decline in immunization rates.

Causes and risk factors

Diphtheria is transmitted through airborne droplets from people who either have the disease or are carriers of the disease. One type of diphtheria known as cutaneous diphtheria affects the skin and can be spread via discharge from skin lesions. Nonimmunized or inadequately immunized individuals are at greatest risk of contracting diphtheria. Typically this includes children under 5 and adults older than 60. People with immunodeficiency disorders and those living in crowded or unsanitary conditions are also at a higher risk.

Symptoms and signs

Within 2–10 days of infection, fever, pharyngitis (inflammation of the throat) and swollen lymph glands develop, which may give a "bull neck" appearance. Symptoms mimic common illnesses such as strep throat (infection with *streptococcus* bacteria) and mononucleosis. However, in severe cases of diphtheria, the heart, nervous system, and kidneys can be affected by a toxin produced by the bacterium, and in some cases a classic grayish membrane may form on the throat, which can cause airway obstruction and death. Left untreated, the infectious period begins at symptom onset and continues for two to six weeks.

Diagnosis and treatment

Diagnosis is made by swabbing the membrane or skin sores and having the bacteria grown (cultured) in a laboratory. Treatment should begin immediately with diphtheria antitoxin and antibiotics (penicillin or erythromycin), followed by diphtheria toxoid vaccine during recovery.

KEY FACTS

Description
Bacterial infection of throat, nose, and/or skin.

Cause
Corynebacterium diphtheriae bacterium.

Risk factors
Contact with respiratory secretions and skin lesions that contain this organism. Also contact with objects contaminated with such secretions.

Symptoms
Fever, pharyngitis (sore throat), swollen lymph glands (lymphadenopathy), nasal discharge, skin sores. Thick, grayish pharyngeal membrane can cause airway obstruction and death.

Diagnosis
Culture of *C. diphtheriae*; positive test for toxin.

Treatments
Antitoxin and antibiotics; vaccine administration.

Pathogenesis
C. diphtheriae has an affinity for the upper airway mucosa, producing a characteristic grayish "pseudomembrane" and causing extensive swelling of tissues.

Prevention
Vaccination.

Epidemiology
Diphtheria is rare in the United States as a result of successful vaccination campaigns.

Pathogenesis

C. diphtheriae multiplies and produces a toxin that can damage the heart, nervous system, and kidneys. Death occurs in 5–10 percent of cases of respiratory diphtheria. Some carry the disease but have no symptoms. Antibiotic treatment usually renders patients noninfectious in 24 hours.

Prevention

Prevention is by vaccination. In children, the vaccine is a combination of diphtheria-tetanus-acellular pertussis (DTaP); in adults it is tetanus and diphtheria (Td). After childhood immunizations, booster doses are recommended every 10 years as immunity can fade.

Rita Washko

See also
- Mononucleosis

Dislocation

A dislocation is a separation of a bone where it meets a joint (joints are areas where two or more bones come together). A dislocated bone is no longer in the normal anatomical position due to trauma to the surrounding ligaments. A dislocation can also cause damage to muscles and skin, as well as vascular and nerve damage. An incomplete dislocation is called a subluxation.

Dislocated shoulders are one of the most common problems in hospital emergency rooms. They represent 50 percent of all major joint dislocations, with nearly 70 percent of all anterior (front) shoulder dislocations occurring in patients younger than 30 years of age. The shoulder joint can dislocate in several ways; a forward and downward dislocation is the most common, resulting from a fall onto an outstretched hand or onto the shoulder itself. Backward dislocation may be caused by a direct blow to the front of the shoulder or violent twisting of the upper arm.

Causes and types of dislocations

Dislocations are usually caused by a sudden impact or external force to the joint. Usually this results from a blow, fall, or other trauma such as a football tackle. Dislocations are classified as congenital (present at birth), traumatic, or pathologic.

Congenital dislocation of the hip is an intra-articular (within the joint) displacement of the head of the thigh bone (femur) from its normal position in the acetabulum (hip socket) that affects the normal development of the joint prior to or shortly after birth.

Traumatic dislocation usually results from a violent encounter. This is clinically classified either as an acute dislocation, which mainly occurs at the shoulder, elbow, or hip; a chronic unreduced dislocation; or a recurrent dislocation. Dislocations are further classified according to the direction of the dislocation of the distal (farthest from the trunk) bone in relationship to the proximal (nearest to the trunk) bone. For example, a dislocation may be anterior (in front), posterior (behind), or inferior (lower).

An acute traumatic dislocation is diagnosed by taking a history and by a physical examination. Acute swelling and pain will be present around the joint as well as gross deformity and distortion. An examination to detect for associated nerve and vascular injuries should be performed and an X-ray taken to confirm the diagnosis and detect other associated fractures. A chronic unreduced dislocation is a dislocation in

which a patient presents him- or herself for treatment weeks to months after the primary dislocation. This can be a difficult problem requiring prolonged treatment. Recurrent dislocations occur when a traumatic dislocation of the joint is followed by subsequent frequent dislocations with minimal or minor trauma. This is commonly seen in the shoulder and kneecap joints.

Pathological dislocations are caused by some disease processes and are common in the hip joint. Usually the head of the femur is damaged, or there

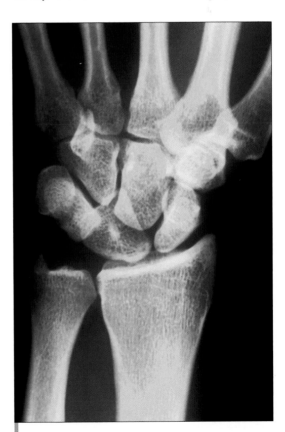

An X-ray confirms the diagnosis of a dislocated wrist. The bone has been displaced from its normal position, which causes pain and restricted movement. Sometimes ligaments around the affected bone are torn during the injury.

is excessive distention (swelling) of the joint capsule by a process such as tuberculosis of the hip or septic arthritis. Dislocation of the head of the femur occurs when the joint capsule is rapidly distended by a collection of fluid or pus.

Symptoms and signs

The clinical signs common to all dislocations are the absence of the end of the bone from its normal anatomical position and the presence of the displaced end of the bone in an abnormal position. Symptoms of a dislocation include discoloration; deformity; a restricted range of movement; swelling and bruising or ecchymosis (black and blue discoloration of the area); intense pain, particularly with use or weight-bearing attempts; and numbness and weakness.

Diagnosis and treatment

Dislocations are diagnosed by taking a complete medical history and carrying out a physical examination along with an X-ray of the injured parts.

The acute dislocation of a joint is an orthopedic emergency requiring immediate manipulation to restore the bone to its correct position under anesthesia or sedation. After the bone has been reset, it is then immobilized until the soft tissue swelling is reduced and the ligaments have healed. After three to four weeks, the joint is then mobilized using specified exercises and physical therapy. Chronic unreduced dislocation is treated by resetting the bone under anesthesia, or surgery may be required.

Pathogenesis

Dislocation of the jaw is most often caused by trauma to the chin when the mouth is open or less commonly when yawning, laughing, or chewing. Dislocation occurs when the hinge joint of the jaw becomes locked. The patient is unable to close the mouth, which means he or she has an open bite, making talking, swallowing, and chewing food extremely difficult.

Elbow dislocation is commonly seen. This is usually a posterior dislocation related to the upper arm that results from a fall onto an outstretched hand. The elbow is held in a bent position with the forearm bone (ulna) visibly out of place. Nerve and artery complications occur in 8 to 21 percent of patients with this injury.

Hip dislocations result from a massive force applied to the joint. Around 90 percent of these dislocations are posterior, occurring behind the hip socket, and just 10 percent are anterior (in front of the socket). If not

---

KEY FACTS

Description

A dislocation is a separation of a bone where it meets a joint. The bone is no longer in the normal anatomical position due to loss of surrounding ligament support. A partial dislocation is called a subluxation.

Causes

Follows a blow, fall, or other blunt trauma to a joint, caused through violence or sudden impact.

Symptoms

Deformity, discoloration, bone visibly out of place. Restricted range of motion, swelling, and increased pain with use or weight-bearing.

Pathogenesis

Patellar (kneecap) dislocation is most common in women. Hip dislocations are 90 percent posterior, 10 percent anterior. Elbow dislocation can cause nerve and artery complications.

Diagnosis

By physical examination, a history of events, and diagnostic X-rays of the injured parts.

Treatment

Dislocations are orthopedic emergencies requiring procedural sedation or anesthesia for immediate resetting or relocation of the bone.

Epidemiology

An anterior dislocation of the shoulder is the most commonly found dislocation of a major joint in the body. Approximately 70 percent of all anterior shoulder dislocations occur in patients less than 30 years of age.

---

manipulated back in less than six hours, there is an increased incidence of loss of blood supply and death of tissue cells in the head of the femur.

Patellar (kneecap) dislocations are most common in women; the kneecap is usually displaced to the outside knee, often with a tear to the inside knee joint capsule.

Prevention

Preventive measures include wearing protective gear when participating in contact sports; avoiding falls by not standing on chairs, countertops, or unstable objects; moving rugs or cords that could entangle the feet and cause a fall; and using a handrail when ascending or descending stairways.

Isaac Grate

See also
- Arthritis • Sports injury
- Tuberculosis

Diverticulitis

Diverticulitis is an inflammatory disease that affects the colon, although it can develop in other parts of the intestine. In this disease, small pouches called diverticula, which can form in the colon wall, become inflamed.

Diverticulitis is the most common noncancerous disease of the colon; it can range in severity from mild to life-threatening and is related to constipation and age. Pockets in the bowel wall known as diverticula become clogged with stools, causing an infection, which may be localized or cause an abscess or rupture of the bowel. Chronic problems include the formation of a stricture, which is a narrowing, or a fistula, which is a tract from the colon to the bladder or vagina. In severe cases, stools leak through a perforation to the abdominal cavity, causing a life-threatening infection.

KEY FACTS

Description
Inflammation in diverticula-containing colon segment.

Causes
Increased pressure inside the bowel from chronic constipation.

Risk factors
Western lifestyle, lack of fiber in the diet, increasing age.

Symptoms
Lower left abdominal pain, fever, elevated white blood cell count. If more severe widespread abdominal pain, dehydration may occur. Rarely a bowel obstruction or fistula to other organs. All symptoms could be mimicked by colon cancer.

Diagnosis
Symptoms, clinical examination, blood tests, CT scan. Once acute episode has resolved colonoscopy or barium enema (X-ray) to rule out cancer.

Treatment
Antibiotics for mild cases. Surgery for more severe, complicated, or recurrent forms.

Prevention
Fiber-rich diet.

Epidemiology
Diverticulosis, the fomation of pouches, occurs in 10 percent of those more than 40 years old, and in more than 60 percent of 80-year-olds. Of these, 15–20 percent develop diverticulitis, and there are 200,000 yearly hospital admissions.

Causes and risk factors

A Western lifestyle lacking in dietary fiber can promote constipation, which means the colon has to work harder to move stools; over time this weakens the bowel wall, resulting in the formation of diverticula. The frequency of diverticulitis increases with age, but even young patients can be affected. Diverticulitis does not increase the risk for colon cancer, but the two diseases share risk factors, have the same age distribution, and may present with very similar symptoms.

Symptoms and diagnosis

Diverticulitis results in fever, pain in the lower left abdomen, and an elevated white blood cell count. Symptoms such as constipation, nausea, and vomiting are less frequent. The diagnosis is based on the patient's history and a physical examination. Additional tests include blood tests, X-rays, and a computed tomography (CT) scan to assess the severity of the inflammation.

Treatment and prevention

Antibiotics cure the majority of mild to moderate episodes of diverticulitis. More severe forms require hospitalization and intravenous fluids. Emergency surgery may be needed for patients who do not recover with antibiotics alone, or have the most severe form of diverticulitis in which pus or feces leaks from the ruptured bowel into the abdominal cavity. Surgery involves the removal of the infected colon segment, and sometimes the patient is fitted with a colostomy bag so that stools pass into a bag on the abdomen. Patients with recurrent episodes of diverticulitis or with a fistula or stricture may need a planned resection of the diseased bowel segment.

Adopting a diet that is rich in fiber and ensuring a high fluid intake are the best means of preventing the development of diverticulitis.

Andreas Kaiser

See also
• Cancer, colorectal

Down syndrome

A common genetic disorder that leads to a variety of symptoms and problems, including mental retardation, Down syndrome occurs when a baby inherits three copies of chromosome 21 instead of the normal two copies. In the past, people with Down syndrome often led dull lives in institutions, but today much more effort is made to help them realize their full potential and improve their quality of life.

Down syndrome is one of the most common genetic disorders worldwide, occurring in 1 out of every 733 live births in the United States in 2006. There are an estimated 350,000 people living with Down syndrome in the United States. The disorder is named after physician John Langdon Down (1828–1897), who supervised an institute for mentally retarded children in England. Based on years of observations, Down was able to distinguish between several forms of mental retardation in children, including what is now called Down syndrome. However, it was not until 1959 that French pediatrician Jerome Lejeune (1926–1994) discovered that most cases of Down syndrome are due to an extra copy of one of the human chromosomes, chromosome 21.

Signs and symptoms

People with Down syndrome are characterized by mental retardation, short stature, abnormal creasing of the skin on the back of the hands, eyes that slant upward at the corners, and a vertical fold of skin over the nasal edge of each eye. More than one in three children with Down syndrome have heart defects. They may have hearing and vision problems, blockage of the intestines, infertility in men, and short fingers and toes. There is also an increased rate of leukemia and a reduced effectiveness of the immune system. Despite these problems, people with Down syndrome, particularly those with good self-help skills, can expect to live into their fifties.

Causes and risk factors

Down syndrome occurs because a baby has three copies of particular genes, instead of the usual two. The genes concerned are those on the smallest human chromosome, chromosome 21. In ways that are still not understood, this genetic imbalance leads to a number of abnormalities.

The most common form of Down syndrome is called trisomy 21 and accounts for around 95 percent of Down syndrome cases. In trisomy 21 there is a complete extra copy of chromosome 21 in every cell of the fetus. In 95 percent of cases of trisomy 21, it was the egg cell from the mother that carried the unwanted extra chromosome. The older the mother, the higher the chance that she will produce eggs with an extra chromosome 21. For women over the age of 40, the chance is nearly 1 in 100 that any children they conceive will have Down syndrome.

A second form of Down syndrome, accounting for around 4 percent of cases, is called translocation Down syndrome, in which a child inherits a large

KEY FACTS

Description
An inherited birth defect.

Causes
A duplication of all or part of chromosome 21.

Risk factors
Age of the mother is the primary risk factor for the most common form of Down syndrome.

Symptoms and signs
Various, including mental retardation, distinct facial features, short stature.

Diagnosis
Can be diagnosed before birth by various screening techniques.

Treatments
There is no treatment for Down syndrome, but complications resulting from it can be treated.

Pathogenesis
There is a risk of a variety of complications appearing as the individual develops.

Prevention
There is no prevention measure available.

Epidemiology
Down syndrome is one of the most common genetic disorders in the United States, occurring in 1 in every 733 live births. There are about 350,000 people with Down syndrome in the United States.

extra section of chromosome 21, but instead of being separate, this chromosomal section is attached or translocated to the end of another normal chromosome, usually chromosome 14. A parent of a translocation Down syndrome baby may carry such a translocation in all of his or her cells already and yet still appear normal; problems occur when the misplaced chromosome is packaged into sex cells (egg or sperm) that may form new individuals. In other cases the translocation may occur during gamete formation, in which case neither parent is a carrier of the translocation. Translocation Down syndrome does not depend on the age of the parents, but any parent carrying such a translocation in his or her own cells has a high risk of producing several children with Down syndrome, so this version of the disorder is sometimes called familial Down syndrome.

The rarest form of Down syndrome is called mosaicism. This can occur pre- or postconception and results from a mistake in cell division within the growing embryo. Consequently, only some of the fetus's cells will have trisomy 21. Depending on how early or late in development the production of cells with trisomy 21 occurred, the effects may be either nearly as severe as other forms of Down syndrome, or they may be much milder.

Diagnosis

Down syndrome is usually obvious after birth. The baby may have a floppy muscle tone and the characteristic facial appearance. Many women, though, wish to know early in pregnancy if they are carrying a Down syndrome baby. Because of the high incidence of Down syndrome, a number of prenatal screening and testing methods have been developed.

Women have their blood screened for trisomal genetic disorders such as Down syndrome in the first trimester of pregnancy. Combined with an ultrasound to check for fluid at the back of the neck, the screen can indicate the possibility of Down syndrome, but fluid at the back of the neck can also be symptomatic of other conditions. Further screening is carried out in the second trimester using what are called triple or quad screens, which measure the levels of certain hormones in the mother's blood and a protein produced in the liver of the fetus. From this test, the risk of the baby having Down syndrome can be calculated. However, the presence of Down syndrome can only be confirmed by a diagnostic test in the second trimester.

A boy with Down syndrome has speech therapy to assist his speech development. Children with Down syndrome usually have a protruding tongue, which can impair speech.

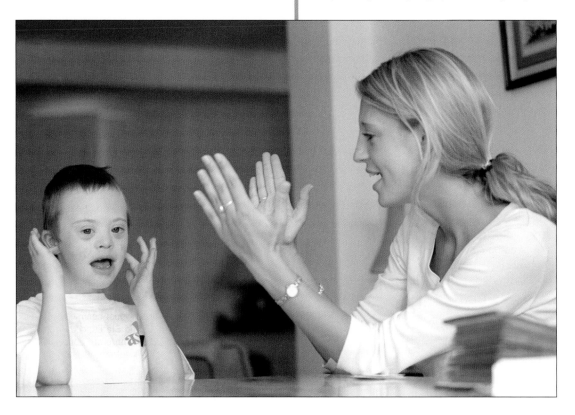

The most commonly used diagnostic method for Down syndrome is amniocentesis. This procedure, also carried out for other reasons, involves the removal of a small amount of the amniotic fluid that surrounds the fetus. The amniotic fluid contains some fetal cells, which can be cultured outside the uterus and analyzed for genetic abnormalities.

Amniocentesis is usually conducted during the fifteenth to eighteenth weeks of pregnancy. It carries a slight chance of producing miscarriage or infection, and so has mainly been performed on women at high risk for having offspring with a genetic disease. However, a newer procedure, chorionic villus sampling (CVS), can be performed earlier in pregnancy (tenth to twelfth week) and provides results faster than amniocentesis. CVS involves the removal of cells of the placenta, the temporary organ that connects the fetus to the mother's blood supply. The cells concerned are derived from the fetus and thus have the same genetic composition as the fetus. During CVS, either a needle is inserted through the abdomen, or a catheter is passed through the vagina and cervix into the area of the placenta, to collect cells for examination.

Treatments and lifestyle

Historically, few attempts were made to treat the mental retardation associated with Down syndrome. One of the main reasons inhibiting the development of effective treatments is the fact that the level of mental retardation varies; some people demonstrate severe problems with mental development, and others display only minor levels. In the past several decades, studies in childhood development have indicated that early intervention programs and special education courses are the key to treating the negative effects of mental retardation in Down syndrome patients. Studies have shown that these programs can help improve the quality of life for patients with the disorder.

In addition to mental retardation, individuals with Down syndrome have a higher incidence of developing congenital heart defects, gastrointestinal disorders, cataract, hypothyroidism, and Alzheimer's disease. Over the past decade the advances in surgical techniques, specifically in the area of open heart surgery, have enabled most of these defects to be corrected. This has effectively increased the life span of Down syndrome individuals. In the 1930s the average life span was nine years; by the year 2000, people with Down syndrome were living into their fifties.

GENETIC BACKGROUND

Most cells of the body contain a complete set of genetic instructions (genes), packaged into 23 pairs of chromosomes. Because the chromosomes are in pairs, each cell has two copies of every gene. Egg and sperm cells, however, have only one set of 23 chromosomes. When an egg and a sperm fuse during fertilization, the new cell has 23 chromosome pairs. When egg and sperm cells form in the body from ordinary cells with paired chromosomes, the chromosomes have to separate so that there is only one of each pair in every egg or sperm cell. Mistakes sometimes happen during this complex process. For example, an unfertilized egg may end up with two copies of a chromosome instead of only one. If the egg is later fertilized by a normal sperm cell, the result will be three copies of that particular chromosome instead of two in the developing embryo. This situation is called trisomy. Trisomy 21, the main form of Down syndrome, is the most common human trisomy.

However, despite developments of surgical techniques, children with Down syndrome often display decreased immune function, resulting in an increased susceptibility to childhood diseases. The classic Down syndrome stereotype of an overweight individual is being combated by nutritionists and exercise physiologists to increase the activity levels and reduce the detrimental effects of adult obesity.

Advances in diagnosis, therapy, and the treatment of associated illnesses in Down syndrome children have resulted in a vastly improved quality of life over the past two decades. It is important to recognize the limitations of individuals with Down syndrome so that they may experience a full and rewarding life. People with Down syndrome who have severe mental retardation may require a significant amount of parental care throughout their lives. As more individuals with Down syndrome are living longer, studies are showing that they are capable of living full, valued lives, and being active members of their families and communities.

Michael Windelspecht

See also
• Alzheimer's disease • Growth disorders
• Obesity

Eating disorders

Eating disorders are complex, chronic illnesses that fill a person's life with obsessions about food and body image. Types of eating disorders include anorexia nervosa, bulimia, binge eating disorder (BED), eating disorders not otherwise specified (ENDOS), disordered eating, and morbid obesity. Eating disorders can lead to hormonal and psychological problems, and even death.

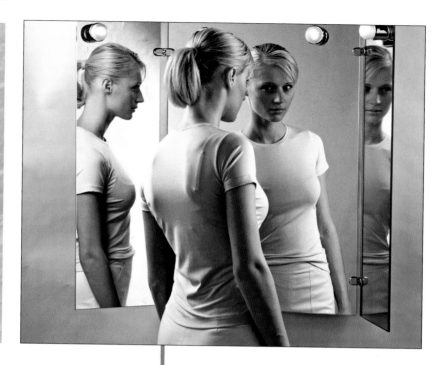

The emphasis on being slim in Western society can put pressure on girls to diet unnecessarily, often the first step to anorexia. An anorexic has a distorted body image whereby she is convinced she is overweight when in fact she is not.

With an obesity epidemic in the developed world and almost daily news about the obesity crisis, attention to healthy eating, exercise, and looking after oneself is important. Television, magazines, and books proclaim that some diets or pills can help everyone lose weight and conquer fat, and society's emphasis on being thin encourages dieting. While it is important to eat healthily, some teenagers, mostly girls, obsess about body image. They go to extremes by skipping meals and stringently reducing food intake. They may exercise frantically and find that they can speed up weight loss by vomiting or using laxatives. Messages about good nutrition and healthy eating are lost in their fear of becoming fat. Eating disorders have many physical, psychological, and social implications. If the disorder continues for a number of years there is a risk of osteoporosis and heart problems. Eating disorders also have the highest death rate of any mental illness. Currently 1 to 4 percent of young women in the United States have an eating disorder.

Causes and risk factors

All cultural and economic groups are at risk. Eating disorders can arise from factors such as a preoccupation with weight, inappropriate eating behavior, and a distorted body image. Studies show that some types of eating disorders are also related to risky activities like smoking tobacco or marijuana, alcohol use, delinquency, unprotected sexual activity, and suicide attempts. Many people with eating disorders suffer with depression, anxiety, or may have been abused as a child.

Anorexia nervosa

Anorexia nervosa is a dangerous condition in which individuals can literally starve themselves to death. Even though they may already be thin, people with anorexia eat very little and have an intense and overwhelming fear of body fat. The individual may refuse to maintain even a minimal normal body weight. The term *anorexia* literally means "loss of appetite," but poor appetite is not a symptom of this eating disorder. People who suffer with anorexia nervosa are constantly suppressing a desire to eat for fear of becoming fat.

According to the American Psychiatric Association's *Diagnostic and Statistical Manual of Mental Disorders*, fourth edition (DSM-IV), anorexia nervosa affects from 0.5 to 1 percent of the female adolescent population with an average age of onset between 14 and 18 years. About 8 million people in the United States have anorexia.

The condition usually appears in bright, attractive young women between the ages of 12 and 25; however, people outside this age group are also at risk. About 5 to 10 percent of victims are male, and body image is becoming an increasing issue in young men.

The condition may arise when a person experiences overwhelming problems. Difficult transitions such as puberty, divorce, family problems, death of a loved one, a new job or school, relationship breakup, sexual or physical abuse, or critical comments may cause a person to feel overwhelmed and out of control.

People with anorexia may possess a certain psychological profile. They are often perfectionists and overachievers who appear to be in control. Often they have been well-behaved, conscientious, hardworking, and able students who have always sought approval and wished to avoid conflict. At the same time, they are self-critical and underneath may feel defective and inadequate. They have low self-esteem but a desire to be special. They feel that by controlling their eating they can gain power and stand out from the crowd by losing weight and being thin. Many people with anorexia are overly engaged with their parents and exclude peer relationships.

In addition to losing a significant amount of weight and continuing to diet although thin, a person with anorexia has an intense fear of weight gain and feels fat even after losing weight. She may have a preoccupation with food and read cookbooks, watch cooking shows on television, and enjoy cooking for others although she will not eat what she has prepared. She may study calories, fat content, and nutrition.

Early signs are excessive exercise and a preoccupation with cooking food for other people, while avoiding eating it. The body reacts to the lack of food by becoming extremely thin, developing brittle hair and nails, dry skin, a lowered pulse rate, and cold hands and feet; there may also be fainting spells, constipation, and diarrhea. Fine hair may grow on the arms, legs, and other body parts, but hair on the head may fall out. In addition, mild anemia, reduced muscle mass, loss of menstrual cycle, and swelling of joints can occur.

The long-term effects of anorexia are the most devastating, and anorexics can suffer from the consequences of the condition throughout their lives, even if they have received treatment. Malnutrition can cause irregular heart rhythms and heart failure, while a lack

of calcium puts the individual at risk of developing osteoporosis during the illness as well as in later life. Clinical depression is present in many people with anorexia, and individuals may also suffer from anxiety, personality disorders, substance abuse, and suicide attempts. Approximately one in ten victims of this eating disorder will die of starvation, cardiac arrest, or other medical complications.

KEY FACTS

Description

A group of illnesses in which a preoccupation with food is displayed. Anorexia is a serious mental disorder involving obsession about body image and food; this illness is a key health issue facing young women and some young men. Although not recognized as a mental disorder, extreme obesity can cause psychological and physical problems in a society where "thin is in."

Causes

No one knows exactly what causes eating disorders, but psychological factors such as low self-esteem are involved.

Risk factors

All socioeconomic, ethnic, and cultural groups are at risk.

Symptoms

Excessive fear of becoming fat; excessive dieting and exercise; refusal to maintain a normal body weight; preoccupation with food, calories, and food preparation. People with morbid obesity overeat dangerously.

Diagnosis

A psychiatrist or psychologist specializing in eating disorders should be consulted; eating disorders are often misdiagnosed and misunderstood.

Treatments

Psychotherapy, diet counseling, and counseling for parents if an anorexic adolescent remains at home; hospitalization may be required. Treatment is more successful if diagnosed early.

Pathogenesis

Eating disorders may last for several years. If untreated, death may occur. More than 6 percent of serious cases of anorexia and bulimia die.

Prevention

Education about the consequences of anorexia, bulimia, binge eating, and disordered eating.

Epidemiology

More than 90 percent of those with eating disorders are women. In the United States, the number of women affected by these illnesses has doubled to at least 5 million in the past 30 years.

Bulimia nervosa

Often called "binge and purge" disorder, bulimia involves eating excessive amounts of food, usually high-calorie sweet foods, followed by self-inflicted behavior, known as purging, to get rid of the food consumed. Purging may involve self-induced vomiting, taking laxatives, diet pills, diuretics or water pills, excessive exercise, or fasting. As with anorexia, people with bulimia are overly concerned with food, body weight, and shape. Binges may occur once or twice a week or several times a day. The illness may be occasional with periods of remission that alternate with reoccurrences of binge eating, or it may be constant.

Because the bingeing and purging is done in secret, the bulimia sufferer may maintain a normal or above normal body weight and in this way may be able to hide the problem for a number of years. This disorder most frequently affects adolescent girls and young adult women, afflicting approximately 1 to 3 percent of this age group.

The psychological profile of a person with bulimia is similar to that of an anorexic, except that bulimics may realize that their eating is abnormal and often become guilt ridden and depressed after binges. Bulimics often have a hard time dealing with and controlling impulses, stress, and anxiety. Bulimia may occur independently from anorexia, although half of all people with anorexia develop bulimia. Some individuals with bulimia have other compulsions, such as addition to alcohol and drugs and compulsive stealing. Others suffer from clinical depression, obsessive-compulsive disorder, anxiety, and psychiatric illnesses.

Bulimia is serious because the individual's actions are disruptive to many aspects of daily life, including work and social life. Purging can have serious effects on the body and can cause a severe imbalance of electrolytes, which are chemicals necessary for normal body functioning. Loss of potassium due to vomiting damages the heart muscle and increases the risk of cardiac arrest. Inflammation of the esophagus is caused by repeated vomiting and exposure to stomach acid, which also damages the enamel of the teeth and eventually causes them to rot.

Treating bulimia involves educating the person about the consequences of bingeing and purging and establishing healthy eating habits through behavior modification. A psychiatrist who is experienced in treating the disorder helps the individual deal with associated problems and low self-esteem. When the condition is out of control and serious health complications occur, hospitalization may be required.

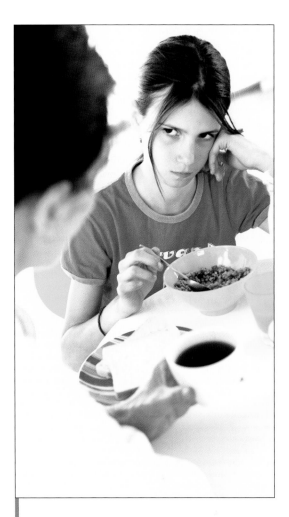

Young girls with an eating disorder are often conscientious and bright but they may come under familial pressure to achieve. By refusing to eat or bingeing they feel that they are able to exert control over one area of their life.

Binge eating disorder

Binge eating disorder (BED) is the newest clinically recognized eating disorder and probably the most common. BED is characterized by episodes of uncontrolled eating in which the individual eats too much to the point where they feel uncomfortably full; they may then experience feelings of embarrassment, disgust, or guilt about the overeating. However, unlike individuals with anorexia or bulimia, they do not use inappropriate behaviors such as vomiting or excessive exercise to purge themselves of the food. It can be difficult for lay people to recognize BED, but the trained physician can diagnose the symptoms of feelings of being out of control and depression. Women are more likely to experience BED than men.

Approximately 2 percent of all adults or 4 million Americans are binge eaters. About 10 to 15 percent of people who are mildly obese and who try to lose weight on their own have BED. They may succumb to yo-yo dieting, which means that they lose weight as a result of dieting and then regain all the weight once they finish the diet.

People with BED are often overweight because they maintain a high-calorie diet without expending an adequate amount of energy. The medical problems of BED are similar to those found in obesity. Individuals are at an increased risk of developing type 2 diabetes, high blood pressure, high blood cholesterol levels, gallbladder disease, heart disease, and certain types of cancers. Researchers have also shown that individuals with BED often have high rates of depression.

EDNOS and disordered eating

A category known as eating disorders not otherwise specified (EDNOS) is named in the DSM-IV as a disorder that does not meet the criteria for any other specific eating disorder. Individuals may engage in some form of abnormal eating but do not exhibit the specific symptoms associated with a particular eating disorder. For example, they may meet most of the criteria for anorexia or they may engage in purging but with less intensity or frequency.

Another category called disordered eating is more common and widespread and is an atypical eating disorder that may include unusual eating habits such as restrictive dieting, bingeing, or purging. This disorder may be a reaction to a stressful life event such as an illness, or the need to improve personal appearance for a special occasion like a reunion or wedding, or in preparation for an athletic activity. Disordered eating rarely requires professional help but may develop into a long-term eating disorder.

Morbid obesity

Obesity is not classified as a disorder in the DSM-IV; however, it may increase a person's risk of developing psychological problems, especially in certain subgroups of obesity. Obesity is defined as an abnormal increase of fat in the subcutaneous connective tissue. Weight classification is determined by body mass index, or BMI, which is calculated by dividing the weight in pounds by the height in inches squared, then multiplying by 703. A person with a BMI of greater than 40 is considered extremely or morbidly obese. Many people who are morbidly obese are binge eaters but do not necessarily feel guilt about their overeating.

Diagnosis and treatment

Some evidence exists that eating disorders tend to run in families, with female relatives most often affected. Family and friends may emphasize the importance of thinness and weight control, which can lead to an eating disorder. Being teased about weight can lower an individual's self-esteem and may create eating disturbances in young people. The many factors are complex; lifestyle choices, activities, environment, and family traditions are all part of the picture, but genes are also possibly involved.

Researchers are looking into brain chemicals and genetics for answers about obesity and eating disorders and have connected biological factors associated with clinical depression with the development of eating disorders. Stress hormones such as cortisol are elevated in eating disorders, while neurotransmitters (chemical messengers) such as serotonin may not function correctly. Although news stories often break about the elusive fat gene that controls weight, in reality not one but a variety of genes affect the weight of a person. Scientists have even located genes thought to control how a person responds to environmental choices such as appetite and overeating. These have been dubbed by the media with names such as the "couch-potato gene," the "stop-eating gene," the "can't-resist gene," and even the "party-platter gene" exhibited by people who follow food trays around at parties. Obesity is not simple but a complex condition controlled by environmental, psychological, and social factors, as well as by a host of interacting genes.

Because of the secretive behavior of many people with eating disorders, treatment is difficult and even controversial as relapse rates are very high. Generally three approaches are used. Cognitive behavioral therapy teaches people how to change and keep track of unhealthy eating habits and how to approach tough situations. It also helps them feel better about weight and shape. Interpersonal psychotherapy helps people examine relationships with friends and family and make changes in any problem areas. Drug therapies, such as antidepressants, may help some people with an eating disorder. Other therapies include medications to regulate behavior, weight loss surgery, self-help books, videos, and support groups.

Evelyn Kelly

See also
• Anemia • Depressive disorders • Diabetes
• Obesity • Osteoporosis

Ebola fever

Ebola fever is categorized as a viral hemorrhagic fever that causes serious abnormal bleeding and can be fatal. It occurs in humans and in nonhuman primates such as monkeys and chimpanzees and is believed to be initially spread to humans via contact with an infected animal. Ebola occurs primarily in Africa, where sporadic outbreaks have been documented since 1976.

Ebola, named after the Ebola River in the Democratic Republic of the Congo (formerly Zaire), first emerged in the area of Nzara and Maridi in the southern Sudan in June 1976. More than 280 people became infected; of those 151 died, more than 50 percent. The virus went unidentified until another outbreak began in nearby Yambuku in the northern Democratic Republic of the Congo that September. This strain, known as Ebola-Zaire, killed 280 people, which was 88 percent of the 318 infected. Ebola outbreaks have been reported sporadically since 1976 with the largest outbreak, known as Ebola-Sudan, in Uganda in 2000 and 2001. More than 400 people were infected, and of those, 51 percent died. Another large outbreak, this time of Ebola-Zaire, was centered on Kikwit in the Democratic Republic of the Congo, in 1995. Eighty-one percent of its 315 victims died.

With just 1,850 infections and 1,200 deaths since 1976, Ebola strikes far greater fear in people than its prevalence warrants, despite the high death rate. This fear is partly due to graphic descriptions of severe internal and external hemorrhaging and the concern that travelers may become infected and spread the disease to other parts of the world.

The Ebola virus is a member of the viral family Filoviridae and has four known strains. Three have origins in Africa and cause disease in humans: Ebola-Sudan, Ebola-Zaire, and Ebola–Ivory Coast. A fourth, Ebola-Reston, appears to have origins in Asia but is only known to cause disease in nonhuman primates.

Ebola-Zaire, the most virulent strain, and Ebola-Sudan are of the most concern because of the mortality rates among their human victims. Ebola-Reston has not been shown to cause disease in humans, and Ebola–Ivory Coast has had only one reported human victim, who was a scientist infected while conducting an autopsy on a dead chimpanzee.

Causes and risk factors

Experts suspect that Ebola has a natural "reservoir," or origin, probably an animal, but this reservoir has not been discovered. The initial human infection in an Ebola outbreak probably stems from contact with the infected animal. The virus then spreads easily from human to human via exposure to secretions, bodily

KEY FACTS

Description
A lethal viral hemorrhagic disease.

Cause
Infection by one of four strains of Ebola virus, of the viral family Filoviridae.

Risk factors
Contact with blood, bodily fluids, or tissues of infected individuals.

Symptoms and signs
Abrupt onset of fever, headache, muscle pain, weakness, and sore throat; early symptoms are followed by diarrhea, vomiting, and gastrointestinal pain, red eyes, rash, jaundice, and internal and external bleeding.

Diagnosis
Examination by experienced medical personnel; blood tests revealing presence of virus or of antibodies to virus.

Treatments
All that can be done is to provide supportive care, especially administration of intravenous fluids and electrolytes (minerals) to maintain blood pressure; providing oxygen if necessary; and treatment of secondary infections.

Pathogenesis
The natural reservoir of Ebola is unknown, but experts suspect it is initially transmitted to humans by contact with an infected animal; the virus then spreads from human to human via contact with secretions and bodily fluids of infected individuals.

Prevention
Wearing protective equipment while caring for infected individuals or while preparing the corpse of an Ebola victim for burial; preventing reuse of contaminated equipment such as needles and syringes so as to avoid infecting others.

Epidemiology
Since 1976, when Ebola was first recognized, there have been approximately 1,850 documented infections; of those more than 1,200 people have died.

fluids, or the tissue of an infected person. As a result, the virus has exacted a heavy toll in caregivers among whom health care equipment is limited. When proper containment measures are taken, outbreaks of Ebola-Zaire and Ebola-Sudan can be controlled fairly quickly.

Ebola-Reston, although yet to cause human disease, is of particular concern due to its means of transmission. The strain, discovered in an outbreak among primates at a laboratory in Reston, Virginia, in 1989, spread from infected cynomolgus monkeys imported from the Philippines to other primates in the laboratory, possibly via the building's ventilation system.

The worst-case scenario for those who study Ebola is that the Zaire and Sudan strains may gain the ability to spread among victims via the air, as Ebola-Reston may be able to do—or that the Reston strain acquires the ability to cause disease in humans.

Symptoms and signs

Ebola has an incubation period of 2 to 21 days. Symptoms begin suddenly with fever, headache, muscle pain, intense weakness, and sore throat. These are followed by gastrointestinal symptoms such as diarrhea, vomiting, and severe pain, as well as impaired liver and kidney function, red eyes, rash, and jaundice. As the virus multiplies, it weakens the body and may prevent an effective immune response. Internal and external bleeding may occur, arguably the most horrific manifestation of Ebola. Lung or gastrointestinal hemorrhaging, hepatitis, or encephalitis are the most common causes of death among Ebola victims.

Diagnosis

Ebola is diagnosed from the symptoms and a blood test to look for the presence of antibodies to the virus. In its early stages Ebola can be difficult to diagnose from its symptoms alone, which are common to other diseases. If Ebola is suspected, then the patient should be isolated and the relevant authorities notified.

Treatment and prevention

Little can be done for Ebola victims other than provide care. The most important step is to replace fluids lost through hemorrhaging, vomiting, and diarrhea to maintain hydration and blood pressure; maintaining electrolyte (mineral) concentrations is also important. Oxygen should be administered if necessary, and secondary infections must also be treated.

There are no vaccines to prevent Ebola infection in humans, although one is being developed that has shown promise in tests on nonhuman primates.

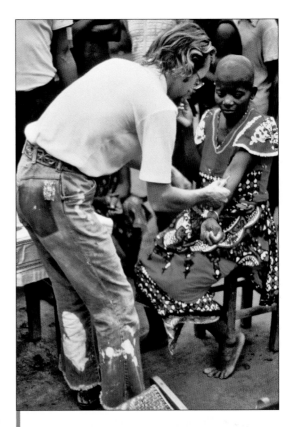

A health care worker takes a blood sample during the 1976 Ebola outbreak in the town of Yambuku, Zaire. The blood sample tests for the presence of antibodies to the virus and can diagnose a case of Ebola within several days.

The best way to prevent the spread of infection is to avoid contact with the secretions, fluids, or tissues of Ebola victims. Quarantine of victims is also important; many African regions practice a sort of reverse quarantine in which people stop visiting villages where infections have occurred.

For medical staff who work with victims, protective equipment, such as gowns, gloves, masks, and goggles, is a must. In some outbreaks the disease was spread by the use of improperly disinfected medical equipment such as needles and syringes. In some African regions the disease spread to family and friends performing ritual washing of the corpses of Ebola victims as they prepared the bodies for burial. Temporarily halting the practice has helped stem some outbreaks.

David Lawrence

See also
• Dengue fever

Ectopic pregnancy

An ectopic pregnancy occurs when a fertilized ovum (egg) implants outside the uterus, usually in the fallopian tube. That occurs in 2 percent of pregnancies. While the pregnancy may naturally terminate, there is a risk that if it continues, the tube will rupture and the patient could bleed to death.

Ectopic pregnancy is a serious disorder and is one of the most common reasons patients die in the first trimester of pregnancy. With modern diagnoses and therapies there has been a decrease in maternal mortality due to ectopic pregnancy. In the 1970s around 35 deaths in 10,000 pregnancies occurred; by 1992, the figure was 2.6 deaths in Western countries such as the United States. In developing countries many women still die from an ectopic pregnancy.

Risk factors

Anything that delays or prevents the passage of a fertilized ovum from the ovary to the uterus may cause an ectopic pregnancy. Factors such as infection of the fallopian tube or damage to the fallopian tube after surgery, as well as the mother smoking, all increase the risk of an ectopic pregnancy. Oral contraceptive therapies reduce the risk of this condition, but intrauterine contraceptive devices may increase its risk.

Diagnosis

Ectopic pregnancies are diagnosed as early as possible. The symptoms are vaginal bleeding and abdominal pain, typically about seven weeks after the last menstrual period. Any woman of childbearing age with symptoms of fainting and bleeding should be suspected of having an ectopic pregnancy. A simple blood or urine pregnancy test is done to measure the hormone beta human chorionic gonadotrophin (beta HCG), then an ultrasound scan of the abdomen to look for a pregnancy outside the uterus. Ultrasound scans combined with a beta HCG test detect 95 to 97 percent of ectopic pregnancies.

Treatments

If the diagnosis is made early enough, ectopic pregnancies might be treated with drugs. Methotrexate, a folic acid blocker, stops cells from dividing. In many cases, this treatment removes the need for surgery.

If there is a sign of a beating heart on the ultrasound scan and the beta HCG level is high, or there is a mass of more than 2 inches (4 cm) in the abdomen, surgery is preferred over drug treatment. If the patient is stable without too much blood loss, laparoscopic surgery (minimally invasive surgery) is done. If the patient is not stable, the abdomen is opened to remove the fallopian tube or to cut out the ectopic pregnancy. Surgery carries a risk of scarring the tube, which may affect future fertility. Once an ectopic pregnancy has occurred, the risk in subsequent pregnancies is higher.

Moeen Panni

KEY FACTS

Description
A pregnancy that develops outside the uterus in a fallopian tube, cervix, or ovary.

Cause
Pelvic infection, abnormality of fallopian tube, damaged tube, intrauterine contraceptive device.

Risk factors
Common risk factors include smoking, infection, and damage to the fallopian tube after surgery.

Symptoms
Severe pain in lower abdomen and vaginal bleeding.

Diagnosis
By ultrasound scan and sometimes laparoscopy.

Treatments
Methotrexate is the common medical drug treatment; laparoscopic surgery is performed if the patient is stable.

Pathogenesis
If one fallopian tube has to be removed, the chance of conception is lessened but still possible. If both tubes are damaged, IVF will be needed to pursue a pregnancy, but IVF has an increased risk for ectopic pregnancies.

Prevention
In any future pregnancies, early ultrasound scan to ensure fetus is developing in the uterus.

Epidemiology
Occurs in 2 percent of all pregnancies. Accounts for 9 percent of pregnancy-related deaths.

See also
• Pelvic inflammatory disease

Emphysema

Emphysema is a progressive, irreversible, and degenerative disease of the lungs. In emphysema, the alveoli, the air sacs in which carbon dioxide in the bloodstream is exchanged for oxygen in the air, become damaged by tobacco smoke and other air pollutants, such as dust.

In emphysema, the alveoli lose their elasticity and break down, eventually destroying the body's ability to acquire sufficient oxygen. As the disease progresses, the ability to exhale becomes more difficult, further undermining the ability to acquire sufficient oxygen.

Causes and risk factors

The primary cause of emphysema is smoking. Although the risk is higher for smokers, nonsmokers chronically exposed to secondhand smoke are also at risk. In the past, men were more likely to develop emphysema than women, but as the number of women smokers has increased, the prevalence rate of emphysema in women has begun to approach that of men.

Other air pollutants besides tobacco smoke will also cause damage to lung tissue that leads to emphysema. For example, the World Health Organization (WHO) reports that there are 400,000 deaths from chronic obstructive pulmonary disease (COPD) caused by burning of biomass fuels (such as wood) each year. It takes years for the lung damage to accumulate before it becomes noticeable; thus more than 90 percent of people diagnosed with the disease are age 45 or older.

Genetic factors influence the risk of developing emphysema in a small percentage of individuals. Research has shown that a hereditary deficiency of the protein alpha-1-antitrypsin, which protects the elasticity of lung tissue, increases the risk of lung damage and leads to emphysema.

In addition, HIV infection and some connective tissue disorders, such as Marfan syndrome, may make affected individuals more susceptible to developing emphysema.

Symptoms and signs

The first signs of emphysema are usually shortness of breath during moderate exercise, such as during walking. Dry or productive coughs and wheezing also indicate the presence of the disease. The symptoms intensify as the disease progresses.

Inability to breathe adequately leads to chronic fatigue. Fatigue while breathing may trigger a loss of

KEY FACTS

Description
A disease of the lungs that reduces the body's ability to get adequate oxygen.

Causes
The alveoli or air sacs in which gas exchange occurs are irreversibly destroyed; as they are destroyed, the lungs' ability to exchange carbon dioxide in the bloodstream for oxygen in the air is reduced.

Risk factors
Tobacco smoking, air pollution, and age all increase the risk of the disease.

Symptoms
Shortness of breath, coughing, wheezing, and reduced ability to exercise are the primary symptoms; they may also include sudden weight loss, swelling of lower limbs, fatigue, and anxiety.

Diagnosis
A physical examination, coupled with tests of breathing efficiency, chest X-rays, or measurements of blood gases.

Treatments
The most important treatment by far is to quit smoking; drugs such as bronchodilators and corticosteroids may boost ease of breathing; supplemental oxygen may be administered; in severe cases, lung reduction surgery or lung transplants may be required.

Pathogenesis
Exposure to tobacco smoke as well as other air pollutants damages the walls of the alveoli, which become brittle and break down; as the lungs lose their elasticity, it becomes more difficult to exhale stale air.

Prevention
Quitting smoking, avoiding tobacco smoke, and limiting exposure to other lung irritants.

Epidemiology
Emphysema develops slowly; thus it is seen most often in older individuals. More than 90 percent of emphysema patients are age 45 or older. Years of exposure to tobacco smoke typically precedes the onset of the disease, but it is also seen in coal miners affected by dust.

PULMONARY EMPHYSEMA

As well as smoking, exposure to air pollution and dust can cause emphysema. (1) shows normal bronchioles and alveoli; (2) shows a distended bronchiole; and (3) shows distended air sacs or alveoli. The distension is typical of pulmonary emphysema suffered by coal miners, who continually breathe in coal dust.

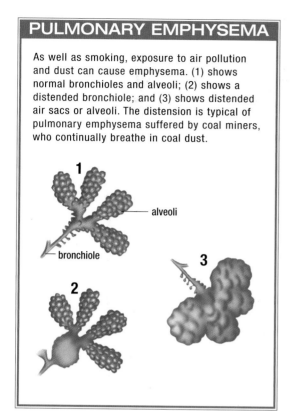

appetite, which in turn leads to weight loss. In advanced cases, even breathing leads to fatigue, since much energy is spent trying to forcibly expel stale air from the lungs. Emphysema may also be accompanied by swelling of the lower limbs and anxiety.

Treatments and prevention

There is no way to reverse the damage to the lungs caused by emphysema; therefore, the best way to treat emphysema is to prevent it. The best way to prevent emphysema is to quit smoking tobacco. Other preventive measures are to find ways to reduce exposures to secondhand smoke and other air pollutants, and to maintain good health and resistance to infection by regular exercise, good nutrition, and adequate rest. Once the effects of emphysema begin to manifest themselves, the symptoms can be managed by a variety of methods. Bronchodilator drugs may be administered to relieve coughing, shortness of breath, and difficulty breathing by relaxing bronchial passages, thus increasing the efficiency of air flow into and out of the lungs. Inhaled or oral corticosteroids may be also administered to help combat inflammation of lung tissues, but long-term use may trigger a number of adverse side effects, such as brittle bones or high blood pressure. Breathing exercises may also help emphysema patients breathe more efficiently.

To prevent infections that may aggravate symptoms, emphysema patients should keep their vaccinations up to date, especially against influenza (which needs to be updated every year) and against pneumonia (which needs to be updated every five to seven years.) Antibiotic treatment may be required to cure existing infections or may be administered as a prophylactic to prevent the onset of secondary infections.

Supplemental oxygen may be administered in severe cases in which a patient's blood oxygen levels are low. The duration and timing of oxygen administration will vary, depending on the severity of disease. Portable oxygen delivery systems make it possible for emphysema patients to engage in many activities once considered impracticable.

In some cases, surgery may be required. Lung reduction surgery, in which portions of the lung are removed, reduces overall lung volume but increases breathing efficiency (at least for some months after the operation). Lung transplants may be the only option in extreme cases of emphysema.

Epidemiology

Global statistics on prevalence of and mortality from emphysema specifically are difficult to obtain. Emphysema is frequently combined with chronic bronchitis and irreversible forms of asthma as COPD. The disease is often described as a contributing factor to the death of a patient but may not be credited as the cause of death. Nevertheless, the World Health Organization (WHO) reports that COPD is the fourth leading cause of death worldwide, with 2.7 million deaths in 2000. Likewise, COPD is the fourth leading cause of death in the United States, claiming more than 120,000 lives annually.

In 2003 about 1.7 percent of adults in the United States (3.6 million individuals) had been diagnosed specifically with emphysema. Nearly 14,000 people in the United States died from the disease that year. Extrapolation of emphysema prevalence rates from nations in which emphysema data are available indicates that more than 40 million persons worldwide may suffer from the disease.

David M. Lawrence

See also
• Cancer, lung • COPD

Epilepsy

A brain disorder in which clusters of nerve cells, or neurons, in the brain exhibit abnormal electrical activity, epilepsy causes disturbance of emotions and behavior and sometimes convulsions, muscle spasms, and loss of consciousness.

When ancient Babylonians or Egyptians saw a person having a seizure, they believed that the condition was of supernatural origin and that the gods were visiting that person. Egyptian papyri show people with a "sacred disease" that is now recognized as epilepsy. However, Hippocrates (c. 460 to c. 380 BCE), disagreeing with these beliefs, scoffed at the idea of a divine origin for epilepsy. In his treatise *On the Sacred Disease*, he sarcastically addressed each of the different gods supposed to produce seizures and declared that there was no evidence for these notions. He insisted that the disease was a disease of the brain. The idea of supernatural causes did persist, however, and during the Middle Ages acquired a demonic twist. Medieval paintings depict people with ghastly demons coming out of the body at the end of a seizure.

Myths and stigmas concerning epilepsy are still prevalent in many places. Epilepsy is feared as a terrible and puzzling disease. But researchers are fitting together pieces of the epilepsy puzzle, and scientists now know that epilepsy is not one disease but many conditions with a common thread.

Epilepsy has been described as an electrical storm in the brain during which groups of nerve cells fire rapid electrical impulses. The type of seizure depends on which parts of the brain are affected.

Types of epilepsy

Hundreds of epilepsy syndromes as well as several types of seizures exist. Each disorder has a specific set of symptoms. While some appear to be hereditary, others are traced to specific events, such as a blow to the head or a stroke. However, for most cases, the cause is idiopathic (unknown). The areas of the brain in which the syndromes originate usually give the conditions their names. The more common types are described below.

In absence epilepsy, people have momentary lapses of consciousness or brief blackouts. At one time called *petit mal* (from the French, meaning "little sickness"), the symptoms begin in childhood or adolescence. The child may not even be aware that he or she has had a seizure; teachers may perceive that the child is staring into space or not paying attention. The child may experience a jerking arm or rapidly blinking eyes. Childhood absence epilepsy usually stops during puberty, but occasionally it may develop into a more serious form of epilepsy. These occurrences tend to run in families, and faulty genes may be responsible.

KEY FACTS

Description
A brain disorder that may cause seizures or other undesirable behaviors.

Causes
An electrical storm in the brain, in which groups of nerve cells rapidly fire electrical impulses.

Risk factors
Some cases appear to be hereditary; some are traced to an event such as a blow to the head or a stroke; most causes are unknown.

Symptoms
Vary with the type of epilepsy and depend on the section of the brain that is affected.

Diagnosis
Electroencephalography (EEG), in which electrodes are attached to the head to study electrical activity of the brain; magnetic resonance imaging (MRI); and computed tomography (CT).

Treatments
No cure exists at present; drug therapies are designed to remedy seizures and control undesirable behaviors; surgery may be recommended when drugs do not control seizures.

Pathogenesis
Can be life threatening, especially if seizures are not controlled.

Prevention
No specific prevention; general caution to avoid injury or blows to the head.

Epidemiology
An estimated 42 million people worldwide are afflicted; around 2.5 million Americans are affected by epilepsy and seizures.

Psychomotor epilepsy is characterized by strange or purposeless movements. This type of epilepsy originates in a region of the brain called the temporal lobe. The child may get up out of his or her seat in school and walk around the room as if in a daze, pulling at clothing or making other unusual movements. This type of epilepsy is also called recurrent partial seizure.

Temporal lobe epilepsy (TLE) is a common type of epilepsy. It usually begins in childhood. An aura—a "warning" sensation—may accompany this seizure. Repeated TLE seizures can cause the hippocampus in the brain to shrink, affecting memory and learning. Recognizing this type for early treatment is critical.

Frontal lobe epilepsy involves a cluster of short seizures with sudden onset and termination. Many types of these seizures exist; the symptoms depend on where in the frontal lobe the seizures occur.

Occipital lobe epilepsy usually begins with visual hallucinations, since this area of the brain is related to vision, rapid eye blinking, and other eye-related symptoms. Otherwise, the symptoms are similar to TLE.

Parietal lobe epilepsy tends to begin in the parietal lobe but spreads to other parts of the brain and closely resembles the symptoms of other kinds of epilepsy.

Lennox-Gastaut syndrome is a type of severe epilepsy that begins in childhood. The syndrome is characterized by sudden attacks resulting in falls. It is very difficult to treat.

Rasmussen's encephalitis is a condition that begins in childhood and is progressive. Half of the brain shows continual inflammation. It may be treated with a radical surgical procedure called hemispherectomy.

Ramsay Hunt syndrome type II is a rare and progressive type of epilepsy that begins in early adulthood and leads to reduced muscle coordination and cognitive ability in addition to seizures.

Infantile spasms is a type of epilepsy that begins in infancy with clusters of seizures before the age of six months. The infant may bend or cry out during an attack.

A complication associated with epilepsy is status epilepticus, which is a severe, life-threatening condition in which the person has prolonged seizures for over five minutes or does not fully regain consciousness between seizures. Rarely, death may occur for no discernible reason in people with epilepsy.

Whereas any type of seizure is a major concern, a seizure in isolation does not mean a person has epilepsy. People exhibit seizures with several other conditions such as high fever, narcolepsy, Tourette's syndrome, cardiac arrhythmia, and eclampsia.

Causes

Recent advances in molecular genetics, molecular biology, and electrophysiology have increased the knowledge and understanding of the basics of electrical discharge in the nervous system that is assumed to underlie epilepsy. Neurotransmitters, the chemicals that regulate electrical charges in the brain, are involved. Alterations in the levels of excitatory neurotransmitters or the inhibitory neurotransmitter gamma-butyric acid (GABA), or both, are believed to play a role in epilepsy. Genes may control the process. Knowing how new nerve cells migrate to their proper locations has led to the identification of faulty genes (mutations) that disrupt the normal pattern. For example, a gene called doublecortin may cause migrating nerve cells to stop short of the destination.

Symptoms and signs

Two major categories, partial and generalized, include more than 30 different types of seizures. Partial seizures occur in only one area of the brain and comprise about 60 percent of all seizures. Partial seizures are divided into simple and complex.

During a simple partial seizure the person remains conscious but may have unusual or unexplainable feelings of joy, anger, sadness, or nausea. They may hear, smell, taste, see, or feel things that are not there.

Complex partial seizures last only a few seconds, and the person just blanks out or has strange movements called automatisms. Violent behavior, such as hitting the wall or throwing a book across the room, may lead others to conclude that the person has a mental illness. The person may have an aura that indicates the seizure is coming. Another term for these partial seizures, especially those centered in the temporal lobe, is *psychomotor seizures.*

Generalized seizures result from abnormal neuronal activity in many parts of the brain, and these are of several types. During absence seizures the person has momentary loss of consciousness and may stare into space for several moments or have jerking or twitching movements. In tonic seizures the victim stiffens muscles of the body, generally the arms, back, and legs. In clonic seizures both sides of the body experience jerking movements. Myoclonic seizures cause the person to experience sudden jerking movements or twitches of the upper body, arms, or legs. In atonic seizures the person loses normal muscle tone and may fall down, nodding the head involuntarily like a rag doll. Tonic-clonic seizures include a mixture of symptoms such as loss of consciousness, stiffening of the body,

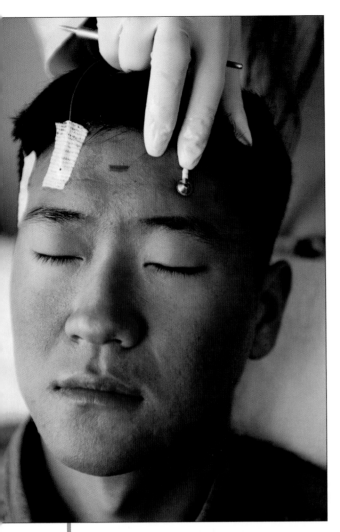

An electroencephalograph can help to diagnose epilepsy. Electrodes are attached to the patient's scalp; these electrodes are connected to a machine that amplifies brain impulses, which are measured as electrical activity. The results are recorded on a monitor. Any abnormal electrical activity is shown on the wave patterns, and different types of epilepsy can be identified.

and repeated jerking of arms and legs. The older name for this type is *grand mal* seizure.

Diagnosis

While some symptoms of epilepsy are obvious, others may be subtle, and discovering which type of epilepsy a patient is suffering from is essential before treatment can begin. The physician begins with an extensive medical history of the patient and family. He or she performs an electroencephalograph (EEG), in which

16 to 30 small electrodes are attached to the scalp with a special paste or with a special cap. A light is flashed in the eyes, and impulses or brain waves are recorded on a moving sheet of paper. Another important test is magnetic resonance imaging (MRI). One new version of MRI called fluid-attenuated inversion recover (FLAIR) may reveal important information about the processes deep in the brain. FLAIR can show abnormalities in the hippocampus and other internal regions. Other tests include blood tests and a spinal tap.

Treatments

Drugs are used to combat convulsions. Several drugs that have been on the market for several years, including phenytoin, valproate, and carbamazepine, are drugs of first choice. For the 30 percent of people with epilepsy who do not respond well to the drugs of first choice, newer drugs called antiepileptic drugs are approved as monotherapy (treatment by means of a single drug) or in combination with other drugs. These newer drugs include tiagabine, lamotrigine, gabapentin, topiramate, levetiracetam, felbamate, zonesimide, and oxcarbamazepine. However, all these drugs are powerful and have side effects.

Intractable epilepsy occurs when a person continues to experience seizures despite treatment with drugs. In such cases, doctors may recommend evaluation for surgery. A team of doctors, usually at a university medical center, looks at the type of seizures and at the brain region involved. Surgery may reduce or halt some seizures, but it is not without risk. Radiosurgery, in which ionizing radiation is used to destroy brain tissue, is being used experimentally in some medical centers to treat epilepsy. Other new treatments include stem-cell transplants and transplanting GABA-producing neurons from the fetuses of pigs into the brains of patients. Future treatments may include gene therapy to counter the effects of faulty genes.

Epidemiology

About 200,000 new cases of epilepsy occur in the United States each year; 10 percent of the population of the United States will have a seizure in their lifetime, and 3 percent will develop epilepsy by the age of 75. Men are slightly more likely to develop epilepsy than women. In addition, African Americans have a higher incidence of the disorder.

Evelyn Kelly

See also
• Head injury

Epstein-Barr infection

Epstein-Barr virus is the most frequent agent of infectious mononucleosis, and it is known to cause cancer of the head and neck in children, especially in Africa. The virus was discovered by Michael Epstein and Yvonne Barr in 1964, while they were researching cancer that primarily affected the head and neck of children.

Epstein-Barr virus (EBV) belongs to the herpes family of viruses; it is also called herpes virus type 4. EBV is transmitted through the saliva of infected people during kissing, sharing food, or other intimate contact. After entry, EBV invades the cells lining the throat (epithelial cells). In the epithelial cells, EBV multiplies, and numerous particles of the virus are released, destroying the epithelial cells in the process. The released viral particles then invade B lymphocytes (a type of white blood cell), which triggers a potent response by "killer" T lymphocytes that attempt to defeat the infection. However, Epstein-Barr infection usually remains inactive in B lymphocytes. The formation of coinlike structures called "episomes" allows EBV to reside in the nucleus of infected cells.

EBV is not spread as easily as some other viruses, such as the virus that causes the common cold, but it is common worldwide. In the United States and Great Britain, 50 percent of the population have positive blood tests for Epstein-Barr infection at the age of five and up to 90 percent in the adult population. Lower socioeconomic groups tend to acquire the virus at an earlier age. However, during early childhood and pre-adolescence the infection does not cause symptoms.

Symptoms and signs

Clinical signs of acute Epstein-Barr infection (mononucleosis) occur mostly in people exposed to the virus after the second decade of life, such as college students and military recruits. Typical signs include sore throat, fever, and swollen glands of the neck. In severe cases, there is also significant spleen enlargement. Although the spleen's primary function is to filter blood, many white cells, particularly lymphocytes, are located in this organ. When there is an inflammatory reaction against the virus, the spleen can become quite large, and there is a risk of rupture. In normal people, the symptoms of acute infection usually resolve in 4 to 6 weeks. However, the virus can remain dormant, establishing a lifelong carrier state. Epstein-Barr infection is spread by the excretion of viral particles in the saliva of people chronically infected with the virus, who are otherwise healthy and symptom free.

Pathogenesis

Epstein-Barr infection remains dormant and chronic in more than 95 percent of infected people. However, in people with altered immune systems, the virus may activate and result in malignancy. Examples include Burkitt's lymphoma, the most common childhood cancer in central Africa, lymphoma after transplant surgery, and leukoplakia (raised white patches in the mouth) in AIDS patients.

Edward Cachay and Sanjay Mehta

KEY FACTS

Description
A type of herpes virus that causes infectious mononucleosis and other disorders.

Causes
A virus invading the lymphocytes.

Risk factors
Epstein-Barr infection is transmitted through exposure to saliva of infected people.

Symptoms
Signs of infection are mostly the result of the body trying to eradicate the virus.

Diagnosis
Clinical symptoms and laboratory tests, such as white cell count and antibody tests.

Treatments
No specific treatment or vaccine is available.

Pathogenesis
In people with weak or abnormal immune systems, the infection may lead to development of cancer.

Prevention
Avoiding close contact with infected people.

Epidemiology
Common worldwide. In the United States 90 percent of adults aged 35 to 40 have been infected.

See also
- Hepatitis infections • Lymphoma
- Mononucleosis

Fetal alcohol syndrome

Alcohol use in pregnancy has a negative effect on the fetus and newborn. In February 2005, the U.S. Surgeon General issued an updated Advisory on Alcohol Use and Pregnancy, asserting that there is no established "safe" level of alcohol consumption in pregnancy. The update recommended that women who are pregnant or are considering pregnancy should not consume alcohol.

Recent studies have shown poor outcomes for children who are exposed to small amounts of alcohol before birth. The amount of drinking in pregnancy that is thought to potentially damage the fetus is typically more than 1 drink per day ($\frac{1}{2}$ ounce), or less if binge drinking occurs (more than five drinks per episode). However, new research indicates that even children prenatally exposed to 0.5 drinks daily may have poor outcomes. Alcohol use in pregnancy results in a known spectrum of disorders. Among these is fetal alcohol syndrome (FAS).

Diagnosis

FAS refers to a set of physical malformations and central nervous system abnormalities seen in the offspring of women who use alcohol during pregnancy. The reported prevalence of FAS in developed countries varies widely, but the average is around 1 in 3,000 live births. Although there is no precise dose response relationship between the amount of alcohol consumed and perinatal outcome, the prevalence of FAS among moderate to heavy drinkers may be as high as 20 to 40 percent.

The diagnosis of FAS is based on three criteria. The first is growth problems, that is prenatal or postnatal height or weight, or both, at or below the 10th percentile, documented at any one point in time. Height documentation must be adjusted for age, sex, gestational age, race, or ethnicity. The second criterion is specific facial features: a smooth area between the nose and upper lip (smooth philtrum), a thin upper lip (thin vermilion border), small eye opening (small palpebral fissures), and underdeveloped mid-face features (hypoplastic midface). The third criterion is central nervous system abnormalities: decreased head circumference, sleep disturbances, attention deficits, decreased response to noise, hyperactivity, and problems with speech development, learning, and visual focus. Other alcohol-related birth defects that may occur are those related to the eyes, heart, ears, kidneys, and limbs. It is important to remember that there is no exact dose-response relationship between the amount of alcohol consumed and infant outcome.

Treatments and prevention

True treatment lies in preventive strategies. Identifying women of childbearing age and screening them for alcohol use is of great importance. No conventional treatment exists because the diagnosis of

---

KEY FACTS

Description

FAS is a specific recognizable pattern of malformations that include prenatal and postnatal growth deficiency, central nervous system abnormalities, and craniofacial abnormalities.

Causes

Alcohol exposure of the fetus.

Risk factors

Maternal alcohol use before or throughout pregnancy, or both.

Symptoms

A spectrum of findings after delivery and as the child develops.

Diagnosis

Diagnosis can be suspected with poor growth in the fetus or other associated ultrasound findings.

Treatments

There is no effective treatment for FAS. As such, every effort should be focused on prevention. All women should be screened for alcohol use in pregnancy.

Pathogenesis

This is complex and incompletely understood. Alcohol and its metabolites easily cross the placenta. Animal models suggest interferences with protein synthesis, and problems with placental transfer of glucose and amino acids.

Prevention

Prenatal and antenatal screening for alcohol use and exposure.

Epidemiology

The reported incidence of FAS varies from 1 in 50 to 1 in 2,500 live births. In the Western world, the incidence has been reported as 0.33 in 1,000 live births. The incidence among those women who are heavy drinkers is significantly greater, possibly as high as 20–40 percent.

FAS is made after delivery. Prenatal ultrasound can only suggest a diagnosis, as most fetuses with FAS appear normal on ultrasound. In addition to growth problems noted above, congenital anomalies that can be seen on ultrasound and that have been associated with FAS include heart defects, central nervous system abnormalities (small head, neural tube defects), facial abnormalities (small chin, cleft lip and palate), truncal and skeletal abnormalities (diaphragmatic hernia, vertebral malformations), and urogenital malformations (small genitalia). The placenta usually appears normal, although the amount of amniotic fluid around the baby may be low. Many of these features may be subtle and may only be seen late in pregnancy.

It is important to note that most of the features mentioned cannot be seen until the late second trimester, and even then, what can be seen on ultrasound may not be so obvious. Additionally, one may not see all of the above features together. Separate findings may be seen, while others may not. Also, any single anomaly may have an alternate cause.

Early recognition is key so that known complications of FAS can be identified and support mechanisms for the family and child can be put into place. Known outcomes include: school failure, difficulties with peers, conduct problems, and mental health disorders. Long-term problems such as crooked teeth, inner-ear tube infections, problems in language, motor, learning, visual-spatial functioning, and cognition have been associated with FAS. Additionally, screening and good follow-up care can help with the identification of newborns at risk for alcohol withdrawal syndrome: symptoms are tremors, agitation, metabolic acidosis, low blood sugar, and seizures. These have been described in the infants of mothers who were intoxicated at the time of delivery. Even in the absence of a history of alcohol use in pregnancy, newborn babies who show symptoms or signs suggestive of possible alcohol withdrawal (such as tremors, agitation, metabolic acidosis, hypoglycemia, and seizures) should be screened for FAS. Treatment lies in recognizing that FAS is present and handling problems noted individually.

Pathogenesis

Exactly how FAS causes these problems is complex and incompletely understood. Alcohol and its metabolites, which are toxic to a fetus, can cross the placenta. How they exert their effects is still unknown. Animal models suggest an interference with protein synthesis, as well as problems with placental transfer of glucose and amino acids. Low blood sugar and a decrease in

fetal thyroid hormones and liver glycogen stores have also been demonstrated; these can all affect overall fetal growth and neonatal growth.

Epidemiology

The 2003 National Survey on Drug Use and Health reported that of women aged 15 to 44 years, 9.8 percent used alcohol and 4.1 percent reported binge drinking in the month before the T-ACE survey (see box, above).

The reported incidence of FAS varies from 1 in 50 to 1 in 2,500 live births. In the Western world, the incidence has been reported as 0.33 in 1,000 live births. The incidence among women who are chronic heavy drinkers is significantly greater, possibly as high as 20 to 40 percent. With screening and counseling of women to avoid alcohol during pregnancy or to stop its use during pregnancy, FAS can be prevented.

Antonette T. Dulay

T-ACE SURVEY

The T-ACE is a survey developed to assess drinking habits. It comprises four questions and takes less than one minute to administer:

Tolerance
Q: "How many drinks does it take to make you feel high?"

Annoyed
Q: "Have people annoyed you by criticizing your drinking?"

Cut down
Q: "Have you felt you ought to cut down on your drinking?"

Eye opener
Q: "Have you ever had a drink first thing in the morning to steady your nerves or get rid of a hangover?"

Scoring: The first question is scored positive if the respondent answers that he or she has had more than 2 drinks. A positive response gets 2 points for this question. The last 3 questions are scored 1 point each if answered affirmatively. A total score of 2 or more is considered positive for risk drinking.

See also
• Alcohol-related disorders • Learning disorders

Fibroids

Fibroids are noncancerous tumors of the uterus. They are the most common pelvic tumors in women. In very rare cases, fibroids may change to a cancerous condition. Fibroids affect women during their reproductive years, beginning as small growths in or attached to the uterine wall.

Fibroids may spread and in severe cases completely fill the uterus. In other cases, the growths may hang outside the uterus via a stalk attached to the outer wall of the organ. They do not usually affect fertility, but may create complications during pregnancy that may require delivery by cesarean section.

Causes

The cause of fibroids is unknown, although a genetic link may be involved in some cases. The growth of fibroids is encouraged by the presence of the female sex hormone estrogen; thus the tumors usually do not begin growing until a girl begins menstruating and estrogen production increases. They will continue to grow until the woman reaches menopause and estrogen production drops. In many cases, fibroids do not cause any symptoms, but in other cases fibroids may be indicated by feelings of abdominal fullness or pressure, severe cramping or pain during periods, heavy menstrual bleeding, or frequent urination.

Risk factors

The growth of fibroids is stimulated by hormonal changes during pregnancy. Fibroids may lead to premature births or may cause complications serious enough to warrant delivery of the baby by cesarean section. Sudden growth of fibroids, especially in postmenopausal women, may indicate changes leading to cancer.

Treatments and prevention

Asymptomatic cases often require nothing more than periodic examinations to monitor the condition of the fibroids. In other cases, the treatment required depends on the nature and severity of symptoms present.

Since the growth of fibroids is encouraged by estrogen, management of hormone levels is often used to treat the tumors, but hormonal therapy must be main-

tained to have lasting effects. Oral contraceptives are effective in reducing menstrual bleeding. Nonsteroidal anti-inflammatory drugs (NSAIDs) may be used to treat pain and cramping caused by the tumors. In severe cases, surgery may be necessary to remove the fibroids, or even the uterus itself.

David M. Lawrence

KEY FACTS

Description
Noncancerous tumors of the wall of the uterus.

Causes
Unknown.

Risk factors
Exposure to the hormone estrogen encourages growth of fibroids.

Symptoms
Fibroids often cause no symptoms, but abdominal fullness or pressure, cramping or pain during periods, heavy menstrual bleeding, or frequent urination may signal the presence of fibroids.

Diagnosis
Pelvic exam, sometimes accompanied with ultrasound imaging.

Treatments
Hormonal therapy to shrink fibroids, oral contraceptives to reduce menstrual bleeding, or nonsteroidal anti-inflammatory drugs to treat pain and cramping; in severe cases, surgery may be necessary to remove the fibroids.

Pathogenesis
Fibroids begin as small growths in or attached to the wall of the uterus, then spread; they may cause complications during pregnancy; in rare cases, they may lead to cancerous conditions.

Prevention
No known means of prevention at present.

Epidemiology
Fibroids affect as many as 20 percent of women of reproductive age, with the percentage increasing to as many as 40 percent of women over the age of 30. African American women are two or three times more likely to develop fibroids than Caucasian women.

See also
• Menopausal disorders • Menstrual disorders

Food intolerance

Food intolerance manifests as an adverse reaction, either physiological or behavioral, or both, in response to certain foods. Reactions can occur in the gastrointestinal, skin, urogenital, musculoskeletal, neurological, or respiratory systems. Unlike food allergies, food intolerances do not involve the immune system, but because symptoms are similar, the two may be confused. Although not life threatening, food intolerance can affect the quality of life.

Food intolerance can develop toward any naturally occurring or artificial food or food ingredient that is ingested. When a particular food item causes irritation in different systems of the body, such as the gastrointestinal, skin, urogenital, musculoskeletal, neurological, or respiratory systems, without the presence of an immune reaction, it is defined as food intolerance. On the other hand, food allergy occurs when the body has an immune reaction, such as the release of histamine, in response to food. Because symptoms of both food intolerance and food allergy are similar, they are difficult to distinguish from each other. For example, peanut ingestion may cause similar symptoms in both conditions, but an allergy to peanuts can be deadly, while intolerance to peanuts may be merely uncomfortable.

Causes and risk factors

Why some foods cause an intolerable reaction in some people is unknown. Common intolerances have been observed to dairy, carbohydrate, gluten, yeast, dyes, flavor enhancers, and preservatives. Carbohydrate intolerance includes intolerance to lactose, the predominant sugar in milk. Those who are lactose intolerant lack the necessary enzyme to digest lactose. Thus, the ingestion of milk products for those people results in digestive discomfort. Lactose intolerance is the most common type of food intolerance. Other substances called sulfites, occurring naturally in red wines or as additives in various foods to prevent mold growth, are another source of intolerance for some people and can cause headaches. A broad group of plant chemicals called salicylates, found naturally in many fruits, vegetables, nuts, coffee, juices, beer, and wine, may trigger other symptoms. Given that aspirin also is a compound of the salicylate family, foods containing salicylates may trigger symptoms in people who are sensitive to aspirin. Furthermore, some people may react psychologically or behaviorally to foods such as caffeine and sugar. Digestive symptoms can also be caused by any food that is consumed in excessive quantities.

Another factor contributing to food intolerances is the quantity of the food ingested; that is, food intolerances are often dose related. People with food intolerance may not have symptoms unless they eat a large portion of the food, or eat the food frequently. For example, a person with lactose intolerance may be able to drink milk in coffee or a single glass of milk, but becomes sick if he or she drinks several glasses of milk or eats a large bowl of ice cream. On the other hand, food allergies can be triggered by even a small amount of the food and occur every time the food is consumed.

KEY FACTS

Description
A physiological or behavioral reaction in response to certain foods.

Causes
Specific foods.

Risk factors
Eating foods that may cause the symptoms of food intolerance.

Symptoms
Digestive problems, runny nose, breathing problems, itching skin, hives, eczema, rash, headaches, insomnia, hyperirritability, anxiety, depression, and concentration problems.

Diagnosis
Eliminating immune involvement that would indicate food allergy rather than intolerance.

Treatment
Depending on the type of food intolerance, enzymes can be taken to aid the digestion of those foods or treatment of symptoms.

Pathogenesis
Unknown.

Prevention
Avoiding foods that cause the symptoms of food intolerance.

Epidemiology
Affects more than 50 million people in the United States.

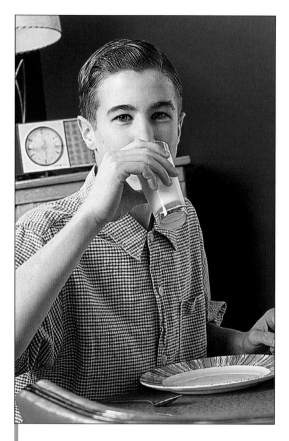

Lactose (the sugar found in milk) intolerance is a common food intolerance. Although someone with a lactose intolerance could probably drink a small amount of milk without ill effect, large quantities would cause digestive problems.

People with food allergies are generally advised to avoid the offending foods completely. Similarly, the highest risk factor for suffering the symptoms of food intolerance is ingesting certain foods.

Food allergies and intolerances are also different from food poisoning, which generally results from spoiled or tainted food and typically affects most people who eat it.

Signs and symptoms

Reactions to foods may be immediate or delayed. Immediate problems may include nausea, vomiting, itching skin, breathing problems, hives, or rashes. Delayed reactions may include digestive problems such as gas, cramps, bloating, runny nose, eczema, headaches, insomnia, heartburn, hyperirritability, anxiety, depression, and concentration problems. All of these symptoms can have a profound effect on the quality of life. Often, if the symptoms are not severe or immediate, the suffering person can rarely distinguish symptoms from some other ailment. For example, dietary components that cause behavioral problems such as irritability and short tempers may not be obvious. Thus, accurate diagnosis is necessary to avoid risk factors and improve the quality of life.

Diagnosis and treatments

Most food intolerances are found through trial and error to determine which food or foods cause symptoms. Keeping a food diary to record what foods are eaten and the symptoms they cause helps to determine what foods are causing problems. Another way to identify problem foods is to go on an elimination diet, completely removing any suspect foods from the diet until a person is symptom free. Reintroducing foods one at a time helps determine which foods cause symptoms. It is important to seek the advice of a health care provider or registered dietitian before beginning an elimination diet to be sure nutritional needs are met. Once it is known which foods are causing problems, treatment is based on avoiding or reducing intake of problem foods and treating symptoms when they arise, such as taking analgesics for headaches. In the case of lactose intolerance, over-the-counter lactase enzyme tablets can be taken to alleviate the symptoms of ingested lactose.

Prevention

Prevention can be simple if certain guidelines are followed. Learning which foods in which amounts cause symptoms, being aware of ingredients and preparation styles while dining out, and reading food labels to check ingredients usually eliminates most symptoms of food intolerance. Prevention of symptoms simply involves avoiding the offending foods.

Epidemiology

The exact number of people who suffer from food intolerance is unknown, but it is thought that the number is greater than those suffering from a true food allergy. Food intolerance affects 1 in 5 people, or 50 million people, in the United States. Lactose intolerance, the most common food intolerance, affects about 10 percent of Americans.

Rashmi Nemade

See also
• Anxiety disorders • Depressive disorders

Food poisoning

Food poisoning is one of the most common illnesses in the United States and worldwide. Food poisoning, which usually arises from contamination of raw foods of animal origin, is characterized by gastrointestinal upsets of varying severity. The illness can be avoided in many cases by following safe food practices.

More than 200 diseases can be transmitted through food. Infectious organisms, present in food through poor hygiene practices, are responsible for most cases of food poisoning. Symptoms, which usually include diarrhea and vomiting, tend to occur suddenly and disappear rapidly, followed by a full recovery. Few people seek medical treatment. However, sometimes more serious illness occurs, leading to widespread symptoms and, rarely, death. People most likely to experience severe symptoms are the elderly, infants and young children, pregnant women, and those whose immune systems are deficient.

Causes

Bacteria, viruses, and parasites can all cause food poisoning. Sometimes illness is caused not by the bacteria themselves but by the toxins they produce, either before or after ingestion.

Worldwide, the leading bacterial cause of food poisoning is *Campylobacter jejuni*, which usually infects raw poultry. One of the most feared food-borne illnesses, called botulism, is caused by bacterial toxins formed by *Clostridium botulinum*. Botulism occurs through improper canning of food and, while rare, is considered a public health emergency. *Salmonella* bacteria are most often associated with eggs; it is estimated that one in 20,000 eggs is contaminated. Infection with *Escherichia coli* (E. coli), a bacterium that produces toxins when it is ingested, is contracted by consumption of contaminated, undercooked ground beef, unpasteurized juice, and raw sprouts. Of particular concern to U.S. travelers is the so-called traveler's diarrhea, caused by a type of E. coli that is transmitted through water or food contaminated with human feces. *Vibrio* bacteria cause food poisoning through contamination of shellfish. Other bacteria responsible for food poisoning include *Staphylococcus*, *Listeria* (particularly found in soft cheeses and prepared foods),

Shigella, and *Toxoplasma*, which is mostly a risk for people with HIV infections.

Two-thirds of reported cases of food poisoning are caused by microorganisms called Norwalk-like viruses. Another common gastrointestinal infection is due to *Crytosporidium*, a parasite that is transmitted by water. An illness called ciguatera poisoning is the result of eating toxins that are sometimes found in large reef fish such as grouper and snapper; similarly, scombroid poisoning can occur when people eat contaminated fish such as tuna and mahi mahi. Hepatitis A, an inflammation of the liver, is a result of eating raw shellfish; and certain fungi contain toxins that produce food poisoning. However, despite an extensive list of potential infectious organisms, the source of most food-borne illnesses is never found.

KEY FACTS

Description

Acute gastrointestinal illness from eating contaminated or toxic food.

Causes

Contamination of food with bacteria, toxins, viruses, or parasites.

Risk factors

Eating food that is improperly washed, stored, or handled.

Symptoms

Stomach upset, nausea, vomiting, diarrhea, and fever; dehydration and death can result.

Diagnosis

Testing of blood and stools for infectious organisms.

Treatments

Anti-infective medicines are given for some bacterial and parasitic infections. Prevention of dehydration.

Pathogenesis

Consumption of food or drink contaminated by toxins or infectious organisms. There is a risk of blood poisoning and, rarely, death.

Prevention

Hygienic handling of food and avoidance of foods that may present a risk.

Epidemiology

In the United States it is estimated that about 76 million people suffer from food poisoning every year; of these, 325,000 require hospitalization and around 5,000 die.

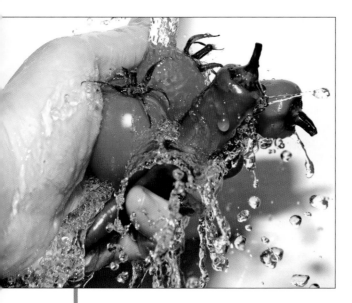

Appropriate handling, preparation, and storage of food are essential to avoid food being contaminated by bacteria. Hygienic practices, such as washing vegetables and fruit under cold running water can help avoid food poisoning.

Symptoms and signs

Stomach pain, nausea, vomiting, diarrhea, and fever are among the most common symptoms of food poisoning; dehydration often follows. In some cases, illness can be severe and even fatal, with widespread symptoms affecting not just the digestive organs but other parts of the body such as the kidneys and nervous system. Hemolytic uremic syndrome, which arises from *E. coli* infection, can result in bloody diarrhea followed by kidney failure and death. Botulism affects the nervous system and can lead to paralysis and death. Food poisoning with *Listeria* bacteria can lead to meningitis or, in pregnant women, spontaneous abortions. Ciguatera and scombroid poisoning produce tingling in the extremities, called paresthesias, and headaches.

The time it takes for symptoms of food poisoning to develop varies, depending on the source of the illness. With bacterial toxins that are formed before ingestion, the onset of symptoms is relatively rapid. Food poisoning caused by bacteria that produce toxins after ingestion, or by organisms that directly infect the gastrointestinal cells, typically takes longer to develop, usually from several hours to a few days. Symptoms of hepatitis A infection may take from 15 to 50 days to appear. The effects of scombroid poisoning appear very rapidly, from only one minute to three hours after ingestion of the toxin.

Depending on the type of poisoning, symptoms can be shortlived or prolonged. In the case of infection with a Norwalk virus, the illness lasts about two days; the symptoms of hepatitis A can continue for weeks.

Diagnosis and treatment

Most cases of food poisoning are never diagnosed because people with this illness often do not seek medical care. Even when they do so, their physician may not order tests to discover the cause. Diagnosis rests on the food history and symptoms followed by specific laboratory testing of suspect foods (if still available), feces, and blood. Treatment in most cases is supportive, involving rest and fluids. Intravenous fluids and hospitalization may be required in severe cases. Some bacterial infections can be treated with antibiotics.

Pathogenesis

Microorganisms associated with food poisoning cause illness by producing toxins prior to ingestion, producing toxins after ingestion, or directly infecting the gastrointestinal lining. When food poisoning is caused by preformed toxins, person-to-person transmission is not possible. *Staphylococcus aureus* food poisoning occurs when a food handler contaminates produce (usually dairy foods, meat, and eggs) with an infected skin sore. With food that has been cooked and left out at room temperature, bacteria can begin to grow in only a few hours. Typically, food infected in this way does not produce any detectable unusual odor or taste.

Prevention

Proper food-handling practices and avoidance of suspect foods such as raw shellfish can reduce the risk of food poisoning. Frozen foods should be defrosted in a refrigerator; raw produce should be thoroughly washed; food should be prepared on clean surfaces with avoidance of cross-contamination of surfaces; meat should be thoroughly cooked. Raw eggs and unpasteurized milk and juices should be avoided. Frequent hand washing is important. Travelers in countries where poor hygiene is likely to be encountered should avoid all raw foods and unbottled water.

Rita Washko

See also
- Diarrhea and dysentery • Toxoplasmosis

Fracture

A fracture is a break in a bone. A bone fractures when bone tissue under stress fails to withstand a break or tear. A bone usually fractures across its width but may also break along its length or at an angle. Fractures can be the result of sudden impact or prolonged tensile, compressive, or shear stress upon bone tissue.

Fractures are classified by their location or break characteristics. Fractures are displaced if the bone fragments have moved away from one another, or nondisplaced if the bone has not moved. A fracture is described as *open* (compound) if the fracture has broken through the skin, or closed (simple) if the skin is intact. A complete fracture is one that has broken through the bone width, separating the bone into at least two separate pieces. An incomplete fracture is a break on one side of the bone, leaving the bone in one piece. Some fractures have specific names; a common wrist fracture resulting from landing on an outstretched hand is a Colles' fracture.

Causes and risk factors

The direction, speed, and applied force are important determinants in whether bone tissue fails and fractures. Fractures can occur as the result of sudden, direct forces. A common cause of fractures is trauma. Low energy trauma, such as catching a toe along an object, can result in minor fractures with limited soft tissue involvement. High energy trauma, such as a motor vehicle accident, can result in severe fractures with extensive soft tissue damage and damage to internal organs.

Fractures can occur as a result of progressive forces. Athletes often experience stress fractures. As muscles fatigue and their ability to support the skeletal system diminishes, energy is transferred to the bone, making the bone more susceptible to injury.

Osteoporosis is the most common cause of fractures in postmenopausal women and people with underlying bone demineralization conditions. Loss of bone density is often a consequence of the aging process, decreased activity level, and osteoporotic conditions. Decreased bone density affects the strength and elastic properties of bone tissue, reducing a bone's ability to tolerate loading (such as the pull of gravity on the stacked weight of the spinal vertebrae) and increasing the likelihood of fracture.

Hip, pelvis, and femur fractures are most often associated with falls; vertebral fractures are often the result of progressive, long-term loading on spinal vertebrae. Risk factors for fractures associated with osteoporosis include advanced age, female gender, low body mass index, low muscle mass, frailty, low activity level, estrogen deficiency, low calcium intake, history of falls, alcoholism, cigarette smoking, and environmental hazards. Individuals more prone to falling are those with vision deficits, balance and gait problems, and functional limitations.

KEY FACTS

Description
A break in a bone.

Causes
Sudden trauma, osteoporosis, or muscle overuse.

Risk factors
Individuals with osteoporosis or bone demineralization are at higher risk for fractures. Athletes are especially prone to stress fractures.

Symptoms
Pain if pressure is applied. Bone fragments may be felt through the skin or may rupture skin. Bruising and inflammation typically present.

Diagnosis
From symptoms; usually confirmed with X-ray.

Treatments
Depending upon severity, location, and type of fracture, surgery may be necessary. Initially, immobilization is used. Rehabilitative therapy may be needed to regain strength and range of motion.

Pathogenesis
Force or load exceeds bone tissue tolerance; result is tissue break or tear.

Prevention
Fall prevention strategies, including home modification, exercise, and proper shoe wear; prophylactic medication; and training modifications to prevent stress fractures.

Epidemiology
The leading cause of death and disability in persons 65 or older is fall-related injuries, especially hip fractures. Of women 65 years or older, white women are more likely to fracture a hip than are black women. Women are more likely to be hospitalized with a fall-related fracture.

BONE FRACTURES

Fractures can occur in many forms, depending on the force applied and the type of injury. Although fractures tend to occur across the bone, they can also occur in the bone in a spiral form, obliquely, or lengthwise.

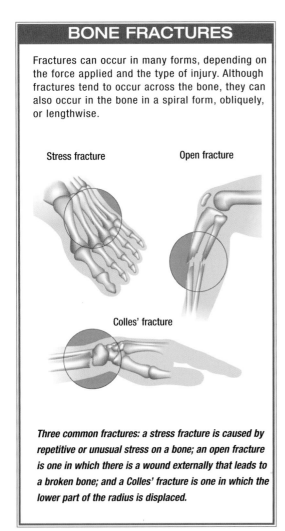

Stress fracture

Open fracture

Colles' fracture

Three common fractures: a stress fracture is caused by repetitive or unusual stress on a bone; an open fracture is one in which there is a wound externally that leads to a broken bone; and a Colles' fracture is one in which the lower part of the radius is displaced.

Signs, symptoms, and diagnosis

Fractures are painful, especially when pressure is applied to the fracture site. Typically, the surrounding tissue is tender, and there is usually swelling within a few hours of injury. With severely displaced bones, there may be limb deformity, a fragment of the displaced bone may be felt through the skin, or the bone may emerge through the skin. Fractures that occur as a result of continuous loading usually cause increasing discomfort. Blood from an injured fracture site may cause a skin bruise, especially with closed fractures. The pooling of blood can cause pain and stiffness in the area around the fracture.

Fracture diagnosis is made based upon signs and symptoms and usually confirmed by X-ray. Hairline or non-displaced fractures are often difficult to confirm by X-ray, and some stress fractures may not be evident by X-ray for several weeks after injury. An MRI (magnetic resonance imaging) scan may be necessary to identify less obvious fractures.

Treatments and prevention

Fracture treatment is highly dependent upon the type, severity, and location of the fracture. Open fractures often require surgery to clean and close the wound and present a greater risk for infection. Closed fractures are usually treated with immobilizers (a cast, brace, or splint) and recommendations for swelling management. The procedure for realigning a bone is called reduction. Surgical reduction for a displaced bone is called open reduction. The nonsurgical reduction of a closed fracture (realigning without penetrating the skin) is called closed reduction. Open reduction is often the sign of a more complicated and severe fracture.

Fixation devices, such as pins and plates, are often necessary to secure bone alignment for proper healing. Fixation devices may be internal (attached to the bone and sutured under the skin) or external (attached to the bone, but with a portion of the fixation device emerging through the skin). Traction may be used to help align bones. After realignment, whether or not surgery is necessary, a period of immobilization is often recommended during the initial healing phases. Immobilization prevents muscle action, helps to keep bones in place, and promotes bone reunification.

During the healing process, there is first tissue inflammation, possibly for several weeks. A hematoma forms, and inflammatory agents respond to the injury. The body cleans up dead tissue and begins to produce collagen for tissue healing. Next, a soft callous forms, often with pain and swelling, owing to increased blood flow to injured areas. Cartilage or early bone tissue begins to form. A natural splint is created to stabilize the fracture. As a result, muscles remain inactive and will often contract into the position of immobilization. Range of motion exercises will lengthen muscles that may have shortened during the immobilization period. Rehabilitation also includes strengthening muscles that have not been used during immobilization.

Bone mineral density assessment using a dual X-ray absorptiometry scan (DXA) can identify those at risk for osteoporosis. For those at high risk, calcium supplements or prophylactic medication. may be indicated.

Patti Berg

See also
• Osteoporosis

Frostbite

Frostbite is injury to body tissues caused by freezing temperatures. It is most common in the winter, in latitudes closer to the North and South poles, and at high altitudes. Risk factors include prolonged activity in freezing temperatures, impaired judgment, such as that due to psychiatric illness or drugs, and an inability to avoid adverse conditions, as might befall very young or old people. Frostbite is more common when the blood supply to the extremities is impaired due to old age, diabetes, peripheral vascular disease, or certain drugs.

Frostbite generally involves parts of the body that are farthest away from the heart, such as the fingers, ears, and nose. The water in the cells becomes frozen and crystallizes, resulting in cell injury or death. Similar to burn injuries, frostbite can be classified by the depth of injury. First-degree frostbite involves the epidermis only and is characterized by redness of the skin. A second-degree or partial-thickness frostbite typically has fluid-filled blisters and is painful. Third-degree frostbite includes all layers of the skin, which is white and has no sensation. Fourth-degree frostbite involves injury to deeper structures such as fat, tendon, and bone and may lead to amputations of the injured toes or fingers. The skin involved is initially pale, firm, cold, and has no sensation. When rewarmed, the area is usually intensely red and painful unless tissue has been destroyed, as evidenced by blisters or gangrene.

Treatment

Treatment should first focus on any life-threatening conditions and include core rewarming if the patient has hypothermia (a low core body temperature). Management of the frostbitten tissue includes initial wrapping in dry clothing, followed by rapid rewarming with water at 104°F to 107°F (40°C–42°C). Rubbing the tissue, dry heat, and hot water should be avoided because they can cause additional injury. Once the injured part is warmed, antibiotic cream can be applied. First- and second-degree frostbite should heal spontaneously, the latter taking 10 to 21 days to form new skin. Third-degree frostbite may require surgical excision of the dead tissue and skin grafting. Fourth-degree frostbite may require amputations.

Prevention

Preventive measures involve protection with appropriate clothing and avoiding risky situations that may lead to prolonged exposure to freezing temperatures. Once numbness of the affected part has developed, the person may not realize that a severe, irreversible injury is occurring.

With adequate precautions, most instances of frostbite are preventable.

David Wainwright

KEY FACTS

Description

Injury to the skin and underlying tissues as a result of freezing temperatures.

Causes and risk factors

Frostbite is caused by prolonged exposure to freezing temperatures. Those at higher risk include outdoor workers, winter athletes, and people with poor circulation. Impaired judgment and an inability to escape from the cold may lead to extended exposure.

Symptoms and signs and diagnosis

The diagnosis is made by the history of exposure and the observed skin changes. The skin is pale, firm, cold, has no sensation, and becomes intensely red and painful when rewarmed. Blisters and gangrene indicate a deeper injury with tissue death.

Treatments

The injured tissue should be rapidly rewarmed and an antibiotic cream applied. When tissue destruction occurs, the skin may need to be replaced with skin grafts, or amputations may be necessary.

Pathogenesis

The water in the cells becomes frozen and crystallizes, resulting in cell injury or death.

Prevention

Avoiding prolonged exposure to the cold; wearing appropriate clothing and protection of body areas when exposure is unavoidable.

Epidemiology

Frostbite is most common in outdoor workers and winter athletes. It is an injury observed most frequently in winter, in areas close to the North or South poles and at high altitudes.

See also
• Burns

Gallstone

Gallstones are concretions of cholesterol or bilirubin that form in the gallbladder. They are common in Western cultures and result in 500,000 to 700,000 cholecystectomies (surgical removal) annually. Gallstones occur in about three women for every man, and are more common in certain Native Americans, Scandinavians, and native Alaskans. Risk factors for gallstone formation include obesity, weight loss, older age, diabetes, pregnancy, liver cirrhosis, and parenteral (outside the intestine, usually by injection) nutrition.

Gallstones come in two main varieties: cholesterol and pigmented stones. Cholesterol stones comprise 80 percent of all gallstones. Pigmented stones are composed of bilirubin (the breakdown product of heme, the iron-bearing pigment of blood) and are typically black or brown. Black stones occur in diseases that cause red blood cell destruction (hemolysis), such as sickle-cell anemia. Brown stones are typically the result of chronic infections in the channels (ducts) regulating bile flow. Rarely, medications can precipitate in bile and form stones.

Signs and symptoms

The mere presence of gallstones in the gallbladder does not cause symptoms. Pain occurs when a stone causes obstruction of biliary ducts. When this happens, patients complain of right-sided abdominal pain that radiates to the back or the shoulder. In more severe instances, nausea, fever, and jaundice can develop and may progress to life-threatening infection.

Diagnosis and treatments

Diagnosis is made by ultrasonography; it often occurs as an incidental finding. Computerized tomography and magnetic resonance imaging can also detect gallstones but are more frequently used to identify complications of gallstone disease. Abdominal X-ray is not helpful because cholesterol stones often lack calcifications and cannot be seen on X-rays.

Treatment depends on symptoms and whether complications develop. Asymptomatic gallstones require no therapy. Chronic gallstone-related pain is usually treated by laparoscopic removal of the gall-bladder. Bile duct obstruction is typically managed by removal of the stone with a nonsurgical endoscope.

Pathogenesis and prevention

Bile is a digestive secretion that is formed in the liver and stored in the gallbladder. A variety of genetic and physiological conditions can result in bile becoming saturated with cholesterol or bilirubin. Gallstone formation begins with deposition of these compounds around a nidus that enlarges over time, especially when the emptying of the gallbladder is impaired. Prevention of gallstones is difficult because many risk factors cannot be modified. When rapid weight loss is anticipated, the bile acid ursodeoxycholate can reduce the incidence of gallstone formation.

Christopher W. Duncan and Stephen D. Zucker

KEY FACTS

Description
Concretions of cholesterol or bilirubin form stones.

Causes
Excess cholesterol or bilirubin in bile, genetic predisposition.

Risk factors
Female gender, race, family history, older age, pregnancy, obesity, hemolytic disorders.

Symptoms
Frequently asymptomatic; abdominal pain, nausea, fever, and jaundice can occur.

Diagnosis
Abdominal ultrasound, computed tomography.

Treatments
Surgery, medication, endoscopy.

Pathogenesis
Precipitation of cholesterol or bilirubin in the gallbladder, poor gallbladder emptying.

Prevention
Medication (ursodeoxycholate).

Epidemiology
More common in women (increases with number of pregnancies), Western cultures, Native Americans, and elderly people. About 11 percent of people in the United States have gallstones.

See also
• Obesity • Sickle-cell anemia

Giardiasis

Giardiasis is an infectious disease of the intestines caused by the microscopic parasite *Giardia lamblia*. Symptoms include diarrhea, stomach cramps, dehydration, and weight loss. In many less-developed countries, most children have had giardiasis by their third birthday.

More than 20,000 new cases of giardiasis are reported every year in the United States alone. The cause is a microscopic, single-celled parasite belonging to the genus *Giardia*. Scientists are still not certain about the classification of this organism, but there appear to be various species, each of which can infect several different kinds of animals. The main species that affects humans is called *Giardia lamblia*.

The symptoms that a *Giardia* infection produces, such as diarrhea, can also be caused by many other disorders. If giardiasis is suspected, examination of a fecal sample or a blood test will discover if the patient has produced specific protective antibodies.

Pathogenesis

Giardia can survive in the environment because the parasite is surrounded by a thick outer coat to form a cyst (an inactive, nonfeeding form). After a person or animal swallows the cysts present in contaminated food or water, the cysts break open when they reach the small intestine, releasing mature parasites that feed and multiply. The parasite does not attack intestinal cells directly. *Giardia* parasites, by attaching to and covering the inner intestinal surfaces, interfere with nutrient absorption and water transport and cause diarrhea, cramps, and sometimes dehydration. As the parasites pass through the small intestines to the large intestines, they form new cysts that pass out of the body. These new cysts, if they infect other people or animals who come in contact with contaminated food or water, start another cycle of infection.

Epidemiology, prevention, and treatments

People get giardiasis when they drink river, stream, or lake water contaminated with fecal matters from wild animals such as bears and beavers. Infection is also possible from drinking insufficiently processed municipal water. Outbreaks sometimes occur in day care centers and nursing homes when caregivers do not wash their hands after a bowel movement. Giardiasis does not spread by exposure to blood or other body fluids, but some people can be infected without apparent symptoms and may spread the infection.

Prevention is mainly a matter of personal hygiene habits such as washing hands after a bowel movement. River, stream, and lake water should be boiled or filtered before it is drunk. Eating uncooked food in countries where giardiasis occurs should be avoided. Nearly four thousand people per year in the United States have giardiasis severe enough to require hospitalization.

Treatment is with drugs such as metronidazole, furazolidone, and nitrazoxanide. Patients take medication for 5 to 10 days. When diarrhea is severe, replacing lost fluids is also important.

Janet Yagoda Shagam

KEY FACTS

Description
Parasitic infection of the small intestine.

Cause
Infection with *Giardia lamblia*, a single-celled microscopic parasite.

Risk factors
Drinking untreated or undertreated water, or eating contaminated raw foods or inadequately cooked foods.

Symptoms
Diarrhea, abdominal cramps, and weight loss.

Diagnosis
Identifying parasites in feces of infected person, or immunological testing.

Treatments
Drugs, plus hydration treatment.

Pathogenesis
Parasites interfere with absorption of nutrients and also cause diarrhea.

Prevention
Good hygiene. Boiling or otherwise treating potentially contaminated water.

Epidemiology
More than 20,000 new cases each year in the United States.

See also
• Diarrhea and dysentery

Glaucoma

A serious eye disorder involving damage to the optic nerve, glaucoma is usually caused by a buildup of pressure within the eye. Because of age, glaucoma is the second most common cause of blindness worldwide after cataracts. As a population grows older, the prevalence of glaucoma rises. It is important to detect and treat the disease as early as possible because damage caused by glaucoma cannot be undone.

Glaucoma is sometimes called the "silent thief of sight" and may be well advanced before individuals become aware that their eyesight is becoming impaired. Typically, vision around the edges of sight (peripheral vision) is affected first. In the United States, an estimated 3 million people have glaucoma; 50 percent of these remain undiagnosed. Glaucoma is the leading cause of blindness in the United States for which treatment is available.

Risk factors

Everyone is potentially at risk. Advancing age is a major risk factor (glaucoma is six times more prevalent in individuals over 60 years), but the disease also occurs in babies and adolescents. It is the leading cause of blindness in African Americans, who are at much higher risk (and at a younger age) than Caucasians. A person's risk of developing the most common form of glaucoma (primary open angle glaucoma) increases if another family member already has it. Normal tension glaucoma (see below) is more common in people of ethnic Japanese origin.

Causes and pathogenesis

Glaucoma is usually caused by a buildup of pressure in the eye. The pressure increase begins in the eye's front chamber, which is filled with a watery liquid called aqueous humor. If too much of the liquid is produced and it cannot drain properly, increased intraocular pressure (IOP) results, which can damage the eye's nerve cells. The most common type of glaucoma is called primary open angle glaucoma (POAG), which develops gradually. In this type, the openings to the drainage tubes for aqueous humor are clear, with blockage occurring farther inside the drainage canals. By contrast, in angle closure glaucoma (also called narrow-angle or closed-angle glaucoma), the drainage openings suddenly become blocked, as with a blocked sink drain. IOP rises suddenly, sometimes just in one eye, resulting in attacks of headaches, nausea, eye pain, and blurred vision. Acute angle closure glaucoma is a medical emergency: the pressure in the eye must be reduced rapidly to prevent permanent loss of vision. More rarely, people can be born with glaucoma or develop it during childhood or adolescence. Glaucoma can also arise from other causes, including eye injuries, infections, diabetes, cataracts, or use of steroid drugs.

KEY FACTS

Description

Partial or complete blindness involving damage to the eye's nerve cells, usually caused by increased pressure within the eye.

Causes

In most cases of glaucoma, overproduction or reduced drainage of aqueous humor is the primary cause.

Risk factors

Increasing age, race, family history, steroid use, diabetes, eye injury.

Symptoms

Depend on type of glaucoma, but can include apparent halos around light, headaches, nausea, blurred or reduced vision, or eye pain. Fifty percent of people with glaucoma show no symptoms until late stage.

Diagnosis

Various procedures, including checking pressure within eye, evaluating quality of vision, and checking damage to optic disk.

Treatments

Drugs or surgery (laser or conventional) aimed at reducing intraocular pressure (IOP).

Pathogenesis

Nerves transmitting information from eye to brain are damaged.

Prevention

Risk can be reduced with eye drops aimed at decreasing IOP, cholesterol-reducing drugs, and regular eye exams.

Epidemiology

Estimated 3 million people in the United States currently affected, 120,000 of whom are blind.

Increased pressure in the eye endangers vision by damaging the optic disk, the area (sometimes called the blind spot) where the cablelike axons that carry messages from the eye's nerve cells to the brain group together. Once their axons are damaged, the nerve cells of the eye die and cannot be replaced. Similar damage to the optic disk sometimes occurs for unknown reasons without increased IOP, in so-called normal tension glaucoma.

Diagnosis

Measuring IOP can be done in various ways. One method (applanation) is to direct a puff of air at the eye, measuring how much force is needed to dent the surface. For best results, the thickness of the cornea should be measured at the same time, because it varies between individuals and can distort readings. A doctor may also carry out a visual perimetry test, in which the extent of vision loss is mapped: Individuals are asked to look ahead and indicate when they detect a moving stimulus introduced into their peripheral vision. Gonioscopy is a technique that uses a mirrored contact lens to examine the angle the iris makes with the cornea, to confirm whether angle closure glaucoma or POAG is involved. Finally, an ophthalmoscope can be used to look into the eye to check whether there is any visible damage to the optic disk.

Treatments

Glaucoma cannot be cured, and dead retinal cells are irreplaceable. Most treatments are aimed at reducing intraocular pressure to prevent or reduce further damage.

Eyedrops or other drugs can be prescribed to lower production of aqueous humor or increase its outflow, or both. A disadvantage of these drugs is that they may have to be taken regularly for life. Laser surgery can be used to clear out the meshwork of drainage canals, inactivate part of the tissue that produces aqueous humor, or open a new hole in the iris. A technique called selective laser trabeculoplasty uses a low-energy laser to make very small disruptions to clogged drainage canals. Because it causes so little damage, the procedure can be used repeatedly.

Nonlaser microsurgery is also used, for example to make a tiny opening in sclera so liquid can drain out. Where necessary, a tiny tube can also be implanted in front of the iris to provide an alternate drainage route. Infection, irritation, bleeding, or scarring may be complications of surgery, although scarring can be minimized with drug treatment.

Alternate treatments like homeopathy, bilberry

CHRONIC GLAUCOMA

In this condition, the fluid that is secreted into the anterior part of the eye, to retain the shape and feed the tissues, cannot flow away normally. A blockage in the drainage angle prevents the release of excess fluid, and the pressure in the eye builds up until there is a loss of vision, by which time the condition is advanced and chronic.

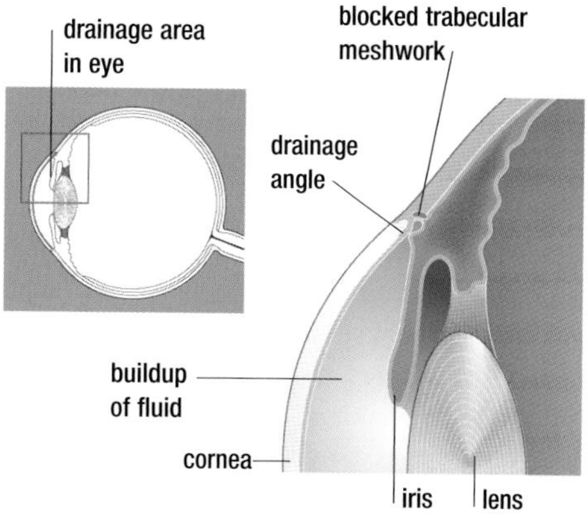

drainage area in eye
blocked trabecular meshwork
drainage angle
buildup of fluid
cornea
iris
lens

In the diagram above of the interior of the eye, the sievelike mesh through which fluid flows out of the eye is blocked, causing chronic glaucoma.

juice, yoga, and use of biofeedback techniques are used by some patients, but there is no clear evidence of their therapeutic value for glaucoma. Earlier tests of medicinal use of marijuana showed some effectiveness in reducing IOP, but safer and more effective drugs are now available. A vaccine that may slow glaucoma progression is currently being developed. Recent research indicates that cholesterol-reducing drugs (statins) may protect against glaucoma.

Prevention

Until recently, no preventive measures were known for glaucoma. However, investigators have now shown that drugs applied to the eye aimed at reducing IOP in individuals who were at risk for glaucoma reduced by 50 percent the chance of developing the disease. With such preventive measures available, screening to detect early symptoms of glaucoma is increasingly important. People can now buy a test kit to measure their IOP.

Sonal Jhaveri

See also
- Cataract • Macular degeneration
- Retinal disorders

Gonorrhea

Gonorrhea is a sexually transmitted disease caused by the bacterium *Neisseria gonorrhoeae*. The bacteria grow and multiply in the warm, moist areas of the reproductive tract, like the cervix, uterus, and fallopian tubes in women, and the urethra (urinary tube) in men and women. Other sites of infection include the eyes, rectum, throat, and mouth; rarely, infection spreads to the blood and joints.

Gonorrhea is the second most commonly reported infectious disease in the United States after chlamydia, another sexually transmitted disease, although it is believed that only about half of all gonorrhea cases are reported. More than 330,000 cases of gonorrhea were reported in the United States in 2004. This was the lowest recorded rate since 1941 when records began and, according to the Centers for Disease Control and Prevention (CDC), a 75 percent fall in rates since 1975, when the national gonorrhea control program began and gonorrhea rates were at their peak. However, while cases have been steadily decreasing, antibiotic resistance has been increasing.

Risk factors

Seventy-five percent of reported gonorrhea cases are in people under 30 years old, with the highest rates occurring in sexually active teenagers, young adults, and African Americans. The greater the number of sexual partners, the greater the risk.

Symptoms and signs

Most women have no symptoms, so many infections go undiagnosed. This can lead to pelvic inflammatory disease and cause chronic pelvic pain, infertility, and ectopic pregnancies. Left untreated in men, gonorrhea may cause epididymitis, a painful inflammation of the testicles that can result in infertility.

When symptoms are present in women, they include vaginal discharge, burning on urination, vaginal bleeding between periods, or only vague symptoms. In men there may be a thick fluid discharge from the penis 2 to 10 days after sexual contact, or as much as 30 days later. An infected mother can pass gonorrhea to the newborn as it passes through the birth canal; the result can be an eye, joint, or life-threatening blood infection.

Diagnosis and treatment

Microscopic examination of a swab sample taken from the infection site may show bacteria, and a urine test or culture can be sent for laboratory analysis. Gonorrhea is curable with antibiotics. In many cases, chlamydia and gonorrhea coexist, so a combination of antibiotics may be used. Sexual partners must be treated to prevent reinfection. Although antibiotics treat the infection, they do not reverse any damage such as scarred fallopian tubes.

Prevention

The best methods of prevention are to abstain from sex, or practice sex in a long-term monogamous relationship with an uninfected partner. Condoms reduce the risk of infection.

Ramona Jenkin

KEY FACTS

Description
A sexually transmitted disease (STD).

Cause
Infection with the bacterium *Neisseria gonorrhoeae*.

Risk factors
Highest rates of infection in sexually active teenagers, young adults, and African Americans.

Symptoms
There may be no symptoms. Men may have burning on urination and a penile discharge; women may have vaginal discharge and bleeding.

Diagnosis
Microscopic examination of a swab from the infection site; urine analysis.

Treatment
Antibiotics; treatment of sexual partners.

Pathogenesis
Gonorrhea increases the risk of contracting and transmitting HIV.

Prevention
Abstinence from sex. Latex condoms can reduce the risk.

Epidemiology
More than 330,000 infections reported in the United States each year.

See also
• AIDS • Chlamydial infections • Herpes infections

Growth disorders

In growth disorders there is disturbance in one or more of the phases of growth during childhood, leading to increased or diminished height. Growth disorders have many causes, including malnutrition, hormonal and genetic abnormalities, and disorders of the digestive tract, bones, kidneys, lungs, and heart.

Before birth, the growth of the developing fetus is determined by factors that include genetics, the mother's health and standard of nutrition, and the functioning of the placenta (the organ that nourishes the fetus in the uterus). After birth, a child's rate of growth is influenced by genetic, hormonal, nutritional, and general health factors. Normal patterns of growth can be monitored at routine checkups by using charts that track height changes throughout childhood.

Growth phases

Growth occurs in three phases: the infantile phase, the childhood phase, and the pubertal phase. The infantile phase occurs during the first two years of life, when growth in height averages 12 to 14 inches (30 to 35 cm). The childhood phase occurs from the age of two until the start of puberty and is characterized by a constant steady height gain of 2 to 2½ inches (5 to 7 cm) per year. The pubertal phase occurs at the onset of puberty, the time of life when sexual development begins. Changes in hormones trigger a rapid increase in height called the pubertal growth spurt, with growth frequently reaching 3 to 5½ inches (8 to 14 cm) per year. In boys, peak growth velocity occurs near the age of 14, with achievement of final height occurring around 19 years of age; in girls, peak growth velocity is near the age of 12, with final height occurring around 16. In growth disorders there is disturbance in one or more of the phases of growth, leading to increased or diminished height.

Growth variations

Some variations in growth are considered normal. Such variations include constitutional growth delay, which occurs when children grow at a normal rate but are small for their age. These children reach puberty later than their peers, and their pubertal growth spurt

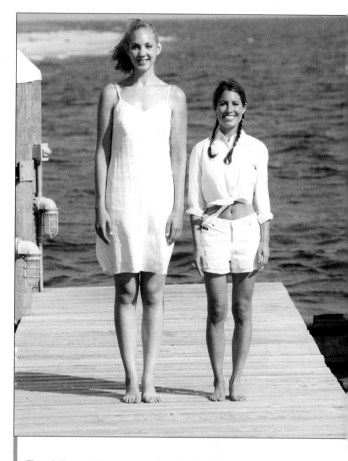

Though they are the same age, there is a big difference in the height of these girls. Many factors can lead to this variation: growth spurts at different times, a familial tendency to a certain height, delayed onset of puberty, or a growth disorder.

is delayed (puberty is considered late if it occurs after 13 in girls and 14 in boys). Frequently, children with constitutional growth delay continue to grow until a later age and have normal adult height. Also normal is short stature in children whose parents are shorter than average. Children with familial short stature enter puberty at a normal age and have normal adolescent growth spurts but have short adult height.

Causes and risk factors

Growth disorders have many different causes, including hormonal and genetic abnormalities, and diseases of the kidneys, heart, gastrointestinal tract, lungs, and bones. Worldwide the most common cause of growth disorders is malnutrition. Having adequate supplies of calories and protein is of critical importance to maintaining growth and development, and if the diet contains insufficient nutrients, short stature is likely to occur.

Hormonal growth disorders are caused by an excess or a deficiency of a hormone. Growth hormone is made by the pituitary gland located at the base of the brain. Low production of this hormone can occur if the gland malfunctions, is damaged, or does not form properly. Tumors, infections, or injury to the pituitary or to adjacent areas can damage or destroy the gland. Radiation therapy used to treat other diseases may also damage the pituitary. Changes in genes that are critical for the development of the pituitary can lead to problems with the growth of the gland.

Rarely, pituitary tumors can produce too much growth hormone. If the tumor develops before puberty, the person grows abnormally and has a condition called gigantism. If the tumor develops once the long bones stop growing, the condition is called acromegaly. Typically, the hands, feet, jaw, and skull become enlarged, as well as some internal organs. Treatment for acromegaly may be the surgical removal of the tumor or drug treatment to try to shrink the tumor.

Thyroid hormone is also essential for normal growth. The thyroid, a gland located in the neck, makes thyroxine, a hormone critical for the growth and development of bones. If too little or too much thyroxine is produced, growth disorders can occur. Another hormone that affects growth is cortisol, which is produced by the paired adrenal glands located near the kidneys. If the adrenal glands produce too much cortisol, children usually have an increase in weight, although their height does not change. This overproduction of cortisol is called Cushing's disease. It is rare in children but may be related to treatment with glucocorticoids, which are steroid medications that act in a similar manner to cortisol.

Precocious puberty is a hormonal disorder that occurs when children enter the pubertal growth spurt early (before 8 years for girls and before 9 years in boys). Initially, most children with precocious puberty are taller than their classmates, but they may stop growing early and be shorter as adults. Growth may also be disturbed by delayed puberty, one cause of which is Turner's syndrome, a genetic disease that affects only girls and occurs in about 1 in 2,500 births. Girls with Turner's syndrome have an abnormal or missing X chromosome, and their ovaries are not properly formed. These children do not undergo puberty normally, which leads to very low levels of estrogen, a hormone that is important for growth in girls.

Down syndrome is another genetic disorder that affects growth. People with Down syndrome are generally shorter than their predicted height. Marfan syndrome is a genetic disease that is associated with a tall stature and very long arms and legs. Marfan, which is the result of defects in connective tissue, may also be associated with eye and heart diseases.

Disorders of the skeleton and cartilage may lead to growth disorders. In these conditions, the bones do not form normally, and children generally are shorter than expected.

Skeletal disorders can be genetic, for example X-linked hypophosphatemic rickets, in which children have bowing of the lower legs and short stature as a result of abnormal metabolism of the mineral phosphate and vitamin D. Vitamin D deficiency through

KEY FACTS

Description

Disrupted growth patterns leading to abnormally short or tall stature.

Causes

Malfunctioning, damaged, or absent pituitary gland; genetic disorders; malnutrition.

Risk factors

Tumors, infections, and injury to the pituitary gland; radiation therapy affecting the pituitary or nearby areas; genetic mutations that interrupt the formation of the pituitary; inadequate maternal diet or poor nutrition after birth.

Symptoms

Short stature with poor growth velocity; or abnormal height.

Diagnosis

Physical exam, laboratory testing, radiological testing, and growth hormone stimulation testing.

Treatments

Hormone replacement with growth hormone; correction of diet in cases of malnutrition.

Pathogenesis

Defects to or absence of the pituitary gland lead to deficiencies of hormones necessary for normal growth.

Prevention

Apart from growth disorders caused by malnutrition, most cases are not preventable.

Epidemiology

Growth disorders appear in an estimated 1 in 10,000 births.

poor nutrition can also cause rickets. Achondroplasia is a disorder of cartilage that is the most common form of disproportionate growth retardation. People with achondroplasia have an average-sized trunk but short limbs because of a progressive decrease in the growth velocity that begins in infancy.

Children with chronic diseases may also have growth disorders. Many different diseases, such as kidney disease, liver disease, sickle-cell anemia, diabetes mellitus, and cystic fibrosis, may slow growth; diseases of the intestines that impair the ability to absorb nutrients from the diet sometimes lead to poor growth. In addition, any disease that is severe, untreated, or poorly controlled can have a negative impact on growth. Severe stress is another possible cause of decreased growth.

Diagnosis

An abnormality in stature is determined by the comparison of a child's height to the average height, plotted on a growth curve, for a child of the same age and sex. If the measured height is not what would be predicted, it is important to evaluate other features of growth. One consideration is the growth velocity, which is based on the change in height estimated to occur in one year. For example, if height measurements are taken four months apart and a 1-inch (2.5 cm) increase in height occurs during that period, the growth velocity is 3 inches (7.5 cm) per year. In children with a suspected growth disorder, it is also important to assess a mid-parental height. For boys, a mid-parental height is calculated by adding 5 inches (13 cm) to the mother's height and averaging this height with the father's height. For girls, 5 inches (13 cm) are subtracted from the father's height, and this height is averaged with the mother's height. A target height can be predicted by (for a boy) adding 3½ inches (8.5 cm) to or (for a girl) subtracting 3½ inches (8.5 cm) from this calculated value. Target heights are considered normal for that family.

Body proportions should also be evaluated. This assessment includes a comparison between the height of the upper body and the height of the lower body, called an upper segment/lower segment ratio (US/LS). Another important measurement is the comparison between the arm span and the height. If either the arm span/height difference or the US/LS is abnormal, the growth disorder may be characterized as disproportionate growth.

Once it is determined that there is a disorder of growth, there should be a physical exam, and possibly laboratory and radiological tests, to look for a possible cause.

Laboratory testing may be used to investigate hormone levels, kidney function, liver function, and chromosomes. Sometimes growth hormone stimulation is performed. In this test, a medication is given to see if the pituitary gland responds appropriately. If a person is suspected of having a pituitary problem, a magnetic resonance image (MRI) might be done. In children with delayed or accelerated growth, a bone age should be obtained. A bone age is an X-ray of the wrist that is done to determine if the skeletal age and the chronological age are the same. If the bone age is advanced, it suggests that there is less time available for growth. If the bone age is delayed, there may be more time for growth to occur. The bone age can be used to predict the final height the child will achieve as an adult, to see if it is expected to be normal for that family (within the target range).

Children with normal growth variants like constitutional growth delay or familial short stature are usually monitored with repeated physical exams and height measurements.

Treatments

There are many different causes of growth disorders, and the specific treatment depends on the cause. In growth hormone deficiency, growth hormone can be given as an injection. Growth hormone injections are also sometimes used to treat people with Turner syndrome and those with chronic kidney disease. If thyroid hormone levels are low, thyroid hormone can be replaced with an oral medication. In short stature linked to nutrition, supplying the proper nutrients leads to improved growth rates and frequently to normalization of height.

Epidemiology

Although acromegaly and gigantism are not strictly growth disorders, they are both caused by an abnormality of the growth process. In the United States only 40 to 60 people per million of the population suffer from acromegaly (which sometimes runs in families), and about 15,000 suffer from achondroplasia (dwarfism).

Mary Ruppe

See also
• Adrenal disorders • Down syndrome
• Thyroid disorders • Vitamin deficiency

Guillain-Barré syndrome

Guillain-Barré syndrome is a form of polyneuritis, in which several peripheral nerves are inflamed. It was initially described by Guillain, Barré, and Strohl in 1916. Guillain-Barré syndrome (GBS) is characterized by loss of myelin covering the nerves, which results in symmetrical and progressive weakness in the limbs, loss of spinal reflexes, and sensory loss.

In two-thirds of patients affected, GBS follows an upper respiratory or gastrointestinal infection, surgery, or immunization. The preceding infection is most commonly intestinal, and it is caused by the bacteria *Campylobacter jejuni*. There may be an associated risk with immunocompromised states, but a clear relationship has yet to be defined.

Symptoms and diagnosis

GBS occurs in people of all ages and can begin with paresthesias (tingling) in the feet and progressive and symmetrical weakness in the legs, causing an ascending paralysis and loss of reflexes over hours to days, for up to four weeks. Diagnosis is made based on the patient's history and physical examination and cerebrospinal fluid analysis, which shows a high content of protein in proportion to inflammatory cells. Electromyography (nerve conduction studies) may be used to assist in diagnosis.

Treatments and prevention

Treatment is based on the severity of the illness and the muscle groups involved. Plasma exchange may be used early in the disease to remove autoantibodies, although alternative treatment is high-dose intravenous immune globulin (IVIG), which is thought to neutralize autoantibodies. These treatments are equally effective, and using IVIG and plasma exchange confers no additional benefit. If respiratory muscles are affected by the ascending weakness, mechanical ventilation may be needed, as well as support for unstable blood pressure and heart arrhythmias caused by involvement of the autonomic nerves. There are no prevention strategies.

Pathogenesis

GBS is thought to be caused by an immune response to an infection, whose molecular signature shares that of the myelin covering peripheral nerves (molecular mimicry). This process results in an autoimmune response causing breakdown of the myelin around peripheral nerves, leading to loss of nerve function and weakness. The illness should peak within four weeks of onset. Up to one-third of patients will need mechanical ventilation; if the person is over 60 years old with rapid progression of GBS, the prognosis is worse. Up to 70 percent of patients recover in the year following the illness.

Epidemiology

Mean annual incidence of GBS is 1.8 per 100,000 population. Men and women are equally affected. GBS has several variants; the most common form in North America and Europe is acute inflammatory demyelinating polyradiculopathy (AIDP). Other variants include acute motor axonal neuropathy (AMAN) and the Miller-Fisher syndrome (MFS).

Meredith Roderick and Robert Daroff

KEY FACTS

Description

A disease caused by progressive breakdown of the myelin in peripheral nerves.

Causes

Post infectious autoimmune response to a virus or often to a gastrointestinal infection.

Risk factors

No known risk factors

Symptoms

Progressive weakness and loss of reflexes.

Diagnosis

Cerebrospinal fluid examination and electromyography (recording of electrical activity in a muscle).

Pathogenesis

Autoimmune attack of the myelin of peripheral nerves.

Prevention

There are no specific preventative strategies.

Epidemiology

Mean annual incidence of 1.8 per 100,000 population with men and women equally affected.

See also
• Paralysis

Gum disease

A potentially serious but preventable disorder, gum disease is a bacterial infection of the teeth and gums that can spread rapidly, causing severe inflammation, tooth loss, and loss of supporting bone. In serious cases, surgery is needed to restore bone in the jaw and prevent further tooth loss.

Gum disease, commonly called periodontal ("around the teeth") disease, involves the breakdown of gums as a result of the buildup of plaque (saliva, food, and bacteria) and tartar on the teeth's surface. It ranges from a mild disease causing moderate gum inflammation to a serious disorder in which bone becomes infected and breaks down. Periodontal disease comes in two forms: periodontitis and gingivitis.

Causes and risk factors

The mouth harbors bacteria which, with mucus and other particles, form an invisible, sticky substance called plaque that coats the teeth; if plaque builds up and hardens, it forms a sticky residue called tartar that is full of harmful bacteria. Tartar can cause gingivitis, a mild form of periodontal disease that causes inflamed and bleeding gums. If untreated, periodontitis can result; this is a serious disease in which the gums pull away from the teeth, forming pockets of infection. As the immune system reacts to fight the disease, both toxins in the bacteria and enzymes released by the body break down the connective tissue and bone that support the teeth. Apart from poor dental hygiene, periodontal disease is caused by stress; tobacco use; hormonal changes during pregnancy, puberty, menstruation, or menopause; diseases such as diabetes, cancer, and HIV; and the use of drugs that reduce saliva flow, which protects gums and teeth. Genetics may play a role since periodontal disease runs in some families.

Symptoms

Symptoms of gingivitis and periodontitis include red, swollen, sore gums that bleed during or after toothbrushing; bad breath; and a bad taste in the mouth. Periodontitis symptoms also include receding gums, the formation of pockets between the teeth and gums, shifting or loose teeth, and changes in the way the teeth fit together.

Diagnosis, treatments, and prevention

A dentist or periodontist checks for pockets among the teeth and gums, and X-rays are taken to determine if the surrounding bone has broken down.

Gingivitis is reversible with daily brushing and flossing and regular cleaning by a dentist or dental hygienist. Advanced gingivitis and periodontitis may be treated with a deep-cleaning method to remove bacteria and rough spots below the gum line; or with antibiotic medications, gels, mouth rinses, and in severe cases, surgery to restore bone. Peridontal disease can often be prevented by not using tobacco, brushing twice and flossing once daily, using toothpaste with fluoride, and drinking fluoridated water.

Lise Stevens

KEY FACTS

Description
Infection of the gums and tissues around the teeth.

Cause
Bacteria in plaque hardens on the teeth.

Risk factors
Crooked teeth, dental work such as bridges that no longer fit and broken fillings, tobacco use, hormonal changes, certain diseases, and some medications.

Symptoms
Frequent bad taste, bad breath, bleeding, red and tender gums, and loose, sensitive teeth.

Diagnosis
Examination of teeth by a dentist or periodontist; jawbone X-ray to detect breakdown of bone.

Treatments
Depending on seriousness: deep cleaning, antimicrobial treatment, bone or gum surgery, gum and bone grafts.

Pathogenesis
Bacteria in plaque break down the gums; teeth loosen; and underlying bone breaks down.

Prevention
Brushing and flossing teeth regularly, a healthy diet, stopping tobacco use, reducing stress.

Epidemiology
In the United States 80 percent of all adults have some degree of periodontal disease.

See also
• Diabetes • Tooth decay

H1N1 influenza

The ability of influenza viruses from different species to swap genetic material and form new, deadly viruses has led to past influenza pandemics. In early 2009, a virus containing genes from swine, birds, and humans became the first pandemic of the 21st century with predictions that it could infect as much as one-third of the world's human population.

Early in 2009, human cases of infection with a novel H1N1 swine flu virus were identified in Mexico. By April, this virus reached the United States and within several weeks became so widespread that the World Health Organization declared that a pandemic was underway.

This new virus had a unique combination of human, swine, and avian (bird) genes, an assortment so different from past circulating flu strains that health authorities predicted up to one-third of the world's population may become infected within 2 years. Because of the presence of swine flu genes, this influenza virus was initially referred to as "swine flu."

Symptoms and signs

Transmission is like that seen with seasonal influenza, occurring by exposure to droplets produced by the cough or sneeze of a person infected with the virus or by touching surfaces that are contaminated with this virus and then touching one's eyes, nose, or mouth. Infectious droplets can survive on surfaces up to 8 hours. Swine flu is not spread by eating pork products.

Symptoms of infection are also similar to those seen with seasonal influenza—cough, shortness-of-breath, sore throat, runny or stuffy nose, fever, chills, headache, body aches, and fatigue. Some people may also experience vomiting and diarrhea. A person infected with swine flu can transmit the disease to others from one day prior to the onset of symptoms up to one week after symptom onset. Antibody that protects against infection from this virus is present in approximately one-third of those older than 60 years of age but absent in the youngest age groups.

Most persons who contract swine flu have a mild illness, require no medical treatment, and recover fully.

Younger age groups (under 25 years of age) and those who have chronic underlying illness or are pregnant or immunocompromised are at greater risk for severe illness and death if infected with this virus. During the 2009 H1N1 outbreak, the highest death rates were found in those under the age of 65 years. In comparison, more than 90% of seasonal influenza-related

KEY FACTS

Description

Acute respiratory infection of swine (pigs) capable of infecting humans.

Cause

Type A influenza viruses.

Risk factors

Contact with pigs infected with swine flu virus or with surfaces that have been contaminated by body fluids or feces of pigs infected with this virus. Human-to-human spread is possible, depending upon the virus characteristics.

Symptoms

Bad cough, shortness of breath, sore throat, fever, head and body aches, fatigue; sometimes nausea and vomiting.

Diagnosis

Testing of respiratory secretions.

Treatments

Antiviral drugs.

Pathogenesis

Most of those infected recover; certain groups are at higher risk of severe complications and death.

Prevention

2009 H1N1 vaccine; cover a cough; hand-washing; avoidance of sick pigs and humans infected with swine flu as well as environments that are contaminated with swine flu virus.

Epidemiology

Influenza viruses are categorized as one of three types: A, B, or C. Influenza A viruses are further divided into subtypes based upon the hemagglutinin (H) and neuraminidase (N) proteins on the surface of the virus. Swine flu virus is a type A influenza virus that was first identified in pigs in 1930. More than four decades later, an isolated outbreak of swine flu occurred among military personnel in Fort Dix, New Jersey, raising fears of a swine flu pandemic. It was not until 2009, however, that a swine flu pandemic materialized.

EMERGENCY WARNING SIGNS

For a person who has H1N1 influenza, medical help should be sought when the following additional symptoms are present.

In children

- Fast breathing or trouble breathing
- Bluish skin color
- Not drinking enough fluids
- Not waking up or not interacting
- Being so irritable that the child does not want to be held
- Flu-like symptoms improve but then return with fever and worse cough
- Fever with a rash

In adults

- Difficulty breathing or shortness of breath
- Pain or pressure in the chest or abdomen
- Sudden dizziness
- Confusion
- Severe or persistent vomiting

Source: Centers for Disease Control and Prevention, *www.cdc.gov/h1n1flu/qa.htm.*

Transmission

Direct transmission of influenza viruses from animals to humans is uncommon. However, if the influenza virus is changed in some way—either by mutation or by combining with genetic segments of other influenza viruses—transmission of this new virus can be facilitated to the extent that a pandemic results. In 2009, a novel influenza A virus was created from gene segments of two swine viruses, an avian virus, and a human influenza virus. Once this novel H1N1 influenza virus was passed from pig to human, widespread transmission was possible since most persons had no immunity to this new virus.

Prevention

Protection against influenza is provided by vaccination and by practicing certain behaviors. H1N1 vaccine became available in 2009; due to expected shortages in availability, public health authorities prioritized who should receive the vaccine first—young children, pregnant women, medical services personnel, and those with chronic health conditions. H1N1 vaccine is available as a shot given by a needle in the arm or as a nasal spray vaccine. The H1N1 shot, which contains inactivated virus, can be given at the same time as any other vaccine including the seasonal flu vaccine. The nasal 2009 H1N1 vaccine, containing live weakened virus, can be given at the same time as other vaccines except for the seasonal nasal influenza vaccine. Although the seasonal flu vaccine does not protect against swine flu, it should be considered since simultaneous or subsequent infection with seasonal influenza is possible. It takes about 2 weeks for a person to produce antibodies that protect against influenza once vaccinated. Antiviral medications are sometimes prescribed as prevention against influenza after an exposure to influenza virus.

Covering a cough with tissues and frequently washing one's hands with soap and water (or using an alcohol-based solution) can protect against influenza. It is also advisable to avoid contact with persons who are ill with respiratory infections. As with other communicable diseases, follow precautions advocated by public health authorities.

Rita Washko

deaths occur in those aged 65 years and older. These early statistics also showed that the hospitalization rate due to H1N1 infection was highest among children up to 4 years of age.

Diagnosis and treatments

Rapid tests that detect influenza viruses, but cannot identify which influenza virus caused the illness, can be performed in an outpatient setting. These results are not as accurate at detecting the presence of influenza viruses as are other tests. Determination of influenza type and subtype (H1N1 versus seasonal flu) requires viral culture or other more sophisticated laboratory tests. Specimens required for testing are respiratory swabs or aspirates.

Medicines effective against the 2009 H1N1 flu include oseltamivir (Tamiflu) and zanamivir (Relenza). Treatment should be started as soon as possible after symptom onset.

See also
- Asian influenza • Avian influenza
- Cold, common • Influenza
- Pneumonia

Hay fever

The disorder hay fever is actually allergic rhinitis caused by grass, tree, and flower pollens in the air. The disorder usually has no connection with hay (mowed grasses), but the name probably developed because most sufferers are affected in the late summer and early fall of the year when hay is being baled. Ragweed, which is in bloom during the same season, has the most commonly identified offending pollen. However, the pollens of other plants may cause an allergic reaction similar to hay fever during other seasons.

Hay fever affects about 20 percent of people in the United States. It is the most common allergic condition. Molds in the air, dust mites, and animal dander or saliva are also frequent causes of allergic rhinitis, so susceptible people may develop symptoms that resemble those of hay fever from a variety of causes throughout the year.

Causes

When the body incorrectly identifies a protein as a potentially harmful invader, or allergen, it responds by producing antibodies to fight the perceived invader. These antibodies cause certain cells of the immune system to release chemicals such as histamine and leukotrienes in the upper respiratory tract, and these chemicals are responsible for producing the symptoms of allergic rhinitis. A type of antibody called immunoglobulin E (IgE) is particularly associated with respiratory allergies.

Exposure to allergens when the immune system is weakened, after an infection, or during pregnancy may increase the chance of an allergic response.

Symptoms

The characteristic symptoms of allergic rhinitis are a runny and sometimes itchy nose, nasal stuffiness, sneezing, watery, itchy eyes, and possibly an accompanying cough. Although very uncomfortable, these symptoms are considered mild reactions.

Because offending pollens are inhaled, symptoms are usually confined to the upper respiratory tract (nasal passages, throat, and voice box). Repeated exposure to inhaled allergens results in chronic inflammation of the lining of the upper air passages and swelling and redness of the protective lining (conjunctiva) of the eyes. Rarely, an extreme response to the offending allergen may result in a life-threatening inability to breathe, along with a severe drop in blood pressure, known as anaphylaxis, which requires immediate emergency treatment.

KEY FACTS

Description
An exaggerated immune response by the body to pollen, causing respiratory symptoms and discomfort.

Cause
Exposure to pollen, incorrectly identified by the body as an invader.

Risk factors
A family history of allergies.

Symptoms
Runny nose, sneezing, nasal stuffiness, and itchy, watery eyes, possibly accompanied by a cough.

Diagnosis
Evaluation of personal history along with intradermal (skin-prick) tests using dilute solutions of common allergens. Various other tests may be done to rule out the possibility of other causes of the symptoms.

Treatments
Medications to reduce the symptoms, such as antihistamines or antileukotrienes. Immunotherapy, or allergy injections, to reduce the body's response to particular, personal allergens identified by skin-prick tests.

Pathogenesis
Once an allergic response has been established, exposure thereafter to the offending pollen or substance (allergen) in the environment results in an inflammatory response, most often involving the upper respiratory tract. Without immunotherapy treatment the allergy is unlikely to disappear. However, children sometimes outgrow symptoms.

Prevention
Avoiding situations where the body would respond to a known allergen. Immunotherapy.

Epidemiology
Hay fever affects about 20 percent of people in the United States. It is the most common allergic condition. Allergies in general are the sixth leading cause of chronic illness in the United States.

ANAPHYLAXIS

Anaphylaxis is a sudden and severe, usually life-threatening, allergic reaction that requires immediate emergency treatment. Although the symptoms may start as the typical symptoms of a mild allergic reaction, within minutes they progress to severe difficulty in swallowing and breathing accompanied by a profound drop in blood pressure resulting in systemic (involving the entire body) shock. Hives (itchy welts), dizziness, and mental confusion may also occur with systemic involvement.

Immediate treatment with IV (intravenous) epinephrine (adrenaline), intravenous fluids, and oxygen is necessary if a fatal outcome is to be prevented. People who survive this type of attack, as well as their families, should be taught by their health care provider how, in the event of an emergency, to administer the necessary medication, usually an epinephrine formulation. They are advised to carry the emergency medication at all times.

Diagnosis

A thorough physical examination and review of an affected individual's personal and family medical history is the initial step for diagnosis. A family history of any type of allergy is significant because it suggests a tendency to be prone to allergy, although specific allergies are rarely inherited.

When allergy is suspected, a series of intradermal (skin-prick) tests using a tiny amount of very dilute solutions of specific common allergens is recommended. After injection of the allergen extract, the site is checked for possible development of redness and swelling. The amount of, or lack of, skin reaction determines the probability of allergy to the injected allergen.

If skin-prick testing is not possible, a RAST (radioallergosorbent blood test) may be done. A RAST test evaluates the amount of antibodies being produced by a person's immune system. In some cases, specific antibodies may indicate particular allergies, but skin tests are usually more accurate.

A complete blood count (CBC) and a differential white blood cell count may be ordered. An increase in the normal number of specific white blood cells (eosinophils and basophils) may suggest that the body is responding to an allergen. Occasionally, various other medical tests may be performed to rule out the possibility of other causes of the symptoms.

Treatments

Over-the-counter (OTC) and prescription antihistamines are the most widely used medications for relief of upper respiratory allergic symptoms. Drugs may be taken orally or as nasal sprays. Some antihistamines, such as diphenhydramine (Benadryl), may cause significant and potentially hazardous drowsiness.

Topical nasal anti-inflammatory steroids and cromolyn sodium may also be prescribed to treat allergic rhinitis, but cromolyn is most effective when taken before symptoms develop.

Decongestant sprays or pills may be used along with antihistamines to relieve nasal congestion, but should be avoided by people with high blood pressure, an enlarged prostate, or glaucoma.

Immunotherapy, or allergy desensitization injections—to reduce the body's response to particular, personal allergens identified by skin-prick tests—is the most effective method of controlling allergic rhinitis in the long term.

Drugs called antileukotrienes, frequently used for allergic asthma, may also be appropriate for treating hay fever, especially if the individual is troubled with large amount of mucous secretions.

Based on the presumption that an allergic attack may not develop if IgE is prevented from attaching to the cells that release the substances that cause allergic symptoms, new treatments using special injectable anti-IgE monoclonal antibodies are under development. However, IgE is not always present in allergic attacks.

Management and prognosis

Managing the environment to avoid exposure to the causative pollen is important in preventing symptomatic allergic rhinitis. Avoiding irritants such as smoke and strong chemical odors should also lessen discomfort.

Inadequately treated allergies may cause difficulty sleeping and fatigue, and possibly lead to more serious conditions such as asthma. The congestion often associated with upper respiratory symptoms may result in sinusitis or middle-ear infections. Without immunotherapy, an allergy is unlikely to disappear. However, children sometimes outgrow the characteristic symptoms.

Nance Seiple

See also
- Allergy and sensitivity • Asthma
- Sinusitis

Head injury

Head injury is a general term used to describe any trauma to the head, including injuries to the brain, scalp, and skull. Traumatic brain injury (TBI) is classified as either closed head injury or penetrating head injury. A closed head injury is any injury to the brain or structures within the skull not caused by a penetrating injury, like a gunshot wound. Brain injuries may be limited to a small area (focal) or may be more widespread (diffuse).

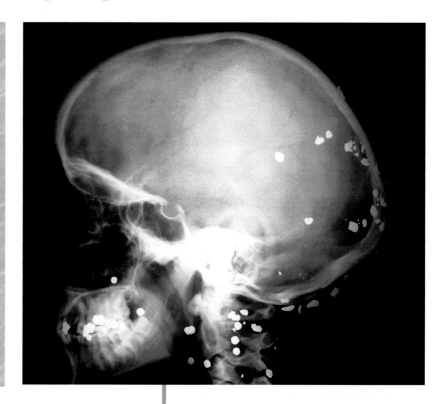

As a result of a hunting accident, this patient was hit by several shotgun pellets. On this colored X-ray of the side of the head, the pellets (white dots) are seen in the neck, around the teeth, and at the back of the skull.

Brain injuries are a common type of head injury. Primary brain injury refers to the initial structural injury to the brain as a direct result of the trauma. Secondary brain injury refers to any subsequent injury to the brain from lack of oxygen, low blood pressure, elevated pressure inside the skull, or as the result of physiological changes initiated by the original trauma. Mild traumatic brain injuries (TBIs) are commonly called concussions. A generally accepted description of concussion syndrome is a traumatically induced alteration in mental status with or without associated loss of consciousness. Injury to brain tissue can occur at the site of impact (coup), at the point opposite the impact (contrecoup), or due to rotational forces resulting in the shearing of axons (fiberlike processes of nerve cells). The direct force at the point of contact may not solely be responsible for the severity of injury if a significant shear effect occurs.

While not a life-threatening injury, concussions can cause both short-term and long-term problems. A mild concussion may involve no loss of consciousness or a very brief loss of consciousness. A severe concussion may involve prolonged loss of consciousness with a delayed return to normal function. Concussions do not include injuries in which there is bleeding under the skull or into the brain.

Diffuse axonal injury (DAI) reflects damage over a widespread area when compared to focal brain injury. Unlike direct brain trauma, DAI is the result of traumatic shearing forces that occur when the head is rapidly accelerated or decelerated, as may occur in auto accidents, falls, and assaults. It usually results from powerful twisting or rotational forces. Unlike concussion, DAI is associated with a high level of debilitation and is a frequent cause of persistent vegetative state.

A skull fracture is a break in the bone encasing the brain, which may or may not be associated with an injury to the brain itself. A linear skull fracture follows a relatively straight line. Depressed skull fractures, which cause dents in the skull bone, are common after forceful impact by blunt objects. Depressed fractures whose depth is equal to or greater than the thickness of the surrounding skull bone have a higher incidence of damage to the brain itself. A basilar skull fracture is a fracture of the bones that form the bottom of the skull and results from severe blunt force. A basilar skull fracture commonly connects to the sinus cavities, which may allow fluid or air entry into the interior of the skull, resulting in possible infection.

Intracranial hemorrhage is bleeding inside the skull, which may exert pressure on the brain. A subdural hematoma is bleeding of the veins between the brain and the dura mater (the brain's tough outer membrane). A subdural hematoma may be acute, developing suddenly after the injury, or chronic, slowly accumulating over a period of 12 days or longer after injury. An epidural hematoma is arterial bleeding between the dura mater and the skull bone, often from a blow to the temple area. Subarachnoid hemorrhage is bleeding into the subarachnoid space, the area between the arachnoid and the pia mater where cerebrospinal fluid flows. Intraparenchymal hemorrhage is bleeding into the brain tissue itself. Without intervention, any persistent increase in pressure on the brain as a result of bleeding will eventually lead to herniation, the pushing of the brain downward out of the skull. Herniation is not compatible with life.

Causes and risk factors

According to the Centers for Disease Control (CDC), the leading cause of TBI is falls (28 percent); rates are highest for children 0 to 4 years old and for adults over 75. Motor-vehicle injuries (20 percent) result in the greatest number of TBI-related hospitalizations. The rate of motor vehicle–related TBI is highest among adolescents 15 to 19 years old. Collisions with moving or stationary objects (19 percent) are the third leading cause of TBI. An estimated 300,000 sports- and recreation-related TBIs of mild to moderate severity occur in the United States each year. Firearm use is the leading cause of death related to TBI. Nearly two-thirds of firearm-related TBIs are suicidal in intent. All assaults comprise 11 percent, which includes child abuse. The male-to-female ratio for TBI is nearly 2:1, and TBI is much more common in persons younger than 35 years. Over half of all TBI incidents involve alcohol use.

Signs and symptoms

Signs and symptoms of head injuries vary with the type and severity of the injury. Some symptoms are evident immediately, while others may only surface days or weeks after the injury. Minor blunt head injuries may involve symptoms of being dazed or a brief loss of consciousness. Common symptoms include headache, confusion, dizziness, altered vision, fatigue, lethargy, altered sleep, mood changes, and trouble with memory, concentration, or thinking. Worsening symptoms indicate a more severe injury. With moderate or severe TBI there may be a loss of consciousness, personality changes, severe or worsening headache, repeated vomiting, inability to awaken, widening of one or both pupils, slurred speech, loss of coordination, increased confusion, and restlessness. Severe blunt head trauma involves a loss of consciousness lasting from several minutes to many days or

KEY FACTS

Description
Any closed or penetrating injury to the head, including bruises and cuts to the scalp, fractures of the skull, bleeding in and around the brain, bruising of the brain and the shearing of axons.

Causes
Falls; motor vehicle accidents; collisions; assaults; weapons.

Risk factors
Alcohol; male; age under 35.

Symptoms
Vary with type and severity. Being dazed; loss of consciousness; headache; dizziness; visual changes; vomiting; lethargy; seizures; cognitive, behavioral and psychological changes; strokelike symptoms; amnesia; coma.

Diagnosis
History; physical exam; X-ray; CT; MRI; angiography.

Treatment
Varies with type and severity. Wound care; observation; antibiotics; seizure medications; ICP monitoring; craniotomy surgery.

Pathogenesis
Varies with type and severity. No residual effects; chronic headaches and dizziness; permanent cognitive and behavioral changes; neurological deficits; coma. Effects over time are cumulative. Repeated TBIs over a short period of time can be catastrophic.

Prevention
Seatbelts; lock up weapons; never drive under the influence; helmets; improve safety of living areas for seniors and children.

Epidemiology
TBIs are responsible for significant death and disability, especially in adolescents and children. TBIs are responsible for over one million emergency room visits and cost $60 billion annually in the United States.

longer. The person may die or suffer from severe and sometimes permanent neurological deficits. Neurological deficits from head trauma include paralysis, seizures, difficulty speaking, seeing, hearing, walking, and understanding. Penetrating trauma may cause death, immediate severe symptoms, or only minor symptoms despite a potentially life-threatening injury. Contrary to Hollywood depictions, amnesia from TBI usually affects memories around and after the incident and not prior to it.

Diagnosis

The patient's medical history, description of the current symptoms, and a physical examination are all important in the diagnosis. In mild TBI, X-rays of the skull may be taken to look for a fracture in the skull bone. Skull fractures are not always associated with brain injury, and the absence of a fracture does not exclude a brain injury. The fracture itself will seldom need treatment, but an underlying brain injury may. In moderate to severe cases, a computed tomography (CT) scan should be obtained, which creates a series of cross-sectional X-ray images of the head; these images reveal bone fractures, hemorrhage, hematomas, contusions, brain swelling, and tumors. Magnetic resonance imaging (MRI) may be used after the initial assessment and treatment of the TBI patient. MRI uses magnetic fields to detect subtle changes in brain tissue content and can show more detail than X-rays or CT. In some cases of bleeding in or around the brain, angiography may be performed by injecting dye into the arteries to visualize the blood vessels and locate the area of bleeding. It is sometimes possible to stop the bleeding during angiography by injecting clot-forming agents. After major falls and car accidents, other imaging and laboratory tests may be performed to rule out other chest, abdominal, or bony injuries. Neck injuries are common in people with severe head trauma. Spine imaging is usually ordered before the head is moved if there is any neck pain or other symptoms of a neck injury.

The Glasgow coma scale (GCS) is used to describe the general level of consciousness of patients with TBI. The GCS is divided into 3 categories: eye opening (E), motor response (M), and verbal response (V). The score is the sum of all 3 categories, with a maximum score of 15 and a minimum score of 3. Mild head injuries are those with a GCS score of 13-15, and moderate head injuries are those with a GCS score of 9-12. A GCS score of 8 or less defines a severe head injury. These definitions should only be considered as a general guide to the level of injury.

Treatments

Treatment varies widely depending on the type and severity of injuries. Minor head injuries are often treated at home if someone is available to watch the person. Ice, bed rest, hydration, and a mild pain reliever may be prescribed. In the event of an open wound, cuts will be numbed, cleansed, and inspected for foreign matter. The wound usually is closed with skin staples, stitches, or special skin glue. An immunization to prevent tetanus is given if needed. People with serious closed head injuries are admitted to the hospital for observation and repeated studies. Seizure medication may be given, though seizures related to a head injury rarely recur. Antibiotics are usually not required in closed head injuries, while antibiotics are sometimes considered in cases of basilar skull fracture. An intracranial pressure (ICP) monitor probe may be surgically inserted into the brain. When there is a closed head injury with bleeding inside the skull, the doctor must consider the location of the bleeding, the severity of the symptoms, other injuries, and the progression of symptoms when determining the treatment plan. Craniotomy surgery may be needed to evacuate the blood and relieve the pressure.

Patients with severe TBI may need a breathing tube placed to protect the airway. Penetrating head injuries often require some sort of surgery, usually to remove foreign material or to stop bleeding. Visualization of the blood vessels (angiography) may also be needed.

Pathogenesis

The outcome of TBI is related to the initial level of injury. While the GCS score provides a description of the initial condition and helps predict death from the injury, it does not correlate tightly with other outcomes. For example, if a patient is older than 60 years, has an initial GCS score of less than 5, presence of an unresponsive dilated pupil, prolonged low blood pressure or low oxygen level, and presence of intracranial bleeding requiring surgery, a poor outcome is likely.

Prognosis varies and depends on the severity of the injury. Even minor head injuries can have long-term consequences (usually psychological or learning disabilities). Serious head injuries can result in anything from full recovery to death or a permanent coma. TBI can cause functional changes in thinking, sensation, language, and emotions. TBI can also cause epilepsy and increase the risk for conditions such as Alzheimer's disease, Parkinson's disease, and other brain disorders. Repeated mild TBIs occurring over an

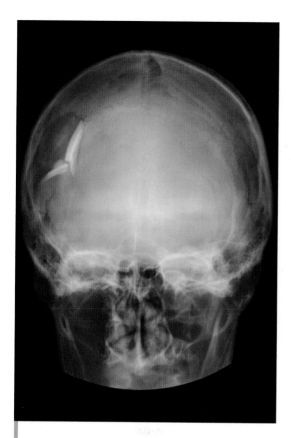

A colored X-ray shows a depressed fracture (red, upper left) in the back of a skull. This type of fracture is caused by a high-energy impact from a blunt object. Brain damage is a high risk for skull injuries such as this one.

extended period of time (months to years) can result in cumulative neurological and cognitive deficits. Repeated mild TBIs that occur within a short period of time (hours to weeks) can be catastrophic or fatal. The cause of the TBI also plays a role in determining the patient's outcome. Approximately 91 percent of firearm TBIs result in death, while only 11 percent of TBIs from falls result in death.

Prevention

There are many ways to reduce the chances of a traumatic brain injury. Firearms and bullets should be stored in a locked cabinet when not in use. Seat belts should be worn whenever driving or riding in a motor vehicle. Children should be buckled into the car using a child safety seat, booster seat, or seat belt. Driving should never occur while under the influence of alcohol or drugs. Helmets must be worn when appropriate, and children should also be asked to wear helmets when appropriate. Living areas can be made safer for seniors by removing tripping hazards, using nonslip mats in washing areas, installing handrails in stairways and bathrooms, and improving lighting throughout the home. Living areas can be made safer for children by installing window guards and using safety gates. Shock-absorbing materials, such as hardwood mulch and sand, can be used under playground equipment to reduce the chance of injury in children.

Epidemiology

TBIs contribute to a substantial number of deaths and cases of permanent disability annually. Of the roughly 1.4 million who sustain a TBI each year in the United States, there are over 50,000 deaths and 450,000 hospitalizations. Greater than one million TBIs are treated and released from an emergency room each year. Among children age 14 years and under, TBI results in an estimated 2,685 deaths, 37,000 hospitalizations, and 435,000 visits to emergency rooms annually.

The mortality rate is high in severe TBI (33 percent) and low for moderate TBI (2.5 percent). About 75 percent of TBIs are concussions or mild TBI; the remaining injuries are divided equally between the moderate and severe categories. An estimated 15 percent of persons who sustain a mild brain injury continue to experience negative consequences one year after the injury.

The cost to society of TBI is staggering, from both an economic and an emotional standpoint. Almost all persons with severe head injury and nearly two-thirds of those with moderate head injury will be permanently disabled and will not return to their previous level of function. The CDC estimates that at least 5.3 million Americans currently have long-term or lifelong need for help to perform activities of daily living as a result of a TBI.

The financial cost is estimated at about $60 billion per year, which includes loss of potential income of the patient and relatives who may need to become caregivers, cost of acute care, and other medical expenses such as continual ambulatory and rehabilitation care. The impact is even greater when one considers that most severe head injuries occur in adolescents and young adults.

Medley O'Keefe Gatewood

See also
• Fracture • Shock

Heart attack

Heart attack, also called myocardial infarction, is sudden death of heart muscle. Heart attack is a major cause of death worldwide. The risk for coronary artery disease (CAD) and heart attack is increased by smoking, high blood pressure, high cholesterol, diabetes, and lack of proper exercise.

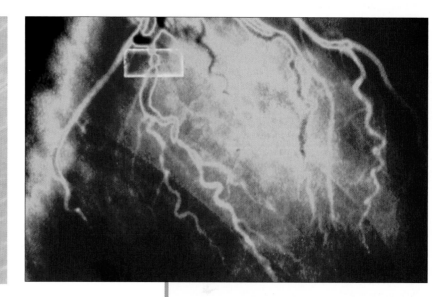

This colored angiogram shows that a coronary artery, which supplies the heart muscle with blood, is narrowed. The box (upper left) highlights the area of narrowing, or stenosis, which is caused by deposits of fatty material on the artery walls, usually as a result of high blood cholesterol levels. This condition can lead to atherosclerosis of the coronary arteries, which in turn impedes blood flow to the heart.

A heart attack, or myocardial infarction (MI), is caused by blockage of one or more of the blood vessels (coronary arteries) that supply the heart. Symptoms may include chest pressure and sweating, or, in about 15 percent of cases, there are no symptoms, in which case it is referred to as a silent heart attack.

Damage to the heart from a heart attack is directly proportional to the muscle mass involved. It may be small enough to be insignificant or it may be massive enough to cause sudden death. It can also cause long-term problems with heart failure and disability. Heart attack is a major cause of death and disability, but attention to proper diet and exercise, as well as control of blood pressure, cholesterol, diabetes, and smoking, may reduce the risk of heart attack.

Causes, risk factors, and pathogenesis

A heart attack is an acute manifestation of CAD. In persons with CAD, plaques composed of fat, cholesterol, calcium, platelets, fibrin, and other materials from the bloodstream build up in the coronary arteries that supply blood to the heart muscle. Plaques may be located in peripheral arteries feeding just a small part of the heart muscle, or in the main arteries responsible for blood flow to large areas of the heart muscle. While these plaques may remain stable or grow gradually in persons with relatively stable CAD, a heart attack occurs if one or more of the plaques ruptures. When a plaque in an artery ruptures, blood flow to the area of the heart supplied by that artery may be blocked in one of two ways: pieces of the plaque (emboli) may flow downstream until they lodge in a smaller segment of the artery, or a clot (thrombus) may develop at the site where the remnant of the plaque is exposed to the bloodstream. Such blockage of one or more coronary arteries prevents the affected area of the heart from receiving nutrients and oxygen, leading to injury or death of the involved heart muscle tissue.

When an area of heart muscle in the ventricle is injured or dies as a result of blockage of an artery, several problems develop soon after. The injured area of the ventricle may generate electrical impulses that are either too fast (ventricular tachycardia) or too irregular (ventricular fibrillation) to allow for proper, coordinated pumping of the heart muscle. Ventricular fibrillation leads to sudden collapse and can lead to sudden death, and ventricular tachycardia can lead either to acute heart failure and pulmonary edema, or sudden death.

If a patient survives an acute heart attack but has permanent damage to part of the heart muscle, the heart may be able to fully recover most of its pumping function, but if a large enough area of the heart muscle is damaged or dies and is replaced by scar tissue, the heart will be unable to pump normally and will eventually develop chronic heart failure.

Risk factors

Risk factors for a heart attack are the same as those for CAD in general. Some risk factors, such as tobacco smoking, high cholesterol, high blood pressure, physical inactivity, obesity, and diabetes, are modifiable and can be controlled or managed to reduce a person's chance of having a heart attack.

Other risk factors, such as age, male gender, and family history and heredity, cannot be changed. Heavy use of alcohol or use of cocaine may also increase a person's risk for CAD or heart attack.

KEY FACTS

Description

Sudden blockage of one or more arteries in the heart, causing injury or death of heart muscle.

Causes

Clots in the arteries that supply blood to the heart causing inadequate blood flow (ischemia) to all or part of the heart.

Risk factors

Tobacco smoking, high cholesterol, high blood pressure, physical inactivity, obesity, diabetes, age, male gender, family history and heredity, heavy use of alcohol, and cocaine use.

Symptoms

Anginal chest pain (squeezing chest discomfort or chest heaviness radiating to one or both arms or to the back), sometimes accompanied by nausea, vomiting, or sweating.

Diagnosis

Based on history of anginal symptoms, specific abnormalities on ECG consistent with ischemia of heart muscle, blood tests when history and ECG are not diagnostic.

Treatments

Oxygen, aspirin, heparin, and interventions to open blocked coronary arteries including fibrinolytic medications, angioplasty, or coronary artery stenting.

Pathogenesis

Rupture of plaques in the coronary arteries, which can lead to clots in the coronary arteries, death or injury of heart muscle due to ischemia, and either sudden death from abnormal heart rhythms or long-term heart problems including heart failure as a result of impaired pumping by a weakened heart.

Prevention

A healthy diet, regular exercise, avoiding smoking, control of high cholesterol levels, and regulating high blood pressure are all important preventive measures.

Epidemiology

Heart attack is a leading cause of death and disability worldwide. It is more common among people who are of lower socioeconomic status, older, male, and have risk factors for CAD.

Symptoms

The most typical symptom of heart attack is new or worsening central chest pain. The pain is often described as squeezing, heaviness, or pressure and may radiate to one or both arms or to the back. It may also be accompanied by nausea, vomiting, or sweating. Less typical symptoms of heart attack include discomfort radiating to the jaw, neck, or ear, and new-onset shortness of breath. Anyone with new-onset chest pain or pressure should be evaluated promptly at an emergency room.

Diagnosis

The first diagnostic step in determining if someone is having a heart attack is a brief physical examination. The initial evaluation focuses on the patient's airway, breathing, and circulation (ABCs). The heart is evaluated for murmurs or gallops, and the lungs are evaluated for crackles or rales that may signal pulmonary edema from acute heart failure. It is also important to evaluate for signs of stroke and for signs or symptoms of shock or hypoperfusion (low blood pressure) such as cool, clammy skin, or a pale or ashen appearance.

The most important diagnostic test in evaluating for heart attack is the 12-lead electrocardiogram (ECG). Electrical activity from the heart produces a trace with peaks called P, QRS, and T, which represent the waves. ST segment connects the QRS and T waves on the trace. Findings on ECG that most strongly suggest a heart attack are ST segment elevation, Q waves, or a new conduction defect such as a left bundle branch block (LBBB). New T wave inversion also suggests a heart attack (see box, page 228). An ECG showing ST segment elevation indicates the patient may be suffering from a heart attack affecting a large portion of heart muscle and may benefit from reperfusion (restoration of blood flow) therapy to open the blocked blood vessel or vessels. This is called an "ST-elevation myocardial infarction" (STEMI), and these patients are at highest risk of death or long-term complications from heart attack. An ECG that shows ST segment depression or no ST segment changes in a

ECG: FINDINGS THAT SUGGEST ISCHEMIA

Ischemia (lack of blood flow) or damage to the heart muscle will produce certain, typical changes on the ECG. A Q wave is an abnormally large "downstroke" at the beginning of the QRS complex, signifying heart muscle tissue that has been permanently damaged or is dead. A block of the right or left bundle conducting systems due to ischemic damage can lead to a prolonged QRS (points on a wave) complex. Acute injury to the heart, such as when a coronary blood vessel feeding the heart is first blocked off with a clot, leads to elevation of the ST segment (the portion of the ECG between the end of the QRS complex and the beginning of the T wave). Chronic ischemia (lack of blood flow that prevents heart muscle from getting enough blood but does not kill that area of muscle) will produce ST-segment depression, or cause the T wave to invert.

patient with chest pain suggests unstable angina or a "non-ST-elevation myocardial infarction" (NSTEMI), due to partial blockages of blood flow or partial damage to an area of heart muscle.

However, absence of ECG changes does not completely exclude heart attack, since up to 6 percent of patients with chest pain and a normal ECG may actually have had a heart attack or unstable angina.

Blood tests can be used to help clarify whether a patient is having a heart attack if the ECG does not definitively show a STEMI. Blood is drawn to measure levels of specific enzymes that are released from damaged heart tissue. Enzymes that are commonly measured are creatine kinase (CK), its MB subform (CKMB), and troponin T (TnT) and troponin I (TnI). Because CK and CKMB are present in both heart and skeletal muscle, elevated levels of total CK or CKMB are relatively nonspecific for heart attack, but CKMB is still the blood test most commonly used when evaluating for heart attack. Cardiac troponins T and I are much more specific indicators of heart damage. Individuals with chest pain and a low-risk history, a normal or near-normal ECG, and normal troponins can safely be further evaluated as outpatients. Overall, CKMB is the most efficient blood test for early diagnosis of heart attack within 6 hours of the beginning of symptoms, while TnT and TnI are much more efficient for late diagnosis of heart attack.

In short, when a patient presents with symptoms of heart attack, the history and ECG are used to decide whether the patient's symptoms are due to: heart attack from STEMI, unstable angina or heart attack from NSTEMI, or noncardiac problems, or CAD that is not causing acute damage to the heart.

Treatments

Any patient suspected of having a heart attack is usually started promptly on oxygen (to prevent death of heart muscle), given by a mask or through small tubes placed in the nose, and is given an aspirin to chew, as aspirin can help prevent blood clots. Heparin (a medication to prevent further blood clotting) is also important and is given either intravenously, or as an injection in the skin. A beta blocker, statin medication, and probably an ACE inhibitor may also be considered. A patient with severe anginal chest pain must be relieved of severe chest pain by powerful analgesics.

ST-segment elevation is diagnosed with STEMI based on history and ECG alone, and typically has complete blockage of one or more coronary arteries. This requires urgent treatment to reopen the blocked blood vessels, in order to minimize damage to the heart muscle and to prevent further complications.

One approach that can be used is to give a medication to break down the blood clot (a "fibrinolytic" medication). Another approach is using angioplasty (in which a catheter is inserted into an artery in the leg and threaded up to the heart) to find the blocked blood vessel or vessels, and to restore blood flow either by opening the blockage with a balloon on the tip of the angioplasty catheter, or by placing a stent in the vessel to keep it open.

A patient who has anginal chest pain and ischemic ECG changes, but no ST-segment elevation, may be having unstable angina or a NSTEMI due to a partially occluding blood clot in a coronary artery. Fibrinolytics are not given in this situation.

Important steps in evaluation of the patient include obtaining ECGs every few hours to look for the development of more severe ischemic changes, obtaining blood tests for heart enzymes such as CKMB, TnI, or TnT, and also evaluating for other nonischemic causes of chest pain. A patient with anginal chest pain and a normal or nondiagnostic ECG is unlikely to be having a heart attack, although CAD cannot be entirely excluded based only on the immediate emergency room evaluation. Evaluation focuses on CAD risk factors and considers further testing to clarify whether there is underlying CAD that has not yet been diagnosed. Exercise or chemical stress testing may be used to further evaluate a patient who has anginal chest pain and is at high risk for CAD but is not suffering acutely from heart attack. Stress tests can help determine the cause of chest pain or other symptoms.

After initial stabilization and treatment, any patient who has had a heart attack or is suspected to have CAD should be assessed for long-term cardiac risk. Advice to avoid smoking is one of the most important preventive measures. Blood pressure and cholesterol levels should be measured, and treated if they are high. Any patient with diabetes requires monitoring, since diabetes greatly increases the risk of CAD and heart attack. Close monitoring of rhythm disturbances and prompt treatment can avert disastrous arrhythmia.

Pathogenesis

If someone has never had a heart attack before and has prompt treatment, the outlook is promising. If there are no complications, the likelihood of another heart attack is reduced. However, the outlook also depends on the extent of damage to heart muscle. Rupture of plaques in the coronary arteries can lead to clots in the coronary arteries, death, or injury of heart muscle due to ischemia. Sudden death can occur if someone has abnormal heart rhythms or long-term heart problems, including heart failure, as a result of impaired pumping by a weakened heart.

Prevention

The prevention of heart attacks depends on controlling modifiable risk factors for CAD: eliminating smoking is essential, and blood pressure, cholesterol, and weight can be improved with a healthy diet and regular exercise. Only moderate amounts of alcohol should be taken, in the region of one to two small glasses of beer or wine a day. Smoking increases the risk of CAD; stopping smoking is the most important step in reducing heart attack risk.

A program of regular exercise and a healthy diet are also important for reducing the risk of CAD and heart attack. All persons should try to get at least 30 minutes of aerobic exercise on most days of the week, such as walking, bicycling, jogging, or swimming. A healthy diet should include at least five servings of fresh fruits and vegetables daily, plus plenty of fiber, and should avoid saturated fats.

A blood pressure above 140/90 is considered high, and for most people the goal is to keep the blood pressure below 140/90. Persons with diabetes or chronic kidney disease should try to keep their blood pressure below 130/80, since they are at much higher risk of heart attack.

An LDL (low-density lipoprotein or "bad") cholesterol level of 160 milligrams per deciliter (mg/dL) or less is acceptable for persons at low risk of CAD or heart attack. Persons at moderate risk of CAD or heart attack should try to keep the LDL cholesterol less than 130 mg/dL. Anyone at high risk of CAD or heart attack due to the presence of multiple risk factors, and anyone with diabetes, should try to keep the LDL cholesterol less than 100 mg/dL. Persons who have previously had a heart attack should also try to keep the LDL cholesterol less than 100 mg/dL.

For persons at risk of heart attack, medications may be needed if exercise and healthy eating are not enough to control high blood pressure or high cholesterol. High blood pressure may be treated with thiazide diuretics, beta-blocker medications, and angiotensin converting enzyme inhibitor or angiotensin receptor blocker medications. High cholesterol is most commonly treated with "statin" medications, although fibric acid derivatives and other medications are sometimes used instead. For men over age 50, taking one aspirin each day may also reduce the risk of CAD or heart attack. All persons with a previous heart attack should take an aspirin each day to prevent further heart damage.

Epidemiology

CAD is one of the most common causes of death worldwide. In 1990, CAD caused 6.3 million deaths worldwide, and in 2003 the rate of death from CAD in the U.S. population was 162 in 100,000. Unstable angina and NSTEMI account for 2.5 million hospitalizations per year. Each year about 900,000 people in the United States suffer a heart attack, and 225,000 of those die. One-half of deaths from heart attack occur within an hour of symptoms (sudden cardiac death). Rates of heart attack are higher among older individuals, are higher in men than in women, and are higher among people of lower socioeconomic status. Heart attack from CAD is a leading cause of death and disability around the world.

Bill Cayley Jr.

See also
• Diabetes • Obesity

Hemochromatosis

One of the most common genetic disorders in the United States, hemochromatosis involves mutations in many different genes, all of which cause the body to be overloaded with iron. The excess iron builds up in various organs, including the heart, liver, and pancreas, leading to serious tissue damage and life-threatening illness.

Iron is an essential nutrient that enables red blood cells to transport oxygen around the body. Normally, only about 10 percent of iron is absorbed from food. A deficiency of iron is fairly common, especially in women, and can cause anemia.

People with hemochromatosis have the opposite problem; they absorb much higher levels of iron than normal. Iron gradually accumulates to toxic levels and is moved into various tissues and organs, which can lead to life-threatening damage. It is not clear exactly how high iron levels damage tissue, but it is probably because of an increase in the production of highly destructive molecules called free radicals.

Causes and risk factors

Hemochromatosis is a genetic disorder that can result because of mutations in at least five different iron metabolism genes. Some of these genes produce proteins responsible for absorbing iron; others are involved in iron transport or storage. Whichever genes are affected, the outcome is always the same: the body becomes overloaded with iron. In most cases, the disease is inherited as an autosomal recessive disorder, meaning that both parents must carry a disease gene for offspring to inherit the disorder. Type 1 hemochromatosis affects about 1 million people in the United States. It is one of the most common genetic disorders, and families of northern European descent are at highest risk; the estimated carrier rate is 1 in 9 people. A rare form, type 4 hemochromatosis, is autosomal dominant. In this case, a single copy of the faulty gene is sufficient to cause disease. Another rare form of the disease, called neonatal hemochromatosis (NH), affects newborns and is usually fatal. Although the inheritance pattern of NH is uncertain, the risk of having a second child with the disorder is 80 percent in women who have had one NH baby.

Gender is an important factor in hemochromatosis. Women, who lose iron through menstruation, typically do not experience symptoms of hemochromatosis until after menopause. Men are five times more likely to develop hemochromatosis than women.

Symptoms

Hemochromatosis type 1 can go undiagnosed for many years, mainly because it has low penetrance (percentage of people with the mutation who show signs of the disease) and because its symptoms mimic so many other disorders. The most common symptoms are joint pain, abdominal pain, heart disease, and fatigue. Some people may also show darkened or

KEY FACTS

Description
A genetic disorder that results in iron overload.

Cause
A mutation in the genes involved in the absorption, transport, or storage of iron in the body.

Risk factors
People with a family history of the disease are at greatest risk. Males are at higher risk of developing symptoms early in life.

Symptoms
Joint pain, darkened skin color, fatigue, abdominal pain, or heart disease.

Diagnosis
Blood tests and a family history.

Treatments
Drawing blood every few months is usually sufficient to maintain normal iron levels.

Pathogenesis
Early diagnosis and treatment needed. Iron overload may eventually damage many organs, leading to complications such as diabetes, liver disease, heart disease, and arthritis.

Prevention
Screening is recommended for any adults with a family history of the disease, so early treatment can prevent serious organ damage.

Epidemiology
The highest rates of the disease are in people of northern European descent. In the United States, roughly 1 person in 10 is a carrier for the disease. About 0.5 percent of people in the United States are susceptible to developing the disease.

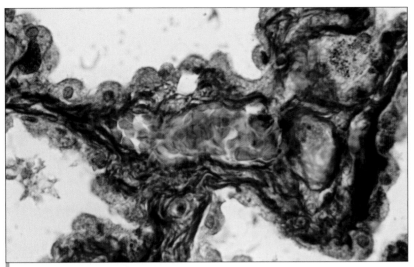

A light micrograph of a section through brain tissue shows a brown area; this patch is as a result of hemochromatosis, an excessive buildup of iron in the body.

bronzed skin tones. The vast majority of patients are not diagnosed until adulthood. In men, symptoms are most likely to appear between the ages of 30 and 50. The disease does not usually become apparent in women until they are past the age of 50.

If hemochromatosis progresses unchecked, iron overload can damage essential organs such as the heart, liver, and pancreas. Liver failure can result from scarring of the tissues (cirrhosis), and untreated hemochromatosis increases a person's risk of liver cancer. Damage to the pancreas can cause diabetes. Hemochromatosis may even affect bones and joints, leading to a type of arthritis.

Diagnosis

Laboratory tests determine the amount of iron in the blood and the level of iron in the liver. In each case, the tests measure the iron bound to iron-transporting proteins (ferritin and transferrin). If iron levels are abnormally high, genetic tests can be used to look for mutations in the most common hemochromatosis gene. These tests cannot identify mutations in the other genes linked to the disorder.

Treatments

The most important way to avoid life-threatening complications from hemochromatosis is to diagnose and treat the disorder early. Once the disease has affected organs, the damage is difficult to reverse. Treatment is simple and safe. Physicians draw blood (perform phlebotomies) until iron levels are restored to normal. It can take up to a year of weekly blood draws to return patients to a healthy iron level. After that, blood is drawn every two to four months. Blood donation may be an option; since 1999, the FDA announced that blood from patients with hemochromatosis was safe to use.

Diet is another key component used in treating hemochromatosis. The aim is to limit the consumption and absorption of iron. Eating foods that contain antioxidants (chemicals that neutralize harmful free radicals) may also be of benefit. Alcohol and large amounts of vitamin C increase absorption of iron and should be avoided. Vitamin C supplements (less than 500 milligrams per day) should be taken between meals. Reducing the amount of red meat in the diet and increasing the amount of fruits, nuts, and vegetables is recommended. Most important, anyone with hemochromatosis should never eat or touch raw shellfish. Shellfish often harbor a bacterium that can be fatal to people with iron overload.

Prevention

Screening for hemochromatosis is controversial, because no definitive and inexpensive test is available. Blood tests can provide misleading results, and not all people with iron overload develop complications, so a positive screening test could have the effect of making it more difficult for a healthy person to get life or health insurance. On the other hand, if there is a family history of the disease, it is important to be diagnosed before symptoms develop to reduce the risk of organ damage. The American College of Physicians has reviewed the possibility of establishing routine screening for hemochromatosis, but lack of information about the risks and benefits means that screening is unlikely to be available in the near future.

Chris Curran

See also
• Diabetes

Hemophilia

Hemophilias are disorders of coagulation characterized by ineffective blood clotting. Hemophilia results from an inherited inability to produce sufficient amounts of one of these clotting factors. The ability of blood to clot or coagulate, that is, to turn from liquid to solid, at the site of damage to a blood vessel restricts blood loss following injury and is the initial step of wound repair.

Blood clotting is necessarily finely regulated through a large number of interacting clotting and anti-clotting plasma proteins, since excessive clotting results in vessel obstruction (thrombosis), ineffective clotting in blood loss. Deficiencies of almost all factors have been described. However, more than 95 percent concern factors VIII (Hemophilia A) and IX (Hemophilia B). Absence of factor VIII stabilizing factor (von Willebrand factor), as occurs in a rare subtype of von Willebrand's disease (type 3), causes severe depletion of factor VIII and may thus manifest with a hemophilia-like phenotype. Depending on the remaining amount of coagulation factor, mild, moderate and severe forms of hemophilia are distinguished; two-thirds of cases are severe.

In hemophilia, as a result of the clotting factor deficiency, blood does not coagulate efficiently. Severe and prolonged external and internal bleeds ensue, often without any significant trauma. Any organ can be affected by such bleeds. Blood loss can be significant, even fatal, if untreated. In addition, bleeding into organs causes damage to the organs. The joints are commonly affected, and accumulated blood leads to destruction of cartilage and joint deformation. Bleeds into the head can be rapidly fatal.

Although relatively rare, hemophilia enjoys a certain public notoriety because of its prevalence among European royalty. Queen Victoria of the United Kingdom (1819–1901) acquired and spread a de-novo mutation in her factor VIII gene, which she passed on to at least three of her children, whose own children in turn spread it through several of Europe's royal families, including those of Russia, Germany, and Spain.

Causes

Hemophilias are inherited diseases caused by mutations in any of the clotting factor genes, which lead to deficiency of that factor. Hemophilia A and B are inherited in an X-chromosomal recessive pattern, since the genes for factors VIII and IX are located on the X chromosome. This pattern of inheritance implies that for males, who have only one X chromosome, inheritance of one defective gene is sufficient to cause (almost) complete absence of this coagulation factor and thus disease. In males, the mutation may either be

KEY FACTS

Description

Hemophilias are disorders of blood clotting, manifesting as prolonged bleeding without (adequate) trauma.

Causes

Inherited deficiency of a blood clotting factor.

Risk factors

The most common types of hemophilia are inherited in an X-chromosomal recessive pattern. De-novo mutations also occur. Because of this pattern of inheritance, most hemophiliacs are male.

Symptoms

Easy bruising or bleeding, spontaneously or after minor trauma, which can affect all organs. Without prompt treatment, patients may bleed to death. Disability frequently results from repeated joint bleeds.

Diagnosis

Suspected from the clinical presentation, a blood sample is required to establish abnormal blood clotting and identify the deficient clotting factor.

Treatments

Replacement of the missing clotting factor through injection into the bloodstream is the mainstay of therapy.

Pathogenesis

A tightly regulated cascade of different interacting protein molecules (clotting factors) regulate the ability of blood to turn from liquid to solid within seconds of an injury at the site of that injury. Severe deficiency in any of the clotting factors leads to impaired clotting.

Prevention

Genetic counseling, abstention of carriers from reproduction.

Epidemiology

The two more common forms of hemophilia, A and B, occur in all races with a frequency of 1 in 5,000 and 1 in 25,000 males, respectively. Females are rarely affected.

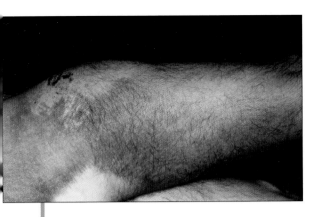

A 55-year-old hemophiliac has a large hematoma (bruise) on his leg after a fall. Because of a deficiency in clotting factors, wounds or injuries bleed into muscles and joints.

inherited from the mother or newly acquired. Hemophilia in females is rare. In contrast to their brothers, who do not inherit a paternal X chromosome and will therefore generally be normal at the hemophilia locus, on average half the daughters of an affected father will carry the hemophilia gene and can pass it on to future generations. Half their sons will again be affected, and half their daughters will be carriers like themselves. In contrast to hemophilias A and B, and with the exception of factor XI deficiency, which follows autosomal dominant inheritance, all the other, rarer hemophilias, as well as type 3 von Willebrand's disease, are inherited in an autosomal recessive mode, that is, two faulty genes are needed to cause abnormality.

Risk factors and symptoms

Since the X-chromosomal hemophilias A and B together make up more than 95 percent of all hemophilias, most hemophiliacs are male. The frequency of factor XI deficiency is very high (around 8 percent) among Ashkenazi Jews, but it is very rare in the general population.

Hemophilia manifests as internal or external bleeding without or with minor trauma. Repetitive and prolonged nosebleeds are as much part of the picture as protracted bleeding from small wounds, bleeding after dental procedures, and bleeds into muscles or joints or any other organ in the body. A frequent cause of disability is ankle or knee joint destruction as a consequence of repeated bleeds. A particularly grave complication is spontaneous bleeding into the brain, which can cause irreversible neurological damage or even death.

Diagnosis

The diagnosis of hemophilia may be suspected from a family or personal history of abnormal bleeding, and is established by blood tests. Absence of a relevant family history does not rule out hemophilia, since approximately 30 percent of mutations are newly acquired. After confirmation of abnormal blood clotting, in subsequent tests the individual clotting factors are quantified. Based on the residual quantity of coagulation factor, mild, moderate, and severe forms of the illness are distinguished. Patients with severe hemophilia have less than 1 percent of normal factor activity. After making the diagnosis, family genetics are frequently studied to identify carriers.

Treatments

There is currently no cure for hemophilia. The principle of hemophilia therapy is to prevent or aggressively treat bleeding. The mainstay of treatment is replacement of the deficient clotting factor by injection into the bloodstream. Lifestyle adaptations, such as avoidance of extreme or contact sports, are also generally recommended. Parental over-protection is a common problem, possibly more so than in many other chronic diseases, because mothers may feel guilty for passing on the causative "bad gene" to their sons. The need for factor injection into the bloodstream, which necessitates frequent needlesticks, adversely affects the quality of life of hemophiliacs, particularly of children, but this discomfort compares favorably with the severe disability and early death occurring in people who are not being treated with substitute clotting factors. Most patients with hemophilia learn to inject themselves and become quite expert at handling their condition in everyday life. The overall clinical management as well as treatment of emergencies belongs in the hands of specialized comprehensive care clinics, if possible. All hemophiliacs should wear emergency bracelets. Joint bleeds are addressed with high-dose factor substitution, rest or immobilization, or both, and external cooling. Head injuries are also treated with high-dose factor substitution. Imaging studies to rule out intracranial bleeds may be indicated.

Most clotting factors used for substitution today are produced in genetically modified cell lines. This has minimized the risk of blood-borne viral infections, such as HIV and hepatitis, associated with older factor preparations that were generated from human volunteer donors. Generally, individuals with less severe forms of hemophilia require factor substitution

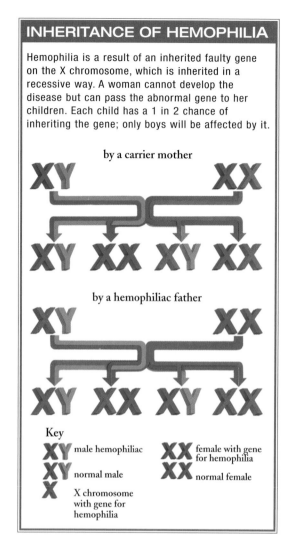

INHERITANCE OF HEMOPHILIA

Hemophilia is a result of an inherited faulty gene on the X chromosome, which is inherited in a recessive way. A woman cannot develop the disease but can pass the abnormal gene to her children. Each child has a 1 in 2 chance of inheriting the gene; only boys will be affected by it.

by a carrier mother

XY   XX

XY   XX   XY   XX

by a hemophiliac father

XY   XX

XY   XX   XY   XX

Key

XY male hemophiliac
XY normal male
X X chromosome with gene for hemophilia

XX female with gene for hemophilia
XX normal female

provided. Irrespective of future results from clinical studies, financial considerations—prophylactic treatment of a hemophiliac costs more than $50,000 per year—will likely remain a major obstacle to the general acceptance of this treatment. Over time a considerable number of patients develop inhibitory antibodies against the injected factor, which may make normal factor replacement ineffective. For such patients, alternative clotting agents are available. These include porcine factor VIII, activated prothrombin complex concentrate, or activated factor VII.

Several considerations, including the fact that as little as 3 to 4 percent normal activity is sufficient for near-normal function, identify hemophilia as a presumably ideal target for somatic gene therapy. Transgenic animals as sources of factor, that is, animals that are genetically engineered to produce human clotting factor, are also the subject of research.

Pathogenesis

A tightly regulated hierarchical cascade of different interacting protein molecules (clotting factors), which is activated by substances released by injured tissue, regulates the ability of blood to turn from liquid to solid within seconds of an injury. Normally, the clotting reaction is normally restricted to the site of injury. Severe deficiency in any of the clotting factors, due to genetic mutations, prevents solidification of blood, leading to easy and prolonged bleeding. Replacement of the missing factor itself or of one of its products further along the cascade allows for coagulation to occur normally.

Prevention and epidemiology

Genetic testing can identify carriers, but global screening in the absence of a relevant family history is not rational, given the low frequency of hemophilia. Abstention of known female carriers from reproduction may be recommended, but will only reduce the number of patients by two-thirds, since one-third of mutations are newly acquired by mother or child.

The two more common forms of hemophilia, A and B, occur in all races with a frequency of 1 in 5,000 and 1 in 25,000 males, respectively. Females are infrequently affected. All other forms of hemophilia are rare.

Halvard Boenig

only after injuries (most hemophiliacs keep factor concentrate in their refrigerator for self-injection) or during surgery. For around two-thirds of hemophilia patients whose disease is classified as "severe," with less than 1 percent residual factor activity, prophylactic factor repletion has been proposed as a better alternative to the on-demand regimen, to prevent pathological bleeding. Since injected clotting factors circulate for very short times, particularly in children, this necessitates frequent injection, such as thrice weekly for factor VIII or twice weekly for factor IX. Such treatment would be initiated after the first year of life and ideally continued lifelong. Many clinicians and the World Health Organization recommendations advocate this prophylactic approach, although a recent Cochrane review concludes that insufficient evidence for prophylactic factor substitution has been

See also
• Anemia • Hepatitis infections

Hepatitis infections

Infectious hepatitis is the inflammation of the liver, usually caused by one of the five hepatitis viruses: A, B, C, D, and E. In the United States viral hepatitis is most commonly due to hepatitis A virus (HAV), hepatitis B virus (HBV), and hepatitis C virus (HCV). Chronic hepatitis, especially from infection with hepatitis C virus, can lead to long-term damage of the liver (cirrhosis) and liver cancer. Vaccines are available to prevent infection with hepatitis A and B viruses.

According to the National Institutes of Health (NIH), viral hepatitis is the leading cause of liver disease in the United States and the world. The mode of transmission and the length and severity of the disease vary in the different types of viral hepatitis, but all five viruses can cause an episode of acute hepatitis. Virus types B, C, and D sometimes can cause chronic lifelong infections that can lead to cirrhosis of the liver and liver cancer.

Symptoms

Symptoms of hepatitis can include fatigue, fever, jaundice (yellowing of the skin and eyes due to bile pigments normally processed in the liver), loss of appetite, vomiting, diarrhea, dark urine, light-colored stools, and headache. In some types of hepatitis there may be no symptoms.

Diagnosis and prevention

Blood tests can be carried out to detect the presence of the virus or of antibodies and antigens that have built up in response to the virus. In some cases a liver biopsy may be done to determine whether there is hepatitis-related damage to the liver, including cirrhosis and liver cancer. There may also be imaging tests that can help assess damage. These include ultrasound, computed tomography (CT), and magnetic resonance imaging (MRI). Vaccines are available to prevent hepatitis A and hepatitis B; as yet no vaccines have been developed to prevent the other types of viral hepatitis.

Hepatitis A

Hepatitis A is caused by infection with the hepatitis A virus (HAV). In the United States, HAV is spread pri-

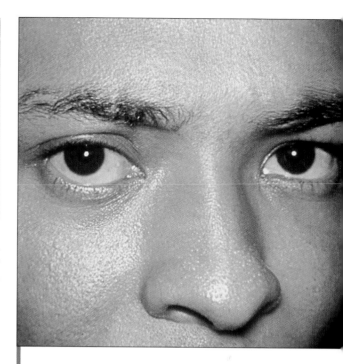

The young man above has infection with hepatitis A virus, which causes jaundice: yellowing of the conjunctiva—the white of the eyes—and facial skin due to bile pigments that are normally broken down by the liver.

marily through the fecal-oral route, whereby the virus from the stool of an infected person is swallowed by another person. This type of transmission can happen when the virus is on surfaces or hands and there is inadequate hygiene and hand washing, or from sexual contact. Localized outbreaks can occur from eating food contaminated with HAV that is uncooked, undercooked, or prepared by HAV-infected food handlers. In developing areas of the world where the water supply may be contaminated with sewage or inadequately treated, drinking water and ice, as well as food, may be contaminated. On rare occasions HAV has been transmitted through blood or blood products taken from infected donors.

Symptoms in people with HAV infection can range from none or mild to severe, and fatal cases are rare. When symptoms are present, they usually last for less than two months. In about 10 percent of people there will be relapses, which can last for as long as nine months. Often children infected with HAV have no symptoms, so they can play a large role in HAV transmission. Hepatitis A is not a long-term illness, and a single episode gives lifelong immunity against the disease. Diagnosis is made with a blood test for the hepatitis A virus.

Rates of hepatitis A in the United States have steadily declined in the last decade, from more than 31,000 reported cases in 1995 to under 6,000 cases in 2004, which is largely due to the introduction of the hepatitis A vaccine in 1995. This vaccine is the best method of prevention for hepatitis A and now is routinely recommended by the Centers for Disease Control and Prevention (CDC) for children age one to 18 years and for all people traveling to risk areas. The risk of infection when traveling outside the United States depends on the sanitary conditions and the rate of infection in the area of travel, as well as the length of the trip and the amount of time spent in rural areas where conditions may be particularly poor. While traveling in risk areas, boiling or cooking food and drinks to 185°F (85°C) for at least one minute inactivates the virus. According to the CDC, hepatitis A is the most common cause of vaccine-preventable infection acquired during travel.

In addition to the hepatitis A vaccine, hygienic measures such as hand washing after using the toilet, changing a baby's diaper, and before preparing food help prevent the spread of HAV. When a person who has not been vaccinated is exposed to the virus, a sterile injection of concentrated antibodies, called immune globulin (IG), can give some protection depending on when the exposure occurred.

Hepatitis B

Hepatitis B is spread through blood or body fluids and is a sexually transmitted virus and a global public health problem. The World Health Organization (WHO) estimates that more than 2 billion people worldwide have been infected with the hepatitis B virus (HBV), and more than 350 million have chronic lifelong infection. These people are at an increased risk of contracting cirrhosis of the liver and liver cancer, two serious disorders that kill about one million people each year.

In the United States it is estimated that more than 1.2 million people have chronic hepatitis B infection, although reported new cases have steadily declined in the United States in the last 20 years, from more than 26,000 in 1985 to 6,000 in 2004. Estimates of the number of new HBV infections have also declined, from about 260,000 each year in the 1980s to about 60,000 in 2004. The highest rate of decline occurred

in children and adolescents, which was a result of the introduction of the hepatitis B vaccine in 1982. Since 2004 more than 90 percent of children aged 19 to 35 months and more than 50 percent of all 13- to 15-year olds have been fully vaccinated with three

KEY FACTS

Description

Inflammation of the liver due to infectious agents that cause acute (short-term) health problems or chronic (long-term) effects.

Causes

The most common cause is infection with one of the five hepatitis viruses: A, B, C, D, or E. In the United States hepatitis viruses A, B, and C are the most common.

Risk factors

For hepatitis virus types A and E, transmission is via the fecal-oral route, which involves fecal contamination of food and water; for hepatitis virus types B, C, and D, spread is through blood or body fluids from an infected person. An infected mother can pass the infection to her baby in the uterus.

Symptoms and signs

These range from none to severe, including fever, flulike illness, jaundice (yellowing of skin and eyes), abdominal pain, nausea, vomiting, poor appetite, and dark urine.

Diagnosis

Blood tests to detect the specific type of hepatitis; liver function tests; biopsy.

Treatment

Depends on infectious agent and ranges from none to a shot of a drug called immune globulin, which increases antibodies against the virus; antiviral drugs are given for hepatitis types B and C.

Pathogenesis

All five viruses can cause acute hepatitis, in which liver cells become inflamed. Hepatitis virus types B, C, and D can cause chronic hepatitis and may result in cirrhosis and liver cancer.

Prevention

Vaccines are available for types A and B. For types B, C, and D, avoid contact with blood or bodily fluids of an infected person; to avoid types A and E, use clean water and practice hand washing, safe food handling and preparation, and general personal hygiene.

Epidemiology

Rates of reported cases have been declining for hepatitis A, B, and C in the last decade. Type E is rare in the United States, and type D only occurs in people with type B.

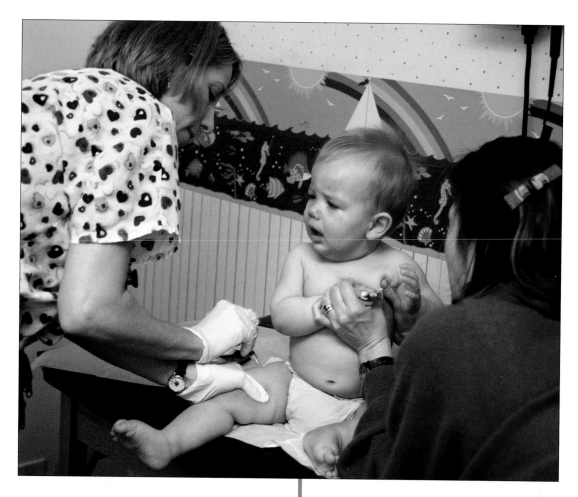

doses of the HBV vaccine. The highest rate of hepatitis B is in the 20- to 49-year age group.

HBV is transmitted through contact with the blood or body fluids of infected people in the same way that the human immunodeficiency virus (HIV), the virus that causes AIDS, is spread—although HBV is about 100 times more infectious. Risk factors include sex with HBV-infected partners; sex with multiple partners; sex with a partner with a diagnosed sexually transmitted disease; men who have sex with men; intravenous drug use; everyday household contact with an infected person; infants born to infected mothers; patients who have hemodialysis for kidney failure; and hospital workers.

Most infants and children with hepatitis B never develop symptoms or signs, and most newly infected adults recover fully from hepatitis B, even though symptoms can be severe. However, when an acute episode does occur, it progresses to a chronic, long-term infection in 30 to 90 percent of infants and children and 6 to 10 percent of adolescents and adults.

In recent years the incidence of hepatitis A and B infections in children has dropped greatly in the United States, due to the introduction of routine vaccination against hepatitis A in 1995 and hepatitis B in 1982.

There are several diagnostic blood tests for hepatitis B. These include a test to check liver function; a test for antigens that indicate current infection; and a test for antibodies that indicates recovery from a prior infection or response to the vaccine. If chronic infection is suspected, a liver biopsy may be performed to establish the extent of the disease. Blood and screening tests may also be carried out to detect the early stages of liver cancer, which can be a complication of chronic infection.

In the United States and many other developed countries, it is now routinely recommended that children and teenagers be vaccinated, as well as people in high-risk groups and people traveling to areas of the world where there is a high rate of HBV. It is also recommended that all pregnant women be screened for HBV. Treatment for chronic hepatitis B includes antiviral drugs. In severe cases a liver transplant may be carried out.

Hepatitis C

The WHO estimates that around 180 million people, or three percent of the world's population, are infected with hepatitis C virus (HCV), and 130 million are chronic carriers at risk of going on to developing cirrhosis of the liver and liver cancer. Each year more than 3 million people are infected with HCV, for which there is no vaccine.

In the United States it is estimated that more than 4 million people, which is about 1.6 percent of the population, have been infected with HCV, and of these more than 3 million have chronic infection. Although the estimated number of new infections each year has decreased from about 240,000 in the 1980s to 26,000 in 2004, HCV infection is sometimes called "a viral time bomb," as about 80 percent of newly infected people have no symptoms and if symptoms do occur they are usually mild. Chronic HCV infection, which progresses slowly over the years, develops in about 75 to 85 percent of infected people with the most common symptom being general fatigue. HCV infection occurs in about one-quarter of all people infected with HIV. This combination can cause higher levels of HCV in the blood and a more rapid progression to liver disease, so all HIV infected people should be screened for HCV.

Like HBV infection, hepatitis C infection is transmitted through virus-contaminated blood. The biggest risk factor is the use of intravenous drugs, which accounts for about 90 percent of cases. Cases associated with blood transfusion or organ transplant occurred before 1992 when screening for HCV began. Although the virus can be sexually transmitted, this is much less common than it is for HBV. A pregnant mother with HCV can pass the virus to her baby, usually while it is in the uterus. Sixty to 70 percent of people with chronic HCV infection develop chronic liver disease, and 1 to 5 percent of people with chronic liver disease die from cirrhosis or liver cancer. According to the CDC, chronic HCV infection is the leading cause of liver transplants in the United States.

HBV is diagnosed by blood tests to check the liver function, and to look for the virus and antibodies to the virus. Unlike many other infections, the presence of antibodies in the blood does not mean that the infection has cleared. Chronic infection is usually treated with a form of an antiviral medication called interferon for several months or longer in combination with another drug. In some people, this helps clear the virus from the liver. Imaging scans may be taken, and a liver biopsy, in which a sample of liver is removed and analyzed, may be carried out to check the progression of the disease.

Hepatitis D

Hepatitis D virus (HDV) is a defective virus that only occurs in people who already have HBV. The WHO estimates that there are more than 10 million people worldwide infected with HDV, although it is thought that the rate of infection in the United States is low. The risk factors and modes of transmission for HDV are the same as for HBV, although the virus is spread more easily by needle transmission and is less likely to be passed on by way of sexual contact, and transmission from a mother to her baby is rare.

When HBV and HDV infect a person simultaneously, it is called coinfection; when HDV infects a person who already has chronic HBV infection, it is called superinfection. In coinfection there is a greater chance of severe acute hepatitis and liver failure and a lower risk of chronic HBV infection. In superinfection there is a greater chance of developing chronic HDV infection, which can progress to chronic liver disease and cirrhosis. Hepatitis B vaccine can prevent coinfection, and chronic HDV infection can be treated with antiviral drugs and, if needed, a liver transplant.

Hepatitis E

Hepatitis E virus (HEV) is transmitted by the fecal-oral route through virus-contaminated drinking water or food. Person-to-person transmission is uncommon. HEV infection usually affects young adults and does not cause chronic infection, but can cause a life-threatening form of hepatitis in pregnant women in their third trimester, with death in about 20 percent of cases. Reported cases of hepatitis E in the United States are rare, with outbreaks more common in developing countries with poor sanitation. There is no vaccine for hepatitis E, and the best way to prevent infection is with a clean water supply, avoiding potentially contaminated water, ice, and food, and practicing good hygiene.

Ramona Jenkin

See also
• AIDS • Cancer, liver • Cirrhosis of the liver

Hernia

The word *hernia* is a Latin term that refers to tissue or an organ in the body pushing through a weak area. In reference to modern medicine, "hernia" is often caused by a weakness of the abdominal wall that allows abdominal contents to protrude from their normal positions outward. This protrusion relates to a visible or otherwise noticeable bulge beyond the point of herniation.

There are many types and causes of hernias, but certain regions of the abdomen are weaker than others and more likely to cause hernias. Hernias result from either a failure of the abdominal wall to close properly during development as a fetus, or more commonly, weakening and enlargement of a defect in the abdominal wall musculature. However, hernias can also occur elsewhere in the body. Examples include hiatus hernia (in which part of the stomach pushes upward through the diaphragm) and hernias in invertebral disks (slipped disk), in the brain as a result of compression by a hematoma, and in the eyelids.

Inguinal hernias

The most common location for hernias to form is in the area of the inguinal canal, leading to what is commonly referred to as a "groin hernia." Other common areas for hernias to develop are at the base of the umbilicus and within the scar tissue of a prior surgical incision.

Visible or painful bulges at the juncture of the lower abdomen and the top of the scrotum in men are typical symptoms in patients who have developed an inguinal hernia. Although identical hernias can also occur in women, they are more common in men as a result of a larger abdominal wall defect present in men that allows passage of the spermatic cord from the abdomen to the testicle. The spermatic cord contains a testicular artery and veins that supply the testicle, as well as the vas deferens, which allows passage of mature spermatozoa from the testicle to the seminal vesicles and prostate within the pelvic cavity. Since the spermatic cord that passes through the inguinal canal is larger in men than the round ligament that passes through the inguinal canal in women, men are more likely than women to develop hernias.

The inguinal canal is a complex anatomical area in the lower abdomen situated between muscular layers of the abdominal wall. The integrity of the anterior abdominal wall is maintained principally by three separate muscle layers. The outermost muscle layer is the external abdominal oblique muscle, the middle layer is the internal abdominal oblique muscle, and the innermost layer is the transversus abdominus muscle. Toward the midline of the abdominal wall, the connective tissues associated with these three muscles, or fascia, fuse into a two-layered sheath containing the rectus abdominus muscle that connects the lower rib cage to the pubic bone. In the lower abdomen a window, known as the internal inguinal ring, below the transversus abdominus and internal abdominal oblique muscles allows passage of the spermatic cord

KEY FACTS

Description
Weaknesses or ruptures of the abdominal wall that allow abdominal contents to protrude.

Causes
Hernias develop at sites of natural defects and weaknesses in the abdominal muscles, which enlarge further when repetitively stressed.

Risk factors
The male gender, chronic coughing, straining, and heavy lifting.

Symptoms
Vague discomfort associated with a bulge in the inguinal region or in the scrotum.

Diagnosis
Physical examination.

Treatments
Surgery.

Pathogenesis
Anatomical weaknesses in the abdominal muscles allow passage of structures to and from the testicle. Repetitive activities increase intra-abdominal pressure, and enlargement of these defects allows hernias to form.

Prevention
Proper lifting techniques may reduce the risk.

Epidemiology
In the United States, 700,000 hernias are repaired annually. Hernias are the most common cause of bowel obstructions in the world.

STRANGULATED HERNIA

Hernias can be pushed back and kept in place with a surgical truss until surgical intervention eliminates the danger of strangulation.

This strangulated hernia has caused part of the intestine (orange) to burst through the abdominal wall. If the neck of the hernia is tight, arterial blood can pass through, but venous blood cannot get back out. Swelling may cause the blood supply to be cut off, leading to a danger of gangrene. Only surgery can prevent this outcome.

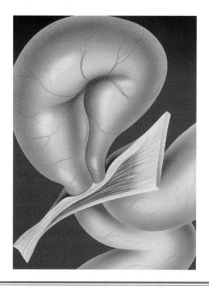

(or round ligament in females) out of the abdomen and into the inguinal canal.

Chronic increases in abdominal pressure, from persistent coughing, straining, or heavy lifting, pushes abdominal contents, such as the small bowel or colon, through the naturally occurring defects of the inguinal canal that enlarge with time and allow hernias to form. In other cases, the inguinal floor represents an area of relative weakness of the abdominal wall. This may become disrupted and allow herniation of abdominal contents through a defect that does not occur naturally. In either case, the protrusion of bowel or other abdominal contents in the inguinal region is perceived by the patient as a noticeable, and sometimes painful, bulge.

Surgical treatment

Inguinal hernias are defects for which the only available treatment is a surgical operation. Numerous approaches to hernia repair have been employed in the past, and they continue to evolve. All types of repair involve strengthening the floor of the inguinal canal and tightening the internal inguinal ring. These procedures ei-

ther pull the lower abdominal wall muscles down toward the pelvic bone or reinforce the area with a sheet of synthetic material.

Umbilical hernia

Another common location for hernias is at the base of the umbilicus. In contrast to most inguinal hernias, which develop later in life, umbilical hernias are frequently present at birth and fail to close spontaneously. During development, the entire small bowel protrudes through a large abdominal wall defect that is centered at the umbilicus. As development progresses and the fetus grows, the bowel returns to the abdominal cavity and the abdominal wall closes. The last area to close is at the base of the umbilicus. When this area fails to close completely, a hernia is present. Treatment of an umbilical hernia depends on the age of the patient. Children younger than five will be observed because the hernia may close spontaneously in the early years of life. After the age of five, however, the likelihood of a spontaneous closure diminishes, and surgical repair with sutures or synthetic material is recommended.

Incisional hernia

A third common area for hernias to occur in the abdominal wall is through a prior incision. After six weeks of healing, muscle layers of an incision approach their maximal strength, which is about 80 percent as strong as the muscle layers prior to the incision. The resulting weakness represents an area of potential herniation as subsequent increases in abdominal pressure, from straining, heavy lifting, or chronic coughing may encourage scar tissue to reopen. As with other types of hernias, an incisional hernia is identified by the presence of a bulge under the incision, particularly when the patient is straining. Surgical repair is recommended.

Incarceration

With hernias the bowel can protrude through the abdominal wall defect and become stuck or incarcerated. Hernias that can be pushed back into the abdomen, or reduced, are not threatening, but hernias that cannot be reduced are surgical emergencies. The blood supply of incarcerated bowel may be restricted, resulting in death of the bowel, which is life threatening and must be urgently treated surgically if the patient is to survive.

Chadrick Denlinger

See also
• Backache • Head injury

Herpes infections

Herpes is a common and usually mild but contagious infection caused by herpes simplex viruses (HSV). HSV can cause repeated outbreaks of blisters and sores on the skin in the area of the genitals or mouth. Unlike many other viral infections, HSV sets up a lifelong hidden presence in the body with recurring outbreaks in or near the area of the original infection when the virus is reactivated.

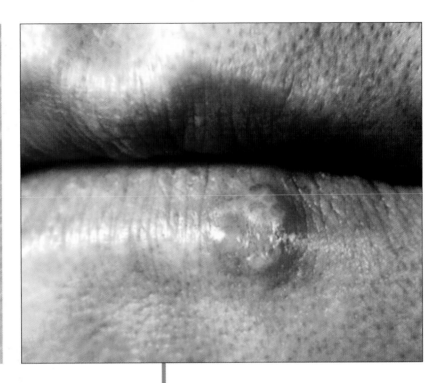

The herpes simplex virus causes painful blisters, usually affecting the mouth and nose, although they can also appear on the cheeks or chin. An attack usually clears up after about 7 to 10 days, but herpes can recur at any time.

According to the National Institutes of Health (NIH), most people in the United States have been infected with oral herpes by the age of 20. Oral herpes is commonly contracted at a young age, by a kiss from a person with oral herpes or from other physical contact, such as in a day care setting, or by sharing utensils, razors, and towels. The Centers for Disease Control and Prevention (CDC) estimates that at least 45 million people in the United States have genital herpes infection, a sexually transmitted disease that is most common in women.

Causes and risk factors

There are two viruses that can cause what is commonly known as herpes: herpes simplex virus type 1 (HSV-1) and herpes simplex virus type 2 (HSV-2). Generally, oral herpes infections, cold sores or fever blisters in the mouth area, are caused by HSV-1. HSV-2 more frequently causes sores in the genital area (genital herpes), although HSV-1 is thought to cause as much as 30 percent of all first-time genital herpes episodes. Another type, HSV-6, tends to affect infants and may be a factor in causing chronic fatigue syndrome.

The risk of contracting genital herpes increases with an increased number of sexual partners, sexual activity starting before age 17, a history of sexually transmitted diseases, HIV infection, multiple sexual partners, and a partner diagnosed with genital HSV infection.

Another virus in the herpes family is varicella-zoster virus, which causes chicken pox. After chicken pox infection, the varicella-zoster virus hides in nerve cells and can be reactivated later in life to cause what is commonly called shingles, a painful outbreak of blisters on the skin. Epstein-Barr virus, which causes mononucleosis, or glandular fever, also belongs to the herpes family.

Symptoms and signs

In genital herpes, symptoms vary greatly from none to severe painful blisters, with fever and flulike symptoms and swollen glands in the groin area. Blisters containing the contagious virus turn into painful ulcers and deep sores in the buttocks, rectum, penis, scrotum, vagina, or cervix, and can make urination painful. Lymph nodes in the groin may swell. However, according to the NIH, more than 80 percent of people in the United States who have genital herpes are not aware of their infection because they have mild symptoms or no symptoms, and may unknowingly infect sexual partners.

In young children a first episode of oral HSV can result in painful blisters and sores inside the mouth on the hard palate (roof of the mouth) and the gums, and lymph nodes in the neck may swell. The child may have a fever and feel ill, but usually recovers in 7 to 14 days. However, as in genital herpes, many people with oral herpes never have symptoms, and the NIH estimates that only 20 to 40 percent of people with oral herpes have recurrent outbreaks as adults. The classic symptom is a single blister or cluster of blisters on the lips or mouth, but they can appear on the nose, cheeks, or chin. A mild infection can appear as a crack or chapped lips or may be mistaken for a bug bite. There may be tingling or pain in the area before the sore breaks out, during which time the virus is already contagious. After blisters form, they crust over and may become itchy as they heal; they usually recur in the same location.

The most noticeable symptoms of herpes infection are usually found in people who have only recently been infected because they do not yet have an immune response to the virus. In recurrent episodes the body's immune response recognizes the virus and responds to it, so the symptoms are usually much milder.

Diagnosis and treatments

A clinical examination can be useful if a typical outbreak with blisters is present, but this is not usually the case. Furthermore, other sexually transmitted infections cause sores in the genital area that can look similar to herpes sores. Viral cultures, in which a swab is taken from a blister or sore and a culture is grown in a laboratory to identify the virus, become less sensitive as the sores heal, but if successful they can distinguish between HSV-1 and HSV-2. Special blood tests can measure the presence of the different HSV antibodies that form in the first few weeks after the first infection, which can be helpful, especially if the viral culture was taken too late and is negative. Since almost all HSV-2 is sexually transmitted, a positive HSV-2 antibody blood test strongly indicates a genital infection. Even though about 30 percent of all new genital outbreaks may be due to HSV-1, recurrent episodes of genital herpes are more likely to be due to HSV-2.

There is no cure for herpes. Cold sores usually heal without treatment in 7 to 10 days. Special medica-

tions, called antivirals, can shorten the duration of an outbreak of genital herpes. When antiviral medication is used to prevent frequent outbreaks, the treatment is called suppressive therapy, although this does not kill the virus or change the frequency or severity of outbreaks once the medication is stopped. Using special

---

KEY FACTS

Description

Lifelong infection caused by two viruses (HSV-1 and HSV-2) that can cause recurrent episodes of blisters on the mouth, face, genitals, or both.

Cause

Infection with the herpes simplex virus.

Risk factors

Skin-to-skin contact, kissing, and sexual contact. For genital herpes infection the risk increases with an increased number of sexual partners, sexual activity starting before age 17, a history of sexually transmitted diseases, HIV infection, multiple sex partners, and a partner diagnosed with genital herpes simplex virus infection.

Symptoms

Most people are unaware that they are infected with herpes simplex virus, as many have no symptoms. Some have outbreaks with recurrent blisters, painful sores, and flulike symptoms. The blisters are located in the genitals or mouth area.

Diagnosis

Clinical examination; viral culture; antibody blood test.

Treatment

No cure. Antiviral medication during breakouts, or suppressive therapy. Local treatment to ease discomfort of sores.

Pathogenesis

After the first infection, herpes simplex virus sets up a lifelong presence in the body by traveling into and remaining in nerve tissue, and later reactivating, causing an outbreak. It can "shed" and infect others even when there are no symptoms.

Prevention

Avoid skin-to-skin contact if blisters or other symptoms are present. Abstinence from sex; long-term monogamous sexual relationship with uninfected partner. To prevent infection in newborns it is necessary to ensure there is no active genital infection in the mother during delivery, or a Caesarean delivery may be necessary.

Epidemiology

At least 45 million people in the United States are thought to have genital herpes infection, and it is estimated that more than half of all adults in the United States have oral herpes infection.

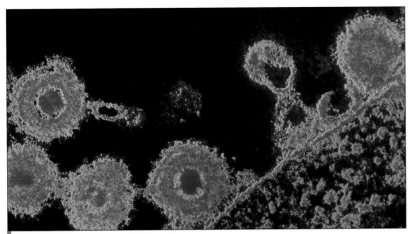

This colored transmission electron micrograph shows a recently discovered strain (HSV-6) of the herpes simplex virus, which may cause chronic fatigue syndrome.

mild soaps to keep the infected area clean, or using ice or warmth, may decrease pain. Rarely, herpes infections can be severe enough to need hospitalization.

Pathogenesis and transmission

HSV enters the body through skin or the soft mucous membranes and multiplies in the skin in the infected area. When the infection heals, the virus leaves the skin and travels along the sensory nerve to its root and remains in the ganglia, a bundle of nerve cells that supply the area of skin where the infection took place. The herpes virus sets up a lifelong presence in the nerve, lying dormant (asleep) and hidden for a period of time. When it is reactivated, the virus travels through the nerve and back to the skin site of the original infection, where it can cause blisters and sores, or it "sheds" (is released through the skin) without symptoms. Reactivation of the virus may be triggered by fever, menstruation, emotional stress, or a suppressed immune system, but often the trigger is unknown.

Genital herpes is easily spread through sexual contact, which can be genital-to-genital or oral-to-genital, either during an outbreak, during or just before an outbreak, or even when there are no blisters, sores, or symptoms, but the virus sheds.

Oral herpes can be transmitted through kissing, oral-genital contact, or other skin-to-skin contact involving the area of the sores, even before they break out. HSV can also be transmitted to other parts of the body, to a finger, for example, when it touches the infected genital area. The finger can then touch and infect other parts of the body like the eye, causing a severe infection.

Usually herpes infection is not dangerous in healthy people. Some people may have severe or prolonged symptoms, or the infection may be in the eye; in these cases a doctor should be consulted. In people with immune system problems herpes symptoms can be more severe. Having genital herpes makes it easier to transmit or acquire HIV, the virus that causes AIDS.

Active genital herpes infection in pregnant women at the time of birth increases the risk of transmission to the newborn as it passes through the birth canal. The risk is higher for women who have a first episode of genital herpes during pregnancy than for women with a history of genital herpes.

Usually, babies of mothers who have active genital herpes are delivered by Caesarean section to reduce the transmission risk. Herpes infection in newborns can be very serious and is almost always treated with antiviral medications.

Prevention

Herpes is a widespread and contagious infection. Prevention may be difficult, especially since most people with HSV-1 and HSV-2 are unaware that they are infected and, even for those who are aware, there may be periods of shedding even when they have no symptoms. The surest way to avoid sexual transmission of genital herpes is to abstain from sex, or to be engaged in a long-term monogamous sexual relationship with an uninfected partner.

People with outbreaks or symptoms should not engage in sex with uninfected partners. Condoms do not always cover the genital areas that may be infected or areas that harbor the infection, so they may not prevent transmission, even with correct and regular use. Daily suppressive antiviral medication can help reduce transmission to sexual partners.

Ramona Jenkin

See also
- AIDS • Chickenpox and shingles
- Gonorrhea • Syphilis

Hodgkin's disease

Hodgkin's disease, or Hodgkin's lymphoma, was first recognized in 1832 by Thomas Hodgkin. Hodgkin's disease is a kind of cancer that originates in lymphatic systems, which are part of the body's immune system.

Hodgkin's disease, in most cases, originates in lymph nodes, especially those in the upper body, such as the chest, the neck, and under the arms.

There are two main types of Hodgkin's disease: the classical type and nodular predominant type. The exact causes of Hodgkin's disease are not yet known, and no major risk factors for the disease have been discovered. However, a few factors, including age, sex, infections, and certain medical conditions such as low immunity, seem to be linked to the disease.

According to the National Cancer Institute (NCI), Hodgkin's disease occurs more often in males than females, and it often occurs in early adulthood (between 15 and 34) and late adulthood (after 55).

According to research done by the American Cancer Society (ACS), people who have had infectious mononucleosis, which is an infection caused by the Epstein-Barr virus, tend to have a higher chance of contracting Hodgkin's disease. People with lower immunity also tend to have higher rates of contracting Hodgkin's disease.

According to the ACS, death rates of Hodgkin's disease have decreased by more than 60 percent since the 1970s. Chemotherapy, radiation therapy, and surgery are, currently, the three main types of treatment for patients with Hodgkin's disease. Chemotherapy uses chemical drugs to stop the growth of cancer cells by killing the cancer cells or by stopping them from dividing. Chemotherapy can be administered orally or by injection, and it can also be placed directly in the areas where cancer cells are found. Radiation therapy uses high energy X-rays to kill the cancer cells. Radiation therapy is either external or internal. External therapy uses a machine outside the body to kill cancer cells, whereas internal therapy uses needles or wires inserted inside the body to kill the cancer cells. Chemotherapy and radiation therapy are often combined in the treatment of Hodgkin's disease. Cancer cells and tissues can also be removed surgically. However, all the treatments for Hodgkin's disease, especially radiation therapy, have significant adverse effects.

Although Hodgkin's disease can strike both adults and children, the treatment for each can be different. For children who are still growing, radiation therapy is generally used with great caution because the radiation could affect bone and muscle growth. Because children tend to tolerate chemotherapy better than adults, doctors often prefer chemotherapy to radiation therapy to treat childhood Hodgkin's disease.

Clinical studies of new types of treatment for Hodgkin's disease, such as high-dose chemotherapy and radiation therapy with stem cell transplant, are ongoing. Because the causes are unknown and the main risk factors are not yet clear, it is currently very difficult to prevent Hodgkin's disease.

Y. Wang

KEY FACTS

Description
A type of cancer originating in lymphatic tissues.

Causes
The exact causes are unknown.

Risk factors
Age, sex, infection, and some medical conditions.

Symptoms
Enlarged lymph nodes, trouble breathing, fever, night sweats, itchy skin, and weight loss.

Diagnosis
Physical exam, biopsy, thoracentesis, chest X-ray, and CT scan.

Treatments
Chemotherapy, radiation therapy, and surgery.

Pathogenesis
Hodgkin's disease can form almost anywhere and can spread through the lymphatic vessels.

Prevention
Because the causes and risk factors of Hodgkin's diseases are not clear, it is very difficult to prevent the disease.

Epidemiology
Hodgkin's disease can strike adults and children. It often occurs between 15 and 34 years of age and late adulthood (older than 55 years of age). About 10 to 15 percent of cases are found in children 16 years old or younger.

See also
• Lymphoma

HPV infection

Human papillomaviruses (HPVs) are widespread in the general population. They produce epithelial lesions of the skin and mucous membranes known as warts, or condylomas, and have been closely associated with cancers of the genital tract.

HPV infects the basal epithelial cells of the epidermis in the skin and of the mucous membranes in the genital tract and leads to the development of lesions known as warts, or condylomas. Infected cells can undergo malignant transformation, replace all the layers of normal cells above, and eventually invade the tissues underneath the epithelium and complete the transition to invasive cancer. Different HPV types cause different disease: cutaneous infections (HPV 1 and 2), genital infections (HPV 6 and 11), and progression of the infected cells to cancer cells, particularly in the cervix (HPV 16 and 18). Cutaneous HPV infections are transmitted through close personal contact, whereas genital HPV infections are transmitted through sexual contact. The three main cutaneous lesions are common warts (about 70 percent of all cutaneous warts), plantar warts (about 30 percent), and flat warts (less than 5 percent) and do not usually progress to cancer. Genital HPV infections can involve both male and female external genitalia (penis, scrotum, vulva) and perianal region and internal genitalia (urethra, vagina, cervix) and anus. Genital lesions range from being small and flat (flat condyloma) to being large and spiked (acuminate condyloma) and are associated with progression to cancer. In women with external genital lesions, cervical lesions are often present as well. Patients with HIV infection are at particular risk of progression to cancer because of their poorly functioning immune system.

Symptoms and diagnosis

Both cutaneous and genital lesions are usually asymptomatic, but they may bleed and be itchy or painful if located over weight-bearing surfaces or areas of friction. About 50 percent of cutaneous lesions clear up on their own, as do 10 to 20 percent of genital lesions. The diagnosis of HPV infection is usually made clinically by physical exam. Women with external genital lesions should all undergo a Papanicolau test (Pap test). Direct visualization of the anal surface with a small camera (anoscopy) should be considered in patients with peri- anal warts, anal symptoms, or a history of receptive anal intercourse. For lesions that are large or that bleed, a biopsy is done to rule out progression to cancer.

Treatments and prevention

Cutaneous lesions are treated locally with preparations containing salicylic acid. Treatment methods for genital lesions are many but unsatisfactory because of their high recurrence rates. Local application of trichloracetic acid, podophyllin, and imiquimod are all valid options. Cryotherapy or laser therapy are indicated during pregnancy and for treatment of cervical lesions. Avoiding contact with infectious lesions is the only method of prevention. Wearing protective footwear in swimming pools protects against foot warts; using condoms confers protection against genital HPV infections. The Pap test is essential for the screening and prevention of HPV-induced intra-epithelial neoplasia and invasive cervical cancer. Vaccines against HPV may be available in the near future.

Corrado Cancedda

KEY FACTS

Description
Viral infection that causes skin and genital warts.

Causes
Human papillomaviruses.

Risk factors
Close contact for cutaneous infections and sexual contact for genital infections.

Symptoms
Lesions usually asymptomatic.

Diagnosis
Physical examination and Pap test.

Treatment
Local applications, cryotherapy, and laser therapy.

Pathogenesis
HPV can lead to the development of invasive cancer.

Prevention
Avoiding contact with infectious lesions.

Epidemiology
5.5 million new cases per year in the United States.

See also
• AIDS • Cancer, cervical • Wart and verruca

Huntington's disease

An inherited genetic disorder, Huntington's disease destroys areas of the brain that affect movement, intellect, and emotional stability. Huntington's disease progresses gradually and can eventually cause the decline of all vital body functions.

Huntington's disease (HD) is a fatal hereditary disease that destroys nerve cells (neurons) in areas of the brain involved in the emotions, intellect, and movement. The course of Huntington's disease is characterized by uncontrollable jerking movements of the limbs, trunk, and face (also called chorea, from the Greek *choreia*, meaning "dance"); progressive loss of intellectual abilities; and the development of psychiatric problems.

Causes and symptoms

Huntington's disease is caused by a mutation in a gene called huntingtin. Normally this gene has up to 26 copies of the DNA sequence CAG; people with HD may have from 40 to more than 100 copies of CAG. It is not known why HD arises from this repeated sequence. The disease is inherited in an autosomal dominant manner; a person with the abnormal gene has a 50 percent chance of passing it on to each of his or her children.

Early signs of the disease vary from person to person. The earlier that symptoms appear, the faster the disease progresses. Usually, symptoms become apparent at midlife. The person experiences mood swings or becomes uncharacteristically irritable, apathetic, passive, depressed, or angry. HD may affect judgment, memory, and other cognitive functions. Early signs might include problems with driving, learning new things, answering questions, or making decisions. Some people may display changes in handwriting. As HD progresses, concentration becomes increasingly difficult. The disease also sometimes begins with uncontrolled movements in the fingers, feet, face, or trunk. Mild clumsiness or problems with balance may occur. Speech may become slurred; swallowing, eating, speaking, and especially walking continue to decline.

Treatments and epidemiology

There is currently no cure for HD, but specific symptoms may be relieved with drugs. Antipsychotic drugs, such as haloperidol, may help alleviate abnormal movements and help control hallucinations, delusions, and violent outbursts. These medications may have severe side effects, such as sedation.

Many community resources are available to help families, including home care services, recreation and work centers, group housing, and legal and social aid. Research is focused on determining how mutation in the huntingtin gene leads to HD. HD affects males and females equally and crosses all ethnic and racial boundaries. One out of every 10,000 Americans has HD. Around 200,000 Americans have one parent with HD, which means that they have a 50 percent chance of developing the disease themselves.

Diana Gitig

KEY FACTS

Description

A genetic disorder resulting in gradual physical, mental, and emotional decline.

Causes

Mutation in a gene.

Risk factors

Having a parent who has either the disease or the genetic mutation that causes it.

Symptoms

Uncontrolled movements, loss of intellectual faculties, and emotional disturbance.

Diagnosis

Typical cases are recognized by the combination of dementia and abnormal movements. Genetic testing confirms the diagnosis.

Treatments

Early symptoms can be managed with antipsychotic drugs and therapy.

Pathogenesis

HD slowly diminishes the ability to walk, think, talk, and reason. Eventually, the person becomes totally dependent upon others for his or her care.

Prevention

None.

Epidemiology

In the United States about 30,000 people have HD; estimates of the disease's prevalence are about 1 in every 10,000 people.

See also
• Dementia

Hyperthermia

Hyperthermia is the abnormal elevation of body temperature, unrelated to fever, as a result of an imbalance between the body's heat production and heat loss. Hyperthermia may be caused by heat-related illness such as heat exhaustion or heat stroke. Heat stroke is a medical emergency; it may lead to organ failure and death.

Hyperthermia can be caused by medications including beta-blockers, diuretics, and antihypertensives. The drugs may reduce sweating, and thus cause a reduced ability to dissipate body heat. Dehydration predisposes to heat illness. Athletes who train vigorously during heat waves are at risk, as are elderly patients or infants who do not have access to fluids. Alcoholics, the morbidly obese, and patients with multiple medical problems are also at risk.

Symptoms and diagnosis

Heat exhaustion and heat stroke occur above 104°F (40°C). Nonspecific symptoms such as headache, nausea, sweating, vomiting, dizziness, or fainting are typical of heat exhaustion. It is differentiated from heat stroke by the absence of central nervous system (CNS) symptoms. Heat stroke has associated CNS dysfunction. Physical findings with heat stroke may include excessively rapid breathing, dry skin, seizures, altered mental status, delirium, coma, and pulmonary edema. Laboratory studies may reveal multi-organ dysfunction. Heat stroke is divided into classic (nonexertional) heat stroke and exertional heat stroke. Elderly individuals with chronic medical problems are predisposed to classic heat stroke. Exertional heat stroke affects young, healthy people who exercise strenuously during extreme heat and humidity. Distinct forms of hyperthermia, not associated with environmental heat stress, include malignant hyperthermia and neuroleptic malignant syndrome. Malignant hyperthermia is a genetically predisposed condition in which patients undergoing general anesthesia experience hyperthermia and muscle rigidity. Neuroleptic malignant syndrome may occur with the use of antipsychotic medications and is associated with hypertension, muscle rigidity, and dysfunction of the autonomic nervous system.

The key treatment for hyperthermia is cooling. Fluid replenishment and rest in a cool environment is usually adequate treatment for heat exhaustion. If heat exhaustion is not treated, it may progress to heat stroke. Treatment of heat stroke involves aggressive cooling and cautious IV fluid replacement. Cooling techniques should be used until the temperature drops to 103°F (39.5°C). Clothes should be removed, fans applied, and water should be sprayed onto the patient. Ice packs to the armpits and groin are also helpful. Cold peritoneal and bladder washing and use of a heart and lung machine are invasive but effective techniques for rapid cooling. Shivering should be abated with the drugs lorazepam or diazepam. Antifever drugs are not helpful. Malignant hyperthermia is treated with dantrolene and the above methods. Treatment of neuroleptic malignant syndrome includes supportive measures and cooling.

Joanne Oakes and Jamie Flournoy

KEY FACTS

Description
Clinical condition due to elevated body temperature.

Causes
Environmental conditions, underlying medical problems, or genetic predisposition.

Risk factors
Advanced age, infancy, chronic illness, physical exertion, medications, alcoholism, obesity, dehydration.

Symptoms
Nonspecific, such as headache, nausea, sweating, vomiting, dizziness, or fainting. Same symptoms for heat stroke but with neurological dysfunction.

Diagnosis
History and physical exam.

Treatments
Cooling.

Pathogenesis
Death from environmental conditions occurs most commonly due to heat-related illness.

Prevention
Adequate amounts of fluids; keep elderly and ill cool; avoid medications that interfere with heat loss.

Epidemiology
Varies: from 1 in 4,500 to 1 in 60,000 cases of malignant hyperthermia have been reported.

See also

• Alcohol-related disorders • Obesity

Impetigo

Impetigo is a common bacterial infection of the superficial layers of the skin. It is characterized by draining inflammatory skin lesions that most commonly occur on the face (especially around the nose and mouth). This condition can become quite severe without appropriate treatment.

Impetigo is always caused by bacteria. *Streptococcus pyogenes* and *Staphylococcus aureus* are the most common causative agents. Other less common types of streptococci can cause impetigo as well.

Impetigo usually occurs in young children. The infection often arises from sites of minor skin trauma such as cuts or abrasions. It is frequently spread from person to person in settings where there is close contact, such as within families and schools. Poor personal hygiene may also promote the spread of infection.

Symptoms and signs

In its classic presentation, the infection begins as localized inflamed lesions over the skin which may enlarge, become fluid-filled, and rupture. Pus may drain from the ruptured lesions. The purulent drainage dries to form a characteristic yellow crust over the skin, described as yellow-amber in appearance. Patients typically have little pain, and fever is usually absent.

Diagnosis and treatments

The diagnosis is typically made based on the characteristic appearance of the skin lesions. Culture of the draining fluid may also grow the bacteria.

In uncomplicated cases, topical antibiotics may be effective. In more severe cases, oral or intravenous antibiotics are recommended. Standard first-line medications include dicloxacillin, cephalexin, and erythromycin. Other antibiotics are equally effective.

The bacteria usually gains entry to the skin through skin trauma, such as a minor cut. Depending on the type of bacteria, it attaches to host cells through various proteins on its surface. It also may produce toxins that damage host tissues and lead to more severe infection.

There is no available vaccine to prevent this infection. Appropriate hygienic measures and avoidance of people who are already affected may prevent the spread of impetigo from person to person.

Epidemiology

Young children are most commonly affected, although all age groups can potentially acquire the infection. Due to crowding and poor hygiene, the condition may also afflict the homeless population. More cases occur during warmer months of the year. Impetigo is a common complaint of patients in outpatient clinics and hospitals, and several million cases occur every year in the United States.

Joseph Fritz and Bernard Camins

KEY FACTS

Description
Bacterial infection of superficial layers of skin.

Causes
Most commonly the bacteria *Streptococcus pyogenes* or *Staphylococcus aureus*.

Risk factors
Overcrowded living conditions, poor hygiene, close contact with those already affected.

Symptoms
Red, inflamed lesions over the skin, usually on the face. The lesions enlarge, become fluid-filled, and eventually rupture and drain pus.

Diagnosis
Based on appearance of skin lesions. Bacteria may be detected by culture of draining fluid.

Treatments
Antibiotics, both topical and systemic, depending on the severity.

Pathogenesis
Entry of bacteria through minor skin trauma; bacteria adhere to skin cells and produces damaging toxins, leading to severe infections.

Prevention
Appropriate hygiene. No vaccine is available.

Epidemiology
Usually affects children of all ages and can be spread person to person through contact. Males and females are affected equally. Several million cases occur annually in the United States.

See also
• Antibiotic-resistant infections

Influenza

A severe viral respiratory infection, commonly called flu, that spreads rapidly from person to person and affects millions of Americans every year. During pandemics (worldwide epidemics), influenza may infect more than 50 percent of the human population. The complications that sometimes arise from flu can be life threatening in high-risk groups of people, including the very young or old and those with preexisting chronic illness.

Every year the flu strikes, causing thousands of deaths and hospitalizing more than 200,000 Americans. The viruses that cause flu in humans have the ability to mutate; that is, they change their genetic material and produce new strains. Public health officials try to stay one step ahead of annual flu outbreaks by producing vaccines tailored to the particular flu strains projected to be circulating. However, the resultant "best guess" vaccine may or may not be a good match. Beyond the minor, continual changes in genetic material, there are major changes leading to drastically different flu viruses to which the human immune system has no resistance. These changes are responsible for the massive pandemics that periodically march through the world's population, taking millions of lives in the process.

Causes

There are three types of flu viruses: A, B, and C. Both A and B cause the flu in humans. Type A is the greatest threat to health; it causes a more severe illness and easily mutates, which makes it easier to infect a human host.

Risk factors

Flu is a highly contagious illness that can be spread by infectious droplets produced by coughs or sneezes. If a person breathes in these infectious droplets, he or she can become ill with influenza.

Flu can also be spread by touch, for example if influenza-infected secretions are picked up on the fingers and then conveyed to the mouth. Anyone infected with the influenza virus is infectious to others from one day before symptoms develop through five days after symptoms first appear.

People with underlying chronic medical illnesses, those living in communities like nursing homes or other chronic care facilities, and those at the extremes of age are more susceptible to the flu and its complications. Also, those who have not received the annual flu vaccine are at greater risk of infection.

Symptoms and signs

Flu symptoms appear suddenly and include fever, cough, headache, weakness, and muscle aches, and sometimes a sore throat. Gastrointestinal symptoms

KEY FACTS

Description
Acute viral respiratory illness.

Cause
Infection by influenza A or B viruses.

Risk factors
Most likely to cause serious illness in people who are very young or old, those with preexisting chronic medical disorders, those who live in nursing homes or other care facilities, or those who have not received an annual influenza vaccine.

Symptoms
Abrupt onset of fever, cough, sore throat, muscle aches, weakness, and headache. Very young children may have nausea, vomiting, and diarrhea.

Diagnosis
Rapid diagnostic tests of nasal or other respiratory secretions; culture of the virus; blood test to check for antibodies.

Treatments
Two classes of antiviral medicines are available, but resistance is increasing to the older class of drugs. Antibiotics are useful only if bacterial complications develop.

Pathogenesis
Contact with secretions infected with influenza. The virus enters cells of the respiratory tract lining, where it multiplies, infecting other cells and ultimately spreading from person to person.

Prevention
Annual influenza vaccine can provide protection from influenza.

Epidemiology
Yearly outbreaks result in more than 200,000 hospitalizations and about 36,000 deaths among United States residents.

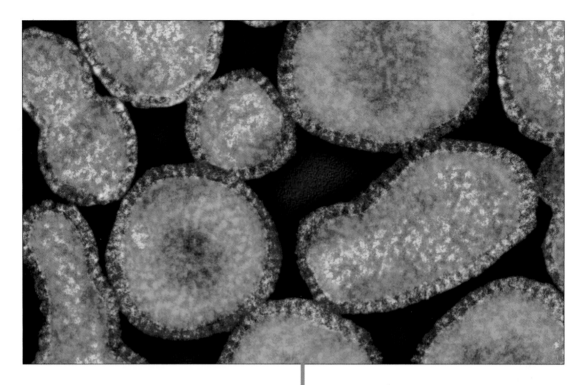

such as nausea, vomiting, and diarrhea may also occur; however, those are more common in children. Flu lasts a few days to a week, although the fatigue that commonly accompanies the illness may continue for weeks afterward, when all other symptoms have cleared up.

There is a possibility of complications, the most common being pneumonia. Pneumonia can arise from the influenza virus itself or from a secondary bacterial infection. Common symptoms of pneumonia are high fever and shortness of breath that, if it worsens, can lead to respiratory failure and death. People with underlying chronic disorders can find that their existing symptoms worsen when they are in the throes of illness from influenza. Dehydration is a potential complication among all age groups with flu, but is more likely in those with gastrointestinal symptoms. In children, a dangerous illness called Reye's syndrome has been associated with the use of aspirin to relieve symptoms of viral infections (see box, page 252). This syndrome is more often seen with influenza B infections and is marked by nausea and vomiting, followed by central nervous system complications that can lead to seizures, coma, and death.

Diagnosis and treatment

During a community outbreak of influenza, some physicians may make the diagnosis of flu based on symptoms common among a population. Rapid diagnostic tests using nasal and respiratory secretions to detect the presence of the flu virus are available for same-day diagnosis. Swabs of the throat, nasal washings, or sputum can be checked for the influenza virus or viral antigens (proteins). Viral cultures in which the organism is grown in nutrient gel can be performed. Cultures take up to 48 to 72 hours to produce results, but they are of value in determining the particular types of viruses that are circulating in a community. Blood testing is also available to look for raised levels of antibodies produced by the immune system to combat influenza; however, these tests will not show results until a person has had the infection for some days.

Two types of antiviral drugs are available for combating the enzymes found on the surface of the flu virus: M2 ion channel blockers (amantadine and rimantadine) and neuraminidase (NA) inhibitors (zanamivir and oseltamivir). Amantadine and rimantadine are effective against influenza A only. Over time, flu viruses have acquired increasing rates of resistance to these drugs. There is less resistance of flu viruses to NA inhibitors, and these medicines are effective against both influenza A and B. Relief of symptoms may include rest, taking acetaminophen for headache and muscle aches, and drinking plenty of fluids. Antibiotics are not effective against viral illnesses such as influenza and can only treat complications caused by bacteria.

Pathogenesis

In addition to humans, influenza A can infect other species such as birds, pigs, sea mammals, and horses. The virus is maintained naturally in the environment by aquatic birds. Various subtypes of this virus exist, identified by the different forms of proteins on the surface of the virus; these proteins are hemagglutinin A (HA) and NA. HA permits the virus to enter host cells. Inside the cells, the virus replicates itself and the new viruses break out (a function facilitated by NA) to infect more cells and ultimately to be passed from person to person. There are 16 subtypes of HA (H1 through H16); and there are nine subtypes of NA (N1 through N9). A specific virus is named for its HA and NA components, for example H1N1.

H1 through H3 viruses have been circulating in the human population for at least a century and were responsible for pandemics in 1918, 1957, 1968, and 1977. By far the most severe pandemic was in 1918.

H5 virus is not recognized by the human immune system, making it a major pandemic threat. The flu strain H5N1, first identified in Hong Kong in 1997, has caused worldwide concern. This strain is responsible for widespread infection in birds, can be transmitted from birds to humans, and has become increasingly resistant to the older class of antiviral drugs. Public health officials are aware that H5N1 may at some point undergo a mutation that will eventually allow it to be transmitted from human to human. Previous pandemics were the result of viruses crossing the species barrier, jumping from an animal host to a human. So far H5N1 meets two of the three criteria that make viruses risk factors for a pandemic: it is a new virus subtype and it can replicate in humans to produce severe illness. At present the virus is not passed easily from person to person.

Small mutations in genetic material, called antigenic drift, continually occur among influenza viruses, especially those of type A. Major changes in the genetic makeup, called antigenic shift, are less common but are more deadly since they lead to epidemics and pandemics. In antigenic shift, a virus evolves for which humans have little or no immunity because the body's defense mechanisms are unable to recognize the new virus. A process termed *reassortment* can likewise

STRUCTURE OF A VIRUS

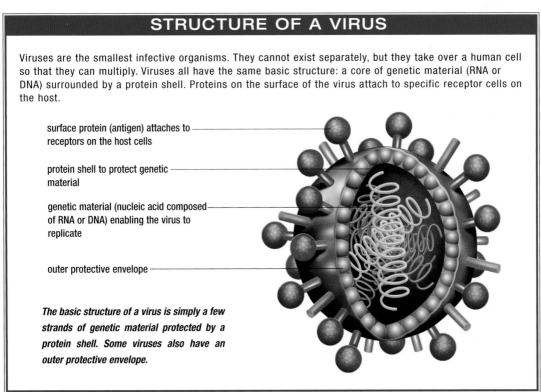

Viruses are the smallest infective organisms. They cannot exist separately, but they take over a human cell so that they can multiply. Viruses all have the same basic structure: a core of genetic material (RNA or DNA) surrounded by a protein shell. Proteins on the surface of the virus attach to specific receptor cells on the host.

surface protein (antigen) attaches to receptors on the host cells

protein shell to protect genetic material

genetic material (nucleic acid composed of RNA or DNA) enabling the virus to replicate

outer protective envelope

The basic structure of a virus is simply a few strands of genetic material protected by a protein shell. Some viruses also have an outer protective envelope.

REYE'S SYNDROME

Children 18 years of age or less should not be given aspirin when they have a viral illness like influenza, chicken pox, or the common cold, because of the risk of developing Reye's syndrome. This dangerous disorder, while rare, is associated with aspirin therapy in children who have acute viral infection. Reye's syndrome causes complications affecting the liver, blood, and brain that can lead to seizures, coma, and death. In children who develop the syndrome, symptoms appear about one week after the viral illness, with sudden and persistent nausea and vomiting. Symptoms can rapidly progress, leading to death in only four or five days. Management in an intensive care unit is required. If recognized and treated early, the child usually recovers without serious consequences, although serious brain injury can result. Since 1980, the incidence of Reye's syndrome has declined, possibly because of increased awareness of its links to aspirin and viral infection. However, the exact cause of the illness is not fully understood.

It is important to check the list of ingredients in over-the-counter medicines since aspirin may be present, particularly in remedies designed to treat a variety of symptoms. Some acceptable alternatives to aspirin include acetaminophen and ibuprofen. An additional preventive measure is for children to receive varicella (chicken pox) and influenza vaccines to reduce the risk of developing these viral illnesses.

produce a virus that is novel to the human immune system. Here, genetic material from one virus combines with that from a second virus. An example would be infection of a pig with both a human virus and an avian flu virus, which then exchange genetic material while in this host. The resultant influenza virus would be very different from others in circulation, making the human population exceptionally vulnerable to widespread infection.

Flu viruses can also be categorized by their pathogenicity, that is, their ability to produce disease in a host. Low-pathogenicity viruses cause mild respiratory symptoms, whereas high-pathogenicity viruses cause more severe illness.

Prevention

One type of antiviral drug used for the treatment of influenza, the NA inhibitor oseltamivir, is also approved for the prevention of flu, but antiviral medicines are not substitutes for the flu vaccine. An annual flu vaccine is available in the form of an inactivated vaccine given as a shot, or a live weakened virus given as a nasal spray. The flu shot is effective only against A and B strains of flu. The Centers for Disease Control collects data on flu strains throughout the world and decides every year which three subtypes of virus are most likely to be in circulation for the upcoming year. If estimates about which flu strains to include in the annual vaccine are accurate, the vaccine provides 50 to 80 percent protection rates. Outbreaks of flu occur during winter months in the Northern and Southern hemispheres, and thus the vaccine should be given in the fall. It takes about two weeks after vaccination for the immune system to produce antibodies against flu viruses.

While all people are encouraged to receive flu vaccine unless there are medical reasons to the contrary, vaccination is recommended for certain high risk groups, including children between the ages of 6 and 23 months; people aged 50 or older; residents of nursing homes and other long-term care institutions; those who have chronic medical conditions such as diabetes, or heart or lung disease; children between the ages of six months and 18 years who are on long-term aspirin therapy (see box, above); women who will be in their second or third trimester of pregnancy during the flu season; and health care workers, who could transmit flu to high-risk, susceptible populations. The nasal spray flu vaccine is approved only for healthy people between ages 5 to 49, and is not given to pregnant women.

Flu vaccine is made from viruses grown in eggs, and people with severe egg allergies should not receive the vaccine. Influenza viruses H5 and H7 are lethal to chick embryos and therefore cannot be grown in substantial quantities, so these viruses remain a serious threat. Flu vaccine should not be given to anyone who has been affected by Guillain-Barré syndrome within the previous six months. Babies aged less than six months and anyone who currently has a moderate or severe illness should not receive the vaccine. For people at high risk of complications from influenza but for whom vaccination is not recommended, antiviral medicines may be considered as a preventive measure.

Rita Washko

See also
• Avian influenza • H1N1 influenza

Irritable bowel syndrome

Irritable bowel syndrome (IBS) is a chronic condition defined by abdominal discomfort or pain that is associated with changes in bowel frequency or appearance of feces. IBS is termed a functional gastrointestinal disorder, because standard medical evaluations of these symptoms fail to identify any laboratory or pathological foundation for the symptoms.

In addition to abdominal pain and changes in bowel patterns, other symptoms of IBS may include bloating, straining, or passage of mucus with bowel movements. People with IBS may also report some pain relief after defecation. Notably, those with IBS typically lack "red flag" symptoms such as blood in their stool, anemia, or weight loss, any of which should alert a physician to the possibility of another diagnosis.

The underlying causes of IBS are not fully understood. Food intolerances, allergies, stress, infection, or overcolonization of the small intestine have all been proposed as factors. However, these may account for symptoms in only some people with IBS, as these factors are not found in all patients with this condition.

For unclear reasons, women report symptoms of IBS more commonly than men. People with anxiety disorders or depression are also more likely to experience IBS. Stress may aggravate symptoms. IBS may be more common following gastroenteritis. Having other family members with IBS may also be a minor risk factor for the development of IBS.

Diagnosis, treatments, and prevention

A detailed account of the patient's bowel symptoms is necessary to make a diagnosis of IBS. The symptoms experienced in IBS are chronic (present for at least 12 weeks). In cases of IBS, previously performed clinical examinations, including laboratory testing, imaging (CT scanning or abdominal X-rays), or colonoscopy, should have ruled out other explanations.

The treatment of IBS depends on which bowel patterns predominate—constipation, diarrhea, or both—and the severity of pain. Dietary fiber supplementation is often used initially and may improve stool consistency and ease of passage. If diarrhea is a major complaint, antidiarrheal drugs can be prescribed. Similarly, if constipation is a predominant symptom, laxatives or newer agents that stimulate colon contractions can be used. Treating constipation or diarrhea often also improves IBS pain. When pain still persists, tricyclic antidepressants may help reduce bowel pain. Psychotherapy and efforts to reduce stressors may also be helpful if psychological factors contribute to symptoms. Avoidance of foods identified by the patient as triggers of symptoms is worthwhile, and minimizing life stressors is often beneficial.

Gregory Sayuk

KEY FACTS

Description
Abdominal discomfort or pain that is associated with changes in bowel frequency or form.

Symptoms and signs
Abdominal pain, changes in bowel patterns, straining, or passage of mucus with bowel movements.

Causes
Theories include intolerances or allergies, stress, and bacterial infection or overcolonization of the small intestine.

Risk factors
Women are more at risk, as are people with anxiety disorders or depression, recent gastroenteritis, or other family members with IBS.

Diagnosis
A detailed account of the patient's chronic bowel symptoms consistent with the syndrome.

Treatments
Dependent on bowel patterns; options include dietary fiber, antidiarrheal medications, laxatives, antidepressants.

Pathogenesis
Not well established; gut motility, intestinal sensitivity, and bowel inflammation are possible outcomes.

Prevention
Avoidance of foods that precipitate symptoms; minimizing stress.

Epidemiology
Affects 10 to 20 percent of adults, onset from adolescence through 50s, more common in women.

See also
- Allergy and sensitivity • Anxiety disorders
- Food intolerance

Kidney stone

Kidney stones, also called renal calculi, are a common health problem affecting about 5 percent of the population. Kidney stones represent a significant U.S. health problem, and an estimated $2 billion is spent on treatment yearly. Effective medical and surgical treatments are available to manage stones and prevent recurrence.

A kidney stone is a solid piece of material composed of mineral crystals, which form on the inner surfaces of the kidney by precipitation of dissolved substances in the urine. Kidney stones usually form when certain substances in the urine are present at higher than normal concentrations. These substances can precipitate and crystallize, become anchored in the kidney, and increase in size to form a stone. Stone composition can vary, and although stones can form from any material that precipitates in the urine, 80 percent of all stones are composed of calcium. Other common stone compositions include uric acid, struvite (magnesium ammonium phosphate), and cystine.

Although several risk factors for developing stones have been identified, a personal history of kidney stones is the highest risk factor. Other risk factors for stone development include metabolic disorders (gout, gastrointestinal, endocrine, or other kidney problems), genetic disorders (cystinuria, primary hyperoxaluria, renal tubular acidosis), and dietary habits (diets high in green vegetables, fat, dairy products, salt and brewed tea, reduced water intake and dehydration, excess intake of vitamins C and D, and excessive alcohol consumption). Certain medications (especially diuretics or calcium-based antacids), recurrent urinary tract infections, and a family history of kidney stones are also risk factors for the formation of stones.

Symptoms and signs

Symptoms are usually caused by the migration and passage of stones from the kidney into the ureter. Many patients have no symptoms, and stones are detected during diagnosis of other medical conditions.

Pain is the most common symptom and can be intense enough to require hospitalization. The pain associated with stones is termed *renal colic* and usually occurs in paroxysms for up to an hour. Persons may present with lower back pain on the same side of the stone, but may also present with lower abdominal and groin pain, depending on the location of the stone.

Blood in the urine is commonly seen in patients with kidney stones. Urine may be visibly red; however, sometimes blood can be seen only microscopically. Other symptoms include nausea, vomiting, painful urination, and a frequent sensation of needing to urinate. Occasionally patients may pass visible gravel or small stones, but if stones become impacted within the ureter, accompanying fevers and chills can result from subsequent infection of the urinary tract.

Diagnosis and treatments

Diagnosis of kidney stones can be based on clinical presentation and laboratory and radiological examina-

---

KEY FACTS

Description
Mineral stones that form in the kidneys.

Causes
High concentrations of certain substances, such as calcium and uric acid, in the urine.

Risk factors
Personal or family history of kidney stones; cetain metabolic disorders, genetic disorders, and dietary habits; recurrent urinary tract infections.

Symptoms and signs
Often no symptoms; pain; blood in the urine; pain on urination; frequent need to urinate; nausea and vomiting.

Diagnosis
From clinical symptoms; radiological imaging, such as CT scanning, or ultrasound.

Treatments
Pain relief; shock wave lithotripsy; removal using endoscope or through the skin.

Pathogenesis
Left untreated can lead to obstruction, infection, and kidney malfunction.

Prevention
Medications; diet changes; drinking lots of fluids.

Epidemiology
Affects about 5 percent of the U.S. population. Generally more common in older people and men. Caucasians are more commonly affected than African Americans.

tions. Classic signs and symptoms, particularly if one has passed a stone, are all useful for the diagnosis of stones. A number of radiological examinations are available, although the gold standard for diagnosis is computed tomography (CT) scanning. Other radiological modalities include plain abdominal films and intravenous pyelogram, which involves injection of contrast dye and provides visualization of the urinary collecting system. Each of these diagnostic procedures involves exposure to radiation; for the pregnant patient in whom avoidance of radiation is desired, ultrasonography is the safest choice.

Most small stones up to 7 millimeters pass spontaneously; treatment is supportive and aimed at pain management and intravenous hydration to increase urine flow and subsequent stone passage. Nonsteroidal anti-inflammatory drugs (NSAIDs) are effective, but occasionally narcotics are required for effective pain control. Patients can usually be managed at home, but if signs suggest infection as a result of an obstructing stone, hospitalization for intravenous antibiotics may be required. Affected patients should strain their urine to collect any passed stones.

Larger stones more than 7 millimeters require removal. The treatment of choice is shock wave lithotripsy, which directs a high energy shock wave toward the stone, to help break it. Other treatment options include removal through the skin (for larger stones that cannot be broken) and telescopic removal of stones by use of a cystoureteroscope. These procedures are performed by interventional radiologists and urologists, respectively. Once a diagnosis of stones is made, further evaluation identifies risk factors. Urine should be examined for blood and crystals, and collected stones should be sent for analysis to determine their composition (calcium, uric acid, or struvite). Blood and urine tests should be done to rule out metabolic abnormalities, which are key to deciding on therapy aimed at preventing recurrence.

Acute stone disease can lead to obstruction and systemic infection if urinary flow is blocked. Struvite stones can grow rapidly over weeks or months, resulting in chronic obstruction, which, if left untreated, can lead to deterioration of kidney function. Recurrence of kidney stones is relatively high. For those who have been affected with one stone, the likelihood of forming a second stone is about 15 percent at one year, 35 to 40 percent at 5 years, and 80 percent at 10 years.

Recurrent stone formers should collect any passed stones, which can be analyzed. Depending on the stone type, medications are available that may help prevent recurrence. Dietary restrictions eliminate

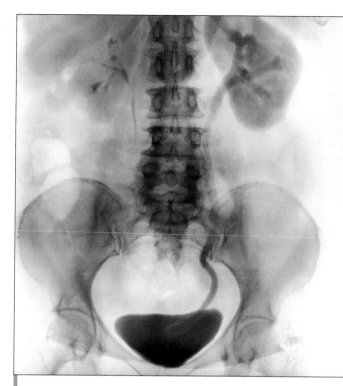

A colored urogram shows a ureter blocked by a kidney stone. The ureter at the right (red) is wide and the renal pelvis that collects the urine is enlarged (red) as a result of urine pooling, unable to pass to the bladder (black).

foods and alter food habits. If the stone type is unknown, it is probably calcium. Regardless of the stone type, patients should be encouraged to drink at least 4 to 6 pints (2 to 3 l) of fluid daily to achieve high urine volume flow. Any infections of the urinary tract should be treated with antibiotics to prevent complications.

The prevalence of stone disease is about 5 percent of the general population, and about 1 in 272 people are newly diagnosed yearly. Kidney stones affect men two to four times more often than women. However, struvite stones, which are typically associated with urinary tract infection, are more common in women. Kidney stones are more common in middle-aged people, and an estimated 12 percent of all men and 5 percent of all women will develop a kidney stone by age 70 years. Caucasians are more commonly affected than African Americans.

Manakan Betsy Srichai
and Matthew Breyer

See also
• Appendicitis

Language and speech disorders

Language and speech disorders are difficulties in communication experienced by children and adults. People with language and speech disorders can have difficulty expressing themselves or understanding others. These difficulties significantly interfere with academic achievement or daily activities that require communication skills. The causes of language and speech disorders can be related to hearing, nerve or muscle disorders, head injury, viral diseases, or physical abnormalities.

Children who have language or speech disorders have difficulty achieving milestones of language development related to expression or comprehension, or both. Verbal communication is vital; if it is delayed, learning difficulties can ensue.

Types of language and speech disorders

There are four main types of language and speech disorders: expressive language disorder, mixed receptive-expressive language disorder, phonological disorder, and stuttering. Standardized tests will usually reveal deficits associated with the area of difficulty. People with language or speech disorders typically have average or above average intelligence.

Expressive language disorder occurs when people have problems expressing themselves using spoken language. Typically, individuals with expressive language disorders have below expected levels in vocabulary, as well as difficulties with the use of tense or production of complex sentences. Language development is usually retarded, and the vocabulary or structure of sentences is limited and simple. Language comprehension in individuals with expressive language disorder is intact.

Individuals with mixed receptive-expressive disorders often have problems expressing themselves using spoken language, and also have problems understanding what people say to them; that is, they have difficulty with language comprehension. This lack of comprehension may result in inappropriate responses, misunderstandings, or failure to follow directions. A child with mixed receptive-expressive disorder often appears to be deaf, but the child does in fact hear.

Individuals with phonological disorders have problems with creating speech at a level expected of their age group because of an inability to form the necessary sounds. The level of severity can range from speech that is completely incomprehensible to speech that can be understood, but in which some sounds are slightly mispronounced.

Stuttering is typically described as a blockage, discoordination, or fragmentations of the flow of speech. Stuttering is often characterized by specific types of disruptions in fluency, such as repetitions of sounds and syllables, prolongation of sounds, and blockages of air flow. Individuals who stutter often show negative reactions to the stuttering, which can make the disorder more severe and difficult.

Causes and risk factors

The brain is divided into various sections that govern different behaviors. Some parts of the brain control the ability to speak, while others control the ability to understand the spoken word or to recognize what words and numbers mean. In people with language disorders, one or more of these areas may not function normally. More specifically, language disorders may be a result of neurological abnormalities that produce impairments in the regions of the brain that control visual and language processing.

Some language disorders may be genetically linked because a person can inherit abnormal brain structure or function. Children from families with a history of language disorders are more likely to develop disorders themselves. Left-handedness appears to increase the risk for expressive language disorder, although the exact reason is unknown.

Structural problems or abnormalities in the areas necessary for speech sound production, such as the tongue or roof of the mouth, can lead to phonological disorders. Neurological problems in which the muscles of the mouth do not work properly can also contribute to phonological disorders.

Finally, in addition to other potential causes, stuttering is often affected by the level of stress present in the environment. An environment that is overly stressful or demanding may cause children to have difficulties developing fluent speech.

Symptoms

In general, the symptoms of language and speech disorders impair an individual's ability to comprehend and produce language, thus making communication with others difficult. The symptoms often vary greatly from one person to the next, but in many cases, individuals are aware of their difficulties in communicating, which can make the disorder even more frustrating and difficult. The presence of language and speech disorders can affect both academic performance and social competence.

Symptoms of expressive language disorders include difficulty in putting sentences together coherently, using proper grammar, recalling the appropriate words to use, and other problems in piecing together conversations. Individuals with expressive language disorder are often not able to communicate their thoughts, needs, or wants at the same level as their peers. Their vocabulary and general sentence structure is generally much more basic and limited than their peers. Individuals with expressive language disorder do, however, understand the material they are trying to communicate to others.

Symptoms of mixed receptive-expressive disorder include those of expressive language disorder. Individuals have difficulty with both producing and understanding spoken language. In addition to problems in expressing language, individuals with mixed receptive disorder also have difficulty understanding what people are saying to them. These individuals may also have difficulty understanding abstract concepts or complex sentences. In addition, individuals with mixed receptive-expressive disorder are more likely to develop other learning disorders, such as reading disorders, so early detection is important.

Individuals with phonological disorders develop speech sounds in the same sequence as their peers, but at a slower rate. Some common mistakes that individuals with phonological disorders will make include omitting sounds (often at the ends of words), distorting sounds, or substituting one sound for another, usually with a sound that is more easily produced.

The primary symptoms of stuttering include excessive problems with fluency in speech, repeating sounds and syllables, and prolonging sounds. Symptoms also include the negative behaviors associated with stuttering that may make stuttering worse.

KEY FACTS

Description

A disorder that involves problems with language expression, comprehension, or a combination of the two.

Causes and risk factors

Thought to involve anomalies in brain structure and function, with various origins. May be also genetically linked or related to different medical conditions. Structural abnormalities related to speech or hearing may also be related.

Symptoms

Diagnosed when performance on standardized tests that measure receptive or expressive language development or sound production is significantly lower than expected for the individual's age, schooling, and level of intelligence.

Diagnosis

After ruling out other medical conditions that may affect performance, such as hearing problems, a series of educational and psychological tests are administered to determine whether achievement is below educational capacity. Diagnosed when a significant discrepancy between standardized scores on expressive or receptive language, or both, and measures on nonverbal intellectual capacity or expected age-appropriate behavior is observed.

Treatments

Usually consists of behaviorally reinforced exercises in practicing basic communication skills, such as vocabulary, sentence construction, sound production, or a combination of all of these necessary skills.

Pathogenesis

Symptoms of language and speech disorders can be present during early childhood. At this time, language develops at a rapid rate, and children with language or speech disorders will appear to fall behind in their development.

Prevention

Because the causes of most language and speech disorders are unclear, there is no obvious way to prevent them.

Epidemiology

For either receptive or expressive language disorders, approximately 1 to 13 percent of school-aged children are affected. Phonological disorders can affect 10 percent of children below 8 years of age and 5 percent of children older than 8 years of age. In the United States the prevalence of stuttering is about 1 percent of the general population, that is, around 3 million people. In all cases, males are almost 4 times more likely to be affected than females.

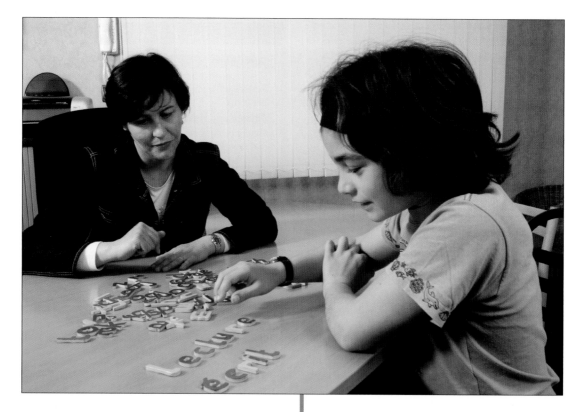

Diagnosis

In order for expressive, mixed receptive-expressive, or phonological disorder to be diagnosed, individuals must be performing or developing at a level below their peers at tasks that require communication. This can be difficult because sometimes an individual may understand the material in a test but have difficulty expressing comprehension. Typically, nonverbal tests are used in addition to tests that require spoken answers. In all cases, hearing should be evaluated.

In order for any of the language disorders to be diagnosed definitively, the communication problems have to create difficulties for the individual in daily life. Finally, when diagnosing stuttering, a speech pathologist will usually collect speech samples from a variety of situations to determine the normal fluency of the individual.

Treatments

Once a language disorder has been diagnosed, one-on-one therapy is usually the preferred treatment. Typically during therapy, the individual will practice basic communication skills repeatedly to develop fluency. For phonological disorders, individuals will practice forming sounds during therapy. Sometimes the individual is shown the physical way the sound is

Children who have language and speech disorders can be helped by a speech therapist, who will devise appropriate exercises and games that include naming or verbal description. For children, early treatment is important because language and speech disorders prevent children from relating to other people and can impinge on learning skills.

made, for example, by showing how to form the lips. In all cases, treatment involves practicing the basic skills necessary for communication (sentence construction, language comprehension, sound production) and also creating an environment at both school and home that is conducive to learning and fluency. This can be done by attempting to minimize stress and being patient with individuals as they learn.

Pathogenesis

Generally, the rapidity and degree of recovery depends on the severity of the disorder, the motivation of the individual to participate in the necessary components of therapy, and how quickly speech and language interventions began. When intervention occurs early, it can sometimes be discontinued by the end of high school. If, however, symptoms are not identified early enough, preferably before school age, or the symptoms are severe, interventions may be necessary into the high school years. With early diagnosis and intervention, the prognosis is usually good, but mild symptoms of language disorders may persist into adult life.

Expressive disorders usually become apparent during early adolescence, when language becomes more complex. By the age of four, most children with expressive language disorder speak in short sentences, but may forget old words or phrases as they learn new ones. With appropriate interventions, however, most children develop normal or nearly normal language skills by high school. In some cases, minor problems with expressive language may never resolve.

With mixed receptive-expressive disorders, the receptive components of the disorder may be apparent between the ages of four and seven. The expressive symptoms may be obvious later as the development of language becomes more complex. If mixed disorder is diagnosed early, it is usually severe in form and will affect the individual throughout life. If the symptoms of the mixed receptive-expressive disorder are milder, the disorder may go undiagnosed for some time, delaying immediate intervention. During this time, other learning disorders may develop, such as reading disorders, which may make the language disorder more obvious but may also hinder intervention.

Phonological disorders are typically diagnosed between the ages of three and six, when speech is developing quickly. Recovery is often spontaneous; those individuals who do not recover before the age of eight will often go on to develop other language and speech problems.

Stuttering usually develops before the age of 12 and peaks during the preschool years when individuals are learning to speak, and later during the elementary school years. During adolescence, stuttering can persist, but usually occurs in response to specific situations, such as reading out loud in class, speaking to strangers, or using the telephone. Fifty to 80 percent of children who stutter will spontaneously recover, but stuttering can continue throughout adult life.

Prevention

There are no known ways of preventing many of the language disorders. In the case of disorders that are caused by damage to the brain, any attempts to avoid any kind of injury could help prevent that type of disorder. In addition, a healthy diet during pregnancy may help prevent neurological or structural problems that can result in a disorder.

Finally, limiting stress during language development may prevent exacerbating already existing disorders and may also encourage development of fluency during therapy for language disorders.

Epidemiology

Language and speech disorders can be relatively common in school-age children and can also be difficult to diagnose. Expressive language disorder is a relatively common childhood disorder, affecting 10 to 15 percent of children under the age of three, and 3 to 7 percent of school-age children. Expressive language disorder is more common in boys than in girls, occurring between two to five times more often.

Mixed receptive-expressive disorder is diagnosed in about 5 percent of preschool-age children and 3 percent of school-age children. It is less common, but more severe, than expressive language disorder. In addition, individuals with mixed receptive-expressive language disorder are more likely to have other types of learning disorders. For example, between 40 to 60 percent of preschool children who have mixed receptive-expressive disorder also have phonological disorder. As many as half of these children may also have some type of reading disorder. They may also be more susceptible to psychiatric disorders, such as attention-deficit hyperactivity disorder (ADHD).

It has been estimated that about 7 to 8 percent of school-age children have phonological disorder. Like the other language disorders, phonological disorders are more common in boys than in girls. Estimates show that boys are up to four times as likely to develop phonological disorders than girls. Children who develop phonological disorders are also more likely to develop some other language problems or disorders.

Stuttering is a relatively low-prevalence disorder. Roughly 1 percent of the general population currently has a stuttering disorder. However, this number differs from the number of individuals who have been diagnosed with stuttering at some point in their lives, which approaches 5 percent. This difference suggests that a significant number of people who develop stuttering problems will often grow out of the problem.

Stuttering is approximately three times more likely in men than in women. This ratio is somewhat lower in childhood, which suggests that females are more likely than men to recover from stuttering problems during childhood.

Lori M. Lieving and
Oleg V. Tcheremissine

See also
• Learning disorders

Learning disorders

Learning disorders are learning difficulties experienced by children and adults of average to above-average intelligence. People with learning disorders have difficulty with reading, writing, or mathematics, or any combination of the three subjects. These difficulties significantly interfere with academic achievement or the ability to carry out daily activities that require any of these three skills.

People with learning disorders have problems collecting new information, remembering and processing that information, and acting on verbal and nonverbal information. The three main types of learning disorders are reading disorders, mathematics disorders, and writing disorders. Standardized tests usually reveal deficits associated with the area of difficulty. Difficulties are due to neurological differences in brain structure or functioning. By definition, people with learning disorders have average or above average intelligence. Thus, they may score poorly on tests, but the low scores are due to a problem with learning, not low intelligence.

Reading disorders

Disorders concerned with reading are the most common type of learning disorder. Individuals with reading disorders have difficulty recognizing letters and words and remembering what they mean (dyslexia). They find it difficult to understand the sounds and letter groups that make up words. Because of these problems, individuals with reading disorders often have impaired performance in reading comprehension.

Mathematic disorders

Individuals with mathematic disorders have problems recognizing numbers (dyscalculia), doing calculations, or understanding abstract mathematical concepts. For example, they may not remember how to use numbers in counting. They have trouble understanding how numbers can apply to everyday situations. A mathematics disorder is present in one of every five cases of a learning disorder. Those with mathematic disorders often have reading or writing disorders as well, or both.

Writing disorders

Individuals with writing disorders have problems with the basic skills of writing, such as spelling, punctuation, and grammar. They have problems with handwriting or with creating sentences that make sense

to others. They often have one other type of learning disorder as well.

Causes

The brain is divided into various sections that control different behaviors. Some parts of the brain control the ability to speak, whereas others control the ability to understand the spoken word or to recognize what words and numbers mean. In people with learning disorders, one or more of these sections may not function normally. Thus, learning disorders may be due to neurological abnormalities that produce impairments in the regions of the brain that control visual and language processing, attention, and planning.

Risk factors

Some learning disorders may have a genetic factor because a person can inherit abnormal brain structure or function. Children from families with a history of learning disorders are more likely to develop disorders themselves. Environmental risk factors for learning disorders include prenatal exposure to a maternal infectious illness, extremely low birth weight, premature birth, birth trauma or distress, or any other factor that can affect the uterine environment, which is so important for healthy brain development. Several factors in early childhood also can contribute to delayed brain development, including neonatal seizures, a poor learning environment, developmental trauma, toxins in the environment, or poor nutrition.

Symptoms

Some individuals earn high scores on intelligence tests, suggesting that they should do well in school, but the grades they receive may be far below what those tests predict. This mismatch may be a sign of a learning disorder. Aside from academic underachievement, other warnings signs that a person may have a learning disorder include overall lack of organization, forgetfulness, and taking unusually long amounts of time to complete assignments. In the classroom, teachers may observe one or more of the following characteristics: difficulty paying attention, unusual sloppiness and disorganization, social withdrawal, difficulty working independently, and problems switching from one activity to another. In addition to these signs related to school and schoolwork, certain general behavioral and emotional features often accompany learning disorders. These include impulsiveness, restlessness, distractibility, poor physical coordination, low tolerance for frustration, low self-esteem, daydreaming, inattentiveness, and anger or sadness.

Symptoms of a reading disorder include difficulty identifying groups of letters, failure to correctly identify the sounds different letters make, reversals and other errors involving letter position, chaotic spelling, difficulty with breaking words into syllables, failure to recognize words, hesitant reading aloud, and word-by-word reading rather than contextual reading.

Symptoms of a writing disorder may often be seen in the kind of written work someone produces. Symptoms include problems with letter formation and writing layout on the page, repetitions and omissions, punctuation and capitalization errors, "mirror writing" (writing right to left), and a variety of spelling problems. Individuals with writing disorders typically take much longer to complete written work than other individuals, often only to produce writing that is large in size and filled with errors.

Individuals with mathematical disorders often cannot count in the correct sequence. They may not be able to name numbers and perform mathematical operations, such as addition and subtraction. Individuals with mathematical disorders may have spatial problems and difficulty aligning numbers into proper columns. They may have difficulty with the abstract concepts of time and direction. For example, they may become confused about the sequences of past or future events. Interestingly, it is common for individuals with mathematical disorders to have normal or accelerated language acquisition, such as verbal skills, reading, writing, and good visual memory for the printed word. They are typically good in the areas of science (until higher-level mathematical skills are needed), geometry (figures with logic, not formulas), and creative arts.

Diagnosis

The first step in diagnosing a learning disorder is conducting a complete medical, psychological, and educational examination. The purpose of this examination is to rule out other conditions with symptoms similar to

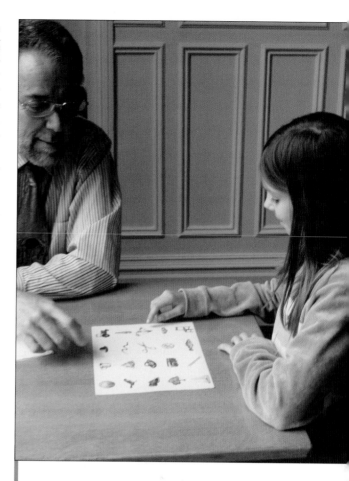

A girl is assessed for dyslexia by an educational psychologist. She is asked to perform a variety of tasks involving words, numbers, and symbols. From her response, the psychologist is able to produce a profile, a unique pattern of strengths and weaknesses, which is then analyzed for evidence of dyslexia.

those of learning disorders. For example, a child with mental retardation, attention-deficit hyperactivity disorder, or an unusually poor educational background may show the symptoms of a learning disorder. These conditions are different from a learning disorder and need to be treated differently. If no medical problems are found, a series of psychological and educational tests is completed. Some of the tests commonly used include the Wechsler Intelligence Scale for Children, the Woodcock-Johnson Psychoeducational Battery, and the Peabody Individual Achievement Test-Revised. These tests measure intelligence and mental achievement. Performance on the standardized tests is compared to actual academic performance. When a significant discrepancy between the two is observed, a specific learning disorder is diagnosed.

Treatments

Once a learning disorder has been diagnosed, special education must be planned, which involves identifying what the individual can and cannot do. After a systematic analysis of learning strengths and weaknesses, an individualized education plan (IEP) is developed that outlines the specific skills that need to be developed. Most effective learning strategies use multiple skills and senses. IEPs may involve special instruction within a regular classroom or assignment to a special-education class. All IEPs also provide for annual retesting to measure the child's progress.

An IEP for an individual with a reading disorder may focus on increasing recognition of the sounds and meanings of letters and words (or phonics training). As training progresses, instruction shifts to improving the ability to understand words and sentences, to remember what has been read, and to learn how to study more efficiently.

Students with writing disorders are often encouraged to keep a daily record of their activities. They often find it easier to express their thoughts by using a computer rather than a paper and pencil. Individuals with mathematical disorders are often given number problems from everyday life. For example, they are taught how to balance a checkbook or compare prices on a shopping trip.

Pathogenesis

In general, although the symptoms of learning disorders may be present before reaching school age, they are seldom recognized or diagnosed prior to the first years of school, when formal education and testing occur. More specifically, the symptoms of a reading disorder may occur as early as kindergarten, but they are seldom diagnosed before the end of kindergarten or the beginning of first grade because formal reading instruction usually does not begin until this point in most schools.

Particularly when associated with high intelligence, individuals may function at or near grade level in the early grades, and reading disorders may not be fully apparent until the fourth grade or later. When intervention occurs early, it can sometimes be discontinued by the end of first or second grade. If, however, symptoms are not identified early enough or the symptoms are severe, interventions may be necessary into high-school years. With early diagnosis and intervention, the prognosis is usually good, but reading disorders may persist into adult life.

Mathematical disorders usually become apparent during second or third grade, or by the age of 8 years. Since the developmental progress of mathematical disorders has yet to be well studied, it is estimated that the symptoms can be diagnosed even into and beyond fifth grade (the age of 10 and later).

KEY FACTS

Description

A developmental disorder that involves problems with reading, writing, mathematics, or a combination of these three disciplines.

Causes and risk factors

Thought to involve anomalies in brain structure and function, with various origins. May be also genetically linked or related to different medical conditions. Toxins *in utero* or in a person's early environment can also cause learning disabilities.

Symptoms

Diagnosed when performance on standardized tests in reading, mathematics, or writing is significantly lower than expected for the individual's age, schooling, and general level of intelligence.

Diagnosis

After ruling out other medical conditions that may affect academic performance, a series of educational and psychological tests are administered to determine whether achievement is below educational capacity. Diagnosed when a significant discrepancy between standardized scores and academic performance is observed.

Treatments

Based on psychoeducational testing, individual education plans (IEPs) are developed that include basic-skill training in the deficient areas, which can be built upon to reach mastery of reading, mathematics, or writing.

Pathogenesis

Symptoms of learning disorders may be present at an early age, but are usually not recognized until individuals reach school age. Typically, reading and mathematical disorders will be recognized before writing disorders.

Prevention

Early intervention may allow prevention of prolonged academic difficulties that may adversely affect family relationships and occupational outcomes.

Epidemiology

Learning disorders affect about 2 million children between the ages of 6 and 17, and one in every seven people in the United States. The male to female ratio for learning disorders is about 5:1. Reading disorders represent four out of every five cases of a learning disorder.

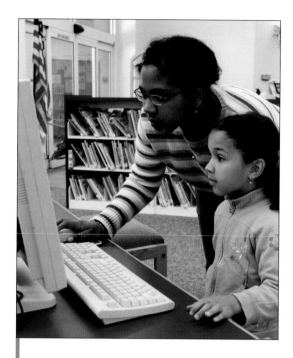

Children who have writing disorders often find that using a computer is easier than writing on paper. They record daily activities to help improve their writing skills.

Because individuals usually learn to speak and read well before writing well, reading disorders are usually diagnosed first, and writing disorders are diagnosed last. Thus, writing disorders are usually apparent by the age of 7 but may not be recognized until the age of 10 or later, with the more severe cases being identified earlier.

As with most other learning disorders, early discovery and intervention is of the utmost importance. Writing disorders may occasionally be seen in older children or adults, but little is known about their long-term prognosis.

Prognosis

The outlook is good for individuals who are diagnosed with learning disorders early in their school years. Early diagnosis allows the development of individualized education plans that will help affected people overcome their disorders. Learning disorders continue into adulthood, but most people who receive proper educational and vocational training can complete college and find a satisfying job.

Studies of the occupational choices of adults with dyslexia indicate that they do particularly well in people-oriented professions and occupations, such as nursing and sales.

Prevention

Although there may be no way to completely prevent the occurrence of a learning disorder, it is important to prevent the symptoms of learning disorders from going undiagnosed. The high school dropout rate for individuals with learning disorders is almost 40 percent. Many of these individuals are never properly diagnosed or given appropriate instruction. As a result, they never become fully literate.

In addition, 10 to 25 percent of individuals with learning disorders also meet criteria for other disorders, such as conduct disorder, oppositional-defiant disorder, attention-deficit hyperactivity disorder, major depressive disorder, or dysthymic disorder.

Learning disorders can lead to other problems. Individuals may become frustrated and discouraged. They may not learn how to get along with other people and become aggressive and troublesome. In addition, learning problems may be stressful for family members and subsequently strain family relationships.

Epidemiology

One in every seven people in the United States has a learning disorder. Learning disorders affect about 2 million children between the ages of 6 and 17, or about 5 percent of schoolchildren. The male to female ratio for learning disorders is about 5:1. More specifically, reading disorders represent four out of every five cases of a learning disorder. Research shows that 60 to 80 percent of individuals with a reading disorder are males. However, the rate of reading disorders in boys may be inflated; boys' reading disorders are usually noticed because of behavioral difficulties in the classroom. As individuals with reading disorders become adults, the sex differences are no longer present.

The prevalence of mathematical disorders has not yet been well established, but is estimated to be about 5 percent. There is an expectation that mathematical disorders are more likely in girls than boys. Similarly, while the prevalence of writing disorders is not well established, it has been estimated to be present in about 3 to 10 percent of schoolchildren.

Oleg Tcheremissine
and Lori Lieving

See also
• Attention-deficit hyperactivity disorder
• Language and speech disorders

Legionnaires' disease

Legionnaires' disease is infection with *Legionella* bacteria, which may cause pneumonia (inflammation of the lungs). Members of the American Legion at a convention in Philadelphia in 1976 suffered an outbreak of a short-term, feverish respiratory illness, which led to the discovery of the disease.

The incidence of Legionnaires' disease depends on the degree of contamination of water reservoirs with *Legionella* bacteria, the susceptibility of the host, and the extent of the exposure to that water. The infection is thought to be contracted through airborne transmission of contaminated water from heat-exchange systems, respiratory therapy devices, whirlpools, shower stalls, and humidifiers. Person-to-person transmission has not been found to occur.

Those at risk for this disease are people who live or work near construction sites, those with long-term lung disease or diabetes, alcoholics, smokers, people with HIV infection, and victims of trauma. Legionnaires' disease can occur at any age.

Symptoms and signs

Legionnaires' disease has two forms: Pontiac fever and *Legionella* pneumonia. Pontiac fever has a one- to two-day incubation period, followed by flulike symptoms of fever, chills, muscle aches, and headaches. This form is usually of brief duration, with full recovery in one week and a low mortality rate. No pneumonia occurs, although there may be a cough and chest pain.

The incubation period for *Legionella* pneumonia is 2 to 10 days. Those affected have fever, chills, headache, malaise, dry cough, and shortness of breath. Half of the patients will have gut symptoms of no appetite, diarrhea, nausea or vomiting, and possibly chest pain and coughing up streaks of blood. The patient looks ill, with rapid breathing patterns and a slow heart rate. Mental status can range from confusion to coma. Complications cam include respiratory failure, shock, coma, and heart problems.

Diagnosis, treatments, and prevention

In infected people, blood tests show a high white blood cell (WBC) count. Blood levels of sodium and phosphorus may be checked because they are commonly low in infected people. Examination of sputum typically shows numerous WBCs with few or no *Legionella* cells.

Most infected people show improvement in 12 to 48 hours after starting antibiotics such as azithromycin. If the source of the disease is the hospital water supply, prevention of hospital-acquired disease is possible. Using monochloramine to disinfect community water supplies has decreased the risk of infection.

Epidemiology

In the United States, between 8,000 and 18,000 people are hospitalized each year with Legionnaires' disease, about 15 percent of whom die from its effects. *Legionella* is more frequent in hospitalized patients, especially those in intensive care units.

Isaac Grate

KEY FACTS

Description
A type of pneumonia.

Causes
Legionella bacteria.

Risk factors
Working or living near construction sites; having lung disease, diabetes, alcoholism, HIV infection, or an injury; smoking.

Symptoms and signs
Fever, headache, malaise, cough, nausea, chest pain, vomiting, diarrhea, blood-streaked sputum.

Diagnosis
Exam of sputum; blood tests.

Treatments
Azithromycin is the drug of choice.

Pathogenesis
People in good health can recover in 2 to 3 weeks; anyone with weakened immunity may die.

Prevention
Monochloramine disinfecting of communities' water supplies has decreased the risk of *Legionella* infection.

Epidemiology
The disease accounts for 2 to 9 percent of community-acquired pneumonia and has a fatality rate of 15 percent.

See also
• Pleurisy • Pneumonia

Leprosy

Leprosy is a chronic bacterial infection that is a worldwide health problem. Also called Hansen's disease, leprosy causes skin lesions and damages nerves, usually in the limbs and face. There has often been stigma associated with leprosy. Although many still remain afflicted, the prognosis of this condition has dramatically improved with appropriate therapy and continuing public health efforts.

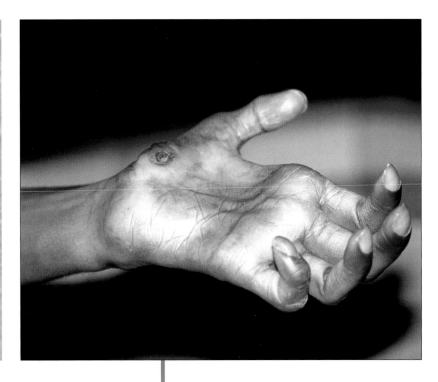

*Nerve damage, as a result of infection with **Mycobacterium leprae**, causes numbness of the hands. The lack of feeling can lead to injury and sometimes loss of the fingers.*

Leprosy is caused by the bacterium *Mycobacterium leprae*. It is a type of bacteria that replicates very slowly and grows best at temperatures of 27°C to 33°C (80.6°F–91.4°F). It is a hardy organism that can survive outside the body for several weeks. It grows well in cooler areas of the human body, such as skin, mucous membranes, and superficial nerves.

Risk factors

The strongest risk factor for leprosy is close contact with infected patients, because the bacterium can be transmitted through the respiratory route, by inhalation of infected nasal secretions. Advanced age and impaired immune function may predispose patients to leprosy. Various poorly defined genetic factors may also increase the risk of developing certain types of the disease. It does not appear that humans acquire leprosy through contact with animals.

Symptoms and signs

The clinical features vary widely. Because the organisms grow slowly, the incubation period ranges from several months to many years. In its earliest form, there may be a localized area of flat skin discoloration. In most people this resolves spontaneously without therapy; however, it can progress to more severe disease in a minority of patients. The area of skin involvement may remain localized but can spread anywhere on the body and often progresses to elevated or nodular lesions. The color of these lesions is usually red, but sometimes they lack pigment. Invasion of the nasal and laryngeal mucosa may also occur, resulting in cartilage erosion and perforation. Another common feature of the bacterium is its ability to infect nerves, typically those closer to the surface of the skin. The affected nerves often enlarge and can be palpated. As a result, there may be progressive impairment in sensation and motor strength, depending on the site of involvement. In severe cases, the organism may infect the nerves of the eyes and lead to blindness. Leprosy is rarely fatal but is a chronic condition that can result in severe disfigurement and disability.

Diagnosis and treatments

The diagnosis of leprosy requires observation of one or more of the three cardinal signs: a characteristic skin patch with loss of sensation, thickened peripheral nerves, and the presence of the bacteria on skin smear or biopsy. The bacterium cannot be grown on laboratory media, and blood tests are not helpful in diagnosis.

There are several different antibiotics available, including rifampin, dapsone, clofazimine, and clarithromycin. A combination of these medications, also called multidrug therapy (MDT), taken over prolonged periods (6 to 12 months), is required for successful treatment. Patients should be monitored closely during therapy for any signs of nerve damage or adverse effects of treatment to try to prevent long-term disability. Treatment also involves an educational element regarding the nature of leprosy and the importance of adhering to prolonged courses of therapy.

Pathogenesis and prevention

The exact mode of transmission is unknown. However, the infection is most commonly spread from person to person through aerosol spread of nasal secretions and inhalation by the uninfected host. Once inside the body, bacteria can spread to distant sites. It grows best at superficial areas including skin and mucous membranes. The bacterium preferentially attacks cells of peripheral nerves. It replicates very slowly, which accounts for the chronicity of the disease. Host cells are damaged by invading bacteria but also by the inflammation that ensues as the human immune response attempts to contain the infection.

People should avoid close contact with leprosy patients until the patient has started on treatment. This includes household contacts. A key to preventing the spread of leprosy lies in early detection of the disease and prompt treatment. Once a person has taken MDT for several days, he or she is no longer infectious to others and does not need to be isolated from society. There is no vaccine that is approved for prevention of leprosy. A vaccine called BCG vaccine, commonly given outside the United States for possible protection against tuberculosis, may provide partial immunity.

Epidemiology

Leprosy is extremely uncommon in the United States and other developed nations. About 100 to 150 cases are reported in the United States annually, and most of these are diagnosed in immigrants. Most cases of leprosy are found in developing countries, particularly in areas of poverty and overcrowding. Leprosy most commonly occurs in tropical and warm temperate areas such as Africa, Asia, and Central America. In 1985, about 12 million people were afflicted with lep-

rosy. The World Health Organization (WHO) has launched a campaign aimed toward the elimination of leprosy. Since that time, the number of leprosy patients has fallen to around 600,000 worldwide. Efforts toward complete elimination are ongoing but unlikely to be achieved in the near future.

Joseph M. Fritz and Nigar Kirmani

KEY FACTS

Description
A chronic bacterial infection that most commonly causes skin lesions and nerve damage.

Causes
Mycobacterium leprae, an organism that can survive outside the body for several weeks.

Risk factors
Close contact with those infected. Age, poor immune function, and genetic factors may also predispose people to develop leprosy.

Symptoms and signs
Typically starts as a localized area of skin discoloration. The skin lesions may progress and can spread anywhere on the body with widely varying appearances. The infection spreads to nerves, and damage results in both motor and sensory impairments. Disfigurement and disability commonly occur with advanced disease.

Diagnosis
Characteristic skin lesions with loss of sensation, thickened peripheral nerves, and identification of typical bacteria in skin biopsy.

Treatments
Multiple antibiotics available. Multidrug therapy (MDT) is required for at least 6 to 12 months.

Pathogenesis
Bacteria living in secretions of those infected spread via aerosol route to susceptible patients and enter new host through respiratory tract. Bacteria most commonly infiltrate cells in skin and nerves.

Prevention
Avoidance of those infected until therapy has been started. Early recognition and treatment of disease also helps prevent spread to others. No vaccine available specifically for leprosy.

Epidemiology
In 2002, about 600,000 patients worldwide. Most cases in tropical and warm temperate areas. Only 100 to 150 cases per year in the United States.

See also
• Antibiotic-resistant infections

Leukemia

Leukemia is the malignant growth of leukocytes (white blood cells). There are four main types of leukemias: acute lymphocytic leukemia (ALL), acute myelogenous leukemia (AML), chronic lymphocytic leukemia (CLL), and chronic myelogenous leukemia (CML). Leukemias are classified according to the particular type of cancerous cell and how quickly the cancer progresses. Current treatments have the potential to cure leukemia.

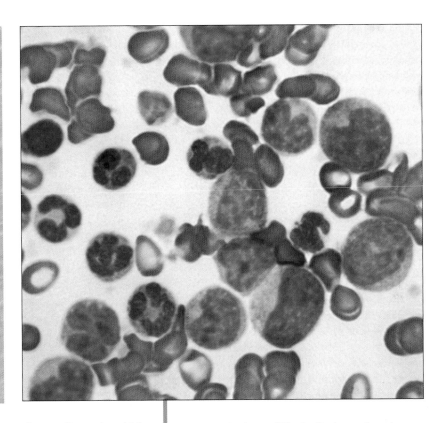

A microscopic picture of blood cells shows a large increase in the number of abnormal white blood cells (purple). These cells do not function properly, and they crowd out the red blood cells (red) and prevent the formation of normal white blood cells. As a result, someone with leukemia is unable to fight off infection, bleeds easily, and tends to become anemic.

Leukemia is an acute or chronic disease in which there is an abnormal increase in white blood cells in the blood and tissues. The word *leukemia* is derived from the Greek *leuk*, meaning "white," and *emia*, meaning "blood."

There are three types of cells in blood: white blood cells (leukocytes), which fight infection and disease; red blood cells, which carry oxygen and carbon dioxide to and from the cells of the body; and platelets (also called thrombocytes), which help form blood clots to control bleeding. When there are genetic changes in the DNA of leukocytes that cause them to grow uncontrollably, the resulting cancer of these cells is called leukemia. Anyone can develop leukemia, and people of all ages and both sexes can be affected.

Blood cells are made in bone marrow, the soft, spongy substance in the middle part of bones. When leukemia develops, the production of white blood cells becomes so rapid that red blood cells and platelets are crowded out and become reduced in number. Impaired white blood cells can lead to serious and life-threatening infections; and fewer platelets can lead to bruising or bleeding. Low numbers of red blood cells (anemia)

can cause weakness and fatigue. When cancerous white blood cells leave the bone marrow and travel through the bloodstream, the cancer may metastasize (spread) to other parts of the body such as the liver, spleen, lymph nodes, testes, and brain. Leukemia is related to lymphoma, which is the cancer of lymphocytes, the white blood cells that circulate in the lymphatic system.

There are two kinds of abnormal white blood cells that cause leukemia. If the cancerous changes have occurred in lymphocytes or in cells that normally produce lymphocytes, the disease is called lymphocytic leukemia. If the cancerous changes are in cells that normally produce neutrophils, basophils, eosinophils, and monocytes, the disease is called myelogenous leukemia. Leukemias may also be acute or chronic. In acute leukemia, cancer cells are blasts (immature cells) that grow quickly, whereas chronic leukemia cells are a combination of immature and mature cells and grow more slowly. There are six types of leukemias, which are identified according to the speed of growth and the type of cancer cell. Acute lymphocytic leukemia (ALL) is the most common leukemia found in children and in some cases adults over the age of 65. Acute myelogenous leukemia (AML) is a type of leukemia that almost always affects adults and is rarely seen in children. It is also called acute nonlymphocytic leukemia (ANLL). Chronic lymphocytic leukemia (CLL) usually affects adults over age 55 and sometimes is found in younger adults, but it almost never affects children. Chronic myelogenous leukemia (CML) is a type of leukemia that almost always affects adults and is extremely rare in children. Hairy cell leukemia and acute promyelocytic leukemia are two forms of leukemia that are extremely rare in both adults and children.

Causes and risk factors

The cause of leukemia is a change in the DNA of leukocytes that causes abnormalities and uncontrolled multiplication of these cells. The cause for this change in DNA is not known. However, there are several known risk factors such as family history, diseases present at birth, exposure to carcinogens, and infection by viruses. Chromosomal disorders present at birth, such as Down syndrome, are associated with a higher risk of leukemia. In addition, chronic and high exposure to industrial carcinogens such as benzene and toluene can lead to leukemia. Furthermore, certain viruses, such as human immunodeficiency virus (HIV, responsible for AIDS) or human T-lymphotropic viruses (HTLV-1 and HTLV-2), are linked to some forms of leukemia. Fanconi anemia, a rare genetic disease, is also a risk factor for developing leukemias.

Although researchers continue to investigate the causes of leukemia, what is already known is that leukemia is not contagious and cannot be transmitted from person to person.

Hematopoiesis is the term for the development of blood cells. Before birth, hematopoiesis occurs in the yolk sac, then the liver, and eventually in the bone marrow. In normal adults it occurs in bone marrow (myeloid tissue) and lymphatic tissues. All blood cells develop from pluripotential stem cells, which are undifferentiated cells that are able to divide and differentiate into other cell types. In other words, stem cells can produce offspring cells to become whatever kind of cell that its environment dictates. Stem cells are not committed to becoming any particular kind of cell, such as

liver or skin cells. Pluripotential hemopoietic stem cells are the precursor cells that give rise to all the blood cell types of both the myeloid and lymphoid lineages.

If a mutation occurs in the genes of hemopoietic stem cells, the result is usually uncontrollable growth of cells in that lineage. For example, a mutation in myeloid stem cells will probably lead to myelogenous leukemia. Leukemia cells ultimately live in the bone marrow, constantly making new cancer cells and suppressing the function of cells that develop into normal blood cells. By circulating in the blood, leukemia cells may also invade other organs, including the liver, spleen, lymph nodes, testes, and brain.

Symptoms and signs

Symptoms of leukemia are general and can sometimes be confused with other disorders or even ignored.

KEY FACTS

Description

Malignant, excessive growth of leukocytes (white blood cells).

Causes

Environmental carcinogens and heredity cause changes in leukocyte DNA that alter its ability to control growth.

Risk factors

Family history of cancer, Down syndrome, viral infection, and exposure to environmental carcinogens, such as benzene and toluene.

Symptoms

Fatigue, weakness, unexplained weight loss, shortness of breath, easy bruising and bleeding, persistent low-grade fever, bone pain, and abdominal pain.

Diagnosis

Examination of blood cells and bone marrow biopsy.

Treatment

Drug therapy or radiation, often in combination with bone marrow transplant.

Pathogenesis

Develops from mutations in stem cells of the bone marrow; likely progression not known.

Prevention

Reduction of contact with environmental carcinogens and in the case of family history, regular visits to the doctor for full physical examinations.

Epidemiology

About 35,000 people in the United States are diagnosed with one of the types of leukemias each year.

Feelings of chronic fatigue, weakness, and shortness of breath from anemia are some of the initial symptoms.

Observation of enlarged lymph nodes, easy bruising and bleeding, pain in joints and bones, recurrent infections, abdominal pain due to an enlarged spleen or liver, and unexplained fever may cause a person to seek medical attention.

Diagnosis

At the present time, there is no definitive screening test for diagnosing leukemia. Routine blood tests such as those for employment, military service, pregnancy, and before surgery are typically the ways in which leukemias are discovered. One of these routine tests includes a complete blood count in which all the cells in blood are analyzed. This test provides information about the white blood cell, red blood cell, and platelet populations. This information includes the number, type, size, shape, and some of the physical characteristics of the cells.

If these results are abnormal, further testing of bone marrow or spinal fluid can be carried out to determine if leukemia cells are present and how far they may have spread. Imaging through X-rays or computed tomography (CT) scans of the chest, abdomen, and pelvis can show whether or not the disease has spread to these areas. Furthermore, chromosome analysis may show certain genetic changes that are associated with leukemia. Based on this combined information, the type of leukemia and the stage of the disease are determined.

Treatments

Treatments for leukemia may include drug therapy, radiation, or bone marrow or stem cell transplant. Both drug therapy (chemotherapeutic or immunological agents) and radiation can begin to kill or slow down cancerous cells, but these treatments rarely cure leukemia. The most effective strategy for curing leukemia involves using drug and radiation therapies in combination with bone marrow transplantation. In bone marrow transplantation, normal stem cells from blood or marrow from a matched donor are injected into the patient's blood. The stem cells enter the marrow and start producing normal blood cells. In some cases, the patient's own stem cells may be used.

The goal of treatment for leukemia is to bring about a complete remission. When a patient is in complete remission, it means that there is no evidence of the disease and the patient returns to good health with normal blood and marrow cells. However, sometimes a relapse can occur, indicating a return of the cancerous cells and the return of leukemia's associated signs and symptoms.

Pathogenesis

The outcome is unpredictable and varies from patient to patient. A patient suffering from chronic lymphocytic leukemia may live with the disease for many years and die from other causes. Alternatively, some people receive many forms of therapy and die of the disease within a few years.

Prevention

In most cases, nothing can be done to prevent leukemia from occurring. Small preventive measures can be taken by avoiding exposure to environmental carcinogens and viruses that are associated with leukemia. In the case of family history, regular visits to the doctor for full physical examinations can help detect early stages of leukemia and initiate treatment.

Epidemiology

In the early part of the twenty-first century, 198,257 people in the United States were living with leukemia, and it is estimated that almost 35,000 new cases of leukemia will be diagnosed yearly in the United States. Most cases of leukemia occur in older adults; more than half of all cases occur after age 67. The most common types of leukemias in adults are acute myelogenous leukemia (AML) and chronic lymphocytic leukemia (CLL).

In children 14 years old and younger, about 35 percent of all cancers are leukemia. The most common form of leukemia in children is acute lymphocytic leukemia (ALL). Nearly 62 percent of new cases of ALL occur among children.

Incidence rates for all types of leukemia are slightly higher among males than among females; in 2005, it was estimated that males accounted for 56 percent of the new cases of leukemia. Leukemia is also more common in Americans of European descent than among those of African descent.

Rashmi Nemade

See also
- AIDS • Anemia • Down syndrome
- Hodgkin's disease • Lymphoma

Lice infestation

Lice infestations occur in every part of the world. Two genera of sucking lice, *Pediculus* and *Phthirus,* are parasitic for humans. *Pediculus humanus* var. *capitis* (head louse) and *Pediculus humanus* var. *corporis* (body louse) are similar flattened grayish insects, 2–4 millimeters in size. *Phthirus pubis* (pubic or crab louse) is round and 2–3 millimeters long.

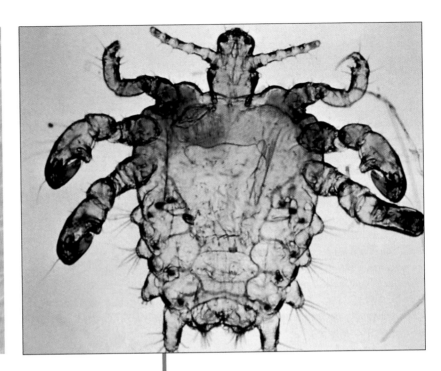

This is a greatly enlarged picture of Phthirus pubis, *the pubic or crab louse. The pubic louse is about 2 millimeters across. It is transmitted through sexual contact and infests the pubic region in adults and the eyelashes of affected children.*

Lice are small insects that live by feeding on human blood. They are wingless and spread by moving from person to person.

Pediculosis capitis

Head lice live on the scalp and can be transferred by close personal contact, as well as sharing of combs, hats, towels, and bed linen. Schoolchildren and their families are affected most often. Infestation is common, but it is not related to personal hygiene.

The adult female lays seven to ten eggs (nits) daily, which are firmly attached to the hair shaft of the scalp and occasionally to the beard. Nits hatch in one week and must feed on blood. Adult lice can survive for two days without a host. Inflammatory responses can cause intense itching of the scalp; a tickling feeling of movement and excoriations (abrasions) from scratching are additional clinical manifestations of infestation, although some children may be asymptomatic. Secondary bacterial infection and cervical lymphadenopathy (swollen glands in the neck) can occasionally occur.

The diagnosis of lice infestation is made by finding the louse or nits. Using a fine toothed nit comb is more effective than visual inspection. Nits that are attached to hairs close to the scalp indicate active infection.

Treatment with topical pediculicides (1 percent premethrin rinse, gamma benzene hexachloride shampoo, pyrethrins, and malathion) is effective in 95 percent of cases. However, resistance is emerging. Scalp application is repeated in one week because nits are more resistant to treatment than adult lice. Lindane shampoo is associated with neurotoxicity in rats and offers no advantage over other agents.

Nits should be removed by applying a solution of equal parts vinegar and water, then combing the hair with a fine-toothed comb soaked in a pediculicide. Taking oral ivermectin, 200 milligrams per kilogram of body weight as a single dose, with a repeat dose two weeks later, is an alternative to using topical agents.

The most common causes of treatment failure are lack of compliance and continued contact with infested individuals. On the other hand, "no-nit" policies in many school districts may be excessive, as many children with nits do not develop active infection.

To prevent reinfection, all clothing and bed linen must be washed in very hot water. To halt the spread of infestation, contacts of the people infected should be traced and alerted to the problem. If found to be infected, close contacts should be treated with a topical pediculicide, which is an agent that destroys lice.

Pediculosis corporis

Body lice are seen where overcrowding and poor sanitation exist, and they are a problem of homelessness and poverty. The body louse lays its nits on the seams of clothing, where they are viable for up to one month. Body lice are a vector for epidemic typhus, trench fever, and relapsing fever.

Itching is the chief complaint. Macules (patches of skin of a different color), papules (small elevations on the skin), and excoriations are seen on the trunk, often as a result of secondary bacterial infection. Generalized hyperpigmentation and thickening of the skin can occur with chronic infestation (vagabond's disease).

The patient should be bathed thoroughly. Clothing and linen should be discarded or laundered in very hot water and then ironed. A rinse of 1 percent premethrin or other pediculicide may be applied to the body if nits are found on body hair.

Phthirus pubis

The pubic (or crab) louse is transmitted by sexual or close body contact, but children can be affected by transmission of the lice from their parents. The life span of the female louse is three to four weeks, and she lays three eggs per day, which are cemented to the base of a hair and hatch after six to eight days. The pubic hair is generally infested, but armpits, chest hair, and eyebrows can also be affected by the lice.

Although some people are unaware of any symptoms, many people notice the signs of pubic lice. Sometimes they leave small spots or tiny specks of blood on the skin, and the brown eggs may also be noticed. However, the primary complaint is marked itching in the affected areas. Macules and papules may be seen but are less severe than in other forms of pediculosis. Small blue spots (maculae cerulae) are the result of injection of an anticoagulant saliva into the skin when the louse feeds. Infestation of the eyelashes causes crusting of the lids and an associated conjunctivitis.

Diagnosis is made by detection of the louse or nits. Evaluation for other sexually transmitted diseases is important, as coinfections are common.

Pubic lice can be treated with 1 percent permethrin cream rinse, 1 percent lindane shampoo, pyrethrins with piperonyl butoxide, or malathion. Ivermectin or 5 percent permethrin cream can be used for treatment failure. It is important to treat all sexual contacts at the same time to prevent cross infection.

Bedding and clothing should be machine washed in water that is hotter than a temperature of 140°F (60°C) and dried in a hot dryer. Eyelid infestation can be treated by applying petrolatum for eight days, or by giving two doses of ivermectin one week apart.

Nigar Kirmani

KEY FACTS

Description

Infestation of the scalp (head lice), seams of clothing (body lice), or pubic hair (crab lice).

Causes

Pediculus humanus var. *capitis* (head louse), *Pediculus humanus* var. *corporis* (body louse), and *Phthirus pubis* (pubic or crab louse).

Symptoms and signs

Itching of the scalp, body, or genital area. Itching leads to macules, papules, and excoriations.

Diagnosis

Detection of the louse or nits.

Treatment

Application of topical pediculicides (1 percent premethrin rinse, pyrethrins, malathion) is used for head and pubic lice. Thorough bathing and washing of clothes and bedding is required for body lice.

Pathogenesis

The adult female lays eggs or nits, which are cemented to the hair shaft on the scalp, pubic hair, or seams of clothing. Nits hatch and must feed on blood to survive.

Prevention

Avoiding the sharing of combs and hats prevents head lice. Improved sanitation and attention to personal hygiene eliminates body lice. Avoidance of sexual or close body contact with infested individuals and treatment of sexual contacts eliminates pubic lice.

Epidemiology

Lice infestation occurs worldwide. Head lice occurs in persons from all socioeconomic backgrounds and is very frequent in school children. Overcrowding and poor personal hygiene lead to body lice. Pubic lice are transmitted by sexual or close body contact.

See also
• Lyme disease

Lou Gehrig's disease

Lou Gehrig's disease is an incurable, debilitating disease in which the nerve cells that control muscular movement die, leading to weakness, wasting and rigidity of muscles, and paralysis. The cause of Lou Gehrig's disease is unknown. One form of the disease is linked to a gene mutation that runs in families.

Lou Gehrig's disease (a type of motor neuron disease), also called amyotrophic lateral sclerosis, is named after the U.S. baseball player who died from the disease. *Amyotrophic* simply means that there is no muscle growth, *lateral* refers to the position in the spinal cord of nerve cells called motor neurons, and *sclerosis* indicates the hardening of tissues that results from cell death. Motor neurons normally control muscle activity. Lower motor neurons, which are found in the spinal cord, directly activate muscles; upper motor neurons, which occur in the front part of the brain, regulate the activity of spinal motor neurons and indirectly influence muscle function. In Lou Gehrig's disease, both types of motor neurons die, and the related muscles stop functioning and waste away.

Symptoms

The onset of Lou Gehrig's disease is gradual, and symptoms, which appear over months, are variable. In the early stages, a person may experience fatigue, muscle twitching, weakness of limb muscles, slurred speech, difficulty swallowing, or uncontrolled laughing and crying. Later symptoms include increasing weakness, rigidity, and wasting of muscles, followed by paralysis. Breathing difficulties can occur if the muscles that control respiration are affected. Some people deteriorate rapidly; in others, there is a spontaneous slowing, or arrest, of the disease. Lou Gehrig's disease does not usually affect the senses or mental faculties. Respiratory arrest or pneumonia are often the cause of death.

Diagnosis

There is no specific test; diagnosis involves tests to rule out other diseases. Comprehensive neurological exams are followed by electromyography, X-rays and MRIs (magnetic resonance imaging) of the brain and spinal cord, nerve conduction tests, testing of blood, urine, and hormones, and muscle and nerve biopsies.

Treatments and epidemiology

There is no cure for Lou Gehrig's disease. The only FDA-approved drug for treating the disease is Rilutek, which slightly slows the progression of the disease. Other drugs, including growth factors to stimulate cell formation, are currently being tested, as are stem cells and gene therapy. Research into genetic factors is underway. Lou Gehrig's disease is diagnosed in 5,600 Americans annually; 93 percent of those affected are of Caucasian origin.

Sonal Jhaveri

KEY FACTS

Description

Also called amyotrophic lateral sclerosis (ALS). The disease causes progressive muscle wasting and paralysis.

Causes

Unknown.

Risk factors

More likely to affect people above the age of 50, particularly men.

Symptoms

Rigidity, twitching, and weakness in limb muscles; slurred speech; tripping; fatigue; difficulty swallowing; trouble with daily activities; progressive paralysis.

Diagnosis

Tests include: neurological exams, electromyography, measuring nerve conduction, spine imaging, nerve and muscle biopsy, spinal tap, and tests of blood, urine, and hormones.

Treatments

Drug treatment with Rilutek provides some relief and slows the progression of the disease.

Pathogenesis

Ongoing degeneration of nerve cells.

Prevention

None. Genetic counseling is offered when Lou Gehrig's disease runs in families.

Epidemiology

About 30,000 people are affected in the United States, of whom 5–10 percent have a genetic form of the disease. Lou Gehrig's disease is 1½ times more common in men than in women.

See also
• Paralysis

Lupus

Lupus is a chronic, complex systemic autoimmune disease that primarily affects young women of all ethnic backgrounds. The signs and symptoms of the disease are highly variable and can affect virtually any organ or tissue in the body. No two cases of lupus are alike, and the pattern of symptoms can change over time in a single individual. About 1 to 4 in every 1,000 women are affected by lupus; rates of the disease are about 10 times lower for men.

The immune system has evolved to eliminate infectious organisms, infected cells, and other abnormal cells from the body by first recognizing the unwanted substances as "foreign" to the body, then mounting an inflammatory attack to destroy the foreign cells. For reasons that remain unknown, the immune system in lupus patients begins to recognize normal, healthy cells and tissues as "foreign" and mounts an immune response against them. It is currently believed that lupus patients inherit genetic predisposition (probably a combination of multiple genes) toward developing the disease, but then another stimulus, likely environmental, triggers the onset of the disease itself. The influence of heredity can be seen in identical twin studies; the risk of developing lupus in an identical twin of an affected patient is nearly 50 percent. However, most cases of lupus occur in people without a family history of the disease. Some possible environmental triggers may include certain viruses like Epstein-Barr infection (which causes mononucleosis) and sunlight. Sex hormones have also been considered as a trigger; however, the exact causes of lupus remain unknown.

Symptoms and signs

Because lupus can affect almost any organ or tissue in the body, there are numerous symptoms that can be present, and these may change over time. Symptoms are generally the result of an inflammatory attack of the tissues. They may range from mild and barely noticeable to severe permanent organ damage or death. The most commonly affected tissues include the skin, joints, blood vessels, blood cells, and lining around the heart and lungs. Patients often experience rashes across the bridge of the nose, extreme sensitivity to the

sun, sores in the mouth, hair loss, and swelling in the joints. Chest pain when breathing deeply and a sensation of shortness of breath may occur if there is inflammation of the lining of the heart or lungs. In more severe cases, the immune response will be directed against the kidneys. Early symptoms may include swelling of the lower legs, headaches, and high blood pressure. When lupus is in remission or is mildly active, there may be no symptoms at all. Physicians rou-

KEY FACTS

Description

A chronic noninfectious autoimmune disease, in which the immune system attacks any variety of organs and tissues in the body.

Causes

Unknown.

Risk factors

Female gender, pregnancy, family members with lupus, and unknown environmental exposures (viruses, sunlight, and hormones).

Symptoms and signs

Rashes on the face and body, hair loss, swollen joints, and sores in the mouth.

Diagnosis

Examination by a specialist in rheumatology; careful assessment of symptoms and blood tests. The diagnosis can take many months to confirm.

Treatments

Many different medications that suppress the immune system can be used, depending on the organs involved.

Pathogenesis

Lupus is characterized by flare-ups and remissions and can range from very mild to more severe. Kidneys are the most common major organ to be affected. Before good treatments were available, kidney failure was very common.

Prevention

No known strategies to prevent the onset of lupus, but flares can be minimized by avoiding direct sun exposure, refraining from smoking, and taking medications as prescribed.

Epidemiology

Prevalence estimates range from 50 to 150 in 100,000 adults. Women are affected nine times more commonly than men. The most common ages at diagnosis are between 15 and 45. About 20 percent of lupus cases are diagnosed before the age of 20.

tinely check blood and urine tests in asymptomatic patients to detect and treat any indications of lupus activity before symptoms become apparent.

Diagnosis

There is no single test that can make a diagnosis of lupus. Experienced physicians rely on a series of 11 criteria, four of which must be present currently or in the past to make the diagnosis. The majority of these criteria are physical symptoms, and only a few are based solely upon laboratory tests. The most frequent screening test for lupus is the antinuclear antibody (ANA) level. This test detects the presence of antibodies (proteins that mark abnormal cells or particles as foreign and subject to attack) in the blood.

Although most people with lupus will have elevated ANA levels, a positive ANA test can be seen in numerous other diseases and in up to 10 percent of healthy people. Because many of the early symptoms can be vague (fatigue, fevers, and joint pains), a definitive diagnosis of lupus may take many months to years as specific signs and symptoms accrue. Additionally, other conditions that can cause similar symptoms, including thyroid problems, anemia, and infections, must be evaluated.

Treatments and prevention

There is no known cure for lupus. The goals of treatment are to relieve symptoms, prevent organ damage, and to restore normal functioning. Treatment for lupus is as varied as its symptoms. The majority of medications used to treat active lupus are immunosuppressive medications that reduce the overall immune system in the body. Steroids (like prednisone) are among the most common medications used to treat lupus, and the doses may range from very low (5 milligrams daily) to much higher (60 milligrams daily), depending on the severity of the lupus. Many lupus medications are the same as ones used after organ transplantation and those used to treat certain cancers.

Doses and types of medications are commonly adjusted depending on the degree of disease activity and the presence of side effects. Treating active inflammation must always be balanced against the risk of potential side effects from medicines, including weight gain, hair loss, abdominal pain, and diarrhea. Among the most serious potential side effect from lupus medications is the increased susceptibility to infections caused by suppressing the immune system. Other side effects of medications—and of lupus itself—are fatigue, depression, and change in physical appearance.

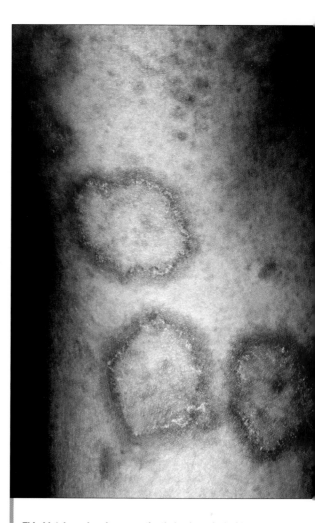

This blotchy red rash on a patient's leg is typical of lupus. It is caused by the immune system attacking connective tissue in the skin and producing inflammation.

These must all be addressed when caring for lupus patients. Another goal of treatment is the prevention of flare-ups. Although it cannot be predicted when flare-ups are going to occur, several factors have been shown to reduce the incidence of and severity of flare-ups, including regular use of sunscreen and sun-protective clothing (even when it is cloudy), adequate sleep, abstention from smoking, taking medications as instructed, and delaying pregnancy until the disease is in remission (quiet).

Eliza Chakravarty

See also
- Anemia • Epstein-Barr infection
- Pleurisy

Lyme disease

An inflammatory disease caused by the bacterium *Borrelia burgdorferi*, Lyme disease is transmitted to animals and humans through the bite of an infected tick. Lyme disease is the most common tick-borne disease in the United States.

Lyme disease was first reported in the United States in the town of Old Lyme, Connecticut, in 1975 and now is reported throughout the United States. Most cases occur in the Northeast (in the states of New York, Massachusetts, Connecticut, Rhode Island, and New Jersey), in the upper Midwest, and along the Pacific Coast. Lyme disease is also found in Europe, China, Japan, Australia, and across the former Soviet Union. There are more than 16,000 cases of Lyme disease each year in the United States.

Causes and risk factors

There are several types of ticks that cause Lyme disease: in the Northeast and Midwest, the deer tick (*Ixodes Dammini*); in the South, the black-legged tick (*Ixodes scapularis*); in the West, *Ixodes pacificus*, the Western black-legged tick. The lone star tick, or *Amblyomma americanum*, is found in several regions.

Risk factors include walking in high grass and heavily wooded areas in the spring, summer, and early fall; wearing shorts and short-sleeved tops; and having a pet that can carry ticks home.

Symptoms

In about 90 percent of cases of Lyme disease there is a characteristic red rash, called erythema migrans, usually occurring at the site of the bite within a few days to weeks, which generally looks like an expanding red ring with alternating light and dark rings. At the same time, flulike symptoms may appear with headache, sore throat, fever, muscle aches, stiff neck, fatigue, and general malaise. Some individuals develop the flulike symptoms without a rash. There may also be a flat or slightly raised lesion at the site of the bite.

If ignored, early symptoms of the disease disappear but are followed in months to years by the more serious complications of joint inflammation (arthritis), neurological symptoms, and sometimes heart, eye, respiratory, and gastrointestinal problems, which may be chronic or intermittent.

Diagnosis, treatments, and prevention

Diagnosis can be difficult because the symptoms can mimic other diseases, and the rash can be confused with that from poison ivy, spider or insect bites, or ringworm. If Lyme disease is suspected, a blood test may confirm the diagnosis, although it is not conclusive. Treated early, the disease can be cured with antibiotics. Recent studies suggest that a single dose of the antibiotic doxycycline after a tick bite can prevent the disease. If the disease remains untreated and complications develop, anti-inflammatory drugs may relieve joint pain and stiffness. Intravenous drugs may be used to treat persistent arthritis or severe heart or neurological symptoms that do not respond to oral antibiotics. For those in tick-infested areas, a vaccine is available that can prevent infection. Other preventive measures include clothing that covers the limbs, light clothing so ticks can easily be seen and removed, and repeated inspection of the body for ticks.

Isaac Grate

KEY FACTS

Description

Inflammatory disease caused by *Borrelia burgdorferi*.

Cause

A bite from an infected tick.

Risk factors

Walking in high grass and heavily wooded areas infected with ticks in spring, summer, and early fall; wearing shorts or short-sleeved tops outdoors.

Diagnosis

Characteristic rash; blood test.

Treatments

Oral antibiotics.

Pathogenesis

A bite from an infected tick releases bacteria into the bloodstream that spread throughout the body; if untreated, symptoms can develop years later.

Prevention

A vaccine helps prevent infection; keeping arms and legs covered; removal of ticks from the skin.

Epidemiology

The most common tick-borne infection in the United States; more than 16,000 cases each year.

See also
• Arthritis

Lymphoma

Lymphoma is a general term for a group of cancers originating in lymphatic tissues. According to the Leukemia and Lymphoma Society, 56 percent of blood cancers diagnosed are lymphomas. Lymphomas are classified as Hodgkin's lymphoma, also known as Hodgkin's disease, and non-Hodgkin's lymphoma.

The main difference between Hodgkin's lymphoma and non-Hodgkin's lymphoma is the type of white cells involved in the cancer development. Under a microscope, the appearances of abnormal white cells in Hodgkin's lymphoma and non-Hodgkin's lymphoma are different, so doctors can differentiate the two types of diseases and make treatment plans accordingly. This article mainly focuses on non-Hodgkin's lymphoma. For information on Hodgkin's lymphoma, see Hodgkin's disease.

Causes and risk factors

The exact causes of non-Hodgkin's lymphoma are unknown. Possible risk factors for non-Hodgkin's disease, which might increase the chances of developing the disease, include age, sex, weakened immune system, genetics, and environmental factors.

The chance of developing non-Hodgkin's lymphoma increases as people get older, and the disease occurs more often in men, especially white men, than women. According to the American Cancer Society (ACS), in the United States about 58,870 people were diagnosed with non-Hodgkin's lymphoma in 2006; among those people, 30,680 were men and 28,190 were women.

Diseases or infections that weaken the immune system increase the incidence rates of non-Hodgkin's disease. Infection with HIV is a common cause of immune system deficiency and is a risk factor of developing certain types of non-Hodgkin's lymphoma. Infection with human T-cell leukemia or lymphoma virus (HTLV-1) is a risk factor of developing certain types of T-cell non-Hodgkin's lymphoma. According to the ACS, HTLV-1, like HIV, spreads through sexual intercourse and contaminated blood supply and can also be passed on to children through breast-feeding.

According to the ACS, some genetic diseases can cause children to be born with a deficient immune system that could increase the risk of developing non-Hodgkin's disease. Environmental risk factors for the disease include radiation and chemicals. Studies have suggested that chemicals such as benzene and insecticides could increase the incidence rates of non-Hodgkin's lymphoma. Confirmational studies are still ongoing. According to the National Cancer Institute (NCI), taking immunosuppressant drugs, having a diet high in animal fat, and a previous treatment of Hodgkin's lymphoma can also increase the risk of developing non-Hodgkin's lymphoma.

Diagnosis and staging

Physical exam is generally the first step of the diagnosis of non-Hodgkin's lymphoma. Because other types of disease can also produce the same signs or symptoms as non-Hodgkin's lymphoma, further diagnosic methods, including imaging and biopsy, are used to confirm the disease. Imaging techniques such as computed tomography (CT), magnetic resonance imaging (MRI), or positron emission tomography (PET) scans are often used to look for enlarged lymph nodes; biopsy is often used to confirm non-Hodgkin's lymphoma. A small part of an enlarged lymph node or a small amount of tissue from the tumor is removed. The biopsy is examined and the type of non-Hodgkin's lymphoma is diagnosed. Once non-Hodgkin's lymphoma is diagnosed, further tests are needed to determine the stage of the disease. Common tests for staging the disease include further physical exam, blood test, imaging test, and sometimes bone marrow aspiration and lumbar puncture. Non-Hodgkin's lymphoma is generally classified into four stages according to the Ann Arbor staging system. In stage I, the lymphoma is found only in one lymph node or a few nodes in only one region. In stage II, the cancer extends from a single lymph node or a group of lymph nodes in one region to lymph nodes in other areas on the same side of the diaphragm. In stage III, the cancer may have extended to both sides of the diaphragm and even the nearby organs or spleen. In stage IV, the cancer has spread outside the lymph system. Depending on how fast the cancers grow and the locations of the affected lymph nodes, non-Hodgkin's lymphomas can also be classified into indolent lymphomas, aggressive lymphomas, contiguous lymphomas, and noncontiguous lymphomas. Indolent lymphomas tend to grow and spread slowly; aggressive lymphomas grow and spread very rapidly. Patients with aggressive lymphomas often have more severe symptoms than patients with indolent lymphomas. In contiguous lymphomas, the affected lymph nodes are next to each other, whereas in noncontiguous lymphomas, the lymph nodes with cancer cells are not.

Treatments

Depending on the type of lymphoma, the stage of the disease, age, and the general health condition of patients, different types of treatment can be used. Radiation therapy, chemotherapy, biological therapy, and watchful waiting are currently the four standard treatment options for non-Hodgkin's lymphoma. Unlike other kinds of cancer, surgery is rarely used as a therapeutic option for non-Hodgkin's lymphoma.

Radiation therapy uses high energy X-rays to kill cancer cells. Depending on whether the source of the X-rays is outside or inside the body, radiation therapy is referred to as external therapy and internal therapy. For external therapy, a machine outside the body produces high energy X-rays toward the area containing cancer cells. For internal radiation therapy, a radioactive seed, such as a wire or needle, is inserted into the affected area to directly kill the cancer cells. Chemotherapy uses chemical drugs to stop the growth of cancer cells, by killing the cells directly or preventing them from dividing. Chemotherapy is often classified into systemic chemotherapy and local chemotherapy, depending on whether the drug travels through the bloodstream or is placed in the affected area. Radiation therapy and chemotherapy are the most common treatments for non-Hodgkin's lymphoma, and they can be given alone or combined.

Biological therapy, also known as immunotherapy, uses materials made either by the body or in a laboratory to stimulate the body's immune system to fight the disease. Watchful waiting is closely monitoring the patient without giving any treatment and it is normally used at an early stage of non-Hodgkin's lymphoma or indolent lymphoma before symptoms appear.

The goal of surgery is to remove confined lymphoma tissues. Unlike chemotherapy and radiation therapy, surgery is rarely used as a therapeutic option for the treatment of non-Hodgkin's lymphoma. It is only used to remove confined cancer tissues unrelated to the lymph nodes, such as stomach tissues.

For some patients, especially those in whom non-Hodgkin's lymphoma has recurred, bone marrow transplantation may also be an option. This treatment provides the patients with stem cells, which are healthy immature cells that produce blood cells, to replace cells damaged during radiation therapy or chemotherapy. In addition to these treatments, new types of treatment for non-Hodgkin's disease, including vaccine therapy and high-dose chemotherapy with stem cell transplant, are currently testing in clinical studies.

Because the causes of non-Hodgkin's lymphoma are unknown and certain risk factors of the disease, including age and sex, cannot be avoided, it is difficult to prevent the disease.

Epidemiology

Around 67,000 people in the United States were diagnosed with lymphoma in 2006. Of these, about 8,000 cases were Hodgkin's lymphoma.

Y. Wang

See also
• AIDS • Hodgkin's disease

Macular degeneration

Macular degeneration is the breakdown or deterioration of the macula, the small, central area in the retina responsible for fine detail in the central vision. Damage to the macula may cause distorted or blurry vision, eventually leading to blank spots and severe vision loss. However, because macular degeneration affects only central vision, peripheral vision is retained, and the condition does not result in total blindness.

The most common form of macular degeneration is age-related macular degeneration (AMD). AMD occurs in two types: dry (atrophic) and wet (exudative). Dry AMD is much more common than wet AMD; it accounts for more than 85 percent of patients with AMD. Dry AMD is caused by the body's natural aging process and slow deterioration of macular tissue, resulting in a gradual loss of vision. Wet AMD is caused by the development of abnormal blood vessels under the retina, which leak blood and fluid, causing the central vision to blur. In wet AMD, vision loss occurs very rapidly.

Risk factors

Age and a family history of macular degeneration are the primary risk factors for developing macular degeneration. Other factors include smoking, obesity, and race (Caucasians have a greater chance of developing macular degeneration), sex (women are more likely to develop the condition), and low nutrient levels. Macular degeneration usually develops gradually and without pain. With dry AMD, early symptoms may include blurriness and the need for greater light. Gradually, a blind spot may begin to develop in the center of the field of vision. In wet AMD, early symptoms generally include a distortion of vision, such as lines appearing wavy or crooked and objects appearing closer or farther away than they should. The symptoms then progress rapidly and involve central vision loss.

Treatments

No treatments are available to reverse dry AMD. Wet AMD has no cure, but treatments are available to slow or possibly stop vision loss. Laser surgery is one option, in which a laser is used to slow or stop the blood vessels that are damaging the macula. Another option is photodynamic therapy, in which a cold laser is used with a drug, verteporfin, to seal off leaky blood vessels. Other emerging treatments are available, including anti-VEGF (vascular endothelial growth factor) therapy, in which drugs injected into the eye target proteins that induce abnormal growth and leakage of blood vessels, and angiostatic therapy, in which a steroid that stops growth of abnormal blood vessels is delivered into the back of the eye. Recent studies show that consumption of omega-3 fatty acids, such as are found in salmon and other fish, reduces the risk of developing AMD.

The number of people over the age of 60 is predicted by the United Nations to grow from 688 million in 2006 to 2 billion in 2050, so people suffering from macular degeneration is also expected to rise. According to the World Health Organization, macular degeneration is the third leading cause of blindness worldwide and the first leading cause in developed nations.

Josephine Everly and Herbert Kaufman

KEY FACTS

Description

Deterioration of the macula, an area in the retina.

Risk factors

Age, family history, race, sex, obesity, smoking, low nutrient levels.

Symptoms

Blurred or distorted vision.

Diagnosis

Eye exam by an ophthalmologist, visual acuity test (Amsler grid), fluorescein angiography.

Treatments

No treatment for dry AMD; laser surgery and photodynamic therapy, as well as some other emerging treatments, are available for wet AMD.

Pathogenesis

Deposits in the choroid area of the eye and growth of new blood vessels.

Prevention

Nutritionally balanced diet, supplemental vitamins, smoking cessation, regular eye exams.

Epidemiology

The third leading cause of blindness worldwide, but leading cause of blindness in developed countries due to the larger populations of elderly.

See also

• Retinal disorders

Malaria

Malaria is one of the world's major infectious diseases, transmitted from human to human by mosquitoes. Each year, there are about 300 million to 500 million cases of malaria and between 1 million and 3 million human deaths, most of them children. Although various treatments and preventive measures are available to tackle the disease, these are often too expensive for developing countries, where malaria is most common.

Malaria has been eradicated from the United States and temperate regions of the world for several decades. Nevertheless, over 40 percent of the human population lives in areas where malaria is endemic (firmly established). In general, these are poor areas in tropical and subtropical regions. There, a number of factors are responsible for the continued presence of this illness, including climate changes, political unrest, and increased resistance of the parasite to drug therapies and of mosquitoes to insecticides.

Cause

Malaria is caused by single-celled protozoa belonging to the genus *Plasmodium*, often referred to collectively as the "malaria parasite." There are about 170 species of malaria parasite, able to infect many different types of vertebrates (backboned animals), but only four of these can cause infection in humans: *Plasmodium falciparum*, *P. ovale*, *P. vivax*, and *P. malariae*. *Plasmodium vivax* occurs in the Middle East, India, and Central America, while the other three species are found mainly in Africa. Of the four species, *Plasmodium falciparum* causes the most serious cases of illness and the majority of deaths.

Malaria parasites are carried from person to person by mosquitoes of the genus *Anopheles*. When an anopheles mosquito pierces the skin to suck blood, it may pick up the parasite from an infected person or, conversely, it may pass on the parasite to someone who is uninfected. It is always female mosquitoes that are involved, because males do not suck blood. Occasionally, a person can become infected with more than one species of malaria parasite at the same time.

Risk factors and epidemiology

Malaria is endemic in many subtropical and tropical regions of the world. Its absence from other regions may be because it has been eradicated but also because the malaria parasite, or the anopheles mosquitoes that transmit it, or both, cannot survive in colder regions.

Children under the age of five years, pregnant women, and travelers visiting regions with endemic malaria are at risk of having a more severe course of illness. In the case of travelers, the risk comes because they have not built up immunity after previous bouts

---

KEY FACTS

Description
A potentially fatal infectious disease involving the bloodstream and internal organs.

Cause
A single-celled parasite transmitted by the bite of infected *Anopheles* mosquitoes.

Risk factors
Children under the age of 5 years, pregnant women, and nonimmune travelers to areas where malaria is endemic are at greatest risk.

Symptoms
Recurrent attacks of flulike symptoms such as fever, chills, and body aches.

Diagnosis
Microscopic examination of blood smears.

Treatments
Various antimalarial drugs, although parasites are developing resistance to these.

Pathogenesis
The parasite's life cycle involves both humans and mosquitoes of the genus *Anopheles*; various stages of the malaria parasite's development occur in both of these hosts.

Prevention
Reducing contact with mosquitoes by using insect repellents and insecticide-treated bed nets. Taking preventive drugs before visiting areas where malaria is endemic.

Epidemiology
Malaria is endemic in many subtropical and tropical regions of the world. It can be spread elsewhere by travelers returning from these regions, at airports, or by infected mosquitoes "hitching a ride" on airplanes.

of malaria, as many local people will have done. About 30,000 people from developed countries contract malaria every year, after visiting regions where the disease is endemic. Pregnant women infected with *P. falciparum* are at higher risk of premature delivery and low birth weight in their offspring. Such infection can also lead to transmission of malaria to the child during pregnancy or delivery.

In endemic areas, risk of malaria decreases at altitudes above 6,560 feet (2,000 meters). The risk increases in the more rural areas. Transmission also varies by season, being highest at the end of the rainy season.

In nonendemic areas, malaria can be introduced, at least temporarily, as long as a mosquito capable of transmitting the disease also lives in the area. In the United States, two species of anopheles mosquitoes capable of transmitting this disease are still present. If, for example, a traveler returns to the United States after having been infected with malaria abroad and is bitten by a local anopheles mosquito on return, this infected mosquito can in turn bite and infect humans. Airport malaria, in which the infected mosquito arrives at an airport and transmits malaria there, can also occur. Of the thousand or so cases of malaria diagnosed each year in the United States, most are acquired outside the country and are referred to as "imported" malaria.

Malaria is not transmitted directly from person to person. It can, however, be acquired through blood transfusions, organ transplants from persons who have the infection, or by sharing needles with someone carrying the infection. Studies have shown that some genetic blood disorders, such as sickle-cell anemia, may actually help protect against malaria, because the alteration in the hemoglobin molecule hinders malarial growth and development.

Symptoms and pathogenesis

In a typical case of malaria, symptoms begin within 10 days to 4 weeks after a bite by an infected mosquito. Characteristic symptoms can be flulike and include fever, shaking chills, or "rigors," headache, and muscle aches. Nausea, vomiting, diarrhea, and jaundice, as well as severe fatigue, may also occur. The symptoms often appear regularly every other to every third day and last for several hours, although there is not always such a regular cycle. The liver and spleen may also become enlarged.

The symptoms of malaria can be related to the life cycle of the parasite (see diagram, page 282). An infected mosquito releases sporozoites (a particular stage

MOSQUITOES AND MALARIA

There are about 430 species of anopheles mosquitoes worldwide, but only 30 to 50 can transmit malaria. In sub-Saharan Africa, the principal carrier of malaria is *Anopheles gambiae*, a mosquito that searches for its human blood meal between dusk and dawn, thus making the evening and night the times of greatest risk of infection.

When an anopheles mosquito infected with malaria parasites bites a human, it can release the parasites into the bloodstream while taking a blood meal.

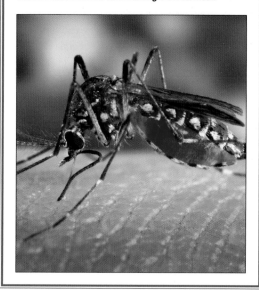

of the parasite's life cycle) into a person's bloodstream while taking its meal of blood. The sporozoites travel to the liver, where they invade the liver cells. There, they multiply asexually (without using sexual reproduction) by the thousands, developing into another stage called merozoites. A person does not usually show symptoms at this stage.

After a few days or weeks, the infected liver cells burst open and release the merozoites into the bloodstream, where they invade red blood cells and multiply further. Typically, infected blood cells tend to burst and release more parasites all at roughly the same time, either every two or every three days depending on the species of parasite. This cycle leads to the repeated flulike symptoms of malaria. Many parasites are released again from red blood cells in the form of more merozoites, ready to invade more red blood cells and continue the cycle of fever. Some parasites, though, are produced in a different form that is able to give rise to sex cells (gametes). If such potential sex cells are sucked up by a mosquito when it drinks an infected person's blood, the parasite undergoes sexual fertilization and multiplication in the mosquito's body until it is ready to be transmitted to another human victim, thus completing its life cycle.

Not all cases of malaria follow the pattern described above. For example, people who have already been infected by malaria before may show few symptoms when they are attacked once again. Where the infection is with *P. ovale* or *P. vivax*, the parasites can remain dormant (inactive) in the human liver and only cause obvious disease at a future date, sometimes as long as several years later. The species *P. malariae* can, in rare cases, remain in the human host for many years without producing symptoms.

An attack of malaria can cause various complications. All four species sometimes cause imbalances in the blood, with lowered blood sugar and increased acidity. Parasites also deform the outer membranes of red blood cells, making the cells more likely to be taken out of circulation by the spleen, further complicating the anemia caused by the bursting of parasite-infested cells. Organ failure involving the respiratory system or heart can occur, as can kidney failure. Dark pigments in the blood resulting from the destruction of large numbers of red blood cells can spill over into the urine, a condition called by the common name *blackwater fever*. The death rate due to severe malaria, even when treated in modern day intensive care units, often exceeds 30 percent, whereas in developing countries with substandard health care, persons with complicated malaria requiring blood transfusions can be at higher risk of contracting HIV and other blood-borne infections.

Of the four malaria parasites that infect humans, *Plasmodium falciparum* is the most common and the most lethal; it causes about 95 percent of deaths from malaria. More so than the other three, this species can infect a much greater proportion of red blood cells, sometimes causing death only a few hours after the rupture of red blood cells begins. In an infection with *P. falciparum*, the central nervous system can be involved, ultimately leading to confusion, seizures, and coma. For those who survive, their nervous system may be severely damaged.

Diagnosis

An active malarial infection can be diagnosed by taking a drop of the person's blood and spreading it on a microscope slide and then staining it with a special stain called Giemsa. These smears are produced as a thick and a thin smear. The microscopist then looks for the malaria parasites within the human red blood cells. Thick smears are useful in making the diagnosis; thin smears allow for species identification. Because parasites are present in the blood at intermittent cycles, smears should be evaluated every 6 to 12 hours over a period of 48 hours to improve diagnostic sensitivity. In 95 percent of cases, however, the first smear is positive for the presence of malaria parasites.

Blood testing using the polymerase chain reaction (PCR) method can also be done to detect the parasite's deoxyribonucleic acid (DNA; genetic material); however, this procedure requires a specialized laboratory, is labor intensive, and is quite expensive. Also, determination of viable versus nonviable organisms is not possible. This method may be useful to monitor the efficacy of drug treatment. A test for antibodies against the malaria parasites is available, but it can only identify prior infection.

Treatments

Various antimalarial drugs are available; however, increasing resistance by the malaria parasites has been noted, particularly to the drug chloroquine. Effective therapies include quinine sulfate, hydroxychloroquine (Plaquenil), the combination drug sulfadoxine and pyrimethamine (Fansidar), mefloquine (Lariam), the combination of atovaquone and proguanil (Malarone), and doxycycline (Doryx, Vibramycin). To improve chances for a cure, it is important to treat early using the correct drug, correct dose, and appropriate length of time. Persons infected with *P. vivax* or *P. ovale* may be treated with a second drug to prevent relapses. For drug-resistance cases, combination therapies involving the artemisinin drugs with other medicines are used, an approach referred to as artemisinin-based combination therapy (ACT).

Prevention

There is no vaccine at this time for malaria. However, because the complete genomes for *Plasmodium falciparum* and *Anopheles gambiae* have been sequenced, there is some hope that treatments such as vaccines or viruses might now be researched.

Most drugs used to treat malaria are also used to prevent it, including antibiotics such as doxycycline and tetracycline. For preventive treatment, the drug is usually started one to two weeks before travel to a malarial country, continues throughout the trip, and is also taken for four weeks after return. Even with such

THE MALARIA CYCLE

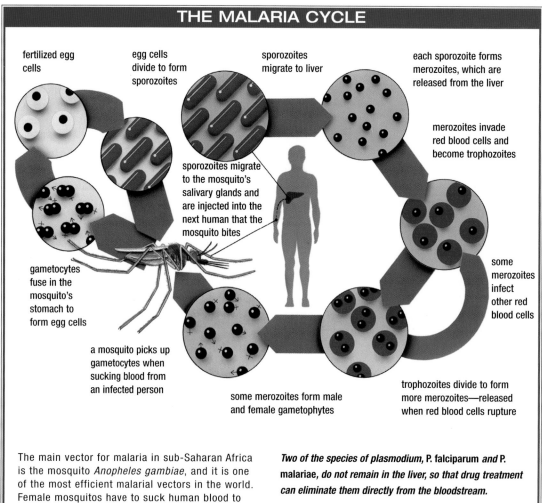

fertilized egg cells

egg cells divide to form sporozoites

sporozoites migrate to liver

each sporozoite forms merozoites, which are released from the liver

merozoites invade red blood cells and become trophozoites

sporozoites migrate to the mosquito's salivary glands and are injected into the next human that the mosquito bites

gametocytes fuse in the mosquito's stomach to form egg cells

some merozoites infect other red blood cells

a mosquito picks up gametocytes when sucking blood from an infected person

some merozoites form male and female gametophytes

trophozoites divide to form more merozoites—released when red blood cells rupture

The main vector for malaria in sub-Saharan Africa is the mosquito *Anopheles gambiae*, and it is one of the most efficient malarial vectors in the world. Female mosquitos have to suck human blood to get protein that they need for egg production. A mosquito carrying malaria parasites pierces human skin with two sharp tubes; one tube injects anticoagulants (and parasites) to keep the blood flowing, the other tube sucks up blood. If another

Two of the species of plasmodium, P. falciparum and P. malariae, do not remain in the liver, so that drug treatment can eliminate them directly from the bloodstream.

mosquito then bites the person some time later, it sucks up infected blood cells. The parasite develops in the mosquito for about 10 days; it can then infect other people. This process is faster in warm, wet tropical countries such as tropical Africa.

preventive measures, it is still possible to acquire malaria, and preventive measures may merely delay the onset of symptoms, making diagnosis more difficult.

Attempts to minimize contact with mosquitoes can reduce the chances of contracting malaria. Insect repellent containing the chemical DEET as its active ingredient is recommended, along with wearing long sleeves and pants to decrease the chance of being bitten by mosquitoes. More recently, insecticide-treated bed nets have been shown to decrease childhood malaria and mortality from the disease.

In the 1950s, programs to eliminate malaria worldwide were implemented. These failed, however, in most malarial regions due to reasons including increased resistance of mosquitoes to insecticides, as well as increased resistance of the parasites to drugs used in treatment and political instability of some of the countries concerned. Furthermore, most people living in these countries cannot afford treatment, even though medicines to treat malaria are inexpensive by U.S. standards.

Rita Washko

See also
• Anemia • Dengue fever • Sickle-cell anemia • Yellow fever

Male-pattern baldness

Male-pattern baldness, or androgenetic alopecia, is a common disorder that affects both men and women. It is characterized by thinning of the hair at the front of the scalp above the temples, so that the hairline recedes and reshapes. Hair loss in women is characterized by a diffusely thinned scalp, particularly from the forehead to the crown, without a receding hairline. Androgenetic alopecia is a cosmetic concern for both men and women. Treatment options have variable results.

Most cases of male-pattern baldness begin during the third or fourth decade, with progression of hair loss over time. Male-pattern baldness has many causes. People who display this condition have a genetic predisposition that is determined by many different genes. Other factors, such as poor diet and lack of exercise, also play a role. Male pattern baldness has increased greatly in Japan since the Japanese diet has become higher in fat and the lifestyle more sedentary.

Hair thins by miniaturization of the hair follicles, not just by decreased density. This process of thinning occurs over time when the combination of genetics with exposure to androgens results in the terminal (mature) hairs of the scalp slowly miniaturizing to intermediate hairs and then finally to vellus (fine) hairs. Androgens, which are the male sex hormones, include testosterone, dehydroepiandrosterone (DHEA), dihydrotestosterone (DHT), and many others. DHT is the chemical most readily linked to male-pattern baldness and is more potent than testosterone. This chemical is amplified in the scalp due to an enzyme called 5-alpha-reductase, which converts free testosterone to DHT. The overall result in those who are genetically susceptible is increased hair loss and male-pattern baldness. If a woman has baldness, she should be screened to ensure that she does not have virilism (high levels of male hormones causing masculinization). Other causes of scalp hair thinning are a thyroid disorder or anemia.

Treatments and epidemiology

Treatment of this condition is difficult, and currently there are only two medications approved by the FDA for androgenetic alopecia. Minoxidil is a topical medication that is thought to work by increasing blood flow to the follicles and increasing the time the hair is in the growth phase (anagen). The medication is best for small areas, or early stages of hair loss. It takes at least four months to start working, and it must be used indefinitely to maintain results. Finasteride is a pill that works to reduce the enzyme 5-alpha-reductase. It is not safe for use in women who can become pregnant because it causes severe birth defects. Finasteride is best used with minoxidil, and it also must be used indefinitely. It does not have any beneficial effect on hair growth in postmenopausal women.

Over the past 40 years, surgical options have become a good alternative but are limited due to high costs. Hair grafting, transfer of 2- to 4-square millimeter "plugs" to one site, is not often performed as the plugs look less natural, resembling a doll's head. In follicular unit transplantation, or micrografting, the donor pieces are individual follicular units containing one to three hairs that are then arranged as individual hair units.

Male-pattern baldness is most common in Caucasian men, then Asians and African Americans, and least often in Native Americans. It is found in more than half of all men worldwide, and up to 75 percent of postmenopausal women.

Maya Kolipakam and Richard S. Kalish

KEY FACTS

Description
Loss of head hair in men and women.

Causes
Multifactorial but mainly genetic.

Risk factors
Poor diet and lack of exercise; increasing age.

Diagnosis
Obvious from characteristic pattern of hair loss.

Treatments
The medications minoxidil and finasteride.

Pathogenesis
Progression of hair loss over time.

Prevention
No known prevention.

Epidemiology
Most common in Caucasian men, followed by Asians and African Americans.

See also
• Alopecia

Measles

Measles is a contagious viral illness that is caused by a ribonucleic acid (RNA) virus. Although measles is a potentially dangerous disease, if children receive the MMR vaccine, the number of cases of measles decreases. Although measles mainly affects children, anybody who has not had the disease can become infected.

Measles used to be one of the most common infectious diseases of childhood before immunization became widespread. Measles virus is a member of the paramixovirus family that includes parainfluenza, mumps, and respiratory syncytial viruses. Measles has existed for many centuries, although its infectious etiology was established only in the nineteenth century. The measles virus was discovered in 1954. In the mid-twentieth century, successful immunization campaigns led to a dramatic decrease in measles cases in the developed world. In contrast, measles remains a significant cause of morbidity and mortality among children in the developing world; it caused an estimated 450,000 deaths in 2004. It is also a leading cause of blindness in African children. The Measles Initiative is a combined effort that aims to decrease morbidity and mortality from measles in the countries most heavily affected by this disease. It was launched by multiple agencies, including the Red Cross, Centers for Disease Control and Prevention, the World Health Organization, and the United Nations Children's Fund The Measles Initiative is vaccinating children at risk in many African countries and is now expanding to Asian countries as well. As a result of this campaign, measles deaths have almost halved. The campaign's goal is to reduce measles mortality by 90 percent by the year 2010. The Pan-American Health Organization has led a campaign to eliminate measles in the Western Hemisphere. The last endemic case in this part of the world was reported in 2002. The remaining reported cases of measles in countries of the Americas have been associated with importation from areas with a higher prevalence of measles.

Pathogenesis and symptoms and signs

This disease is only transmitted among humans by large air droplets. The air droplets containing the virus can survive in the environment for several hours. The person with measles remains contagious from the first day of the symptoms until approximately four to five days after the rash develops. Damage from the measles virus results in compromised function of the mucosal epithelial cells and the development of bronchitis and pneumonia.

The symptoms usually develop 10 to 14 days after exposure (incubation period), but they can start as early as 7 days or as late as 21 days after the virus enters the human body. Children less than 5 years of age or adults older than 20 years, as well as malnourished and immunocompromised individuals, are at risk for

KEY FACTS

Description

Measles (rubeola) is a highly contagious acute infection caused by a virus.

Causes

Measles is caused by an RNA virus that belongs to the family of paramixoviruses.

Risk factors

It is a highly contagious disease and almost everyone without previous immunity to measles is susceptible.

Symptoms

The symptoms of measles are fever, cough, coryza (runny nose), conjunctivitis, and a rash.

Diagnosis

Diagnosis is usually based on typical clinical symptoms and a history of contact if this information is available.

Treatments

Fluids and relief of fever.

Pathogenesis

The disease spreads through the air in droplets containing the virus from an infected person. The virus enters through the upper respiratory tract and invades the epithelial cells that line the respiratory tract.

Prevention

The best way to prevent measles is to maintain specific antibody protection against measles. This is commonly achieved by immunization.

Epidemiology

Measles is one of the major causes of childhood mortality in many developing countries. It is a leading cause of blindness in African children.

more severe illness and a higher chance of complications. Patients with measles develop high fevers up to 104°F–105°F (40°C–40.5°C), cough, runny nose and conjunctivitis. A typical rash helps identify measles. It develops after several days of fever and starts on the face and descends down the body and then the extremities. The rash is erythematous (red) and maculopapular; it can change its color to brown and scale before resolving. It lasts for several days and then slowly clears, starting from the face. Another very specific finding for patients with measles is Koplik's spots, white-gray patches found on the buccal mucosa of the oral cavity. They develop one to two days prior to the appearance of the rash. These are easy to miss and not always present in all the patients. Measles usually resolves on its own in an average of 14 days. The general prognosis for measles is good. Infection with measles results in lifelong immunity. Mortality from measles is associated with poor nutritional status and immunocompromised states such as HIV and cancer. Pneumonia accounts for the majority of deaths from measles.

The most common complications of measles include superinfections of the respiratory tract, such as bronchitis, pneumonia, and otitis media (ear infection). Another dangerous but rare complication of measles is encephalitis. It typically develops five to six days after the rash and results in headache, vomiting, and fever. It can also result in seizures and coma. Another illness associated with measles is subacute sclerosing panencephalitis, which is a chronic, debilitating neurological condition. It is very rare and develops years after the episode of measles.

Diagnosis and treatments

Diagnosis of measles is mostly based on the clinical presentation. In addition, a blood test called serology could be used to diagnose measles. It detects a specific immune response to the invasion of this virus: measles antibodies. Other methods, like virus isolation and detection of antigen in the mucosal cells, are also available. Another typical laboratory feature of measles is a low leukocyte count in the peripheral blood (leukopenia).

For treatment, supportive measures such as provision of fluids and relief of fever are usually necessary.

Prevention

There are two ways to prevent measles: active and passive immunization. For active immunization, a live attenuated (weakened) virus is used for vaccination in a

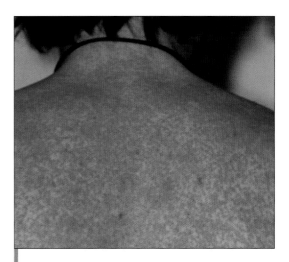

This adult male has measles and is exhibiting the typical red, blotchy rash. The symptoms are more severe in adulthood.

combined vaccine called MMR (measles-mumps-rubella). It is given twice, first at 12 to 16 months of age and later in childhood at 4 to 6 years of age. The vaccine is not given prior to 12 months of age because there are circulating maternal antibodies that are passed to the baby via the placenta. MMR vaccine is well tolerated; among the most common side effects of the vaccine are low grade fever and rash that resolve spontaneously in several days. There is no real scientific evidence to support an association of MMR with the development of autism, as some reports have suggested in the past. MMR vaccine should be given to adults born in 1957 or later if there is no evidence of specific immunity against measles. MMR vaccine should not be given if there is a history of an allergic reaction to a prior dose of MMR or allergy to the components of the vaccine (like gelatin and neomycin).

Passive immunization is achieved by the administration of specific immunoglobulin to persons exposed to measles who are not already immune. This is especially important for individuals at high risk of severe measles. Passive immunization is only indicated to prevent the disease in the event of exposure to a person with measles. In order to be effective, immunoglobulin should be given within six days of exposure to the disease.

Diana Nurutdinova

See also
- Chicken pox and shingles • Conjunctivitis
- Diphtheria • Mumps

Melanoma

Melanoma is the deadliest form of skin cancer. Although it accounts for only 4 percent of all skin cancers, melanoma causes more than 75 percent of all deaths from skin cancer. Melanoma cases are increasing; the rate doubles every 10 to 20 years, which is consistent with increased leisure time and the public's attraction to a tanned body. In the United States, the male death rate for melanoma has risen from 2.4 in 100,000 in 1959 to 3.8 in 100,000 in 2000.

The top layer of the skin is called the epidermis, and it is within this structure that a melanoma forms. It arises from the melanocyte, which is the pigment-containing cell responsible for skin color, located in the deepest layer of the epidermis. As in other forms of skin cancer, most melanomas are the result of the harmful effects of ultraviolet (UV) radiation, which is cumulative over a lifetime. It is the combination of the ultraviolet light injuring the deoxyribonucleic acid (DNA) in the melanocyte and the cell's inability to repair the damage that leads to uncontrolled growth.

Risk factors

Risk factors for developing melanoma include exposure to UV radiation (sun or tanning beds) and a family history of dysplastic nevus syndrome. The latter is an inherited condition in which family members develop many unusual pigmented skin lesions, which can often change and potentially progress to melanoma. Other risk factors include burning easily in the sun, a history of severe sunburns, a tendency to freckle rather than tan, and living in areas with high-intensity sunlight, such as Florida and Australia. It is also more common when an individual has irregular or unusual moles, or more than 50 moles, has xeroderma pigmentosum (a hereditary condition in which the skin cells cannot repair the DNA damage from the sun), or has an impaired immune system, from drugs or disease (HIV).

Melanoma can occur in all individuals but is more common in Caucasians, especially those with a fair complexion, light-colored eyes, and red or blond hair. When it occurs in dark-skinned individuals, it generally occurs on unexposed areas such as palms, soles,

KEY FACTS

Description

A melanoma is a dark-colored skin cancer arising from the pigmented cells of the skin (melanocytes).

Causes

Most melanomas are the result of ultraviolet radiation damage to the skin.

Risk factors

The leading risk factor is a long history of unprotected exposure to UV radiation. It is more common with advanced age, in Caucasians, and when a large number (more than 50) or unusual moles are present. Individuals with certain inherited diseases (dysplastic nevus syndrome, xeroderma pigmentosum) and immune deficiencies are also at higher risk.

Symptoms

Melanoma is heralded by the change in a preexisting mole or the development of a new dark skin growth. Worrisome signs include asymmetry of the growth, irregular borders, variation in the color, a diameter of more than 6 mm, and elevation of the lesion above the surrounding skin. The cancer can also be itchy or have a tendency to bleed or have an open sore.

Diagnosis

The diagnosis of melanoma is suspected when the above characteristics are observed and confirmed by the microscopic examination of the tissue removed.

Treatments

Surgical excision is the treatment for the primary skin lesion of melanoma. Other methods, such as chemotherapy, are used for advanced disease.

Pathogenesis

Melanoma develops from unrepaired UV radiation damage to the DNA of melanocytes. It can quickly spread to other organs through the lymph system or blood vessels.

Prevention

Limiting harmful sun exposure, protective clothing, and sunblock can prevent skin cancers. Regular skin examination and prompt treatment of suspicious lesions prevent spread and reduce the risk of death.

Epidemiology

Most commonly seen in Caucasians, especially those with fair complexions, blue eyes, and red or blond hair. It is more prevalent in areas with high-intensity sunlight. The incidence doubles every 10–20 years.

and mucous membranes. Unlike other forms of skin cancer, which occur almost exclusively in older age groups, melanoma can occur in younger people and is the most common cancer in adults under the age of 30.

Symptoms

An individual should suspect a melanoma with any changes in a preexisting dark skin lesion or development of a new mole. The "ABCs" of warning signs for melanoma are as follows: asymmetry, in which the growth is not of a uniform shape, without two similar halves; borders, in which the edges of the lesion are irregular; color (the dark color of the mole varies from one area to another); diameter, which depicts a pigmented lesion that is more than 1/4 inch (6 mm) in diameter; and elevation, which is a growth that is higher than the surrounding skin. Other signs for concern include skin growths that are constantly itchy or bleed or darkly pigmented streaks or areas beneath a nail or on the palm or soles of the feet.

Diagnosis

A diagnosis can be made from the appearance of the melanoma, which can appear in many forms. The most common form is an enlarging, irregularly shaped black or dark brown patch (superficial spreading melanoma), usually located on the back of males and the back and lower legs of females. In the elderly, a slowly growing tan patch on sun-exposed areas may represent a lentigo maligna melanoma. It can also present as a dark raised nodule (nodular melanoma), which has the worst prognosis. There are also forms that appear on the palms or soles of the feet (acral lentiginous) and others that are not pigmented (amelanotic melanoma).

When a melanoma is suspected, it is important to remove the lesion in a timely fashion, since cure rates are very good with early detection and proper treatment. A sample or biopsy of the suspicious area is removed to be examined under a microscope. Characteristics of the appearance of the tumor, such as the location, the diameter, the presence of ulceration, and the microscopic features (tumor thickness, depth of extension, invasion of lymphatics or blood vessels) help the physician determine the best treatments and the patient's prognosis from their tumor.

Treatments and prevention

Unlike other forms of skin cancers that can be treated by a variety of methods, treatment of melanomas requires surgical excision with a margin of a normal tis-

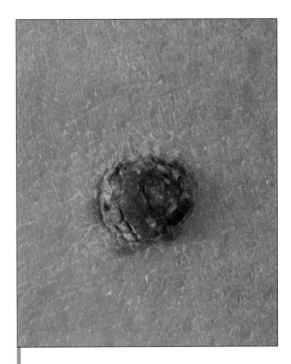

Melanomas usually grow from an existing mole, which becomes lumpy and irregular, changes shape, darkens, and sometimes bleeds or ulcerates. The mole may be itchy or tender and painful.

sue. If an enlarged lymph node is present, it may be biopsied through a needle or excised. Melanoma has a high mortality, since it can rapidly spread through the lymph system or bloodstream to other internal organs, a process called metastasizing. The addition of chemotherapy, radiation, and other modalities is used for tumors that have spread. Cure rates can approach 95 percent if detected and treated early.

Similar to other skin cancers, preventive measures include limiting the exposure to the damage inflicted by the sun's rays and tanning booths. Limiting the time of exposure (especially between the sun's peak hours of 10 AM to 4 PM), wearing protective clothing, and use of sunblocks with a sun protection factor (SPF) of 15 or greater are the standard methods. Individuals should also regularly check their skin for new moles or changes in existing ones. Those with a family history of dysplastic nevus syndrome need to have their skin examined by a dermatologist annually.

David Wainwright

See also
• Cancer, skin

Meningitis

Meningitis is an inflammation of the meninges, the thin membranes that surround the brain and spinal cord. Between the meninges is the subarachnoid space, which contains cerebrospinal fluid (CSF). Meningitis develops when the subarachnoid space becomes infected, usually from outside organisms carried in the bloodstream. This infection typically involves the entire surface of the meninges.

Inflammation of the meninges—meningitis—can be caused by various infectious agents, most commonly viruses and bacteria. It may occur as a complication of another infectious illness such as syphilis, Lyme disease, or tuberculosis. Other microorganisms such as protozoa and fungi may also cause meningitis. In addition, certain medications, cancers, and other diseases can inflame the meninges—but these are very rare occurrences.

Pathogenesis

Many of the bacteria or viruses that can cause meningitis are fairly common and more likely associated with other everyday illnesses. At other times they spread to the meninges from an infection elsewhere in the body, such as the heart and lungs. The infection can start in the skin, gastrointestinal tract, or urinary tract. From there, the microorganism enters the blood and travels through the body and enters the central nervous system. Bacteria can also spread directly to the meninges from a nearby severe infection such as a serious ear infection (otitis media) or nasal sinus infection (sinusitis). Bacteria can also enter the central nervous system (CNS) from head surgery or after blunt head trauma, such as skull fracture.

In otherwise healthy individuals, the subarachnoid space is relatively resistant to microorganisms even during persistent bacteremia (presence of viable bacteria in the bloodstream). Cell-mediated immunity and antibody-mediated destruction of bacteria are the predominant defense mechanisms in the central nervous system. Once infection in the subarachnoid space is established, the invading microorganism can rapidly multiply to high levels, resulting in severe inflammation of the meninges.

Viral meningitis is relatively more common and far less serious than bacterial meningitis. It often remains undiagnosed because the symptoms are similar to those of the viral infection influenza. Most cases of viral meningitis are caused by a group of viruses called enteroviruses, which are viruses that can affect the stomach. These viruses account for 80 to 92 percent of

A mother is testing her young daughter for meningitis. Because a meningitis rash is blotchy and does not fade under pressure, a simple test is to press a glass against the skin. If the rash does not fade, medical help must be called at once.

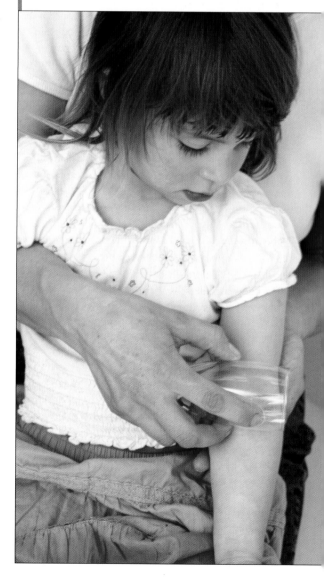

all cases of viral meningitis. Anyone can get viral meningitis; however, it occurs most often in children during the summer and fall months and resolves spontaneously after 7 to 10 days. Many other types of viruses, such as herpes viruses, lymphocytic choriomeningitis virus, Epstein-Barr virus (which causes mononucleosis), varicella-zoster virus (which causes chicken pox and shingles), and paramyxovirus (which causes mumps), can also cause meningitis.

Bacterial meningitis is less common than viral meningitis, but it is much more serious and can be life threatening if not treated promptly. Many types of bacteria, such as streptococcus, E. coli, and *Listeria monocytogenes*, are common causes of meningitis in newborns. *Streptococcus pneumoniae* and *Neisseria meningitidis* are more frequent in children older than two months of age. *Hemophilus influenzae* type B (Hib) was the leading cause of meningitis in children in the United States, but the widespread use of Hib vaccine as a routine standard immunization has dramatically reduced the frequency of this type of meningitis since the 1990s. In developing countries, *Mycobactrium tuberculosis* is a common cause of bacterial meningitis. Bacterial meningitis can occur in adults or children, but is more common in the very young (infants and young children) and elderly people (those more than 60). College students and teenagers are at a relatively higher risk for the disease due to time spent in close contact in dormitories with their peers.

Symptoms

Symptoms of meningitis vary but often include the classic triad of headache, fever, and stiff neck. Other symptoms include sensitivity to light (photophobia), nausea, vomiting, drowsiness, body aches, and confusion. Weakness, loss of appetite, shaking chills, profuse sweats, cranial nerve palsies (weakness of 3rd, 4th, 6th, and 7th cranial nerves) occur in between 10 and 20 percent of patients with meningitis. Generalized seizures occur in up to 40 percent of patients. Kernig's sign, in which extension of the knee with hips flexed is met with strong passive resistance, and Brudzinski's sign, in which passive flexion of the neck causes flexion of the leg, are observed in up to 50 percent of patients and are suggestive of meningitis. The presence or absence of the signs, however, does not make a definitive diagnosis of meningitis.

Symptoms in very young children may be particularly difficult because they often lack the classic signs mentioned earlier. Babies with meningitis may be irritable, less active, vomit, and refuse to eat. Normally, infants who are not feeling well are comforted when their mother picks them up. However, a baby with meningitis may show increased irritability when picked up and gently rocked when an attempt is made

---

KEY FACTS

Definition

Meningitis is an inflammation of the meninges, the thin membranes that surround the brain and spinal cord.

Causes

Meningitis is triggered by microorganisms that cause inflammation of the meninges.

Risk factors

Extremes of age, alcoholism, severe liver disease, renal disease, HIV and AIDS, malignancy, non-functional spleen due to sickle-cell disease, and diabetes. Living in close quarters, prolonged or close contact with a patient with meningitis, and direct contact with a patient's oral secretions (kissing or coughing) are considered increased risks for acquiring the infection.

Symptoms

Classic triad of headache, fever, and stiff neck in adults. In children, symptoms may include irritability, decreased activity, vomiting, refusal to eat, fever, jaundice, rashes, weak sucking, and bulging fontanelles (soft spots on an infant's skull).

Diagnosis

Analysis of cerebrospinal fluid (CSF) for signs of infection; clinical presentation suggestive of meningeal inflammation.

Treatment

For viral meningitis, treatment is relief of symptoms, bed rest, and analgesics. For bacterial meningitis, there must be prompt early diagnosis, broad-spectrum antibiotics given early, and treatment of complications, such as shock and abnormal electrolyte levels in the blood.

Pathogenesis

Microorganisms enter the blood and travel through the body and enter the central nervous system or spread directly to the meninges from a nearby severe infection.

Prevention

Routine immunization of young children and adolescents with vaccine against *Pneumococcus*, *Hemophilus*, and *Neisseria* (Hib, Menactra T, and pneumococcal vaccine).

Epidemiology

20,000 to 25,000 cases of bacterial meningitis in United States yearly; about 2,000 Americans die of meningitis each year; greatest group at risk for meningitis are children between 1 and 24 months.

to comfort him or her (paradoxical irritability). Other symptoms of meningitis in infants can include jaundice (a yellow tint to the skin), stiffness of the body and neck (neck rigidity), a lower than normal temperature, poor feeding, a weak suck, and a high pitched cry, and bulging fontanelles (membranous junction between two surfaces of the skull bones).

Meningitis can also lead to skin rashes (50 percent of meningococcal meningitis), seizures, and loss of consciousness in the latter stages of the disease. Viral meningitis has similar symptoms to bacterial meningitis, such as fever, headache, nausea, vomiting, and body aches. These signs and symptoms are preceded by several days of a nonspecific, acute febrile (feverish) illness with malaise and loss of appetite.

Diagnosis

The most important diagnostic test for meningitis is to examine a sample of cerebrospinal fluid. The fluid is removed from the spinal canal with a needle in a procedure called a lumbar puncture. The classic symptoms and a lumbar puncture analysis that shows purulent spinal fluid (sign of inflammation) are usually all that is required for diagnosis.

Cerebrospinal fluid is examined for numbers and types of blood cells (complete blood count), for levels of substances such as glucose and protein, and for presence of microorganisms, which may be cultured, or propagated, for identification. In meningitis, the white blood cell count is elevated with a predominance of immature forms. Conversely, severe infection can be associated with a low white blood cell count. The results of glucose and protein analyses will depend on the severity of the disease.

Treatments

Treatment for meningitis depends on the cause of the infection. Viral meningitis comprises the majority of cases, with most people getting better in about two weeks. Mild cases of viral meningitis may only need home treatment, including fluids to prevent dehydration and control of pain and fever.

Bacterial meningitis will require hospital admission and a course of intravenous antibiotics. The disease is regarded as a medical emergency because death can occur within hours if bacterial meningitis is not treated promptly.

Broad-spectrum antibiotics should be started before test results become available, on the presumption that all cases are bacterial in nature until proven otherwise. Appropriate antibiotic treatment can reduce the mor-

tality rate of meningitis to below 15 percent. Corticosteriod drugs can reduce or prevent complications, such as hearing loss, that are associated with *Hemophilus influenzae* meningitis.

Prevention

Routine immunization of young adolescents will help prevent this rare but serious infection. Vaccines against the most common causes of bacterial meningitis (*Streptococcus pneumoniae* and *Neisseria meningitidis*) are recommended for people at high risk of infection. These include older adults and children, those with a weakened immune system, and those with a nonworking spleen. People traveling to areas, such as sub-Saharan Africa, where meningitis is prevalent should receive the *Neisseria meningitidis* vaccine.

The Centers for Disease Control and Prevention (CDC) now recommends the new vaccine Menactra T for protection against certain strains of *Neisseria meningitidis* for children age 11 and 12 years, teens entering high school, and college freshmen living in dormitories. Children between 2 months and 5 years should be vaccinated against *Hemophilus influenzae* type B bacteria. Pneumococcal conjugate vaccine (pneumovac) is part of the regular immunization for all children younger than 2 years in the United States. CDC recommends pneumovac for children 2 to 5 years with chronic heart disease, lung disease, or cancer. It is also recommended for adults older than 65, as well as those with chronic heart disease, diabetes, or sickle-cell anemia.

Epidemiology

There are 20,000 to 25,000 cases of bacterial meningitis in United States each year, and 2,000 people die of meningitis each year. There is an incidence of 4 to 10 cases per 100,000 people in the United States. The people at greatest risk for acute bacterial meningitis include children who are between 1 and 24 months of age. Adults older than 60 years account for 1,000 to 3,000 cases of acute bacterial meningitis each year in the United States and for more than 50 percent of all deaths related to meningitis. Worldwide, bacterial meningitis accounts for about 1.2 million cases annually.

Isaac Grate

See also
• Lyme disease • Syphilis
• Tuberculosis

Menopausal disorders

A set of symptoms and disorders commonly associated with menopause, a natural event that occurs in a woman's life as part of the aging process. Menopause is defined as 12 consecutive months without menstrual periods that is not due to an unrelated disease or other condition.

Menopause is either natural, with the gradual cessation of menstrual periods, or it can be induced or surgical, which is the cessation of ovarian function due to the surgical removal of the ovaries or as a result of chemotherapy or radiation therapy. There are more than 40 million menopausal or post-menopausal women in the United States, of whom almost half are over 65 years old. As life expectancy increases, most women will spend one-third of their life postmenopausal. Many women experience a relatively trouble-free menopause with just mild symptoms, but some women are seriously affected with symptoms and disorders that impact severely on their lifestyle.

Causes and risk factors

In the ovaries about 600,000 eggs are present at birth, 300,000 at the onset of menstruation, and fewer than 10,000 at the time of menopause. This normal decline is caused by the genetically programmed death of the eggs. Follicle-stimulating hormone (FSH) is one of the hormones the brain sends to the ovaries to develop the eggs. When a healthy egg is stimulated, it grows and produces estrogen. As the number of viable eggs declines, the level of FSH rises. When there are no viable eggs left, no more estrogen is produced by the ovaries, and FSH levels become even higher in an effort to stimulate the ovaries.

These hormonal changes and the irregular menstrual cycles that are associated with menopause typically start at about age 47, with menopause being completed by about age 52. This time period between the beginning and completion of menopause is called the climacteric.

About 1 percent of women are affected by premature menopause, which is the spontaneous cessation of menstrual periods before the age of 40 years. Factors associated with earlier menopause include a woman's mother's age when she experienced menopause,

KEY FACTS

Description
A set of symptoms associated with menopause, which is the cessation of menstrual periods due either to the natural loss of ovarian activity between the ages of 45 and 55, the surgical removal of the ovaries, chemotherapy, or radiation therapy, or the spontaneous cessation of periods prior to the age of 40, called premature menopause.

Causes and risk factors
Early menopause is linked to a woman's mother's age at menopause, nulliparity (never having delivered a baby), current cigarette smoking, genetic abnormalities, early onset of puberty, living at high altitudes, left-handedness, lower education and socioeconomic status, type 1 diabetes, and blindness. Late menopause is associated with having delivered many babies, obesity, prior use of oral contraceptives, and higher socioeconomic status.

Symptoms
Hot flashes, night sweats, sleep disturbances, vaginal dryness, pain and problems with intercourse, urinary incontinence (leaking urine unintentionally), mood changes, or problems with memory or concentration.

Diagnosis
There is no single perfect test for menopause. The diagnosis is confirmed by an elevated level of the hormone FSH (the signal the brain sends to the ovaries to tell them to make eggs), which rises dramatically when the ovaries do not respond because there are no longer any viable eggs. Menopause may also be suspected from the associated symptoms.

Treatments
Treatments are geared toward the specific medical issue or symptom.

Pathogenesis
The genetically programmed normal loss of ovarian function results in an estrogen-deficient state that affects many different systems or body parts, including bones, brain, breasts, skin, colon, urogenital (urinary and genital tract), and cardiovascular systems.

Prevention
There is no accepted way to delay or prevent menopause, although there are interventions and drugs that can help treat symptoms.

Epidemiology
There are more than 40 million menopausal and postmenopausal women in the United States.

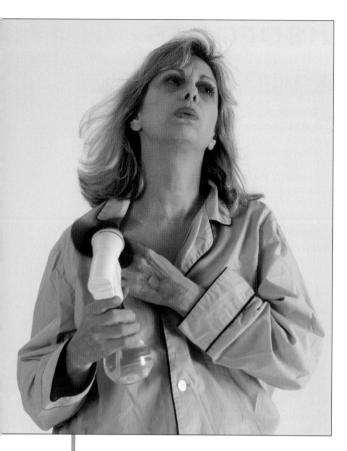

The most common complaints of menopause are vasomotor symptoms. These include hot flashes and night sweats—temporary reddening of the upper body with a sensation of heat, followed by sweating.

nulliparity (having no children), current smoking, genetic abnormalities (which may limit ovarian function), abnormally early puberty, living at high altitudes, left-handedness, lower education and socioeconomic status, type 1 diabetes, and blindness. Late menopause is associated with having given birth to several children, obesity, prior use of oral contraceptives, and higher socioeconomic status.

Symptoms and diagnosis

Vasomotor symptoms, which include hot flashes and night sweats, remain the most common and bothersome complaints faced by menopausal women, with up to 85 percent of menopausal women affected. Other associated symptoms include sleep disturbances, vaginal dryness, pain and problems with sexual intercourse, urinary incontinence (leaking urine unintentionally), mood changes, and problems with memory or concentration.

Although there is no perfect way to diagnose menopause, measuring the FSH level in the blood is the best single test. Menopause may also be suspected from the associated symptoms.

Pathogenesis

As the ovaries produce fewer hormones, including estrogen, many organ systems may be affected, including the cardiovascular and vasomotor systems, which are concerned with the constriction and dilation of blood vessels, the brain, breasts, urogenital tract (bladder and vagina), bones, colon, and skin.

Treatments and prevention

Treatments exist for each system affected by menopause. Cardiovascular disease, which includes heart attacks and stroke, is the leading cause of death in postmenopausal women, killing more women than all cancers combined. Treatment is geared toward lifestyle measures such as stopping cigarette smoking, managing weight and fat distribution, ensuring good nutrition, checking blood pressure, increasing physical activity, and lowering cholesterol.

Hot flashes usually go away (regardless of treatment) within five years in most women. About one-quarter of menopausal women will have flashes for up to ten years, and an unfortunate 10 percent of women can experience hot flashes for even longer. Treatment includes lifestyle modification such as dressing in layers of clothing, which can be sequentially removed when a flash comes on, and avoiding triggers such as spicy food. Various drugs or herbal preparations may help; hormone replacement therapy, which boosts the estrogen levels in the body, is the most effective medical treatment, and black cohosh the best herbal preparation. Estrogen creams may also be used to treat other menopausal symptoms such as vaginal dryness.

Osteoporosis, which is the loss of bone (and bone density) from the skeleton, is one of the biggest health problems in older women following menopause; it commonly leads to brittle bones and fractures of the hip, spinal column, or other bones. Exercise, calcium supplementation, and drugs are the mainstay to minimize this age-related disease.

Roxanne Vrees and
Gary Frishman

See also
- Diabetes • Fracture • Menstrual disorders
- Obesity • Osteoporosis

Menstrual disorders

Menstrual disorders include any interference with the normal menstrual cycle, menstrual pain, unusually heavy or light bleeding, and delayed or missed menstrual periods. A regular menstrual cycle occurs between 21 to 35 days, with 3 to 10 days of bleeding. Interruptions in this cycle can result in amenorrhea (cessation of menstruation), oligomenorrhea (infrequent menstrual cycles) menorrhagia (heavy bleeding), menometrorrhagia (irregular heavy bleeding) and dysmenorrhea (severe menstrual cramps).

Most women experience a form of menstrual disorder at some time. A regular menstrual cycle begins between the ages of 12 and 13 years. Most cycles occur between 21 and 35 days, with 3 to 10 days of bleeding and 1 to 1½ fluid ounces (30 to 40 ml) of blood loss. A typical menstrual cycle occurs about every 28 days, unless a woman is pregnant or moving into menopause. When the menstrual cycle is abnormally disrupted, a menstrual disorder may be occurring.

Menstrual disorders include amenorrhea (the cessation of menstruation), oligomenorrhea (infrequent menstruation), menorrhagia (heavy bleeding), menometrorrhagia (irregular heavy bleeding), dysmenorrhea (severe menstrual cramps), and premenstrual syndrome (PMS); emotional symptoms a week preceding menses. The physical and emotional symptoms accompanying these irregularities in the menstrual cycle may cause serious anxiety and distress for patients and their families and diminish the quality of life.

Symptoms and signs

Symptoms of menstrual disorders vary depending on the cause. Most menstrual disorders are caused by a hormonal imbalance or a dysfunction that is related directly to the female reproductive organs. A common cause of menstrual irregularity is polycystic ovary syndrome (POS), in which there is anovulation (lack of ovulation), which can result in oligomenorrhea or menometrorrhagia. The lack of progesterone associated with anovulation in POS can predispose a woman to endometrial cancer. In primary amenorrhea, the only symptom is delayed menstruation; in secondary amenorrhea, menstruation stops for at least three months.

Heavy bleeding and fatigue due to the loss of iron-rich blood are the symptoms of menorrhagia. In this type of menstrual disorder, blood flow soaks through a tampon or pad every hour for several hours, or a period lasts more than seven days. Symptoms of primary dysmenorrhea include severe cramping, pelvic pain, nausea, and vomiting and diarrhea. The symptoms may be stronger on one side of the body than the other. In secondary dysmenorrhea, the pain might feel like regular menstrual cramps but lasts longer than normal and occurs throughout the month. Another

KEY FACTS

Description
Painful menstruation; too light or too heavy bleeding during menstruation; frequent or infrequent menstruation; premenstrual syndrome.

Causes
Hormonal imbalance; the most common is polycystic ovary syndrome.

Risk factors
Excessive exercise, eating disorders, stress, and medical conditions such as fibroids, bleeding disorders, or diabetes.

Symptoms
Too much or too little blood flow or lower abdominal and pelvic pain radiating to the thighs and back during menstruation; debilitating emotional symptoms the week before menses.

Diagnosis
Laboratory tests for hormone levels, MRI or ultrasound imaging.

Treatments
Hormone replacement therapy or treatment of pain.

Pathogenesis
Fluctuation of ovarian hormones leading to irregular or ceased menstrual cycles.

Prevention
Healthy exercise and nutritional program, as well as dietary supplements and vitamins.

Epidemiology
Amenorrhea affects 2–5 percent of childbearing women; menstrual cramps or painful periods affects up to 90 percent of all women; heavy bleeding occurs in about 9–14 percent of all women. About 13–18 percent of women have symptoms severe enough to interfere with work and daily activities.

menstrual disorder is PMS, which is used to describe emotional symptoms like mood swings in the week preceding menses. If PMS is severe and debilitating, it is also known as premenstrual dysphoric disorder (PMDD).

Causes and risks

Since *menstrual disorders* is a general term to describe pathological variations in the menstrual cycle, the causes of each component are different. Lifestyle choices such as excessive exercise or low body weight can lead to primary amenorrhea. Medical conditions causing amenorrhea include Turner's syndrome, a birth defect related to the reproductive system, or ovarian problems. Secondary amenorrhea can be caused by pregnancy, breast-feeding, sudden weight loss or gain, intense exercise, stress, endocrine disorders affecting the thyroid, pituitary, or adrenal glands, and surgical procedures affecting the ovaries, including removal of the ovaries, cysts, or ovarian tumors. Amenorrhea is common in athletes or dancers and is frequently associated with two other disorders—reduced bone mass and eating disorders. This combination is sometimes called the female athlete triad.

Heavy or irregular bleeding during menstruation is a symptom of an underlying condition rather than a disease itself. It is usually related to a hormonal imbalance but can be caused by fibroids, cervical or endometrial polyps, the autoimmune disease lupus, pelvic inflammatory disease (PID), blood platelet disorder, a hereditary blood factor deficiency, or possibly, some reproductive cancers. Having these other conditions may increase the risk of menstrual disorders in a particular individual.

Dysmenorrhea is usually related to the production of prostaglandins, naturally occurring chemicals that cause an inflammatory reaction. Women with severe menstrual pain have higher levels of prostaglandin in their menstrual blood than women without such pain. In some women, prostaglandins can cause some of the smooth muscles in the gastrointestinal tract to contract, resulting in the nausea, vomiting, and diarrhea that some women experience. Other causes of dysmenorrhea include fibroids, PID, an intrauterine device, uterine, ovarian, bowel, or bladder tumor, uterine polyps, inflammatory bowel disease, scarring or adhesions from surgery, and endometriosis or adenomyosis, conditions in which the endometrial lining grows in other areas of the pelvic cavity. As in menorrhagia, having any of these conditions increases the risk for menstrual disorders. The likely causes of PMS or PMDD are hormonal imbalances.

Diagnosis and treatments

Menstrual disorders are diagnosed by considering family and medical history, eating and exercise habits, lifestyle, stress levels, changes in body weight, and a pelvic exam. Routine blood tests are done to measure hormone levels and to check for pregnancy. A diagnosis may include an endometrial biopsy in which a small amount of tissue is scraped from the lining of the uterus for examination. An ultrasound of the pelvic area typically allows visualization of any internal structural anomalies. Similarly, surgical procedures may include laparoscopy, in which a thin tube with a camera attached is inserted through a small incision below or through the navel, or a hysteroscopy, in which a thin tube with a camera attached is inserted into the vagina and up through the cervix; these allow internal views of the abdominal cavity and uterus, respectively.

Treatments for menstrual disorders depend on which type of disorder is diagnosed. In the case of amenorrhea, simple changes in lifestyle such as reducing the intensity of exercise, maintaining an appropriate weight, and reducing stress levels may solve the problem. Surgery is recommended only in rare cases in which amenorrhea is linked to ovarian cysts, vaginal blockage, or uterine anatomical abnormalities. It is essential to determine the cause before treating menorrhagia. Medical therapies may help, but occasionally surgery is indicated. In most cases, surgery involves removing the lining of the uterus temporarily or permanently. There are a number of procedures that can achieve this goal, such as a dilation and curettage, endometrial biopsy, endometrial resection, and endometrial ablation. Primary dysmenorrhea is handled with drugs and nonmedical treatments. Drugs include either over-the-counter nonsteroidal anti-inflammatory drugs (NSAIDS) or prescription medications such as oral contraceptives that provide cycle control and reduce menstrual blood flow.

Nonmedical treatments include using a heating pad on the abdomen or taking warm baths to reduce discomfort. Taking B vitamins, magnesium, and omega-3 fatty acid supplements may also help. Menstrual disorders are diverse and complicated and require medical consultation.

Rashmi Nemade

See also
• Anemia • Cancer, ovarian • Cancer, uterine • Fibroids • Menopausal disorders

Migraine

Migraine is characterized by intense pulsing or throbbing pain in one area of the head, accompanied by extreme sensitivity to light and sound, nausea, and vomiting. Some people can predict the onset of a migraine because it is preceded by an "aura," a type of visual disturbance that appears as flashing lights, zigzag lines, or a temporary loss of vision. Migraine is three times more common in women than in men.

Migraine headaches are a legitimate biological disease consisting of severe, painful headaches and extreme sensitivity to light and sound. Migraines can often be recurring and disabling. These types of headaches are also associated with nausea and vomiting. Some migraine sufferers also experience an aura, a warning in which visual disturbances appear as flashing lights, zigzag lines, or even a temporary loss of vision that forecast an oncoming migraine.

Typically, people with migraine tend to have recurring attacks triggered by eating certain foods, a lack of food or sleep, exposure to light, or hormonal irregularities (only in women). Anxiety, stress, or relaxation after stress can also be triggers.

About 13 percent of the U.S. population—28 million Americans—suffer from migraines. Migraine is more common than asthma, diabetes, and coronary artery disease combined. It afflicts both women and men, but three times more women experience migraine. The first attack usually occurs before the age of 30, but even children as young as 2 years can be affected by migraine. Migraine is a chronic, recurrent disease. Although some people have attacks several times a month, sufferers typically experience an average of two attacks per month, which can last any duration between 4 and 72 hours.

Causes

Although the cause of migraines is unknown, there are many theories put forward by the medical and research communities. For many years, it was believed that migraines were linked to the dilation and constriction of blood vessels of the dura mater (the outer covering of the brain). However, recent evidence has led investigators to believe that migraine is caused by inherited abnormalities in genes that control the activities of certain cell populations in the brain. A predominant theory is that migraines are caused by functional changes in the trigeminal nerve system, a major pain pathway in the nervous system, and by imbalances in brain chemicals such as serotonin, which regulates pain messages passing through this pathway. During a migraine, serotonin levels drop. Researchers believe this causes the trigeminal nerve to release substances called neuropeptides, which travel to the dura mater. There, they cause blood vessels to become dilated and inflamed. The result is a headache. Because levels of magnesium, a mineral involved in the functioning of neurons, also drop right before or during a migraine, it is possible that low amounts of magnesium may cause nerve cells in the brain to misfire.

KEY FACTS

Description
A headache of intense pulsing or throbbing pain in one area of the head.

Causes
Unknown but there are many theories.

Risk factors
Family history and being young and female, along with a number of triggers including hormonal changes, certain foods, stress, sensory stimuli, changes in the environment or schedule, and certain drugs.

Symptoms
Recurring attacks of severe pain on one or both sides of the head, nausea, vomiting, and sensitivity to light and sound.

Diagnosis
Medical history; physical exam; CT or MRI scan.

Treatments
Drugs for pain relief and prevention.

Pathogenesis
Drop in serotonin thought to cause the trigeminal nerve to release neuropeptides, causing inflammation of the brain's outer covering (dura mater).

Prevention
Avoiding migraine triggers.

Epidemiology
More than 28 million Americans—three times more women than men—suffer from migraine headaches.

Risk factors

Whatever the exact mechanism of migraine headaches, a number of factors may trigger them. Common migraine headache triggers include hormonal changes, sensory stimuli, foods, stress, changes in the environment or schedule, and certain drugs. Although the exact relationship between hormones and headaches is not clear, fluctuations in the hormones estrogen and progesterone seem to trigger migraine headaches in many women. Women with a history of migraines often have reported headaches immediately before or during their menstrual periods. Others report more migraines during pregnancy or menopause. Hormonal drugs, such as contraceptives and hormone replacement therapy, also may worsen migraines. Sensory stimuli such as bright lights and sun glare can produce headaches, as can pleasant scents, such as perfume and flowers, and unpleasant odors, such as paint thinner and secondhand smoke. Certain foods appear to trigger headaches in some people. Common offenders include alcohol, especially beer and red wine; aged cheeses; chocolate; fermented, pickled or marinated foods; aspartame; caffeine; monosodium glutamate, which is a key ingredient in some Asian foods; certain seasonings; and many canned and processed foods. However, skipping meals or fasting also can trigger migraines. Behavioral aspects such as stress, intense physical exertion, including sexual activity, changes in sleep patterns (too much or too little sleep), or changes in the weather, season, altitude, barometric pressure, or time zone may provoke migraines as well. Also, certain drugs can aggravate migraines. Thus, there are many aspects to migraine triggers. Triggers are not the same for everyone; what causes a migraine in one person may relieve it in another.

The definite risk factors for developing migraines are family history and being young and female. Migraine is often hereditary. In fact, a child has a 50 percent chance of becoming a sufferer if one parent suffers and a 75 percent chance if both parents suffer. The fact that young women are more likely to suffer from migraines possibly reflects the puzzling relationship between migraines and hormones. Many people find that their attacks of migraine lessen and are not as severe as they get older.

Signs and symptoms

Migraine headaches are characterized by throbbing head pain, usually located on one side of the head and often accompanied by nausea and sensitivity to light or sound or both. The combination of disabling pain and associated symptoms often prevents sufferers from performing daily activities. Symptoms, incidence, and severity vary by individual. Less than a third of sufferers experience what is called an aura. They may see flashes of light, blind spots, zigzag lines, and shimmering lights and may experience vision loss and numbness prior to the head pain and other symptoms.

Diagnosis

Typically, diagnosis of migraine is simple, involving only a medical history and physical examination. Occasionally, CT (computed tomography) or MRI (magnetic resonance imaging) scans and lumbar puncture are conducted to rule out underlying causes.

Treatments

Drugs are the primary treatment for migraine. Drugs for migraines fall into two classes: pain-relieving drugs that stop pain once it has started, and preventive drugs that reduce or prevent a future migraine headache.

Pain-relief drugs such as nonsteroidal anti-inflammatory drugs (NSAIDs) can treat the inflammation in the dura mater, whereas drugs called triptans and ergots can treat the blood-vessel dilation in the brain and dura mater, and others still can treat nausea and vomiting.

Preventive drugs can reduce the frequency, severity, and length of migraines and may increase the effectiveness of pain-relieving drugs used during migraine attacks. Preventive drugs include cardiovascular drugs, antidepressants, NSAIDs, antiseizure drugs, and cyproheptadine, an antihistamine. Overall, there are many treatment options for people who suffer from migraine headaches.

Epidemiology

Sources from the American Medical Association report that approximately 6 percent of men and 18 percent of women suffer from migraine in the United States. The age range of those people most likely to report migraine is 24 to 44 years. People who suffer from migraine typically have 24 to 35 attacks each year.

Rashmi Nemade

See also
• Alcohol-related disorders • Allergy and sensitivity • Anxiety disorders

Miscarriage

A miscarriage, also known as a spontaneous abortion, is a pregnancy that spontaneously ends before the fetus is able to live outside the uterus. *Therapeutic abortion* is the equivalent term for an elective termination of pregnancy, which lay people often refer to as an abortion. About 15 to 20 percent of women who know they are pregnant will spontaneously miscarry. However, many pregnancies end before women even realize they are pregnant. Miscarriages generally occur before 20 to 22 weeks of pregnancy and most take place in the first trimester (first three months of pregnancy). Miscarriage is the most common problem in early pregnancy.

Genetic abnormalities, such as too few or too many chromosomes, are the most common reason for miscarriages. This is especially true during the early part of a pregnancy. Less commonly, a medical problem with the mother can lead to a miscarriage. These problems include uncontrolled diabetes mellitus or the uterus being abnormally structured, which prevents the normal growth and development of a pregnancy.

The single biggest risk factor for miscarriage is the increasing age of the mother. This probably relates to a higher risk of chromosomal abnormalities, and a woman more than 40 has a risk of miscarriage of 40 percent or more. Smoking more than 10 cigarettes each day or consuming more than 30 ounces (880 ml) of alcohol per month also increase the chance of a miscarriage. Taking in 500 milligrams or more of caffeine per day has been linked to an increased rate of miscarriage. One cup of coffee contains 0.003 to 0.005 ounces (100 to 135 mg) of caffeine. Infections, such as herpes, may be linked to miscarriage. Contrary to popular belief, abdominal injuries in early pregnancy, such as falling down stairs or having a motor vehicle accident, are unlikely to result in miscarriage.

If a woman has had one previous miscarriage, the probability of miscarriage during her next pregnancy is not significantly elevated and remains at about 20 percent. After two miscarriages, the probability of miscarriage is 28 percent, but it rises to 43 percent after three previous miscarriages. However, the majority of pregnancies still result in the delivery of a baby, even in women who have had three miscarriages.

Symptoms

The most common symptoms of miscarriages are vaginal bleeding or abdominal cramping, or both, similar to a very heavy period. The vaginal bleeding can vary from light spotting to (rarely) hemorrhaging requiring a blood transfusion. There are different types of miscarriages. Passing all the pregnancy tissue is known as a complete miscarriage. If some of the pregnancy tissue is not passed and remains in the uterus, this is known as an incomplete miscarriage. A threatened miscarriage is when a woman has bleeding but the pregnancy is ongoing. Threatened miscarriages occur in up to 50 percent of pregnancies, but only half of these will miscarry. An inevitable miscarriage is one

KEY FACTS

Description
Spontaneous ending of a pregnancy before the fetus is able to survive outside the womb (uterus).

Causes
Usually genetic (chromosomal) abnormalities of the fetus. Less commonly, medical problems with the mother such as uncontrolled diabetes or structural abnormalities.

Risk factors
Advancing age, previous miscarriages, smoking, alcohol or drug use, high caffeine intake.

Symptoms
Vaginal bleeding or abdominal pain, or both.

Diagnosis
Pelvic examination; blood tests; ultrasound.

Treatments
Surgical procedure (dilatation and curettage); drugs that cause the uterus to pass any remaining tissue; observation.

Prevention
Treat any correctable causes, such as malformation of the uterus; avoidance of tobacco and drugs.

Epidemiology
15 to 20 percent of women who know they are pregnant have a miscarriage. Many miscarriages occur before women know they are pregnant.

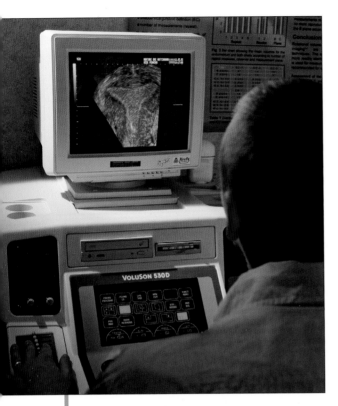

A gynecologist performs an ultrasound scan on a woman's uterus. The uterus shows a congenital deformation called uterus arcuatus; it has a Y shape instead of a rounded top. This malformation may result in infertility or miscarriage.

in which the cervix (the lower opening of the uterus) is open. Although the pregnancy is still inside the uterus, a miscarriage cannot be avoided.

Septic miscarriages are uncommon, accounting for less than 2 percent of all miscarriages. Septic miscarriages result from an infection in the uterus, often due to a foreign object being placed in the uterus, such as during an illegal abortion. In addition to bleeding and pain, symptoms of septic miscarriage include fever, chills, and possibly a thick, yellow-green, foul-smelling vaginal discharge. A septic miscarriage can be very dangerous if not treated in a timely manner.

Diagnosis

The most helpful blood test in early pregnancy is the beta human chorionic gonadotropin (B-hCG) test. This test confirms the presence of a pregnancy, and serial measurements can help determine whether it is healthy. An ultrasound uses sound waves without radiation to examine pregnancies for their location and health and is very useful in diagnosing miscarriages. A

pregnancy cannot usually be seen with an ultrasound until about five weeks of age. If the pregnancy is more than six weeks old, a fetal heartbeat may be seen. Obversation of a fetal heartbeat on ultrasound is a reassuring sign that the pregnancy is likely to continue.

Treatments

Treatments for miscarriages include surgery, drug treatment, or observation. Surgical treatment consists of a dilatation and curettage (D and C) or, later in pregnancy, a dilatation and evacuation (D and E). Both of these involve gently dilating the cervix and removing the pregnancy contents inside the uterus. Surgery is the fastest way to treat a miscarriage and is the preferred choice for women who are bleeding heavily or have a septic miscarriage. Although very safe, the risks of this surgery include damaging the uterus or causing an infection. These complications may diminish future fertility. Management with drugs is an option for women whose pregnancy is less than 12 weeks and who wish to avoid surgery. Currently, misoprostol is the drug most commonly used to treat miscarriage in the United States. The most common side effects from misoprostol are nausea, vomiting, and severe cramping. This treatment results in successful expulsion of the pregnancy 70 to 90 percent of the time. A dilatation and curettage may need to be done if the treatment with misoprostol is unsuccessful. Observation, or expectant management, is the third option for women without significant bleeding, cramping, or signs of infection. Most miscarriages will be naturally expelled within the first two weeks after diagnosis. If this does not happen, the woman can then undergo surgery or treatment with drugs.

Emotional impact of miscarriage

Grieving and a profound sense of loss often accompany a miscarriage, with the intensity of these symptoms varying among patients. Frequently, women blame themselves for their loss. It is often helpful to explain to patients that most miscarriages are due to genetic abnormalities and reassure them that they did not cause the miscarriage. Also, it is important to explain that one miscarriage does not lessen a woman's chance of having a successful pregnancy in the future.

Emily White and
Gary Frishman

See also
• Diabetes • Ectopic pregnancy

Mononucleosis

Also called the "kissing disease," mono, and Pfeiffer's disease in North America and glandular fever in other countries, mononucleosis is characterized by sore throat, fever, and enlarged lymph nodes, particularly those in the neck. The disease most commonly affects people between the ages of 12 and 20 years.

Mononucleosis was first described in Germany in 1889 as *drusenfieber*, meaning "glandular fever." In 1920, the term *infectious mononucleosis* was applied to six college students who developed an illness that was characterized by fever and an increased count of white blood cells called lymphocytes. Since then, research has shown that 90 percent of mononucleosis syndromes are a result of infection with the Epstein-Barr virus (EBV). Other infections that have symptoms that may resemble mononucleosis include acute toxoplasmosis, a protozoan infection obtained from cats or from eating raw meats; acute cytomegalovirus (CMV) infection, a viral infection of white blood cells; hepatitis B, a viral infection that can cause liver inflammation; and infection with human immunodeficiency virus (HIV), which in its early stages has symptoms similar to those of mononucleosis.

Herpes family of viruses

EBV is a virus in the herpes family that has a predilection for infecting B lymphocytes. Once inside these cells, the virus can become a persistent, lifelong (but generally silent) infection, reactivating when the immune defenses weaken. EBV is nearly ubiquitous in humans, with 90 to 95 percent of adults harboring evidence of past infection. The virus is transmitted by intimate contact, often through saliva, hence the nickname "kissing disease." Asymptomatic carriers can shed the virus in their saliva for over a year and sometimes intermittently throughout their life.

Symptoms and signs

Mononucleosis occurs in a wide range of ages from childhood to adulthood, but in developed countries the disease most commonly affects preadolescents and adolescents. Young children often do not have symptoms. Classically, adolescents with mononucleosis have the triad of moderate to high fever, sore throat, and enlarged lymph nodes. These symptoms occur after a four- to seven-week incubation, during which people may have milder symptoms, such as headache, fatigue, and a slightly raised temperature. Other symptoms that may occur include rash, enlargement of the spleen, swelling around the eye, yellowing of the white of the eyes (jaundice), anemia, and neurological syndromes. There is an interesting phenomenon in which patients who are treated with the antibiotic amoxicillin for the possibility of a streptococcal throat infection, but who actually have Epstein-Barr infection, develop a rash.

KEY FACTS

Description
A syndrome characterized by fever and enlarged lymph nodes caused by a number of different pathogens.

Causes
Predominantly caused by the Epstein-Barr virus, but also by HIV, *Toxoplasma* protozoa, hepatitis B virus, and the cytomegalovirus. Transmitted by intimate physical contact, including via passage of saliva during kissing.

Risk factors
Close contact with someone suffering from mononucleosis.

Symptoms and signs
Fever, sore throat, enlarged lymph nodes, fatigue, malaise, enlarged spleen, rash. Complications include splenic rupture, tonsil enlargement, persisting fatigue, and neurological syndromes.

Diagnosis
Blood tests, including a complete blood count and finding a heterophile antibody. Serology may be done to help confirm the diagnosis.

Treatments
Supportive care.

Pathogenesis
May result in chronic fatigue syndrome.

Prevention
Physical activity limited to prevent splenic rupture and to allow the body to recover from fatigue.

Epidemiology
Nearly all humans infected by adulthood. Once infected, the virus can persist in an individual in a silent state, reactivating when the immune system weakens.

Diagnosis

Mononucleosis should be suspected in patients who display the classic triad of symptoms. The addition of blood tests help confirm the diagnosis. A complete blood count and a smear of blood may show an elevated lymphocyte count and a small percentage of atypical lymphocytes. These abnormal lymphocytes are large, with generous cytoplasm, and often are seen to be sticking to nearby cells. Liver enzymes may also be elevated on blood tests. Serology studies, the measurement of a person's immune response against an antigen, can be helpful in diagnosing the specific cause of mononucleosis.

In about 90 percent of patients with a mononucleosis syndrome due to EBV, the diagnosis can be made by finding a heterophile antibody. This is an antibody found in infected people that has the ability to clump sheep red blood cells. In the same blood sample, specific antibodies against EBV can also be screened for.

If evidence of EBV cannot be confirmed, further serological tests can be carried out to look for the other potential causes of mononucleosis, including tests for HIV, CMV, *Toxoplasma*, and hepatitis viruses.

Treatments

Therapy for mononucleosis is mainly supportive. Providing adequate rest, fluids, and nutrition, along with pain control with acetaminophen or nonsteroidal anti-inflammatory drugs such as ibuprofen, are usually all that is needed.

Complications

A rare, but potentially life-threatening complication of mononucleosis due to Epstein-Barr infection involves the spleen. About 50 percent of people with mononucleosis due to EBV will have splenic enlargement. Very rarely, this enlargement can lead to rupture and disastrous internal bleeding. Although half of these cases are spontaneous, it is important that infected individuals, especially those with an enlarged spleen, limit participation in contact sports.

Recovering from the tiredness brought on by mononucleosis may take several weeks or even months. Experts recommend limiting activity for at least three weeks after the start of the illness for noncontact sports, and a minimum of four weeks for contact sports such as football. However, if the spleen is still enlarged after four weeks, it is prudent to continue to limit activity. Athletes should return to activity gradually, as the fatigue from the illness may prevent them from reaching preinfection activity levels until several months later.

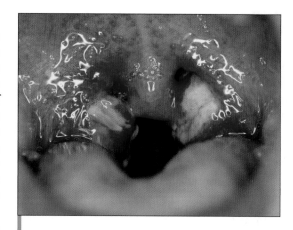

This inflamed throat, with the tonsils covered in a thick white coating, is a typical symptom of mononucleosis. This infection is usually caused by the Epstein–Barr virus, which belongs to the herpes virus family.

Another potentially dangerous complication of mononucleosis is the extreme enlargement of the tonsils, lymphoid tissue located on both sides of the back of the throat. These can grow and touch one another—a condition that is often called "kissing tonsils"—which can lead to airway obstruction that requires placement of a mechanical airway.

A more common complication often seen by physicians is fatigue and sleepiness that persists for months after the acute illness. Usually these individuals improve, and their symptoms will resolve in less than six months, but some continue to have fatigue for over a year. It is thought that EBV triggers chronic fatigue syndrome in these people.

Other rare complications of mononucleosis due to Epstein-Barr infection include encephalitis (infection and inflammation of the brain) and a rare syndrome known as Guillain-Barré syndrome. In this syndrome the coating of the nerve axons is destroyed, starting from the toes, and gradually progresses up the body, resulting in an ascending paralysis. However, most people do make a complete recovery from the syndrome, although some suffer repeated attacks and have a residual weakness.

Edward Cachay and
Sanjay Mehta

See also
• Epstein-Barr infection • Guillain-Barré syndrome • Hepatitis infections • Herpes infections • Paralysis • Throat infections

Mood disorders

Mood disorders, also known as affective disorders, are a group of disorders that display an abnormal range of moods that fluctuate between extremes of lows and highs and result in impairment in social and occupational functioning. They are one of the most ancient and common mental disorders affecting the general population.

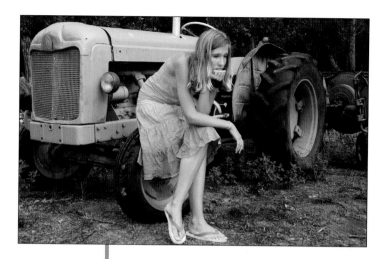

Mood disorders are defined by their patterns of mood episodes. Depressive disorders include major depression and dysthymic disorder. Bipolar disorders consist of bipolar I, bipolar II, and cyclothymic disorder.

People who have affective disorders, such as bipolar disorders, may feel elated and depressed at the same time. Two chemicals in the brain, serotonin and norepinephrine, are imbalanced and are believed to influence mood swings.

Causes of mood disorders

The exact causes are unknown, but genetic, biochemical, psychosocial, and environmental factors each may contribute. The genetic factor for depressive disorder suggests that first-degree relatives are 2 to 3 times more likely to have a major depressive disorder. Twin studies reported 50 percent of identical twins and 10 to 25 percent of fraternal twins are affected with depressive disorders.

First-degree relatives of patients with bipolar disorder are 8 to 18 times more likely to develop the illness. Twin studies reported 75 percent of identical and 5 to 25 percent of fraternal twins are affected with bipolar disorders.

Biochemical causes of mood disorders include a decrease in certain neurotransmitters (brain chemicals) such as serotonin, norepinephrine, and dopamine. Individuals with bipolar disorder may have increased norepinephrine, serotonin, and dopamine in the central nervous system (CNS).

Stressful life events more often cause a first episode of mood disorders (major depressive disorders and bipolar I disorders). The loss of one parent before age 11 most often causes depression at a later age. Environmental stressors, for example, the death of a relative or of a spouse, are most often associated with the onset of depression.

Risk factors

In addition to the above factors, certain medical conditions, including thyroid diseases, adrenal diseases, and hormonal imbalance are risk factors for developing a mood disorder. Other known risk factors are certain medications, such as antihypertensive medications, bronchodilators, and levodopa. The abuse of central nervous system (CNS) depressants such as alcohol and sedative-hypnotics or CNS stimulants such as amphetamines and cocaine, viral infections such as mononucleosis, and HIV infection can all increase the chance of developing a depressive disorder.

Major depression

The symptoms of major depression include feelings of intense sadness that cause daily life to become very difficult. A person with major depression tends to be in a depressed mood most of the day, loses interest in pleasurable activities, has changes in appetite or body weight (increased or decreased), has feelings of worthlessness or excessive guilt, insomnia or hypersomnia, decreased concentration, restlessness or slowness, fatigue or loss of energy, recurrent thoughts of death, and suicidal ideations or attempts.

The criteria for diagnosis of major depression are that a person must have at least two weeks of either a depressed mood or the loss of interest or pleasure in nearly all activities. The individual must have at least five of the symptoms. These symptoms cannot be due to substance abuse or medical conditions, and they must cause social or occupational impairment.

Hospitalization is indicated if the patient is at risk of suicide or unable to care for him- or herself. Selective serotonin reuptake inhibitors (SSRIs), tricyclic antidepressants, and atypical antidepressants are types of antidepressant medications. Electric shock treatment is recommended for a person with a severe form of depression that is not responsive to medications. Psychotherapy (counseling) for major depression includes supportive, cognitive, and behavioral therapy. The natural course of depressive episodes is

from 6 months to 13 months, and if left untreated, depressive episodes are self-limiting.

There is a 50 percent risk of having a subsequent major depressive episode within the first two years after the first episode. About 15 percent of patients will eventually commit suicide.

Antidepressant medications significantly reduce the length and severity of symptoms. To reduce the risk of subsequent episodes, antidepressants could be used prophylactically between major depressive episodes. Approximately 75 percent of patients are treated successfully with medications.

The average age of the onset of major depression is 40. Women are twice as likely to be affected with this disorder as men. Lifetime prevalence is 15 percent; in the elderly the prevalence is from 25 to 50 percent. There are no ethnic or socioeconomic differences associated with this disorder.

Dysthymic disorder

Symptoms consist of someone having a depressed mood for the majority of the time on most days, poor concentration, difficulty making decisions, change in appetite (loss of appetite or overeating) and sleep (insomnia or excessive sleep), low energy or fatigue, low self-esteem, and feelings of hopelessness.

For a diagnosis of dysthymic disorder to be confirmed, the person must have at least two of the above symptoms for two years or more, and must never have been without the symptoms for more than two months at a time. There is no major depressive episode.

Cognitive therapy and insight-oriented psychotherapy are most effective. Antidepressant medications are given that are similar to those prescribed for major depression, except that the treatment is of shorter duration for dysthymic disorder. These treatments are useful when they are used concurrently.

Twenty percent of patients will develop major depression, 20 percent will develop bipolar disorder, and 25 percent will have lifelong symptoms.

Medications and psychotherapy similar to those used for major depression are commonly used. Daily exercise and stress management could be helpful.

Lifetime prevalence is 6 percent. It is 2 to 3 times more common in women. The onset of this disorder is before age 25 in 50 percent of patients. It is a chronic and less severe form of major depression.

Bipolar I disorder

Also known as manic depression, a person with bipolar disorder tends to alternate between periods of high ac-

KEY FACTS: DEPRESSIVE DISORDERS

Description
Depressive disorders are mood disorders with both severe and mild forms of depression.

Causes
Unknown, but genetic and bio-psychosocial factors may each contribute.

Risk factors
Genetic factors, medical conditions, stressful life events, and a decrease in brain chemicals, such as serotonin and dopamine.

Symptoms
Depressed mood, decreased interest, change in appetite, sleep disturbances, poor concentration, worthlessness or guilt, and suicidal ideation.

Diagnosis
Evaluation by a psychiatrist.

Treatments
Antidepressants and psychotherapy are usually recommended.

Pathogenesis
Affects people of all ages and is recurrent. The usual duration of major depression if untreated lasts for 6–13 months. Suicide rate is about 15 percent with major depression.

Prevention
Antidepressant medications, which can also be given prophylactically between episodes of illness, reduce the length and severity of symptoms.

Epidemiology
Around 15 million people in the United States suffer from depression in a given year, which is about 7 percent of the population. Women are twice more likely to have depression than men.

tivity or mania and low energy levels with abnormal depression. Manic symptoms also include inflated self-esteem or grandiosity; increase in goal-directed activity (occupational or social or both); easy distractibility; decreased need for sleep; racing thoughts or ideas; hypertalkative or pressured speech (rapid and uninterruptible); excessive involvement in pleasurable activities that have a high risk of negative consequences, for example spending sprees, hypersexuality, and driving while under the influence of drugs and alcohol.

To be sure of a definitive diagnosis for bipolar I disorder, the patient must show a period of abnormally and persistently elevated, expansive, or irritable mood, which lasts at least one week and which includes at least three of the symptoms above. These symptoms should not be a result of general medical conditions or substance abuse, and they must cause impairment in social and occupational functioning.

Medications (mood stabilizers) such as lithium, carbamazepine, or valproic acid can help. Supportive psychotherapy, group therapy, and family therapies are used when the patient is well controlled with medication. Electroconvulsive therapy (ECT) is usually used only for patients who do not improve with medications.

Untreated manic episodes generally last about three months. The course is usually chronic with relapses. More frequent relapses are associated with a longer history of manic symptoms. Bipolar I disorder has a worse prognosis than major depressive disorder. Lithium prophylaxis between episodes helps to decrease the risk of relapse of bipolar I disorder.

Onset is usually before age 30. Women and men are equally affected with this disorder. Lifetime prevalence is 1 percent. There are no ethnic differences associated with bipolar I disorder.

Bipolar II disorder

Hypomanic (an abnormality of mood resembling mania) symptoms include elevated mood, inflated self-esteem, decreased need for sleep, hypertalkative, racing thoughts or ideas, distractibility, and hyperactivity with high potential for painful consequences. The depressive symptoms exhibited are similar to those of major depression.

The criteria for a definitive diagnosis of bipolar II disorder are that the person is required to have a history of one or more major depressive episodes—and at least one hypomanic episode of abnormal mood that lasts for 4 days. During these episodes, the person has no impairment in either social or occupational functioning.

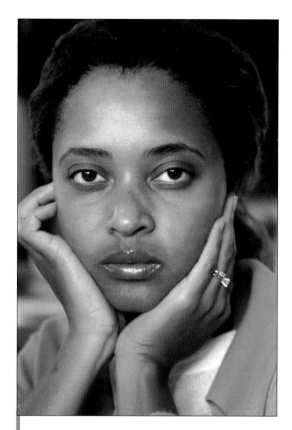

Many mood disorders are more common in women and they often begin at a crucial period in someone's life. However, they do vary in severity. Mood stabilizers and psychotherapy can help many people.

Medications and psychotherapy are the treatment of choice and are similar to the treatment of bipolar I disorder. Caution must be taken for patients on antidepressants, because there is a possibility of a switch to mania with tricyclic antidepressants and some SSRIs.

Bipolar II disorders tend to be recurrent and chronic, requiring long-term treatment. Mood stabilizers such as lithium and psychotherapy are helpful in preventing bipolar II disorders.

Lifetime prevalence for bipolar II disorders is 0.5 percent. The disorder is slightly more common in women. The onset of this disorder is usually before age 30. There are no ethnic differences associated with this disorder.

Cyclothymic disorder

This is a milder form of bipolar disorder consisting of recurrent mood symptoms associated with hypomania (like mania but of lesser intensity) and dysthymic mood. There are numerous periods of hypomanic symptoms and periods of dysthymic disorder symptoms for two years. However, the symptoms are less severe than bipolar I, bipolar II, and major depression. Cyclothymic disorder is not diagnosed if a person has had a manic episode or a major depressive episode. Mood stabilizers such as lithium, valproic acid, and carbamazapine are usually helpful.

KEY FACTS: BIPOLAR DISORDERS

Description
Bipolar disorders are mood disorders with episodes of mania and major depression, hypomania, and mild to moderate depression with low grade mania.

Causes
Both genetic and environmental factors appear to play a role.

Risk factors
Decrease in brain chemical such as dopamine and serotonin; stressful life events; genetic factors, and certain medical conditions.

Symptoms
Elevated mood; decreased need for sleep; inflated self-esteem; racing thoughts or ideas; distractibility; hyperactivity; hypertalkative; risk-taking behavior; may or may not have an episode of major depressive symptoms. Hypomanic symptoms with bipolar II; mild manic and depressive symptoms with cyclothymic disorder.

Diagnosis
Evaluation by a psychiatrist.

Treatments
Medications (mood stabilizers and antidepressants) and psychotherapy.

Pathogenesis
Untreated manic episodes usually last for 3 months with bipolar I disorder. The course is usually chronic with relapses for all types of bipolar disorders.

Prevention
Mood stabilizers such as lithium and valproate. Psychotherapy may help prevent bipolar II disorders. For bipolar I disorders, lithium as a prophylactic between episodes helps decrease risk of relapse.

Epidemiology
Bipolar disorder affects about 6 million people in the United States, that is, about 2.5 percent of the U.S. population who are 18 years or more in a given year.

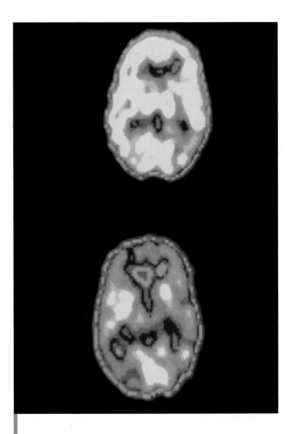

These axial PET scans are of a normal brain (top) and the other from a patient with a depressive illness. The brain of the person suffering from depression shows a markedly lower brain activity than that of the normal brain. The activity in the brain is processed to produce color coded images; areas of activity in these scans are yellow.

This disorder has a chronic course. About one-third of cyclothymic patients are eventually diagnosed with bipolar disorder (I and II). A person with cyclothymia may seldom feel the need to seek medical attention for their mood symptoms.

The lifetime prevalence of this disorder is less than 1 percent. The onset is usually between the ages of 15 to 25. Cyclothymic disorder occurs equally in men and women.

Nurun Shah

See also
- Adrenal disorders • Anxiety disorders
- Bipolar disorder • Depressive disorders
- Post-traumatic stress disorder
- Psychotic disorders • Schizophrenia
- Sleep disorders • Thyroid disorders

Motion sickness

Motion sickness, seasickness, and airsickness are all essentially the same condition: unease followed by nausea and vomiting during motion or travel. For reasons that are unclear, some people are more prone to motion sickness than others.

For a person to be able to balance, the brain must receive sensory input from three very different sources. Input from the eyes tells the person where the horizon is and the position of the head and the body in space. Input also comes from the muscles, tendons, and joints of the lower extremities (the so-called proprioceptive system) and from motion sensors in both inner ears. The inner ear comprises the organ of hearing, or the cochlea, and the organ of balance, which includes structures called the utricle, saccule, and semicircular canals. Electrical impulses from these three distinct inputs are processed in the part of the brain called the cerebellum, and the patterns of these impulses are integrated in the brain. This information tells a person exactly his or her position in space. In simple terms, the brain can be compared to a computer receiving simultaneous information from three different sources and matching them for symmetry. Should there be a mismatch between these inputs, conflicting information reaches the brain. The confusion results in dizziness, or giddiness, or even vertigo. This sensory conflict is thought to be the cause of motion sickness.

For example, a person sitting at the back of a bus reading a book does not see any movement, and his or her eyes send information to the brain that his or her head is stationary. However, as the bus moves, the inner ears are unconsciously informing the brain that the head and body are in motion. As a result, the brain becomes confused, and this confusion is thought to be the underlying cause of motion sickness.

Symptoms and signs and prevention

Motion sickness is often characterized by a feeling of dizziness and fatigue, which may progress to headache, nausea, and vomiting. Stopping the motion stops the symptoms of motion sickness.

Prevention is best performed by sitting in an area of a vehicle that pitches and rolls the least, such as over the wings in an airplane. On boats or ships, staying above deck in midship and facing forward, in the direction of travel, appears to be efficacious for seasickness. To prevent motion sickness in an automobile, sitting in the front with eyes open is preferable to sitting at the back in a car with eyes closed. When these strategies do not work, medications may be required.

Over-the-counter (OTC) medicines such as promethazine, dimenhydrinate, and meclazine are all effective when taken an hour before a short trip. For longer trips, scopolamine patches may be worn behind the ear for three days at a stretch. There is some evidence that ginger root may be as effective as some of the OTC medications. Acupressure may be helpful, but its true effectiveness has yet to be studied in a systematic fashion.

Arun Gadre

KEY FACTS

Description
Nausea and other symptoms induced by motion.

Causes
Conflicting sensory information from the eyes, inner ears, and proprioceptive system.

Risk factors
Road, sea, and air travel.

Symptoms
Dizziness (or giddiness); vertigo; fatigue; nausea and vomiting; headache.

Diagnosis
From symptoms.

Treatments
Stopping the motion; OTC preparations such as promethazine, dimenhydrinate, and meclazine (for short trips), and scopolamine patches (for long trips); ginger root; possibly acupressure bands.

Pathogenesis
Conflicting sensory information in the brain results in nausea and other symptoms.

Prevention
Sitting in the least rocky part of a moving vehicle and facing forward with eyes open.

Epidemiology
Very common, affecting millions of people in the United States.

See also
• Migraine

Multiple sclerosis

Multiple sclerosis (MS) is a progressive disease of the central nervous system (CNS). The CNS is composed of the brain and spinal cord, and within are numerous nerves. Each nerve is composed of a nerve cell body and its processes, called axons. Nerves are like electrical wiring that transmits electrical impulses by which the brain and spinal cord control the function of many body parts. Myelin is a fatty substance that acts as insulation for many of the axons of the CNS. The myelin sheath helps speed the pace of electronic impulses in the CNS so that signals are sent rapidly over relatively long distances.

In MS, there is a selective destruction of the myelin sheath, a process called demyelination, resulting in significant impairment of transmission of electrical impulses. Demyelination probably results from inflammation, a process caused by the accumulation of immune cells like T- and B- lymphocytes and macrophages. These cells can directly injure myelin, the cell that produces it in the CNS (called the oligodendrocyte or the underlying axon), or may indirectly cause similar injury via the secretion of inflammatory substances.

Clinical symptoms of MS depend upon which area of the CNS is affected. For example, if the optic nerve, which supplies the eye, is affected, there can be loss of vision. If the connections for movement of the eyes are affected in the brainstem, then there can be double vision. If damage occurs in the spinal cord, there can be paralysis and numbness of the legs.

A definite cause for MS is not known, but there are a few hypotheses. Infection is a possible cause. For decades, viruses and bacteria have been implicated in MS. Viruses like human herpes virus-6, Epstein-Barr virus, retroviruses, and bacteria such as *Chlamydia pneumoniae* have been implicated but never clearly shown to be the cause.

Autoimmunity is another likely possibility. There are several such diseases of the body, affecting many different organ systems. It is believed that some factor turns the immune system against the body; possibly triggered by one of the infectious agents above.

MS has been shown to be hereditary, but many genes may be involved, so the risk of vertical transmission is still quite low, in the order of 3 to 5 percent.

Risk factors

The mean age of onset of MS is 30 years. The onset is usually between 18 to 60 years, but there are many instances in which MS has occurred in children, adolescents, and the elderly.

Gender is a factor. Women tend to be affected slightly more frequently than men, with a female-to-male ratio of 1.77 to 1 (an oddity peculiar to most autoimmune diseases).

Geographical and racial distribution are relevant factors. MS is common in Europe, Canada, northern United States, New Zealand, and southern Australia. However, race is a major determinant of MS risk. Caucasians have the highest risk. Persons of African, Asian, and Native American origin have the lowest risk. However, persons migrating from a place of higher risk to a place of lower risk carry their risk with them, especially if they migrate before the age of 15 years. The same applies to persons of lower risk migrating to high-risk areas.

There is a genetic influence. The risk of MS is highest for siblings (2 to 5 percent) and decreases for children, aunts, uncles, and cousins. Among siblings, the risk is the highest for identical twins (monozygotic): up to 20 to 25 percent.

Environmental factors such as climate, diet, and toxins have been implicated as risk factors. According to a few studies, persons residing in areas with low exposure to the sun, resulting in vitamin D deficiency, may be at higher risk of MS.

Symptoms

Clinical symptoms reflect the areas of CNS that are damaged. Typically, patients will experience loss or blurring of vision, double vision, facial pain like an electric shock (called trigeminal neuralgia), slurring of speech, loss of sensation, tingling sensations, discomfort like an electric shock on bending the neck forward, paralysis, stiffness of the limbs, loss of balance, tremulousness, loss of coordination, bladder or bowel disturbances, impotence, change of personality, and poor mental functioning, such as memory disturbances. A common unexplained symptom is severe fatigue, which may be out of proportion to other clinical symptoms or signs. Depression is also quite common.

There are two typically common phenomena associated with MS. The first is Uhtoff's phenomenon, in which symptoms worsen with an increase in body temperature or exposure to heat and improve with reduction of the temperature. The second is l'Hermitte's sign, in which the patient experiences a shocklike sensation, usually running from the head down the back of the spine, upon bending the neck forward.

There are four types of multiple sclerosis, depending on symptoms and the course it follows.

KEY FACTS

Description
Autoimmune inflammatory demyelinating disease of the CNS.

Causes
Unknown, but genetic loading, environmental triggering, and autoimmunity all play a role.

Risk factors
None proven, but being a white female in the 20 to 30 age range, growing up and living in high-risk areas are clear risk factors. There are no clear dietary or other risk factors.

Symptoms
Most typical symptoms are episodic loss of neurological function with recovery, such as: unilateral loss of vision, numbness or tingling, paralysis, bladder or bowel disturbances, and lack of coordination or loss of balance.

Diagnosis
Primarily a clinical diagnosis involving the demonstration of clearly separate areas of the CNS being affected at different times. Diagnosis supported by MRI findings of white matter lesions and cerebrospinal fluid findings of increased immunoglobulin-G with the presence of oligoclonal bands.

Pathogenesis
An autoimmune inflammatory disease that attacks multiple ares of the CNS, causing the degradation of myelin, followed by loss of axons.

Treatments
Symptomatic therapy to improve quality of life and disease-modifying drugs to alter the natural disease course leading to slowed progression.

Prevention
Nothing proven.

Epidemiology
Most common in Caucasians and in high risk areas like Europe, northern United States, Canada, New Zealand, and southeastern Australia.

Relapsing remitting MS. The patients experience attacks of neurological symptoms, usually with new signs, that last for at least 24 to 48 hours before subsiding. Typically, an MS attack evolves over hours to days and can build over several days, lasting several weeks. Recovery from attacks is variable, in some cases complete, but in others there is residual deficit. Steroid treatments help to reduce the duration of attacks, but seem to have no influence on the outcome.

Primary progressive MS. From the onset, there is gradual worsening of the neurological symptoms and signs over months to years. There is generally no improvement, but at times the course might waver. Patients do not experience any attacks. Though progression is generally unstoppable, the rate of deterioration is quite variable, and very slow protracted courses are not atypical.

Secondary progressive MS. Evolving from the relapsing-remitting course, attacks start to diminish, residual deficits build, but between any perceived attacks or in the complete absence of relapses, there is steady progression, not unlike that which is seen with primary progressive disease.

Progressive relapsing MS. A rarer condition, but usually patients appear to be primary progressive disease, then they begin having attacks. The course seems to follow that of primary progressive disease.

Pathologically, there have also been four subtypes of MS described, but there does not seem to be a particular association with any clinical subtype.

It is important to know the particular type of MS since the management differs for each group. Patients with relapsing remitting MS tend to have more inflammation and therefore do better than the other types with regard to treatments.

There are some variants of MS, which are conditions somewhat similar to MS and often grouped with MS.

Optic neuritis. This is a condition involving the optic nerve, resulting in loss of vision and pain on moving the eyes. One or both eyes may be affected. Patients may have only recurring episodes of optic neuritis, while others clearly evolve into typical MS.

Neuromyelitis optica. Also called NMO (Devic's disease), this condition often involves devastating bilateral optic neuritis and large demyelinating destructive spinal cord lesions. Although originally described as a monophasic illness, more typically it is a relapsing condition that can be quite disabling, with each attack building on the other. Patients most often have a measurable specific antibody in their blood that characterizes the condition. Patients often have loss of vision in one or both eyes in a progressive pattern, usually with paralysis of or loss of sensation in the limbs, and bladder disturbances. A form of MS in Japan called optico-spinal MS is most commonly NMO.

Slow progressive myelopathy. There is demyelination of the spinal cord and it progresses slowly. Patients may present with stiffness and weakness of the lower limbs and bladder disturbances. There are still such cases that evolve with or without a history of transverse myelitis; they lack all the features of primary progressive MS.

Acute tumorlike (tumorigenic) MS. The patients present with confusion or paralysis similar to that seen with brain tumors. The cause, however, is large-scale demyelination of areas of the brain that have the appearance and presentation of a brain tumor. Despite the presentation, these lesions tend to recover well, and the course is no different from typical MS.

Marburg variant of MS. A severe progressive widespread demyelinating condition often leading to death. This condition is still quite rare, but many individual cases have been reported.

Diagnosis

The diagnosis of MS must be established prior to considering any therapy. Diagnosis is based primarily on clinical presentations and is supported by laboratory findings. An international committee have recently published revised criteria focused on making an accurate diagnosis. They are based on the ability to demonstrate a condition that affects at least two separate areas of the CNS on at least two separate occasions (dissemination in place and time). Patients should have suffered at least two attacks of neurological symptoms lasting at least 24 to 48 hours in the absence of flu or fever (see Uhtoff's phenomenon, above). These attacks should be verified by a physician to ensure that separate areas of the CNS have been affected. For example, one attack could be the loss of vision and another numbness of the legs, indicating that as a minimum there are lesions both in the optic nerve and spinal cord. The symptoms should be accompanied by findings on clinical examination involving two separate parts of the nervous system. The current appearance of clear new lesions on magnetic resonance imaging (MRI) remote from a first episode would qualify for evidence of new activity over time.

If there is only one attack or clinical finding of involvement of only one part of the nervous system, additional tests of cerebrospinal fluid (CSF) and radiological investigations like MRI are advised in

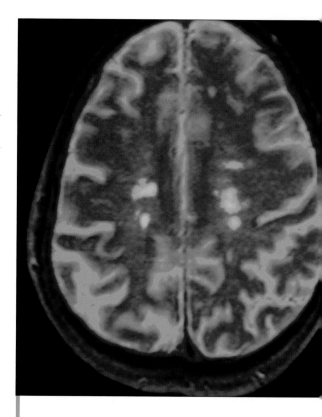

An MRI scan of a brain of someone suspected of having multiple sclerosis shows some damaged areas (pink). These are the result of plaques or damaged patches in the myelin sheath that surrounds nerve fibers.

order to ascertain the risk of the attack evolving to MS. Patients who have "silent" lesions on their MRI after only one attack (areas of involvement that do not correspond to symptoms or signs) are termed *clinically isolated syndrome*; this is most likely an early form of MS.

In patients with MS, typically there is an increase in immunoglobulin G in the spinal fluid that resolves as bands on protein separating gels (electrophoresis). These bands have been termed *oligoclonal* (*oligo* is a Greek word meaning "few"; *clonal* pertains to a clone, that is, one or a few genetically identical cells). They are not specific for MS, but in the absence of CNS infections, they are supportive of an MS diagnosis. There is still no specific test for MS, but many potential leads in serum and spinal fluid are being examined.

MRI is used increasingly in the diagnosis of MS. Some believe a normal MRI virtually rules out MS, even if the MRI is done early. During an MRI, the brain and spinal cord are subjected to a magnetic field that stimulates water molecules to become excited. When the magnetic field is removed, the water molecules relax and the energy they emit is measured. The computer converts this energy to an image. Areas containing more water will give off more energy. Typically, areas of inflammation contain more water, and this is the case with most MS plaques of demyelination. Demyelinated areas of the brain and spinal cord have a characteristic appearance on MRI that differentiate them from other conditions. They appear predominantly in the CNS white matter, and their number, distribution, and evolution over time are characteristic of MS. There are specific areas in the brain that typically harbor MS plaques. These are the periventricular region (area surrounding the CSF spaces in the brain), corpus callosum (white matter connecting the left and right hemispheres of the brain), and the centrum semiovale (white matter above the ventricles of the brain). In computed tomography, a dye called gadolinium can be used to enhance newer lesions.

Pathogenesis

The cause of MS is unknown, but the main evidence that MS is an autoimmune disease comes from pathological studies showing the presence of T cells and macrophages within MS lesions. These cells are vital to protect the body from infections. What causes immune cells to attack CNS myelin is unknown, but a popular theory suggests this could be due to molecular mimicry. This refers to the introduction to the body of a foreign protein (usually from an infectious agent such as a virus) that is similar in structure to a protein in myelin. The immune system becomes primed to locate the foreign protein, but instead launches an attack against CNS myelin, leading to chronic demyelination (MS). Removing the myelin exposes the underlying axons to inflammatory substances. It is this progressive loss of axons that probably represents the progression seen in all forms of MS. Destruction of myelin may or may not be followed by some regeneration or repair.

Treatments

There are now several proven effective treatments for some forms of MS.

Acute attacks. Typically a short course (3 to 5 days) of high dose steroids (oral or intravenous) can shorten the duration of an attack, but does not seem to impact on the final disability. For more severe attacks, plasma exchange has been shown to be effective.

Relapsing remitting MS. There are now five approved and proven effective immunomodulatory treatments that reduce the number of attacks and also slow MRI activity. Some, but not others, have been shown to slow disease progression. First line agents are the interferons and glatiramer acetate; second line agents (because of potentially more toxic side effects) are mitoxantrone and natalizumab. Interferon beta-1a and beta-1b have both been shown to reduce attacks and MRI activity and to slow disease progression. Glatiramer acetate reduces attacks and MRI activity. Mitoxantrone reduces attacks and MRI activity and slows progression, but it is a chemotherapeutic drug with potential toxic effects that can cause irreversible heart damage and increase the risk for leukemia. Natalizumab, a newly approved humanized mouse monoclonal antibody, reduces attacks, slows MRI activity, and slows progression, but it is also associated with a rare irreversible brain disease called PML, caused by a virus.

Secondary progressive MS. There are no approved or proven treatments for this form of MS, though for years immunosuppressive agents have been used with varying and limited success. It seems that timing is key; if these agents are used when there is still evidence of ongoing inflammation, they will be more effective. Once a slow progressive course ensues, they seem to be of limited benefit. Agents such as cyclophosphamide, azathioprine, methotrexate, and others have all been tested.

Primary progressive MS. No effective therapy has been shown to alter the course of this form of MS.

Prevention and epidemiology

There is no way of preventing MS, although studies have been initiated that focus on correcting activated Vitamin D levels.

The highest prevalence of MS is 30 to 60 in 100,000 or more in Europe, northern United States, Canada, New Zealand, and southeastern Australia. In the United States the prevalence is 0.1 percent, or a total of 250,000 to 400,000 persons. A lower prevalence is seen in the southern United States, northern Australia, the Mediterranean basin, South America, and the white population of South Africa. The lowest prevalence is seen in Asia, Africa, and parts of South America and Mexico. Race is an important predictor of susceptibility to MS and may be reflective of genetic differences. MS is most prevalent in Caucasians and affects Africans, Asians, and to a lesser degree, Amerindians.

Monica Badve and
Mark Freedman

See also
• Paralysis

Mumps

Mumps is a viral infection that usually occurs in children, resulting in swelling of the cheek area. However, a vaccine has been in use since the 1960s, so actual cases are fairly rare. If an adult becomes sick, mumps may cause mild cases of meningitis, encephalitis, or orchitis.

The term *mumps* is an old English word for either "bumps", "grimace," or "mumble." It always involves swelling of the cheeks. Mumps was also commonly referred to as epidemic parotitis before the vaccine was introduced and the prevalence of the virus was significantly reduced.

Causes and risk factors

Mumps is an acute systemic viral infection, which occurs mainly in children. The virus is a member of the paramyxovirus family, which includes parainfluenza and the measles viruses in humans as well as animal pathogens such as the Newcastle disease virus and simian viruses. The virus is passed through contact with droplets from sneezing, coughing, or any personal contact with infected saliva. Although contagious, it is not as easily spread as chickenpox or measles. Most children are vaccinated against the disease, but children in school or day care settings are most likely to come in contact with the virus.

Symptoms, signs, and diagnosis

The virus usually incubates for 14 to 24 days. Symptoms include a loss of energy and little appetite, chills, headaches, and a fever as high as 104°F (40°C). Once symptoms appear, within 12 to 24 hours the patient will probably have painful swelling of the parotid area (saliva glands in the cheeks just in front of the ears). The skin over the gland will usually be hot and flushed, but there will not be a rash. Sometimes only one side will be swollen, and as it shrinks, the other side will swell, or both sides may swell at once. The parotitis usually lasts three to four days.

An infected person is infectious from three days before the symptoms start until nine days after the symptoms appear.

It is estimated that 30 percent of patients have subclinical symptoms needing no treatment. In adult cases of mumps, complications are more common. One complication is a mild case of meningitis, an inflammation of the brain and spinal covering causing a stiff neck, headache, vomiting, and lack of energy. It usually resolves within seven days. Mumps meningitis only occurs in about one in 20 cases of mumps.

Another complication is encephalitis, an inflammation of the brain that can cause seizures, a high fever, or even an inability to feel pain. Encephalitis may cause permanent brain damage. In normal cases, encephalitis is usually resolved within one or two weeks,

KEY FACTS

Description
A short-term viral infection best known for causing parotitis.

Causes
A paramyxovirus transmitted through contaminated saliva.

Risk factors
Close proximity to unvaccinated children such as at schools or day care centers.

Symptoms
Parotitis, chills, headache, loss of appetite, loss of energy, fever, and complications in adults may cause meningitis, encephalitis, or orchitis.

Diagnosis
Examination by experienced medical personnel; lab tests of saliva.

Treatments
If uncomplicated, the infection is self-limiting and will be allowed to run its course. Antibiotics may be prescribed for complications.

Pathogenesis
The virus causes an infection of the upper respiratory tract that spreads to the lymph nodes. Infection of the lymphocytes causes a blockage of the ducts in the salivary glands.

Prevention
Childhood immunization from 12 to 15 months along with the measles and rubella vaccine.

Epidemiology
Before the vaccine was licensed in 1967, there were approximately 200,000 cases each year in the United States. Currently there are less than 1,000 cases reported each year in the United States.

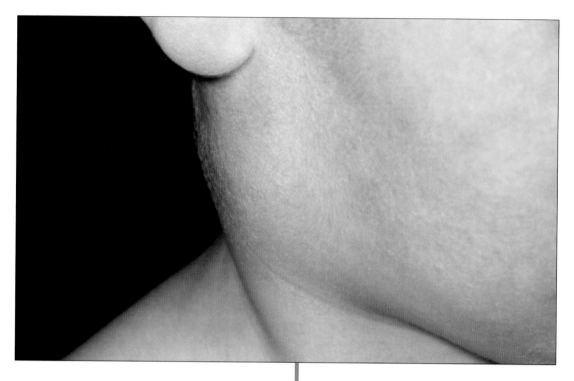

A young child with mumps (infectious parotitis) has an inflamed parotid gland. The swelling can cause difficulty chewing, and swallowing may be painful. Sometimes a child will have fever and headache, but many children will merely feel slightly unwell.

and it only occurs in one or two cases out of 10,000. Finally, orchitis, which is relatively common in post-pubertal males, is a swelling of the scrotum that causes severe pain, fever, and nausea. One out of four men with mumps will have orchitis, but it does not cause any sterility and will usually subside after five to seven days. Most cases of mumps can be diagnosed by a trained medical professional on physical examination, but confirmation of the presence of the mumps virus may require additional lab tests of saliva, urine, or cerebrospinal fluid.

Treatments and prevention

There is no treatment for mumps. However, a vaccine for mumps has been licensed and administered to the public since 1967. The vaccine contains live, attenuated mumps virus and is administered usually when children are 12 to 15 months of age in combination with the measles and rubella vaccines (MMR vaccine).

The World Health Organization, the British Medical Association, and the American Academy of Pediatrics all endorse the vaccine and its safety. However, some parents choose not to have their children vaccinated because of personal beliefs or fear of a connection between the immunization and autism.

Pregnant women should avoid getting vaccinated until after they give birth because of the risk of birth defects or miscarriage.

Before the vaccine was licensed, 200,000 cases of mumps were reported every year in the United States. The virus usually peaked between January and May, with epidemics occurring at two- to five-year intervals. Since the advent of the vaccine, the occurrence of mumps has decreased substantially.

In the event that the vaccine does not build up a sufficient quantity of mumps antibodies, most children will recover from the illness in several days and be immune to further illness after having it once. The most important thing in normal cases of mumps is to keep the patient fed and hydrated since swallowing and chewing will be painful. Citric beverages should be avoided because they will sting the swollen cheeks. Blended foods can help keep the patient nourished. Painkillers may help reduce the pain of the swollen parotid glands.

Graeme Stemp-Morlock

See also
• Meningitis

Muscular dystrophy

Muscular dystrophy is used to describe more than 30 different inherited diseases in which the muscles weaken over time and the muscle cells are unable to repair themselves after being damaged. Although each type of muscular dystrophy has a unique genetic cause, it is difficult to distinguish between them because many of the different types have similar clinical features. Important factors that help differentiate the types of muscular dystrophy include the age of onset and types of symptoms, which muscle groups are affected, and whether other members of the individual's family are affected or show signs of muscular dystrophy.

The muscular dystrophies are genetic diseases. They have been shown to be inherited in an autosomal dominant manner (in which only one copy of the defective gene is necessary to cause abnormality), in an autosomal recessive way (in which a pair of abnormal genes, one from each parent, causes the defect), and in X-linked recessive patterns (caused by defects on the X chromosome). It is therefore important to determine which type of muscular dystrophy affects an individual in order to know who else in the family is at risk.

Causes

Some muscular dystrophies are caused by a deficiency in the protein dystrophin, which provides stability to the muscle fibers. Dystrophin is reduced in Becker muscular dystrophy (BMD) and completely absent in Duchenne muscular dystrophy (DMD). The gene for dystrophin is located on the X chromosome, so these conditions show X-linked inheritance. Mothers and sisters of boys with these disorders have up to a 50 percent chance of having an affected son.

Myotonic dystrophy (DM) results from changes to a protein that is involved in the regulation of muscle cells. DM is inherited in an autosomal dominant pattern and affects both males and females equally.

There are 16 subtypes of limb girdle muscular dystrophy (LGMD). They are caused by changes to many different proteins that are associated with muscle stability and maintenance. Some types of LGMD are inherited in an autosomal dominant manner, while some of the others show an autosomal recessive pattern of inheritance.

There are other, more unusual types of muscular dystrophy, for example Emery-Dreifuss muscular dystrophy (EDMD). Around 300 cases have been identified in the United States. Oculopharyngeal muscular dystrophy (OPMD) causes weakness in the eyes and throat. It is prevalent in French Canadian families in Canada and in Spanish-American families in the southwestern United States.

Distal muscular dystrophy (DD) begins in middle age or later. It is most common in Sweden and rare elsewhere in the world.

The term *congenital muscular dystrophy* (CMD) refers to a group of inherited disorders. Muscular dystrophy is present from birth. It has a slow progression with generalized weakness. A variation is more common in Japan; this is called Fukuyama CMD.

Symptoms and disease progression

All muscular dystrophy types are characterized by progressive muscle weakness in different muscle groups. Onset of symptoms can range from infancy to adulthood. The rate of disease progression is dependent on the type of muscular dystrophy. Some types are mild, with slower progression of muscle weakness over an individual's life span. Other types are more severe, with rapid progression of muscle weakness resulting in death in infancy or childhood.

Signs of DMD usually present in early childhood. Symptoms include delays in sitting, walking, gait problems, muscular-looking calves (called pseudohypertrophy), and curvature of the spine (scoliosis). Affected boys are usually wheelchair-bound by early adolescence, and respiratory failure and cardiac problems result in death by their early twenties.

BMD is a milder form of DMD. The onset of symptoms is later than in DMD, and progress takes place at a slower rate. Many boys with BMD can still walk in their teens, and some even into adulthood. The average age of death in individuals with BMD is in the mid-forties.

Although BMD is associated with milder muscle weakness than DMD, heart failure is the most common cause of death for individuals with BMD. DM

KEY FACTS

Description

The term *muscular dystrophy* refers to more than 30 diseases characterized by progressive muscle weakness and wasting. Some of the more common muscular dystrophies include Duchenne muscular dystrophy (DMD), Becker muscular dystrophy (BMD), limb girdle muscular dystrophy (LGMD), and myotonic dystrophy (DM).

Causes

The muscular dystrophies are genetic diseases with various modes of inheritance. Many different genes have been implicated.

Risk factors

A family history of muscular dystrophy may indicate that other individuals in the family are at risk, depending on the mode of inheritance associated with the specific muscular dystrophy.

Symptoms

All muscular dystrophies are characterized by progressive muscle weakness. This may present as frequent falls, uncoordinated movements, or difficulty walking. However, which muscle groups are affected, the age of onset and severity of symptoms, and the rate of progression vary depending on the specific type of muscular dystrophy.

Diagnosis

Elevated creatine kinase levels in the blood, muscle biopsy, electromyography (a measurement of electrical activity in the muscles), and genetic testing.

Treatments

There is no cure for muscular dystrophy. Treatments such as physical therapy and orthopedic surgery may be used to slow the progression of disease and improve quality of life.

Pathogenesis

Changes in the DNA (mutations) lead to abnormal proteins that play important roles in muscle maintenance, stability, and structure. When damage occurs to the muscle cells, they are unable to repair themselves as they normally would. Muscle cells are eventually replaced with connective tissue and fat.

Prevention

There is no known prevention for any of the muscular dystrophies.

Epidemiology

The incidence differs with the type of muscular dystrophy. The most common, DMD, occurs in 1 in 4,600 to 5,618 male births. BMD is less common and occurs in approximately 1 in 30,000 male births. DM affects approximately 1 in 20,000 individuals. Other types of MD are much rarer.

generally has an onset of symptoms anywhere between 10 and 30 years of age. Infants who suffer from the disorder are likely to have limp limbs, without normal tension and tone, and fail to reach milestones in development. This type of dystrophy is characterized by muscle weakness in the face and digestive tract, an inability to relax muscles (for example, unable to let go of someone's hand after shaking it), cardiac and respiratory problems, and cataracts, endocrine problems, and mental retardation. The average age of death for these individuals is in their early fifties. The onset of DM tends to occur earlier and the symptoms are generally more severe with each generation of affected individuals in a family.

A more severe form of DM (called congenital DM) can present at birth in some individuals. These infants have severe muscle weakness, which leads to difficulties with feeding and breathing. Approximately 25 percent of these infants die in the first 18 months of life. For those that survive past the first several years of life, 50 to 60 percent have mental retardation. Congenital DM is most often inherited from the individual's mother.

All types of LGMD show symptoms of weakness of the muscles closest to the body, such as in the arms and legs. The bones of the shoulders abnormally protrude, known as scapular winging. Cardiac problems due to weakness in the cardiac muscle have also been identified in some types of LGMD. The severity of muscle weakness and the rate of progression of disease is variable, depending on the subtype of LGMD.

For some autosomal recessive types, symptoms can appear in childhood and clinically resemble DMD. However, onset of the autosomal dominant types of LGMD is often in adolescence or adulthood with slower progression of muscle weakness.

Diagnosis

For both DMD and BMD, a diagnosis can be made by seeing reduced or absent dystrophin on a muscle biopsy. For all types of muscular dystrophy, significant signs on a muscle biopsy include the breakdown of muscle tissue, and muscle cells replaced with connective tissue and fat. Individuals with DMD, BMD, and several other types of muscular dystrophy also have elevated levels of creatine kinase. This is a substance released into the bloodstream when the muscle cells break down, and it is a sign that there is muscle damage. Although both of these tests are useful for diagnosis of DMD and BMD, they are not as helpful for identifying female carriers of these diseases.

Electromyography is a test that measures the electrical activity of the muscles when they are at rest and contracted. Tiny needles with electrodes are inserted through the skin into the muscle. These electrodes then record the electrical activity. In muscular dystrophy, the electrical activity of the muscles is abnormal.

Genetic testing is currently available for DMD and BMD, DM, and certain types of LGMD in which the involved gene is known. Once a genetic mutation is identified in an affected individual, then carrier and prenatal testing can be made available to other family members to determine who else is at risk.

Treatments

There is currently no cure for MD. Treatments target the symptoms associated with the specific type of muscular dystrophy and aim to improve an individual's quality of life. Physical therapy helps maintain flexibility and allows patients to remain ambulatory (walk unaided) as long as possible.

Several types of medication have also been found to be effective in treating the symptoms associated with specific muscular dystrophies, such as pain and inflammation. For example, muscle relaxants are used in the treatment of DM. Another medication, prednisone, has been shown to delay the progression of disease and increase muscle strength in boys with DMD.

Orthopedic surgery is an option that can also be used to correct scoliosis or increase a patient's range of motion. Researchers are currently exploring the possibility of replacing the absent dystrophin through gene therapy in DMD and BMD.

Epidemiology

The incidence differs with different types of muscular dystrophy. The most common, DMD, occurs in 1 in 3,500 male births; it affects around 8,000 boys and young men in the United States. A few female carriers show mild symptoms.

BMD is less common and occurs in about 1 in 43,000 male births; this type of dystrophy tends to affect older boys and young men. BMD produces milder symptoms than DMD.

LGMD is difficult to diagnose, and estimates of the prevalence are not easy to produce, but it is believed that the number of people affected in the United States is in the low thousands.

DM affects about 1 in 20,000 individuals. Other types of MD are much rarer and tend to be common to certain areas of the world.

Brian Brost

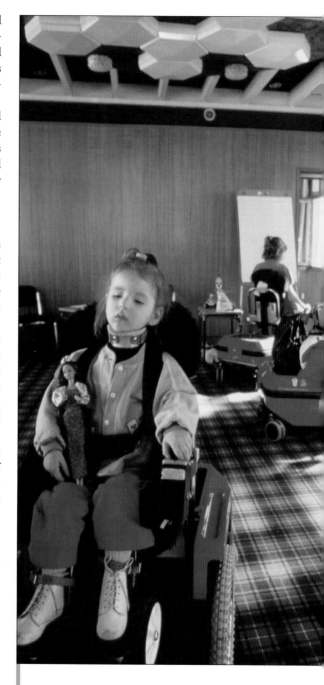

A young girl who suffers from muscular dystrophy attends a support center. She wears a neck brace and sits in a specially adapted wheelchair, in which she is securely strapped. The aim at the center is to maintain muscles not yet affected.

See also
- Learning disorders • Paralysis
- Spinal curvature

Neuralgia

Neuralgia is pain that is often sharp, severe, and typically unilateral along an affected nerve. There are various types of neuralgia; trigeminal neuralgia and post-herpetic neuralgia are the most common, but neuralgia can arise from any sensory nerve root in the body. Other common forms of neuralgia include: glossopharyngeal neuralgia, geniculate neuralgia, and occipital neuralgia.

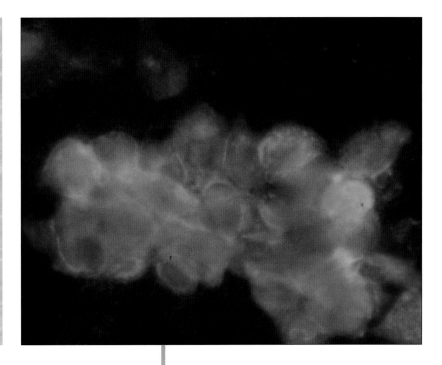

A colored photomicrograph shows the varicella-zoster virus magnified 200 times. After this type of infection, post-herpetic neuralgia sometimes develops in older people.

The cause of trigeminal neuralgia is thought to be vascular compression of the nerve root near its entry into the brain with subsequent focal demyelination (breakdown of fatty insulation around nerve fibers). Multiple sclerosis may cause trigeminal neuralgia; other causes are rare, but include tumors in the posterior fossa compressing the trigeminal nerve. The biggest risk factor for trigeminal neuralgia is advancing age, with female gender as a lesser predisposing factor. The cause of post-herpetic neuralgia is related to inflammatory changes that occur in the nerve and nerve root after infection (often decades earlier) with the virus that causes chicken pox and herpes zoster. The risk factors for post-herpetic neuralgia include preceding herpes zoster infection, advanced age at the time of infection, and location in the trigeminal nerve root.

Symptoms, signs, and diagnosis

The trigeminal nerve is responsible for sensation over the skin of the face and so, when individuals suffer from trigeminal neuralgia, they will complain of severe, paroxysmal pain in one side of the face. The pain is often reproduced by gentle stimulation of that area of the face, such as chewing or sometimes cold air. It lasts a few seconds to minutes in duration. Typically, trigeminal neuralgia is diagnosed based on the charac-

teristic history and normal examination. There are no laboratory, electrophysiologic radiologic abnormalities except in atypical cases associated with a structural lesion: demyelination or tumor. Pathological diagnosis of trigeminal neuralgia is not typically made, but when examined, histological changes can be seen in the gasserian ganglion.

Post-herpetic neuralgia (PHN) is diagnosed when pain continues more than three months after a herpes zoster infection (shingles). Herpes zoster infection is reactivation of a varicella virus (chicken pox) that remains dormant (inactive) in nerve cells. Herpes zoster manifests itself as a painful vesicular rash (fluid filled) in the distribution of the affected nerve root. The pain may be described as an unpleasant burning or tingling sensation in the distribution of the affected nerve root. Compared to trigeminal neuralgia, the pain is usually persistent. Most people who have a zoster infection will not develop PHN, but the older individuals are when they develop zoster, the greater the chances of PHN. Development of PHN is determined by the location of herpes zoster infection, with involvement of trigeminal and brachial plexus sites highest, followed in descending order by jaw, neck, sacral, and lumbar. The diagnosis is typically made based on the history of a painful herpes zoster eruption (shingles), with resolution of the vesicular rash but continued pain. Laboratory testing is not required, but examination of cerebrospinal fluid will often show an elevated number of lymphocytes and elevated protein due to inflammation in the nerve roots.

Other neuralgias such as glossopharyngeal neuralgia have symptoms similar to those in trigeminal neuralgia, but the symptoms occur in the distribution of the corresponding nerve root (that is, the pharynx).

Treatments and prevention

Medical treatment is generally the first line treatment for trigeminal neuralgia. The drug commonly used is carbamazepine. Other anti-epileptic drugs can also be used to treat neuralgia. A combination of two drugs may be required. Surgical options include local injections to anesthetize affected nerves or decompression of the nerve root in the case of trigeminal neuralgia.

Post-herpetic neuralgia is usually treated with anticonvulsants such as gabapentin, tricyclic antidepressants, analgesics, corticosteroids, or antiviral agents. These agents typically alleviate the neuropathic pain, allowing most people to function normally and participate in daily activities. In very severe and unremitting cases, surgical intervention with sectioning of the dorsal root ganglion may be helpful.

Pathogenesis

Trigeminal neuralgia is thought to result from vascular compression of the nerve as it enters the brain; age is therefore a risk factor. Trigeminal neuralgia may have typical exacerbations and remissions through life, but usually worsens with time and may require additional medications or surgical interventions as it worsens. Many individuals learn to avoid activities such as shaving, extreme temperatures, or smiling, or any conditions that worsen or bring on attacks. In extreme cases, the severe pain causes depression and suicidal tendencies.

Post-herpetic neuralgia is thought to result from inflammatory changes that occur in the nerves related to a prior herpes zoster infection. The inflammation affects and changes nerve fibers secondary to the preceding varicella virus infection. This manifests itself as a misperception of temperature or light touch. These pain sensations can be spontaneous or elicited with a light, nonpainful stimulus. Postherpetic neuralgia usually remits over time, but may occasionally worsen.

KEY FACTS

Description
Intermittent, severe pain in a single nerve.

Causes
Trigeminal neuralgia is thought to be due to vascular compression, but has not been definitively proven. PHN is due to inflammatory changes in the corresponding nerve and root.

Risk factors
Age and female gender are risk factors for trigeminal neuralgia. The risk factors for PHN include preceding herpes zoster infection, and advanced age at the time of the skin eruption.

Signs and symptoms
Unilateral pain in a nerve root such as the trigeminal, facial, or spinal nerves. A healing vesicular and painful rash is strong evidence for a post-herpetic neuralgia.

Diagnosis
History typical of a classic syndrome and corresponding exam findings.

Pathogenesis
Trigeminal neuralgia is lifelong but may have spontaneous exacerbations and remissions and is responsive to medical and surgical therapy. PHN occurs about one month after a herpes zoster skin eruption and typically persists indefinitely.

Prevention
No know prevention strategies for trigeminal neuralgia, but a recent vaccine can prevent zoster eruptions in those over the age of 60.

Epidemiology
More common in women over the age of 40. Affects about 5 in 100,000 people. PHN is reported in 3–15 percent of people.

Epidemiology

Trigeminal neuralgia is more common in women over the age of 40, and the incidence is estimated to affect 5 in 100,000 people. It is 200 times more common in patients with multiple sclerosis. PHN is reported in 3 to 15 percent of individuals after a herpes zoster infection, with an incidence of 500 in 100,000 in those over 50 years old; this more than doubles in people who are more than 80.

Meredith Roderick
and Robert Daroff

See also
• Chicken pox and shingles • Depressive disorders
• Herpes infections • Multiple sclerosis

Obesity

Obesity is increasing at a rapid rate throughout both the developed and developing nations of the world. The World Health Organization (WHO) estimates that there are as many as 300 million obese people worldwide.

Obesity may be defined as an excess of body fat. WHO defines overweight as a body mass index (weight in kilograms divided by height in square meters) of at least 25 and obesity as a BMI of at least 30. Morbid obesity is defined as a BMI of 40 or greater. Both overweight and especially obesity are associated with increased risk of disease and death.

Epidemiology

In the United States, obesity afflicts approximately 33 percent of adults (28 percent of men and 34 percent of women) aged 20 to 74 years; this has more than doubled over the past two decades. Almost 10 percent of U.S. children between the ages of 5 and 17 are classified as obese. In Canada obesity rates have climbed to approximately 15 percent of adults, an increase of 150 percent since 1985. In Europe, most countries report adult obesity rates of more than 10 percent, with the United Kingdom, Ireland, Germany, Cyprus, Finland, Slovakia, Malta, and Greece reporting rates above 20 percent. The most rapid increase has been reported in England, where adult obesity rates tripled from 1980 to 2001. Rates for overweight and obesity (BMI of 25 or greater) among adults are as high as 65 percent in the United States and 60 percent in England. Although overweight and obesity levels are lower in most developing nations, WHO suggests that excess adiposity is a problem there as well.

Childhood overweight and obesity is also increasing in the United States and among European nations. Data from the United States and England suggests that 15 percent of children and adolescents are obese and almost 30 percent are included in the categories of overweight and obese. Children in other European nations show slightly lower levels but still show levels approaching 20 percent.

Causes

Most researchers agree that multiple factors contribute to obesity. These include a complex interface among genetic, physiological, metabolic, hormonal, sociocultural, environmental, behavioral, and psychological influences. More simplistically, there is an interaction between an individual's genetic heritage and an environment that promotes excessive food consumption and a sedentary lifestyle. Thus, weight gain and, ultimately, obesity result from positive energy balance in susceptible individuals, that is, consuming more food energy than is utilized throughout the day.

Other factors influence the cause of obesity. Genetics most influences the risk for obesity. Theories include: possessing a thrifty gene, causing individuals to burn less energy at rest and during activity; maintaining weight at a predetermined set point, making it difficult to lose weight or maintain the loss; and alterations in various hormones, such as leptin, which influence energy intake. However, some people with overweight parents do not become obese themselves.

Overeating and eating foods that are highly calorific and contain a large amount of fat, as well as too little exercise, are contributory factors in causing obesity.

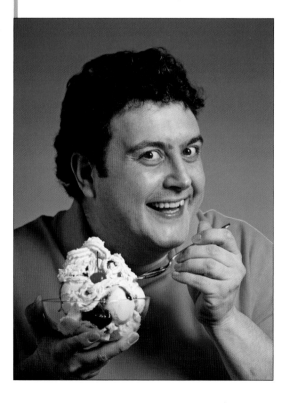

Risk factors

Beyond the genetic risk factor, a number of modifiable risk factors for obesity exist. Being overweight as a child can lead to adult obesity. It is estimated that about one-half of obese children will become obese adults. Substantial weight gain during gestation, early infancy, in the early schoolage years (five to seven years), and the adolescent period all increase the risk of adult obesity.

Lack of physical activity has been linked with greater body weight. Children and adults who watch excessive amounts of television or spend too much time in front of a computer have a greater risk of obesity. That, combined with eating a high-caloric diet, which causes increased storage of energy as body fat, has proved a potent risk factor for increased adiposity.

Psychological factors also influence the likelihood that an individual will become obese. In some, the sight or smell of foods may overstimulate the pleasure centers of the brain and trigger appetite and overeating, even when the individual is not very hungry.

Additionally, a number of social factors, including pressure to eat from family and friends, easy access to inexpensive and high-fat foods (often found at fast food restaurants), smoking cessation, excessive alcohol consumption, and an increased number of meals eaten away from home, often at establishments that serve large portions, are all linked to obesity.

Signs and symptoms

The most obvious sign of obesity is an individual who is overweight. However, excessive body weight does not necessarily correlate with obesity. Individuals who are very muscular (football or rugby players) may be overweight but may still be within recommended ranges for body fat. A measurement of stored fat will give a better indication of whether a person is obese.

A number of symptoms are associated with obesity. Those apparent with the onset of obesity include reduced physical agility, increased risk of accidents and falls, impaired heat tolerance (inability to stand or do well in hot weather), and in women menstrual irregularities and infertility.

Symptoms that are related to long-term obesity include: increased surgical risk attributed to increased anesthesia needs and greater risk of wound infections; pulmonary disease because of excess weight over the lungs and respiratory tract; type II diabetes as a result of insulin insensitivity of enlarged fat cells; hypertension (high blood pressure) owing to increased blood volume and increased resistance to blood flow

---

KEY FACTS

Description

An excess of body fat.

Causes

Multifactorial, including genetics, excessive food consumption, and sedentary lifestyle, coupled with sociocultural and psychological influences.

Symptoms

Excess body weight seen as abnormally large waist, hips, buttocks, and thighs. Obesity is associated with increased risk for many disorders, including high blood pressure, heart disease, type II diabetes, and some types of cancers.

Diagnosis

BMI more than 30 or body fat levels greater than 25 and 32 for males and females, respectively.

Treatments

Decreased food intake, regular exercise, and behavior modification. Drug therapy as an adjunct to diet, with surgery as a last resort.

Prevention

Lifestyle modifications include selecting limited amounts of nutritious foods, incorporating regular vigorous exercise into one's life, and practicing healthy food-related behaviors.

Epidemiology

Nearly one-third of U.S. adults and more than 20 percent of British adults are obese. Slightly lower or similar figures are found in most developed nations. The trend for overweight and obesity is increasing in both developed and developing nations.

---

throughout the circulatory system; cardiovascular disease as a result of increases in LDL-cholesterol (bad cholesterol) and triglycerides with concomitant decreases in HDL-cholesterol (good cholesterol) and physical activity; bone and joint disorders, including gout and osteoarthritis caused by increased uric acid levels and excess pressure on the hip, knee, ankle joints, respectively; gallstones due to increased cholesterol content of bile; skin disorders as a result of trapping of moisture and possibly microbes in tissue folds; various cancers (of the breast, colon, pancreas, and gallbladder) as a result of increased estrogen production by fat cells and possibly excess energy intake that encourages tumor development; pregnancy risks including more difficult delivery, increased number of birth defects, and increased toxemia of pregnancy; increased psychological problems associated with societal stigma attached to obesity; and increased mortality. The greater the degree of obesity, the more likely it is that someone will develop health problems.

CHILDHOOD OBESITY

Childhood overweight and obesity is increasing dramatically among U.S. children. It is estimated that around 18 percent of children between the ages of 5 and 18 are overweight, a number that has tripled since the late 1970s. Additionally, more than 10 percent of children between the ages of two and five are overweight or obese. Overweight in children and adolescents is generally caused by unhealthy eating patterns and lack of physical activity, with genetics and lifestyle both playing important roles. Being overweight or obese as a child is directly correlated to adult obesity. Childhood obesity has also been linked to increased and earlier onset of a number of diseases, including type II diabetes and heart disease, as well as premature death in adulthood. Prevention of obesity is of paramount importance. Ideally, parents and caregivers should offer a selection of nutritious food, while allowing children to decide how much they eat. Providing the opportunity for children to engage in physical activities that are fun, rather than competitive, should be a goal for both parents and schools. Modeling appropriate food- and exercise-related behaviors would also be quite useful in managing the childhood obesity epidemic.

Diagnosis

Obesity is commonly diagnosed by using BMI. However, body composition assessments that estimate the proportion of an individual's body fat, muscle mass, bone, and body water give a more accurate indication. Body composition methods commonly used include underwater weighing, skinfold measures, bioelectrical impedance analysis, near infrared reactance, dual-energy X-ray absorptiometry (DEXA), and computerized axial tomograpohy (CT or CAT scans). Although some disagreement exists, acceptable body fat ranges for adults are between 8 to 25 percent and 10 to 32 percent for males and females, respectively. Additionally, the location of body fat stores is quite important. Fat concentrated in the abdominal area (apple shape) is thought to be more problematic than that around the hips and thigh area (pear shape). Apple-shaped people have a higher risk for diabetes, hypertension, high blood cholesterol, and heart disease. Thus, some researchers assess obesity using the waist-to-hip ratio. Ratios of greater than 0.80 and 0.90 for women and men, respectively, are thought to increase the risk for health problems. Other researchers use waist circumference as an indicator of potential problems. A waist circumference of more than 40 inches (101 cm) in men and more than 35 inches (89 cm) in women is problematic.

Treatments and prevention

Weight loss treatment involves decreasing energy intake, increasing physical activity levels, and modifying behavioral problems. For success, the above triad must be coupled with a desire for change and self-acceptance (within reason) of body size. Diets should generally include a restriction of 500 to 1,000 kilocalories/day from the normal intake. This would allow for a weight loss of 1–2 pounds (0.5–1 kg) per week. Many nutritionists advocate total dietary fat intake below 30 percent of kcals, carbohydrate at 55 percent or more of kcals, and the balance from protein. Reducing saturated fat, cholesterol, and sodium are important, as well as eating foods high in fiber. Moderate exercise, initially 30 to 45 minutes three to five times per week (if tolerated), should later be increased to 30 to 60 minutes on most days.

Drug therapy has also been tried. A number of drugs, including orlistat (xenical), which blocks absorption of dietary fat, and sibutramine (meridia), which inhibits appetite, have met with some success.

Surgery should be used as a last resort due to the increased risks involved. A number of procedures, such as gastric bypass surgery, vertical banded gastroplasty, and laparoscopic adjustable gastric banding, are available to reduce the size of the stomach and limit the amount of food that can be eaten. Some individuals also use liposuction, a cosmetic procedure that removes fat deposits from the thighs, hips, arms, back, or chin. Both types of techniques are expensive and carry the risk of infections or other complications.

The rate of success for treating obesity is quite low, therefore prevention is the preferred strategy. Since little can be changed in terms of genetics, lifestyle changes are the keys to success. An eating plan that focuses on healthy nutritious foods, daily physical activities that are fun rather than competitive, and practicing healthful food-related behaviors would dramatically reduce the number of obese children and adults.

Alan Levine

See also
• Diabetes • Eating disorders

Osteoporosis

Osteoporosis is a systemic disorder characterized by loss of bone tissue and bone density, leading to skeletal fragility and an increased risk of insufficiency fractures. A fracture that results from a standing position is considered an osteoporotic fracture.

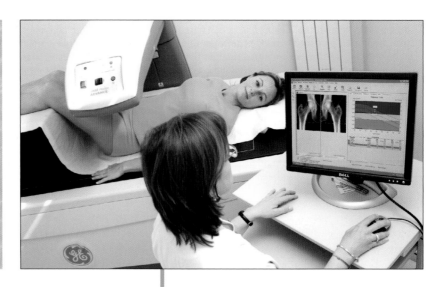

A doctor uses a bone densitometer to measure the optical density of the neck of the femur of a female patient to confirm a diagnosis of osteoporosis.

Risk factors that are associated with osteoporosis include: female gender; postmenopausal status; Asian or Caucasian race; weight less than 127 pounds (57.6 kg); history of fracture in a parent, sibling, or child; and personal history of a fracture as an adult. Modifiable risk factors associated with osteoporosis include tobacco use, alcohol abuse, low calcium or vitamin D intake, or both, and physical inactivity. Certain medical conditions predispose to osteoporosis: malabsorption states, such as celiac disease; prior gastric bypass; inflammatory disorders such as rheumatoid arthritis; primary hyperparathyroidism; and hyperthyroidism. Medications associated with bone loss include corticosteroids, intravenous heparin, lithium, depakote, and suppressive doses of thyroid replacement. Any condition that increases the risk of falls, such as decreased vision or Parkinson's disease, is associated with osteoporotic fractures.

Symptoms and diagnosis

Usually a patient does not suspect that she has osteoporosis. There is no pain unless a fracture occurs. Height loss of more than two inches may suggest vertebral compression fractures. Thoracic kyphosis (curvature) may also be a sign of multiple compression fractures and osteoporosis. Many vertebral fractures are asymptomatic when they occur and are noted incidentally on a lateral chest X-ray.

The diagnosis of osteoporosis is made after a dual X-ray absorbtiometry (DXA) scan is performed. This is the standard imaging technique that analyzes bone density (BMD, literally, "bone mass density"). It is painless and exposes a patient to less radiation than a chest X-ray. The World Health Organization (WHO) has defined osteoporosis as a T-score of 2.5 standard deviations (SD) below that expected for a gender- and race-matched control. A T-score -1.0 to -2.4 SD below that expected indicates osteopenia (decrease in bone mass). If the T-score is within one SD of that expected, the bone density is normal. The Z-score compares the patient to an age-, gender-, and race-matched control. If a patient has one or more insufficiency fractures and the bone density is not suggestive of low bone density, consideration of abnormal bone quality or of a falsely elevated BMD must be considered. Osteomalacia refers to abnormal bone resulting from vitamin D deficiency, which is associated with a higher fracture risk. Osteoarthritis of the spine or improper positioning on the bone density table can result in falsely elevated BMD results.

If the Z-score is more than one SD below that expected for age, the cause of low bone mass should be determined. Modifiable risk factors should be corrected, such as ongoing tobacco use or alcohol abuse. If a patient is on medications associated with bone loss, alternatives should be considered. If a patient is on glucocorticoids, the lowest possible dose should be prescribed. It may be necessary to do a laboratory evaluation to look for an etiology of low bone mass. Tests to consider include TSH, ESR, SIEP/UIEP, intact PTH, 25 Vitamin D, celiac antibodies, urine calcium, phosphorus, and bone alkaline phosphatase. If a cause of low bone mass is identified, it is evaluated and treated.

The urine N-telopeptide (NTX) is a test that measures bone breakdown products. The second urine sample of the morning is the most useful. A value of 40 to 50 bone collagen equivalent/millimoles (BCE/mmol) suggests ongoing bone loss and predicts loss of BMD and fracture. A value less than 10 BCE/mmol suggests a low bone turnover state and perhaps an increased risk of microdamage and a tendency toward stress fractures.

Treatments

All patients with low bone mass should be advised to take 1,200 to 1,500 milligrams (mg) calcium per day, divided into two to three servings, by diet or supplements. Calcium carbonate is associated with a small risk of kidney stones. When this concern exists, calcium citrate may decrease this risk. The recommended vitamin D intake is being reevaluated. Patients should get 800 to 1,000 international units (IU) per day. The level can be measured and dose adjusted when necessary. Patients should strive to participate daily in a weight-bearing exercise program with emphasis on balance and falls prevention.

The National Osteoporosis Foundation (NOF) recommends treating postmenopausal women with a T-score of -2.0 or greater or -1.5 or greater if other risk factors for osteoporosis are present. Care must be based on a patient's bone density results and other comorbid medical conditions.

Surgical procedures are being explored to attempt correction of vertebral deformities. These procedures include vertebroplasty and kyphoplasty. In vertebroplasty, cement is injected into the compressed vertebral body. In kyphoplasty, a balloon is inserted into the compressed vertebra, and polymethyl methacrylate is injected. Both procedures are indicated for pain relief. Long-term studies to evaluate benefit and safety are needed. Primary risks include neurological impairment as a result of extrusion of cement near the spinal cord and increased risk of vertebral fractures above and below the surgical site. Early treatment of hip fractures reduces morbidity and mortality associated with hip fractures. Ideally, repair is within 24 hours.

Pharmacological treatments are either antiresorptive (they inhibit bone loss caused by the activity of osteoclasts—cells associated with bone removal) or anabolic (they increase production of osteoblasts—cells associated with production of bone). Antiresorptive therapies reduce osteoclast resorption. Anabolic therapies increase osteoblast function. The FDA mandates that new therapies demonstrate reduction in fracture risk.

There has been recent concern of a small risk of avascular necrosis of the jaw with bisphosphonate therapy. It appears most commonly in patients treated with monthly intravenous zoledronic acid for metastatic cancer, in patients with poor dental hygiene, and in patients with low bone turnover. All of these agents appear to be associated with increased bone density and a reduction in vertebral and nonvertebral fractures.

Hormone replacement therapy (HRT) has come in disfavor for the treatment of osteoporosis due to the associated risk of stroke, myocardial infarction, and breast cancer. The Women's Health Initiative (WHI) study was the first randomized double-blind study to

KEY FACTS

Description

A systemic disorder characterized by skeletal fragility and an increased risk of insufficiency fractures.

Causes

Bone density declines with age. Certain medical conditions predispose to bone loss.

Risk factors

Include female gender, postmenopausal state, Caucasian and Asian race, low adult weight, family history of osteoporosis, and personal history of a fracture as an adult.

Symptoms

Include loss of height and thoracic kyphosis.

Diagnosis

Dual energy X-ray absorbtiometry (DEXA) and evaluation by experienced medical personnel.

Treatments

Calcium and vitamin D supplementation, weight-bearing exercise program, and medications to preserve or improve BMD.

Pathogenesis

Without treatment, there is a progressive decline in bone density associated with increased fracture risk.

Prevention

Appropriate intake of calcium, vitamin D and weight-bearing exercises throughout a lifetime.

Epidemiology

In the United States, there are 700,000 vertebral fractures, 300,000 hip fractures, and 250,000 wrist fractures annually. As the population ages, the incidence is expected to increase.

demonstrate a reduction in hip fracture with the use of HRT. If a woman chooses to take HRT, it may well prevent postmenopausal bone loss. Generally, the bisphosphonates are more potent in the prevention of osteoclast resorption than HRT.

The selective estrogen receptor modulator (SERM) FDA-approved for the treatment of osteoporosis is raloxifene. This agent has been shown to reduce the risk of vertebral fractures but not of hip fractures. Side effects include hot flashes, leg cramps, and an increased risk of thrombosis.

Teriparatide is the only anabolic agent FDA-approved for the treatment of osteoporosis. It is a self-injection given daily for two years. It improves BMD and reduces the risk of vertebral and hip fractures. Early on, it may be associated with orthostatic hypotension. There has been an increased risk of osteosarcoma in rats treated with this agent. This has not been seen in humans, dogs, or monkeys. It is useful in patients with severe osteoporosis, patients not responding to bisphosphonate therapy, and in patients with a low bone turnover state.

Calcitonin is of questionable efficacy in bone density improvement and fracture reduction and therefore is not considered a mainstay of osteoporosis treatment.

Pathogenesis and prevention

Bone is composed of matrix and mineral. The matrix consists of type I collagen and a cellular component called osteoblasts, which form bone and osteoclasts, which resorb bone. Bone remodeling is a dynamic process. Peak bone mass is achieved by age thirty. Thereafter, osteoclast function outweighs osteoblast function, and there is a 0.5 to 1 percent loss of bone each year. In women, for the two years before menopause and up to five years after menopause, there can be a 5 percent loss every year. Most Caucasian women become osteoporotic at age 70.

Mineral is composed of hydroxapatite containing calcium and phosphorus. If a patient does not consume or absorb enough calcium, secondary hyperparathyroidism occurs. Calcium is then removed from the skeleton to maintain appropriate serum levels. As a result, bone loss occurs. Both primary and secondary hyperparathyroidism is a cause of osteoporosis.

It is critical that children, teens, and young adults get regular exercise and have adequate calcium and vitamin D intake so that they reach a maximal peak bone mass. Patients should avoid behaviors known to contribute to osteoporosis such as tobacco use and alcohol excess. Falls prevention should be a goal for all

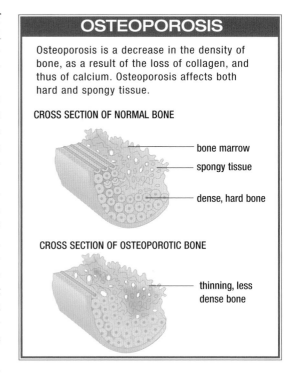

OSTEOPOROSIS

Osteoporosis is a decrease in the density of bone, as a result of the loss of collagen, and thus of calcium. Osteoporosis affects both hard and spongy tissue.

CROSS SECTION OF NORMAL BONE

— bone marrow
— spongy tissue
— dense, hard bone

CROSS SECTION OF OSTEOPOROTIC BONE

— thinning, less dense bone

patients. Physicians must screen all patients at risk for osteoporosis and treat those with indications for pharmacological therapy.

Epidemiology

Osteoporosis is an increasingly prevalent condition that accounts for more than 700,000 vertebral fractures, 300,000 hip fractures, and 250,000 wrist fractures annually in the United States. This results in significant morbidity and mortality and a large economic burden on society due to the costs of caring for these individuals, who often fail to regain their pre-fracture functioning state. Many patients must live in nursing homes either temporarily or permanently after a hip fracture. Osteoporotic fractures are more common in women, but the mortality rate after hip fracture is higher in men. The risk of mortality within the first year after a hip fracture is up to 20 percent.

Severe osteoporosis is associated with a loss of confidence, a fear of falling, and often social isolation, as patients go out less. As a result, depression becomes common. Once a patient becomes severely kyphotic, little can be done to correct the deformity.

Linda A. Russell

See also
• Fracture

Paralysis

Paralysis is a general term used to describe an inability to move one or several parts of the body. A lesser degree of weakness is termed *paresis*. Paralysis can be congenital or acquired and has many causes, including cerebral palsy, trauma, tumor, or stroke; or autoimmune, toxic, infectious, musculoskeletal, or metabolic compromise of the motor pathways in the nervous system.

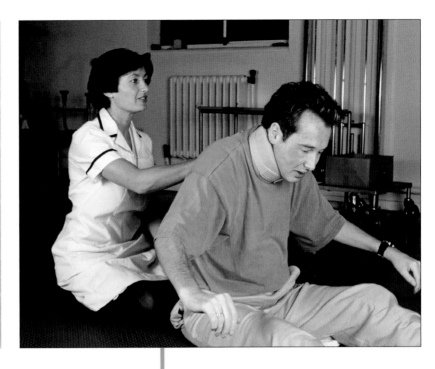

A physiotherapist assists a man with paralysis of all four limbs (quadriplegia) to balance in a supported "long sit position." The patient has a broken neck and has to relearn how to balance in this particular position.

Paralysis can occur at any level of the nervous system and may also be due to psychiatric conditions. Paralysis may be partial (paresis) or complete (plegia), mild or life threatening. It may involve one side of the body (hemiparesis or hemiplegia); all four limbs (quadriparesis or quadriplegia); the lower limbs (paraparesis or paraplegia); a single limb (monoparesis or monoplegia); or an isolated muscle group supplied by a single motor nerve (mononeuropathy). Paralysis can develop suddenly or slowly over time. Paralysis is an important cause of disability in the United States because the limitation in movement prevents individuals from carrying out activities of daily living. The diagnosis, prevention, and treatment of paralysis are determined by its etiology (cause).

Causes and risk factors

Some common causes of paralysis include stroke, cerebral palsy, multiple sclerosis, Guillain-Barré syndrome, spinal cord injuries, central nervous system tumors, and various neuropathies (for example, Bell's palsy). Risk factors are variable and are based on the causative disease process. For example, the risk factors in stroke include heredity, high blood pressure, sex, diabetes mellitus, and age. In multiple sclerosis, the risk factors relate to geographical location in that the farther an individual lives from the equator in the first fifteen years of life, the greater his or her chance of developing the disease. Women are also at a higher risk. The etiology is presumed to be autoimmune, but the precise cause is unknown.

In some parts of Asia and Africa, the polio virus remains endemic and continues to be an important cause of paralysis due to one of its complications, poliomyelitis. However, it has been eradicated in most industrialized parts of the world through vaccination.

Symptoms, signs, and diagnosis

Paralyzed individuals will usually complain of loss of movement or weakness in the affected part of the body. The loss of strength may also sometimes be associated with numbness or paresthesias (abnormal touch sensation, such as burning or prickling). The symptom of weakness is verified on neurological examination, which focuses on isolated testing of the major muscle groups. When paralysis is caused by damage to the central nervous system, there may be associated symptoms, such as trouble producing speech (aphasia) or numbness. In many cases, these associations can aid in determining the anatomical location of the disease process.

In stroke or in certain infectious or metabolic conditions, an individual may not be able to describe weakness, but an examiner may find decreased muscle tone, absent reflexes, pathological reflexes, muscle atrophy, increased muscle tone, or spasticity.

Alternatively, if paralysis is caused by damage to the peripheral nervous system, there may be associated pain. Metabolic abnormalities such as electrolyte imbalances tend to cause more widespread weakness. An infectious cause may be suggested if there is fever, diarrhea, vomiting, mental status changes, neck stiffness, insect bites, or another affected person who ate the same food.

Diagnostic testing is guided by a physician's assessment of the pattern and chronological development of the paralysis and associated symptoms. If these factors lead to suspicion of a disease process in the brain or spinal cord, computed tomography (CT) or magnetic resonance imaging (MRI) of the brain, spinal cord, or brachial plexus is used to examine the tissue in detail and to look for evidence of stroke, tumor, infection, or demyelination. If the lesion is suspected in the peripheral nervous system, such as the peripheral nerves, neuromuscular junction or muscle, electromyography (EMG) is used. Diseases of the muscle that cause paralysis are sometimes diagnosed using a muscle biopsy. When the cause of paralysis is thought to be a metabolic disorder or to be systemic in nature (autoimmune), then blood tests are used to aid in diagnosis. These tests may include investigation for antibodies known to be associated with certain conditions, such as acetylcholine receptor antibodies found in myasthenia gravis, or genetic mutations associated with specific conditions (amyotrophic lateral sclerosis and superoxide dismutase) or metabolic disturbances (hypocalcemia, hypokalemia).

Treatments and prevention

Dynamic preventive treatments such as widespread vaccination for polio virus have essentially eradicated poliomyelitis as a cause of paralysis in industrialized parts of the world, although it remains an important cause of paralysis in parts of Africa and India.

In the United States and most of Europe, stroke is treated in the first three hours of onset with drugs designed to break up the clot obstructing an artery. Close monitoring and control of blood pressure, glucose

KEY FACTS

Description

Paralysis is a general term used to describe an inability to move a part, or parts, of the body. Weakness, as distinct from paralysis, is designated *paresis*, and has the same causal factors as paralysis.

Causes

There are multiple causes of paralysis that originate from different levels of the nervous system; some more common examples are: stroke, tumor, neuropathy, amyotrophic lateral sclerosis, trauma, and Guillain-Barré syndrome.

Risk factors

Reduction of modifiable risk factors is based on the specific disease process causing paralysis. In stroke, these include lowering blood pressure, smoking cessation, lowering cholesterol, tight glycemic control in diabetes mellitus, and treatment of obstructive sleep apnea.

Symptoms

The pattern of weakness, associated symptoms, and time course of onset are essential features that aid in characterizing the type of paralysis, its cause, and treatment.

Diagnosis

Aimed at the suspected part of the body affected, it may include MRI, CT, EMG, X-rays, or blood tests in conjunction with a detailed medical history and physical examination.

Pathogenesis

Mechanisms of paralysis vary based on the underlying disease process. In stroke, the process is vascular due to inadequate blood supply or bleeding into the brain. Tumors cause mass effect and compression of important anatomical structures. Demyelinating diseases, such as multiple sclerosis, are caused by disruption or loss of the myelin sheaths in the central nervous system. The result is impaired signal transmission.

Prevention

Strategies are aimed at the disease process responsible for paralysis. In stroke, prevention consists of medical and dietary modifications that will lower blood pressure and cholesterol and will optimize glucose control. A healthy diet, exercise, and smoking cessation are also important preventive factors for stroke. In polio, vaccinations are powerful prevention strategies. In diseases such as primary central nervous system tumors or multiple sclerosis, there are no known prevention strategies.

Epidemiology

Strokes are one of the leading causes of paralysis; in 2000, around 1 million people had some form of paralysis after a stroke.

TYPES OF PARALYSIS

Depending on where the damage occurs in the nervous system, paralysis can affect one side of the body, the lower half of the body, or the trunk and all four limbs.

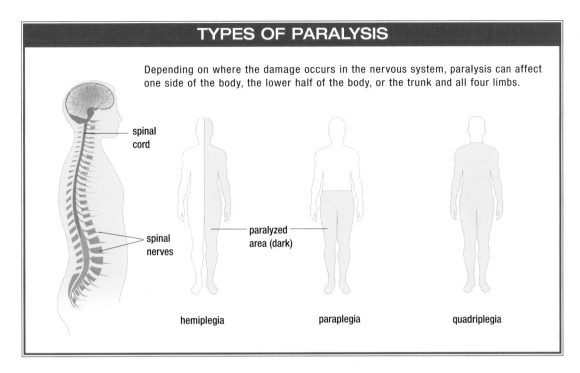

spinal cord

spinal nerves

paralyzed area (dark)

hemiplegia

paraplegia

quadriplegia

level, and temperature are also important treatments in the acute setting of stroke. However, most of the treatment is aimed at primary and secondary prevention of stroke, which entails reducing modifiable risk factors such as high blood pressure, high cholesterol, poor glucose control in diabetes, and obstructive sleep apnea.

In demyelinating diseases, such as multiple sclerosis, immunomodulating agents or immunosuppressant agents are used, as well as filtering of blood to remove pathogenic antibodies (plasma exchange).

Although treatment is usually directed at the specific disease process causing paralysis, paralysis of any etiology is treated with aggressive physical therapy and rehabilitation because immobility, in and of itself, can lead to atrophy, deconditioning, contractures, and other morbidity. There are some new therapies, such as constraint-based therapy, which is aimed at restricting the functional parts of the body so that an individual is made to use the dysfunctional limb, rehabilitating it into function.

Pathogenesis

Mechanisms of paralysis vary depending on the cause. There are two broad types of stroke, hemorrhagic (bleeding) and ischemic (blocked vessel). Paralysis in ischemic stroke occurs as a result of rupture of a cholesterol plaque or embolization of clot material from the heart that clogs a cerebral artery. The blocked artery leads to inadequate perfusion of brain tissue and subsequent cell death and edema. Often, the tissue that dies involves the motor fibers of the nervous system, which control strength and movement. If these areas of the brain are affected, the appropriate signals required for coordinated muscle movements are not transmitted to the spinal cord, nerves, and muscles. As a result, the patient experiences paralysis.

Paralysis can be reversible or permanent, depending on the cause. In general, paralysis from stroke and multiple sclerosis is permanent, with rehabilitation potential occurring over a period of months after the initial event. Other causes of paralysis, such as amyotrophic lateral sclerosis or tumors, are progressive in nature. Paralysis from an electrolyte or endocrine abnormality can be completely reversible.

Epidemiology

The incidence of cerebral palsy is 2 in 1,000 in developed countries; in 30 percent of cases, the spastic form is found. In 2005, polio, another cause of paralysis, was endemic in six countries; worldwide, there were around 2,000 cases of polio.

Meredith Roderick
and Robert Daroff

See also
- Diabetes • Multiple sclerosis • Sleep disorders
- Stroke and related disorders

Parkinson's disease

Parkinson's disease (PD) is a chronic, slowly progressing neurodegenerative movement disorder. Its main pathological hallmark is the death of nerve cells (neurons) in a specific region of the brain (substantia nigra pars compacta).

The neurons that are lost in PD are nerve cells that produce dopamine. Dopamine is a chemical neurotransmitter that transmits nerve signals between the substantia nigra and a brain region called the corpus striatum. These signals typically produce normal muscle activity. The loss of dopamine allows striatal neurons to discharge action potentials (fire) without regulation and leaves the afflicted person unable to control his or her muscle movements. It is apparent that 50 to 80 percent of neurons in the substantia nigra may be lost before disease symptoms appear. The symptoms of PD have been known for centuries. It was not until 1817, however, that the disorder became a recognized disease entity.

Causes and risk factors

Parkinson's disease is the most common form of a disease cluster, called parkinsonism, all forms of which share the primary symptoms. Parkinson's disease is classified in two general categories: familial and sporadic. The familial forms of the disorder are caused by gene mutations in any one of about eight identifiable genes. The causes of sporadic or idiopathic Parkinson's disease are unknown but are most likely the result of environmental risk factors acting on genetically susceptible individuals when aging.

Many environmental risk factors have been identified. Decreased risk appears to be associated with such factors as diet (vitamin E, multivitamins), smoking, alcohol, and caffeine. Increased risk appears to be related to such factors as aging, gender (men are at higher risk than women), race (whites are at higher risk than others), family history, life experiences (trauma, stress, and depression), infectious agents (encephalitis and herpes), environmental exposures (heavy metals, well water, farming, and pesticides). A compound that was produced in an attempt to synthesize street heroin called MPTP (1-methyl 4 phenyl 1, 2, 3, 6-tetrahydropyridine) also causes PD-like symptoms and is used, in fact, to study possible mechanisms of neuronal destruction in various disease models.

Aging is a risk factor for Parkinson's disease. It usually affects people over fifty, and the average age of onset is around sixty years. Some people, however, especially those with familial PD, manifest an "early onset" form of the disease before their fortieth year.

Symptoms

The loss of striatal neurons and decreased striatal dopamine concentrations lead to the typical characteristics of PD. These include altered muscle function that negatively impacts many bodily activities that involve movement. Altered muscle function results in the cardinal symptoms of resting tremor in the limbs, hands, and face, including the jaw; muscle (cogwheel) rigidity; slow voluntary movement (bradykinesia); and postural instability, with impaired balance and coordination. As the disease progresses, patients usually have difficulty with speech and with walking, and in advanced cases there may be loss of movement. These collective symptoms are caused by excess muscle contraction due to decreased dopamine production. More subtle, non-motor consequences include cognitive impairment, mood disorders, sleep disturbances, sensation disturbances, altered autonomic function, changes in sensation, and minor problems with language.

Resting tremor is usually one of the earliest symptoms. It presents on one side, is most severe in the resting state, and decreases in intensity with movement. It is estimated, however, that perhaps as many as 30 percent of patients have barely detectable tremor (akinetic tremor). Cogwheel muscle rigidity, or jerky, alternating resistant or nonresistant movements, or both, is observed when a limb is moved passively by the examiner. Bradykinesia and postural instability also result from poor muscle control, owing to the lack of adequate dopamine production and the loss of dopaminergic neurons. This leads to impaired balance and altered postural reflexes that often result in loss of balance and subsequent falls.

PD patients often experience other motor symptoms, such as changes in gait, especially in more advanced cases. The patient may be observed "shuffling," using short steps with minimal foot elevation, accompanied by a shuffling sound as the footwear scuffs along the floor. These patients often fall, especially on a cluttered walking surface. They will often have a decreased arm swing due to the short steps and bradykinesia. Even turning is difficult and is done in a series of small steps without flexing the trunk and neck. Another motor symptom of the advanced patient is a stooped posture, which can become so severe that the upper torso may be at right angles with the rest of the trunk. Eventually, the patient may experience festination, an increasing gait that, when combined with postural changes and poor balance, results in a fall. Akinesia, or "freezing," is also experienced by the advanced PD patient. The patient cannot move his or her feet, especially in confined or obstructed places or when first initiating a step from a standing position.

Other motor effects include alterations in speech and swallowing. Problems with speech include hypophnia, a soft, hoarse, and monotonal speech; and festinating speech, an excessively rapid, usually soft and unintelligible style of speaking. Weak swallowing (dysphagia) and a stooped posture often lead to drooling. In these patients, salivary or food aspiration can lead to poor lung clearing and pneumonia. About 50 percent of patients experience fatigue. Often, patients blink infrequently and can acquire a masklike facial appearance (hypomimia) with a blank expression. Decreased motor activity also impairs the patient's ability to shift positions in bed and to rise from a sitting position. It impairs fine motor coordination and causes an overall loss or severe decrease in movements such as the walking arm swing. These more advanced patients tend to make small letters when handwriting (micrographia).

As the diseases progresses, most patients develop motor symptoms even though they have been treated successfully for symptoms over many years. Motor symptoms begin to manifest with the normal treatment regimen. This is known as "wearing off." Initially it is treated by more frequent administration of levodopa (a drug that increases dopamine levels). "On-off" is another complication that arises over time. The effectiveness of levodopa suddenly disappears and the patient becomes rigid and may have tremors and slow movement. An additional dose of medication can usually, with a little time, overcome this effect. Apomorphine injection also can be used, and it is effective in just a few minutes after administration.

Patients can develop mild to severe uncontrolled movements (dyskinesia) with spasms, writhing, twitching or contraction of muscles, and chorea (involuntary jerky movements) that may often occur as a side effect at the peak of levodopa effect. As the disease progresses, it becomes more difficult to control. Many PD patients also experience nonmotor effects. Cognitive impairment includes executive dysfunction, memory loss, and ultimately dementia in a significant number of cases. Executive dysfunction implies that the patient has problems with planning, abstract thinking, mental agility, initiating appropriate actions within a framework of rules including determining appropriate and inappropriate reactions to environmental circumstances, and appropriately processing sensory input information. These symptoms may be the early stages of dementia, which affects 20 to 40 percent of patients. Dementia often manifests with difficulty in abstract thinking, memory deficits, and behavioral abnormalities.

Depression is a notable mood disorder in PD patients. Because there are no tools to assess depression specifically in PD, it is difficult to determine the degree to which this disorder permeates the afflicted population. It is felt, however, that it is very common and may affect 50 percent or more of people with the disorder. Depression often goes undetected in this population because it is assumed the behavior may be an unavoidable consequence of the disease. A skilled professional can distinguish depression from the effects of PD since people without PD present with a different profile.

KEY FACTS

Description
A chronic, progressive neurodegenerative disorder.

Causes
Gene mutations and environmental factors.

Risk factors
Aging, diet, race, ethnicity, gender, exposure to chemicals, and infectious agents.

Symptoms
Tremor in the hands, limbs, and face. Poor balance and coordination. Depression, memory loss, and dementia.

Diagnosis
Based on the symptoms. PET can help diagnosis.

Treatments
Increasing dopamine levels.

Pathogenesis
Cognitive impairment, dementia in some cases.

Prevention
None as yet.

Epidemiology
Statistics are variable; best estimates are that around 1 million people in the United States have been diagnosed, and three times that number are believed to be undiagnosed.

During the course of PD and the related parkinsonian disorders, sleep disturbances affect most patients. Altered sleep patterns can profoundly influence the patient's quality of life, affecting performance at work and activities such as driving. Sleep can also be altered by the medications prescribed for PD, especially those that act on dopamine systems. Studies of sleep in this population have found disrupted night sleep, greater leg movements, sleep apnea, drug-independent sleepiness, and REM sleep behavior disorder. In REM sleep behavior disorder, the normal muscle paralysis (atonia) that occurs during REM sleep is disturbed in a way that allows the patient to retain muscle tone. Thus, the patient can respond to dreams in an often violent manner, potentially causing severe injury to himself or herself or another person in the same bed. PD patients also frequently experience restless leg syndrome, a neurological consequence characterized by strange, unpleasant sensations in the legs. Significant disruption in normal sleep patterns can lead to exhaustion.

The senses can be affected in this neurological disorder. Visual function, such as detecting differences in contrast, spatial orientation, color discrimination, binocular vision, and oculomotor control may be impaired. Other disturbances include a decreased ability to properly modulate blood pressure changes in response to changes in body position; dizziness; altered proprioception (awareness of movement and spatial orientation of body parts to each other), reduction (microsmia) or loss (anosmia) of smell acuity, and pain related to the demands placed on the musculature.

Seborrheic dermatitis (oily skin) is fairly common in PD. Later in the course of the disease, urinary incontinence, constipation, altered sexual function, and weight loss can occur.

Diagnosis and treatments

There is not a definitive diagnostic test or combination of tests for PD. The diagnosis of the disease is based mainly on the hallmark symptoms discussed above and the unified PD rating scale. In combination with these, positron emission tomography (PET), an instrumental test that is useful in observing organ function, greatly increases diagnostic accuracy. Good specificity for the test is provided because radioactive test substances that mimic dopamine can show that dopamine uptake is decreased.

Treatment of symptoms with medications is often the first approach to managing the disorder. Usually, the type of medications, the dose and frequency of ad-

ministration, and the combinations of medications must be adjusted over time during the course of the disorder. Many of the medications have significant side effects; the patient's physical well-being and mental health must be closely monitored. Most of the medications primarily control symptoms by increasing available dopamine levels. The most widely used drug for the treatment of PD tremor is levodopa. However, only a small portion, probably not more than 5 percent, of the levodopa gets into the brain. The remaining material is metabolized in other tissues and eventually causes significant side effects. Also, the administered levodopa inhibits the normal production of levodopa, so doses must be increased over time. In addition to levodopa, inhibitors (carbidopa and benserazide) of the nonbrain enzymes that convert levodopa to dopamine can be administered in "combination therapy" with levodopa to decrease the amount of levodopa that is metabolized before it reaches the brain. These inhibitors also decrease the side effects experienced by the extraneural metabolism of levodopa.

When symptoms are not controlled by medication, surgery, such as deep brain stimulation, pallidotomy, and thalamotomy, may be tried. Speech therapy and exercise may improve quality of life for the PD patient.

Pathogenesis and epidemiology

There is no cure for PD, but medications or surgical procedures give significant symptomatic relief for extended periods. Because the disease follows a chronic course, long-term management is important. Adjustments in medications, family and patient education, the use of support personnel and groups, maintenance of well-being, exercise, and nutrition all help.

An estimated 0.37 percent, or 1 million people, in the United States suffer from PD, and an estimated 3 to 4 million people with PD remain undiagnosed. Around 15,000 per year in the United States die from PD. Some data has associated increased PD mortality with countries using agricultural pesticides. The incidence of PD may depend on gender, age, and ethnicity. Men have a higher incidence of PD than women; the incidence in both genders increases over the age of 60; and Hispanics have the highest rate of the disease, followed by non-Hispanic whites, Asians, and blacks.

David Ullman

See also
• Dementia • Paralysis

Pelvic inflammatory disease

Pelvic inflammatory disease (PID) is an infection of the female reproductive tract, which causes sickness and infertility worldwide.

PID is caused by infections, usually chlamydia and gonorrhea, and these bacteria are the targets for treating the disease. If left untreated, 18 percent of women will have chronic pelvic pain, 9 percent will have an ectopic pregnancy, and 20 percent will be infertile. The organisms causing PID usually spread up the female reproductive tract from the vagina, through the cervix, and can infect the uterus, fallopian tubes, and peritoneum. PID is complex because there are many ways it can present in women. In the United States more than 1 million women develop PID yearly.

Causes and risk factors

Common organisms that cause PID are chlamydia and gonorrhea, and possibly bacteria that lead to bacterial vaginosis. Many women do not have any symptoms, but most experience pelvic pain and may also have vaginal discharge or bleeding. Women at increased risk for PID are those with STDs (sexually transmitted diseases), PID in the past, early age sexual activity, those not using good barrier contraception, and those with many sexual partners. Other risk factors include vaginal douching or using an intrauterine contraceptive device. Using oral contraceptive pills may reduce the risk of PID.

Diagnosis and treatments

It is recommended that all women with abdominal pain be examined and tested for STDs. Tests that are helpful in diagnosing infection are the presence of white blood cells (WBC) in a vaginal swab or increased blood WBC counts. Ultrasound scans of the reproductive tract are also useful and can show thickening of the fallopian tubes in women with PID. Other changes related to inflammation may be seen with magnetic resonance imaging or computed tomography scans. Biopsy samples taken from the uterus can show inflammation changes under the microscope, and laparoscopy may be needed to confirm the diagnosis.

Tests include radiological examinations and exploratory surgery to look for the disease, if treatment with medications are not effective. The most effective way to reduce the incidence of PID is to prevent it from developing. Screening women for chlamydia and gonorrhea who do not have symptoms and treating those women with antibiotics that can act against chlamydia and gonorrhea and possibly bacterial vaginosis are effective measures in preventing PID. There are different patterns of drug resistance of these organisms in different parts of the world, so regional variations may decide which antibiotic is chosen. Early treatment of those with PID will also prevent the development of complications. Whether the treatment is given in the hospital or at home depends on the severity of the PID.

PID is a serious condition and causes medical issues for women worldwide. Early screening and treatment can prevent many long-term complications.

Moeen Panni

KEY FACTS

Description
An infection of the female reproductive tract.

Causes
Caused by chlamydia and gonorrhea.

Risk factors
Sexual activity at an early age, many sexual partners, IUCDs, previous PID, and an STD.

Symptoms
Pelvic pain, vaginal discharge, and bleeding.

Diagnosis
Examination, blood tests, ultrasound, radiological examinations, and exploratory surgery.

Treatments
Early screening and treatment can prevent many of the long-term complications. Antibiotics.

Pathogenesis
If left untreated, the disease can lead to chronic pelvic pain, ectopic pregnancy, and infertility.

Prevention
Regular checkups, prompt treatment of infection.

Epidemiology
Around 1 million cases of PID yearly in the United States.

See also
- Chlamydial infections • Ectopic pregnancy
- Gonorrhea

Peritonitis

Infection of the peritoneum may be primary (without evident cause), secondary (related to an intra-abdominal process), or a complication of peritoneal dialysis.

Primary or spontaneous bacterial peritonitis (SBP) occurs in adults with cirrhosis and ascites and children with kidney damage or cirrhotic livers with large nodules. Risk factors for SBP include advanced cirrhosis, prior episode of SBP, coexisting gastrointestinal bleed, and low protein concentration in the fluid in the peritoneal cavity. The microorganisms causing SBP include E. coli, Klebsiella, *Streptococcus pneumoniae*, and *Streptococcus* species (19 percent). Fever, abdominal pain, nausea, vomiting, diarrhea, and altered mental status are common symptoms, but many patients are asymptomatic. Diagnosis of SBP requires paracentesis, in which a needle is used to puncture the body cavity, to take fluid for culture, to relieve the pressure of excess fluid, or to inject medication. Treatment of suspected SBP should be started as soon as cultures are obtained. Empiric antibiotics should be given—that is, without definite knowledge of the disorder but based on the fact that they were effective in similar cases. Clinical improvement occurs within 48 hours. Treatment for five days is as efficacious as longer courses. Mortality has declined from 95 percent to 40 percent since 1924. In high risk patients, antibiotic prophylaxis decreases the recurrence rate of SBP.

Secondary peritonitis

Perforation of the gastrointestinal or urogenital tract caused by infection, trauma, or surgery leads to secondary peritonitis. A large number of microorganisms spill into the peritoneal cavity, leading to polymicrobial infection with anaerobes (especially *Bacteriodes fragilis*), enterobacteraceae, streptococci, enterococci, and clostridia. *Neisseria gonorrhoeae* may be present in female genital tract infection. Activation of the immune system by the protein cytokine can cause inflammation, toxins can be released when bacteria die, and anaerobic and aerobic bacteria can cause sepsis and abscesses. Abdominal pain aggravated by motion is a predominant symptom. Anorexia, nausea, vomiting, fever, and abdominal distension are seen. Marked abdominal tenderness with rebound tenderness, rigidity, and hyperresonant or absent bowel sounds are other signs. High heart rate, fast breathing, and low blood pressure signify septic shock. An increase in white cells and elevated serum amylase levels are frequent. Dilated bowel loops or free air may be seen on radiographs. Ultrasonography or computed tomography scans of the abdomen detect lesions and guide drainage of fluid or abscess. Surgery to control the contamination, remove necrotic tissue, and drain abscesses is essential. Antibiotics should be started immediately after obtaining blood cultures. Supportive measures to maintain circulation, oxygenation, and nutrition are critical. Survival depends on the age of the patient, co-morbid conditions, duration of peritoneal contamination, and the microorganisms involved. Peritoneal dialysis carries a risk of peritonitis.

Nigar Kirmani

KEY FACTS

Description

Infection of the peritoneum may be primary, secondary, or related to peritoneal dialysis.

Causes

Primary: enteric gram negatives and streptococci. Secondary: bowel anaerobes and gram negatives. Peritoneal dialysis: gram positive bacteria.

Symptoms

Fever, abdominal pain, nausea, vomiting and diarrhea. Abdominal tenderness, rebound tenderness, and hypoactive bowel sounds.

Diagnosis

Elevated cell count in fluid in peritoneal cavity and positive culture are diagnostic.

Treatment

Broad spectrum antibiotics are needed. Surgical drainage and anaerobic coverage are essential for secondary peritonitis.

Pathogenesis

Translocation of intestinal bacteria, spillage of bowel contents and infection of catheter exit site.

Prevention

Antibiotic prophylaxis prevents recurrences of SBP.

Epidemiology

SBP occurs in cirrhotics with ascites and children with nephrotic syndrome. Secondary peritonitis occurs after bowel perforation, trauma, or surgery.

See also
• Cirrhosis of the liver

Personality disorders

Personality disorders are a group of disorders described by the *Diagnostic and Statistical Manual of Mental Disorders*, fourth edition (DSM-IV), as "an enduring pattern of inner experience and behavior that deviates markedly from the expectations of the individual's culture, is pervasive and inflexible, has an onset in adolescence or early adulthood, is stable over time, and leads to distress and impairment." Personality disorders are notoriously difficult to treat.

Although personality disorders have their onset in adolescence or early adulthood, they are considered adult disorders. Personality disorders are pervasive and maladaptive patterns of human behavior. These enduring patterns of inflexible and aberrant behavior are not a consequence of another psychiatric disorder, medical condition, or substance abuse.

Causes and risk factors

Numerous factors may contribute to the development of personality disorders. Some of these factors are biological, while others are environmental. The interactions between biological and environmental factors are complex. For instance, Cluster A personality disorders are more common in the biological relatives of patients with schizophrenia. Depressive disorders are common in the family backgrounds of patients with borderline personality disorders.

A strong association has been demonstrated between individuals with histrionic personality disorders and patients with somatization disorder, in which people think they have a physical illness, but no cause can be discovered for the symptoms. Parental alcoholism and antisocial behavior are prevalent in the families of individuals who have antisocial personality disorder.

Since children's behavior is shaped by their family environment, personality disorders are often viewed as direct results of these interactions, or they may serve as adaptation strategies to their specific families. For example, very active children may be restrained in their activities by overly protective and controlling parents. Consequently, those children might develop coping strategies that predispose them toward avoidant behavior.

Individuals at high risk for the development of personality disorders are often abused children, children raised in chaotic family environments, children with close relatives diagnosed with personality disorders and major psychiatric illnesses, and children whose parents are alcohol and substance abusers.

Diagnosis

The assessment of the symptoms and patterns of behavior should be based on as many sources of information as possible. From the diagnostic point of view, it is also advisable to conduct more than one clinical interview with an individual prior to a diagnosis being given. In addition to the fact that the ethnic, cultural, and social background of the individual must be taken into account, it is important to assess the stability of symptoms in a variety of contexts. With the exception of one type of personality disorder, antisocial personality disorder, the diagnosis of personality disorders can be applied to adolescence and young adults; however, in order to diagnose a personality disorder in an individual prior to age eighteen, the symptoms must be present for at least one year. When individuals meet the criteria for more than one personality disorder, each of them should be diagnosed separately. Personality disorders are coded on Axis II of DSM-IV, as opposed to any other psychiatric disorders, which are coded on Axis I.

Based on the DSM-IV, a diagnosis of personality disorder requires that an individual must experience significant problems in two or more of the following general areas in addition to the number of specific symptoms. These general diagnostic criteria are cognition, affectivity, interpersonal functioning, and impulse control. It has previously been noted that the general concept of the category of personality disorders is mostly based on Western understanding of personality and the definition of "normalcy."

Symptoms

The personality disorders are grouped into three clusters in the DSM-IV, based on their symptom similarities. Cluster A covers the paranoid, schizoid, and schizotypical personality disorders. Individuals from this cluster often appear to be odd or eccentric. Cluster B is made up of the antisocial, borderline, histrionic, and narcissistic personality disorders. Individuals from this cluster are often described as emotional, dramatic, and unpredictable. Cluster C includes the avoidant, dependent, and obsessive-compulsive personality disorders. Individuals from this cluster are often described as anxious. There is an additional DSM-IV category of personality disorder: not otherwise specified (NOS). This category is usually applied in the clinical cases in which an individual is considered to have a personality disorder that is not included in the DSM-IV (for example, passive-aggressive personality) or an individual exhibits symptoms of more than one type of personality disorder.

Cautionary note

Although the cluster system has proved helpful for research and educational purposes, the DSM-IV adds a warning note that there are limitations to the system, not least because some people have co-occurring personality disorders from different clusters.

Cluster A personality disorders

Paranoid individuals with paranoid personality disorder are often suspicious of others and preoccupied with doubts regarding the motives of other people. Those individuals have major difficulties in establishing close relationships because of their fear that the information they share can be used against them. Such people are also prone to bear grudges and have difficulty forgiving insults or other real or perceived injuries. Because they lack trust in other people, these individuals have an excessive need to be self-sufficient and have a strong desire to control their environment.

Schizoid individuals with schizoid personality disorder often demonstrate a lack of desire for intimacy. They often have a restricted affect in emotional situations and appear to be disinterested in developing close relationship with others. They rarely experience or display emotions such as anger or excitement.

Schizotypical individuals with this disorder are characterized by a marked discomfort concerning close relationships as well as cognitive and perceptual distortions. It is not uncommon for these individuals to have ideas out of reference or even have some paranoid ideations. Their affect is usually restricted. Under stressors, these individuals may experience transient psychotic episodes with a duration from a few minutes to hours.

Cluster B personality disorders

Antisocial individuals with this disorder are characterized by a pervasive pattern of disregard for, and viola-

KEY FACTS

Description
Pervasive and maladaptive patterns of behavior that lead to the significant impairment of functioning in major areas, in the clear absence of other psychiatric or medical conditions or changes in personality related to alcohol or substance use.

Causes and risk factors
Personality disorders may be the result of multiple interactions between the individual's characteristics, such as temperament, and environmental factors, for example cultural and social norms and family upbringing.

Diagnosis
The diagnosis of personality disorder is usually made by a clinician based on the results from clinical evaluations. There are no laboratory tests or other procedures available that can provide a definitive diagnosis.

Symptoms
Based on the similarity of symptoms, personality disorders are grouped into three clusters in the DSM-IV. Cluster A covers the paranoid, schizoid, and schizotypical personality disorders. Cluster B is made up of the antisocial, borderline, histrionic, and narcissistic personality disorders. Cluster C includes the avoidant, dependent, and obsessive-compulsive personality disorders. There is also a DSM-IV category of "personality disorder not otherwise specified" (NOS) for those individuals who do not clearly fit into any of the described personality disorders.

Treatments
The types of treatments depend on the particular subtype of personality disorder, severity of symptomatology, and comorbid conditions (that is, substance use disorders, eating disorders, and anxiety disorders). Treatment is typically successful when it is individualized and may include both psychotherapy and pharmacotherapy.

Pathogenesis
The outlook varies. Some personality disorders diminish during middle age without any treatment, while others persist throughout life despite treatment.

Prevention
Early identification and treatment of individuals at high risk.

Epidemiology
Varies across different personality disorders.

tion of, the rights of others, which begins in childhood or early adolescence and continues into adulthood. For this diagnosis to be given, the individuals must be at least 18 years of age and must have been diagnosed with conduct disorder prior to the age of 15. Lack of empathy, arrogance, superficial charm, and self-assurance are hallmarks of this disorder.

Borderline individuals with this disorder are characterized by a pattern of instability in their personal relationships, self-image, marked fluctuation of affect, and impulsivity at least in two areas (for example, unsafe sexual practices, gambling, binge eating, or substance abuse). Their dysphoric mood is often disrupted by episodes of anger or extreme anxiety and despair. Under stress, some of these individuals are prone to psychotic-like symptoms, such as ideas out of reference, body-image distortions, and hallucinations. Histrionic individuals with this disorder are characterized by excessive emotionality and attention-seeking behavior. These individuals often become depressed and upset if they are not the center of attention. They are novelty driven and become easily bored with their usual routine. Their appearance and behavior can be inappropriately sexual and seductive.

Narcissistic individuals with this disorder are characterized by a need for admiration, a lack of empathy, a sense of self-importance, and exploitative attitudes toward others. They often believe that they are superior and expect others to recognize it as well. These individuals are very sensitive to criticism and may become extremely agitated or angry because of it.

Cluster C personality disorders
Avoidant individuals with this disorder are usually preoccupied with feelings of inadequacy and hypersensitivity to rejection or negative evaluation in social situations. They prefer to have minimal social interactions because of their fears of criticism or humiliation. There are often shy, quiet, and isolated. In many cases, individuals with this disorder also fit the criteria for social phobia.

Dependent individuals with this disorder are characterized by marked difficulties with the decision-making processes of everyday life. These individuals often lack the initiative to take control of major areas in their lives. They tend to form a close relationship in order to obtain the care and support they need. They rarely question authorities and usually display compliant behaviors to avoid displeasing other people.

Obsessive-compulsive individuals with this disorder are preoccupied with orderliness, perfectionism, and a

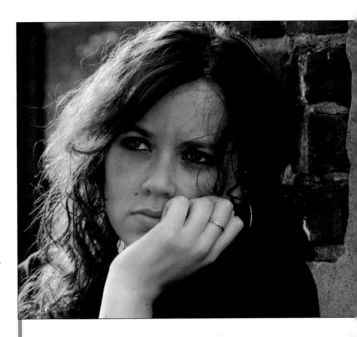

For someone who has a personality disorder, poor social functioning and an inability to adapt to changing circumstances can cause distress in everyday life. It can impinge on all relationships and cause occupational problems.

need for mental and interpersonal control. Their everyday relationships have a formal and serious quality, and their interpersonal style is often described as stiff or rigid. They are preoccupied with concerns that things have to be done a specific, "correct" way; subsequently, they have difficulties accepting ideas or suggestions from other people.

Treatments
The treatment of personality disorders is complicated by the fact that affected individuals rarely seek help on their own. Most of the patients view their problems as part of their self-image, which explains their reluctance to participate in treatment. Subsequently, the type of treatment depends on the willingness of the affected individuals to accept a need for change, the severity of the symptoms associated with specific personality disorders, and comorbid conditions. A growing body of evidence supports the notion that a biopsychosocial approach to the treatment of personality disorders provides a foundation for integrating diagnosis and treatment modalities. Based on this approach, psychotherapy and pharmacotherapy can be matched to meet the individual needs of patients. A variety of psychotherapeutic methods have been tried for personality disorders. Each of them provides inter-

ventions based on the theoretical understandings of the development of personality disorders. On a practical level, different schools of psychotherapy are not mutually exclusive, but rather overlap and complement each other. The psychotherapeutic modalities are often aimed at examining the psychodynamic aspects of the patient's relationships, enhancing problem-solving skills and the ability to tolerate frustrations, stressors, and the uncertainty of daily life, and improvement of cognitive skills.

Each personality disorder subtype requires specific modifications of therapeutic goals, and objectives and must be based on realistic expectations of how much character change can be achieved by the particular patient.

The pharmacotherapy of personality disorders is not organized around different subtypes, but rather targets symptom domains such as physical aggression, hyperactivity, impulsiveness, transitory psychotic symptoms, anxiety, and mood reactivity. For example, it is not uncommon to prescribe antipsychotic medications to patients with paranoid and schizotypal personality disorders during a brief psychotic episode.

Patients with borderline personality disorder can be also given antipsychotics during episodes of transient paranoid ideations or dissociative symptoms. Mood stabilizers such as lithium, carbamazepine, lamotrigine, and valproate can be used to improve impulsiveness, anger outbursts, and sudden mood changes. Antidepressants and anti-anxiety medications are also clinically effective therapeutic agents in the manage-

ment of depressive symptoms, episodic dysphoria (feeling sick or unhappy), irritability, sleep problems, and anxiety.

Pathogenesis

Although personality disorders are lifelong patterns of maladaptive behavior with an onset in adolescence or early adulthood, most of the individuals experience periods of remissions and exacerbations. Positive life experiences and major life events, such as the death of a parent or spouse, marriage, birth of a child, and retirement can modify the course of personality disorders and the age of diagnosis.

Prevention

The preventive strategy involves the early identification of children and young adolescents who are at high risk based on family histories and significant environmental variables, such as chaotic family upbringing. Once an at-risk individual is identified, therapeutic measures aimed at the prevention of the development of full-blown disorder are implemented.

Epidemiology

The prevalence of personality disorders varies in different population samples. It is estimated that 0.5 to 2.5 percent of the general population meet the criteria for paranoid personality disorder, about 2 percent for schizoid, and about 3 percent for schizotypical. The prevalence of antisocial personality disorder is about 3 percent in men and 1 percent in females in community settings, but the prevalence of this disorder is 10 times higher in prisons or other forensic settings. About 2 percent of the general population carry a diagnosis of borderline personality disorder; about 75 percent of those patients are women. It is estimated that histrionic personality disorder occurs in about 2 percent of the general population. Fewer than 1 percent of the population have narcissistic personality disorder, and 75 percent of them are men. About 1 percent of the population have avoidant or obsessive-compulsive personality disorders, and between 0.5 and 1 percent have dependent personality disorder.

Oleg Tcheremissine

If a person has a narcissistic personality disorder, he or she feels an unrealistic sense of self-importance. The person needs a lot of praise but cannot accept criticism and so tends to have unsatisfactory relations with other people.

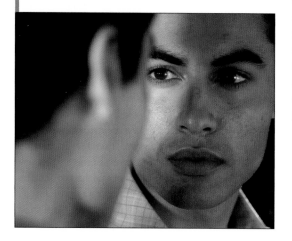

See also
• Alcohol-related disorders • Anxiety disorders • Asperger's disorder • Autism • Bipolar disorder • Depressive disorders • Psychotic disorders • Schizophrenia

Plague

Plague is an ancient disease that has killed hundreds of millions of people. It is one of the most deadly diseases humans have ever known. The disease never completely disappears, and the world has experienced three major outbreaks, or pandemics, of plague.

The first pandemic of plague was in 541 C.E. The outbreak began in Egypt and then moved across Europe, killing over 100 million people. Seven hundred years later, a second outbreak killed one in three people in Europe. During this time, people began calling plague the Black Death or the great pestilence. A third pandemic swept around the world in 1855. It eventually spread to every inhabited continent and killed more than 12 million people in China and India alone. There are still approximately 1,000 to 3,000 cases in the world each year. Now, however, the chances of a pandemic are very low. Plague used to kill about 90 percent of the people who got sick, but thanks to antibiotics, now only one out of seven cases of plague is fatal.

Causes

Plague is a zoonosis, that is, a disease that can spread naturally from animals to humans. Plague is caused by an infection with the bacterium *Yersinia pestis*. The bacteria live in animals such as rats, prairie dogs, marmots, and other rodents. Fleas bite these animals and pick up the bacteria. The fleas then jump onto humans and bite them, giving them the infection.

Plague has two main forms. One is bubonic plague, which results from fleabites. It gets its name from the large, swollen, and tender lymph nodes, called buboes, which it causes. These swollen lymph nodes are usually in the neck, under the arms, or at the top of the legs. The other main form of the disease is pneumonic plague. This occurs when the infection is in the lungs.

Bioterrorism

Naturally occurring plague is not the only form of the disease; several countries have found ways to turn plague into a biological weapon. Many countries conducted research with plague, and a few actually created weapons. The Japanese army used plague as a weapon against the Chinese in 1940. In this particular

KEY FACTS

Description

A disease of animals that can infect humans. Bacteria called *Yersinia pestis* cause plague. It occur in two forms: bubonic plague and pneumonic plague.

Causes

A bite from an infected flea causes bubonic plague. Pneumonic plague occurs in some people with bubonic plague when the bacteria travel to the lungs. Other people get pneumonic plague when exposed to airborne droplets from a person with pneumonic plague. Some biological weapons can also cause plague.

Risk factors

Yersinia pestis lives on every continent except Australia. The infected fleas usually come from rats, prairie dogs, marmots, and other rodents.

Symptoms

A patient with plague feels very ill. People with bubonic plague will develop large painful masses of lymph nodes, called buboes, usually in the armpit or at the top of the leg. Those with pneumonic plague may have chest pain, trouble breathing, and a cough that brings up bloody material from the lungs.

Diagnosis

Doctors will make their initial diagnosis based on the patient's symptoms. Special laboratories can perform tests to verify the diagnosis.

Treatments

Health care providers treat plague with intravenous or oral antibiotics.

Pathogenesis

In bubonic plague, bacteria grow in the lymph nodes and release toxins that make the patient very ill.

Prevention

Anyone exposed to plague should begin taking antibiotics as soon as possible to reduce the chance of becoming infected. People with pneumonic plague can spread the disease to others not infected. They should be isolated and health care workers must use protective equipment when caring for these patients.

Epidemiology

If untreated, bubonic plague kills 30 percent of its victims in around four days. Untreated pneumonic plague kills 95 percent of its victims in three days. In rural areas of the United States, 10 to 15 cases occur annually. Worldwide, 1,000 to 3,000 cases occur annually, in countries such as Africa, Asia, and South America.

case, the attackers dropped plague-infected fleas from an aircraft. This attack caused 120 deaths. After World War II, both the United States and the Soviet Union were able to create a weapon system that spread the bacteria directly, without the need for fleas. The United States never took this project very far, but it is believed that the Soviet Union did a substantial amount of work in this area.

Plague is a problem only in extremely unsanitary conditions in poorer areas of the world where there are regular small outbreaks; there are only occasional outbreaks in developed countries. As living conditions improve around the world, the number of people who develop plague continues to fall. However, because plague is well-established in wild rodents, it probably will never be totally eradicated. Rat extermination should be carried out in both developed and undeveloped countries.

Diagnosis

Plague is not very difficult to diagnose in the laboratory. It has a distinct appearance under a microscope. A scientist in a laboratory can use several tests to examine samples of blood or other body substances from a patient to make certain the disease is plague. A patient with plague also produces antibodies to the bacteria. Laboratory tests that show elevated antibody levels would also confirm that a person was infected.

Treatments

Doctors can treat plague with antibiotics. For quite some time, the antibiotic of choice was streptomycin. This particular medication is not always widely available, and pregnant women should not use it, so doctors may use another medication, such as gentamicin. Health care providers will usually give these medications as an injection, either into the muscle or into a vein. If there are many people who develop the disease at one time, it may not be possible to start intravenous lines on everyone. Doctors may treat patients with oral medications. In this case, the preferred medications are doxycycline or ciprofloxacin, which are acceptable for both adults and children. Plague can be prevented if an exposed person is treated with antibiotics. A vaccine can prevent plague but may not be available in sufficient quantities if plague were used as a biological weapon.

Prevention

Pneumonic plague causes special problems because it spreads from person to person, in droplets that spray

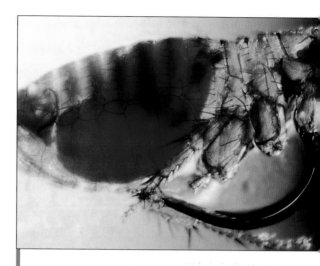

This greatly magnified picture shows a plague-infected oriental rat flea (Xenopsylla cheopsis) after feeding on an inoculated mouse. This flea is known to transmit the bacterium Yersinia pestis, the causative agent of plague.

with each sneeze. Because of this, doctors and nurses must isolate individuals with pneumonic plague so that they do not infect others. People who take care of those with plague must wear personal protective equipment, including a face mask.

In areas where plague is enzootic (known to exist in a locality), preventive measures should be taken. These include eliminating any sources of food or shelter for rodents near homes; ensuring that rodents do not have any means of access to homes; treating pets, such as dogs and cats, with insecticides; avoiding touching dead or sick rodents; and taking care not to handle sick domestic animals, especially cats. Hunters in affected localities should wear gloves before touching dead animals. Hikers and campers must use an appropriate insecticide on clothing and avoid rodent nests. Any pets accompanying hunters, hikers, or campers should also be sprayed with an appropriate insecticide.

Epidemiology

In 2003 the World Health Organization reported 2,118 cases of plague in nine countries. Of these cases, 182 of the victims died.

Richard Bradley

See also

• Anthrax • Avian influenza • Malaria
• Rabies • Rickettsial infections • West Nile encephalitis

Pleurisy

Pleurisy is an inflammation of the lining of the lungs that causes pain on breathing or coughing. Pleurisy most commonly results from an infection (pneumonia, viruses, or TB), but can also be caused by chest trauma, rheumatic diseases, lung cancer, and other disorders.

The lungs and inner chest wall are lined by a thin, smooth, self-lubricating tissue called pleura. When a person has pleurisy, this lining becomes inflamed and roughened, such that each breath can produce a grating sound called a "friction rub," which can be heard with a stethoscope. Pleurisy is usually caused by lung infections, but other conditions can also cause pleural inflammation. In some cases, the inflammation causes the accumulation of pleural fluid in the potential space between the pleural surfaces just outside the lung.

Symptoms and diagnosis

The main symptom of pleurisy is sudden pain in the chest, made worse with deep breathing, coughing, and chest movement. Pain may be referred to areas away from the site of origin, such as the shoulder, lower chest, neck, or abdomen, which can be confused with intraabdominal disease. If sufficient pleural fluid accumulates, it can compress the underlying lung, causing rapid or difficult breathing.

Pleurisy is easily diagnosed when the characteristic pleuritic pain occurs. A pleural friction rub is diagnostic but may be transient in nature. Chest radiographs are useful to demonstrate pleural fluid. Analysis of the pleural fluid when present is the most helpful diagnostic test in establishing a diagnosis in most cases of pleurisy. This is done using a procedure called thoracentesis, in which a fine needle is inserted into the chest to reach the pleural space and extract fluid.

Treatments

The pain of pleurisy is controlled with acetaminophen, nonsteroidal anti-inflammatory drugs, or occasionally with narcotics, depending on the severity of the pain. Treatment of the underlying cause of pleurisy is essential. Bacterial pneumonia is treated with antibiotics. Viral infections are usually self-limiting and do not require medication other than symptomatic relief.

Alternative treatments can be used along with traditional therapy to heal pleurisy. Acupuncture and botanical medications may alleviate pleuritic pain and breathing problems. Contrast hydrotherapy and homeopathic treatment can also be efffective in relieving the pain.

Pleurisy can be prevented depending upon the cause. Early treatment of pneumonia can prevent the accumulation of fluid (pleural effusion).

Isaac Grate

KEY FACTS

Description
Inflammation of the lining of the lungs that causes roughening of the lining and acute pain with breathing and coughing.

Causes
Pleurisy is caused by a number of conditions, including bacterial and viral infections, tuberculosis, cancer, trauma, certain systemic diseases, and other conditions.

Symptoms
Sudden pain in the chest, made worse with deep breathing, coughing, and chest movements.

Diagnosis
A diagnosis of pleurisy is made when a patient is experiencing the characteristic pleuritic pain, or the pleural friction rub can be heard through a stethoscope, or both. Chest radiographs may show accumulated fluid.

Treatments
Depends on the cause of the pleurisy. Bacterial infections are treated with antibiotics; viral infections are self-limiting and run their course without medications.

Epidemiology
None available.

Risk factors
None known.

Prevention
Early treatment of pneumonia with antibiotics, or treatment of the underlying disease.

See also
- Bronchitis • Cancer, lung
- Legionnaires' disease • Pneumonia
- Rheumatic fever • Tuberculosis

Pneumonia

Pneumonia is a common respiratory illness, affecting millions of people annually. It ranges in severity from mild to serious and can even be fatal, depending upon the type of infecting organism, the victim's age, and underlying health status. People at higher risk for pneumonia include the elderly, smokers, young children, and people with anatomic problems, chronic conditions, or compromised immune systems.

Pneumonia is caused most often by bacteria and viruses and less often by fungi and parasites. Pneumonia may also occur because of various lung injuries or other medical issues. More than one hundred strains of microorganisms can cause pneumonia, yet only a few are responsible for most cases. The smallest airways of the lungs are surrounded by alveoli (air-filled sacs), which are vital to oxygen and carbon dioxide exchange. Destructive, invading microorganisms trigger an immune system response, causing inflammation and interruption in gas exchange. The symptoms of infectious pneumonia are caused by both destructive, invading microorganisms and the immune system's response. Lobar pneumonias involve only a single lobe or lung section; multilobar pneumonias involve more than one lobe and are often more serious.

Bacterial pneumonia

In adults and children over five years of age, bacterial pneumonias are typically the most common and most serious. The term *atypical pneumonia* refers to pneumonia caused by certain bacteria: *Legionella pneumophila*, *Mycoplasma pneumonia*, and *Chlamydophila pneumoniae*. Atypical bacteria and viruses are the most common causes of interstitial pneumonia, which involves the areas between the alveoli (interstitial pneumonitis). The word *atypical* is used because healthier people are commonly affected and the pneumonia is generally less severe and responds to different antibiotics from other bacteria. An exception is *Legionella pneumonia*, which can be severe, with high mortality rates. Although bacteria are typically inhaled, they can also reach the lungs through the bloodstream, if there is an infection elsewhere in the body. Many of the types of bacteria that cause pneumonia can be found in the nose or mouth of healthy people. *Streptococcus pneumoniae* (pneumococcus) is the most common pneumonia-causing bacterium in all age groups except newborn infants and is the most common cause of lobar pneumonia. Another important cause of pneumonia is *Staphylococcus aureus*. Less common bacterial causes include *Hemophilus influenzae* and *Pseudomonas aeruginosa*. Many of the less common causes of bacterial pneumonia live in the gastrointestinal tract and may enter the lungs if vomit is inhaled.

Viral pneumonia

Besides damaging lung tissue, viral pneumonias can affect other organs and disrupt many body functions. Although respiratory syncytial virus (RSV) is the major pathogen in viral pneumonias, these types of pneumonias can also be caused by other viruses, including influenza, parainfluenza, adenovirus, cytomegalovirus (CMV), and herpes simplex virus. Herpes simplex virus is a rare cause of pneumonia, except in newborns. People who have compromised immune systems are at risk for CMV pneumonia. Viral pneumonias are the most common types of pneumonias in children less than five years of age.

Community-acquired pneumonia

Community-acquired pneumonia is infectious pneumonia in a person who has not recently been hospitalized. It is the most common type of pneumonia; its most common causes, which differ by age group, include *S. pneumoniae* (the most common cause worldwide), the atypical bacteria, *H. influenzae*, and viruses. The term *walking pneumonia* has been used to describe a type of community-acquired pneumonia of less severity, usually caused by an atypical bacterium or virus.

Hospital-acquired pneumonia

The more serious hospital-acquired pneumonia (nosocomial pneumonia) is acquired during or after hospitalization for another illness or procedure. Its causes, microbiology, treatment, and prognosis, are different from those of community-acquired pneumonia. Up to 5 percent of patients hospitalized for other causes subsequently develop pneumonia. Many have risk factors for pneumonia, like mechanical ventilation, prolonged malnutrition, underlying heart and lung diseases, decreased amounts of stomach acid, and compromised immune systems. The microorganisms a person is exposed to in a hospital are often different from those at home and they are more dangerous; they include resistant bacteria such as methicillin-resistant *S. aureus* (MRSA) and *P. aeruginosa*.

Aspiration pneumonia

Aspiration pneumonia (aspiration pneumonitis) is caused by inhaling oral or gastric contents while eating or as a result of reflux or vomiting. The resultant lung inflammation can contribute to infection, since the material aspirated may contain anaerobic bacteria. Aspiration is a leading cause of death among hospital and nursing home patients.

KEY FACTS

Description
Infection of human respiratory tract.

Causes
Infection by either bacteria or viruses, less commonly by fungi and parasites. Can also be caused by lung injury.

Risk factors
African Americans, newborns, elderly, people who smoke, and people whose immune system is compromised are at more risk. People who are hospitalized and on mechanical ventilators, those suffering from malnutrition, or those who have underlying heart or lung diseases are also at risk.

Symptoms
Dry or productive cough, fatigue, loss of appetite, chest pain, sore throat, fever, nausea, vomiting, diarrhea, aching muscles and joints.

Diagnosis
Physical examination and chest X-ray. Examination of blood and sputum for microorganisms.

Treatments
Antibiotics and supportive care.

Pathogenesis
Sepsis or septic shock can occur, leading to liver, kidney, brain, and heart damage.

Prevention
Treating underlying illnesses; quitting smoking; vaccination of vulnerable groups.

Epidemiology
In the United States, around 5 million cases occur each year; about 1 million will need hospitalization. Pneumonia is the fifth leading cause of death in people older than 65 in the United States. In 2000 around 8 percent of patient deaths were a result of pneumonia.

Less common pneumonia classifications include fungal pneumonia, which can occur in people with compromised immune systems; parasitic pneumonia, in which parasites typically enter the body through the skin or by swallowing, then travel to the lungs through the blood; and chemical pneumonia, which is caused by chemical toxins that enter the body through inhalation or skin contact. Often, pneumonias are classified as acute (less than three weeks duration) or chronic. Chronic pneumonias tend to be either noninfectious or mycobacterial, fungal, or mixed bacterial (caused by airway obstruction). Acute pneumonias are further divided into classic bacterial pneumonias (*S. pneumoniae*), atypical pneumonias (*M. pneumoniae* or *C. pneumoniae*), and aspiration pneumonias.

Symptoms of pneumonia

The symptoms of pneumonia include cough (dry or productive), chest pain, respiratory distress, and fever. Increased respiratory rate is the most consistent clinical manifestation. Headache, stiff and aching muscles and joints, loss of appetite, fatigue, sore throat, and gastrointestinal complaints (nausea, vomiting, diarrhea, abdominal distention) may also be present. Infectious pneumonias are often preceded for several days by symptoms of an upper respiratory infection. Less common forms of pneumonia can also cause anemia, rashes, and neurological syndromes. In the elderly, pneumonia may manifest itself atypically, with new or worsening confusion or unsteadiness leading to falls. Infants with pneumonia may experience the above symptoms but may also have a decreased appetite and be increasingly sleepy.

Diagnosis

People with suspected pneumonia should undergo a medical evaluation that includes a thorough physical examination and a chest X-ray, since pneumonia shares symptoms with other conditions and can be difficult to diagnose in people with other illnesses.

A physical examination may reveal the above symptoms, as well as low blood pressure, increased heart rate, or low blood oxygen. People with respiratory distress, confusion, or low blood oxygen need immediate medical attention. Listening to the lungs with a stethoscope reveals diminished breath sounds and crackling sounds or wheezing. Feeling the way the chest expands, tapping the chest wall, and palpating for increased chest vibration can also help to identify affected lung areas. Chest X-rays can reveal affected lung areas, confirm the pneumonia diagnosis, and in-

PNEUMONIA

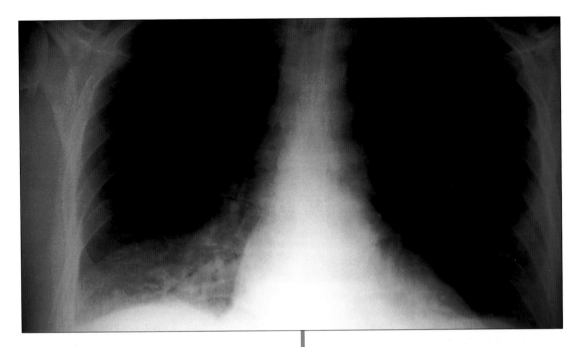

A chest X-ray reveals basal (the base of the lung) pneumonia in the right lung (lower left of image).

dicate certain complications. They are not diagnostic alone and must be considered in combination with other clinical features. By evaluating the location, distribution, and appearance of affected areas, chest X-rays can distinguish between pneumonia types and help predict the course of illness, though they cannot determine the microbiological cause. A chest computed tomography (CT) scan or other tests may be useful.

The diagnostic evaluation and microbiological classification may include a sputum culture, blood tests (blood cultures, a complete blood count, and blood tests for antibodies to specific viruses), bronchoscopy, urine tests, throat swab, and even an open lung biopsy, if the case is particularly serious and the diagnosis evasive. The definitive diagnosis of a bacterial infection requires isolation of an organism from the blood, pleural fluid, or lungs. The sample can then be cultured to look for infection and test for antibiotic sensitivities. Since cultures typically take a few days, they are mainly used to confirm sensitivities to an antibiotic already in use or as an epidemiological tool to define incidence and prevalence. A white blood cell count may be useful in differentiating viral pneumonia from bacterial pneumonia. The definitive diagnosis of a viral infection rests on the isolation of a virus or detection of viral antigens in a sputum sample.

Treatments

Treatment of suspected bacterial pneumonia is based on the presumptive cause and on the patient's clinical appearance. Antibiotics are the mainstay of treatment. Antibiotics are not effective in the treatment of viral pneumonias, though they are often used to prevent or treat the secondary bacterial infections that can occur in lungs damaged by viral pneumonia. The more serious forms of viral pneumonia can be treated with antiviral medications, although these treatments are often beneficial only if started within 48 hours of symptom onset. Supportive care for pneumonia may include treatment for the relief of associated symptoms, increased fluids, incentive spirometry (to show if the airways are narrowed), oxygen supplementation, and chest clearance therapy. Most cases of pneumonia can be resolved within one to three weeks without hospitalization using oral antibiotics, rest, fluids, and home care. However, the elderly and those with respiratory distress or other medical problems may need more intensive treatment. If the pneumonia does not improve, symptoms worsen, or complications occur, hospitalization and intensive care may be needed. Serious infections can result in respiratory failure requiring noninvasive or invasive mechanical ventilation.

The antibiotic choice depends on the nature of the pneumonia, the area's most common pneumonia-causing microorganisms and their sensitivities, and the age and underlying health of the victim. Pneumonia treatment is ideally based on the causative microor-

340

ganism and its antibiotic sensitivities, but specific causes are identified in only 50 percent of cases, even after extensive evaluation.

The duration of treatment is traditionally seven to ten days, but shorter courses may be sufficient. A combination of antibiotics may be administered in an attempt to treat all possible causes.

Complications

Complications of pneumonia are usually the result of the spread of infection within the body. Occasionally, the microorganisms infecting the lungs will cause fluid (effusion) to build up in the pleural cavity (the area between the lungs and chest wall). If the microorganisms themselves are present, the fluid collection is called an empyema. When pleural fluid is present in a person with pneumonia, the fluid can often be collected with a needle and examined. Depending on the examination results, complete drainage of the fluid may be necessary, often requiring a chest tube. In severe cases, surgery may be required because, if the fluid is not drained, the infection may persist, since antibiotics do not penetrate well into the pleural cavity. The treatment for empyema is based on its stage, which can be ascertained by imaging studies.

Sepsis or septic shock most often occurs with bacterial pneumonia when microorganisms enter the bloodstream and the immune system responds. Individuals with sepsis or septic shock need hospitalization and intensive care; intravenous fluids and medications help keep their blood pressure from dropping. Sepsis can cause liver, kidney, brain, and heart damage, among other problems, and often causes death.

Rarely, bacteria in the lung will form a pocket of infected fluid called an abscess that can usually be seen on a chest X-ray or chest CT. They typically occur in aspiration pneumonia and often contain several types of bacteria. Antibiotics are usually adequate to treat a lung abscess, but the abscess may have to be drained.

In the United States, about 1 in 20 people with pneumococcal pneumonia will die. In cases where the pneumonia progresses to a bacterial blood infection, 1 in 5 will die. Pneumonia caused by *M. pneumoniae* is associated with few deaths; however, about half of those who develop MRSA pneumonia while on a ventilator will die. In regions of the world without advanced health care systems, pneumonia is much more deadly. Limited access to health care, X-rays, antibiotics, and the inability to treat underlying conditions contribute to higher death rates. Ultimately, an individual's prognosis depends on the type of pneumonia, symptom severity, appropriate treatment, complications, their age, and underlying health.

Prevention

Appropriately treating underlying illnesses can decrease a person's risk for pneumonia. Smoking cessation is important, not only because it limits lung damage but because cigarette smoke interferes with the body's natural defenses. Testing pregnant women for Group B *Streptococcus* and *Chlamydia trachomatis* and then giving antibiotic treatment, if needed, reduces pneumonia in infants. Suctioning the mouth and throat of infants with meconium-stained amniotic fluid decreases the rate of aspiration pneumonia.

Vaccination of infants against *H. influenzae* type B has led to a dramatic decline in cases. Vaccinations against *H. influenzae* and *S. pneumoniae* in the first year of life have greatly reduced their role in pneumonia in children. Vaccinating children against *S. pneumoniae* has led to a decreased incidence in adults, since many adults acquire infections from children. For adults in the United States, the vaccine against *S. pneumoniae* is currently recommended for all healthy individuals older than sixty-five and any adults with chronic conditions or compromised immune systems. A repeat vaccination may be required. Vaccines against RSV are available for high-risk populations. Influenza vaccines should be given yearly to health care workers, nursing home residents, and pregnant women.

Epidemiology

Pneumonia is a major cause of death among all age groups. In children, the majority of deaths occur in the vulnerable newborn period, with over 2 million deaths each year worldwide (1 in every 3 deaths). Mortality from pneumonia generally decreases with age until late adulthood, though it is a leading cause of death among the elderly and chronically ill. More cases of pneumonia occur during the winter months than at other times of the year; it occurs more commonly in males than females and more often in African Americans than Caucasians. Hospitalized people are at higher risk for pneumonia, and those with chronic health conditions or compromised immune systems are at risk for repeated episodes.

Julie A. McDougal

See also
- Antibiotic-resistant infections
- Cold, common • Influenza

Poliomyelitis

There is evidence suggesting that poliomyelitis existed since ancient times. Although its contagiousness was established in the nineteenth century, the viral etiology of poliomyelitis was confirmed in the early twentieth century. Since the discovery of the virus, tremendous efforts led to a successful vaccine development. Such urgent need was dictated by continued increase of worldwide polio epidemics that peaked in the mid-twentieth century. It was important to prevent an illness that could cause significant disability and death.

In the United States the effort to create an effective vaccine began with the support of President Franklin D. Roosevelt and the establishment in 1938 of the National Foundation for Infantile Paralysis (now the March of Dimes), which supported both scientists conducting research on this disease and patients affected by this illness. Polio has been eradicated from the Western Hemisphere. In the rest of the world, the majority of cases are reported from several countries in Africa and the Indian subcontinent (such as Nigeria, Somalia, Afghanistan, Pakistan, and India). The Global Polio Eradication Initiative was launched in 1988, when poliomyelitis crippled an estimated 1,000 children per day. The initiative aims for global polio eradication in the first decade of the twenty-first century. The initiative uses several strategies involving surveillance of paralytic polio cases, supplemental immunizations on national immunization days, and ensuring universal vaccine coverage with oral poliovirus vaccine (OPV) for children in the first year of life.

Poliomyelitis is caused by serotypes 1, 2, and 3, polioviruses that are members of the enterovirus group. Type 1 poliovirus was responsible for most of the paralytic polio cases in the pre-immunization era. Since the introduction of the first polio vaccine in 1957, the number of cases steeply declined in the developed world; in the United States the last naturally occurring case of poliomyelitis was in 1979. In the rest of the world, the incidence of polio has reduced by 99 percent from 350,000 cases in 1988 to 1,918 cases reported in 2002 as polio vaccines became more widely available.

Pathogenesis

Poliomyelitis is transmitted from human to human through the fecal-oral route via contaminated hands, food, or water. People with subclinical forms of polio can shed the virus with feces for several weeks, thus becoming a source of the infection for others. Incubation period for poliomyelitis is 7 to 14 days

KEY FACTS

Description
Poliomyelitis (or polio) is a highly contagious viral infection that is known to invade the nervous system and cause paralysis.

Causes
By poliovirus, which is a virus that includes 3 distinct groups called serotypes (serotypes 1, 2, and 3).

Risk factors
It is a contagious disease; anyone who has no prior specific immunity (antibodies) is susceptible. Children younger than 5 years are at risk for contracting polio. Male and female genders are equally at risk for the infection.

Symptoms
Polio can present with several different clinical symptoms, including fever, headache, and stiff neck; the most serious one is paralytic polio.

Diagnosis
Diagnosis is made by recovering the virus from the body fluids or by the measurement of specific antibodies against polioviruses.

Treatment
As for many viral illnesses, there is no antiviral medication active against poliovirus.

Pathogenesis
The disease spreads through direct contact with infected body fluids; the virus invades nerve cells.

Prevention
The best way to prevent polio is to maintain specific antibody protection against the virus. This is commonly achieved by vaccination.

Epidemiology
Due to aggressive immunization campaigns and the Global Polio Eradication Initiative led by the World Health Organization, poliomyelitis has been eliminated in most of the world, apart from parts of Asia and several countries in Africa, where there is a high burden of endemic cases.

(range 5 to 35). The virus enters through the nose or mouth into the digestive system, where it multiplies and spreads to the lymphatic system and blood. Polioviruses have a specific preference for invading and destroying nerve cells (neurons) in the brain and spinal cord. The nerve cells regulate the function of various muscles; as a result of the destruction of nerve cells by polioviruses, muscles cannot function.

Symptoms and complications

The spectrum of clinical manifestations of polio ranges from subclinical (unapparent polio) to paralytic polio. In 90 to 95 percent of cases the infection with polioviruses results in subclinical or unapparent polio with minimal or no symptoms. Abortive poliomyelitis, which is another clinical presentation of this infection, has nonspecific features typical for many viral illnesses (fever, headache, sore throat, and abdominal pain) and no evidence of nervous system invasion. Nonparalytic poliomyelitis has typical features of any enteroviral infection, with symptoms such as fever, headache, and meningeal irritation. Both nonparalytic polio and abortive polio typically resolve without any residual complications. Around 0.1 percent of polio infections result in paralytic poliomyelitis distinguished into spinal and bulbar forms. In very rare cases, paralytic polio can evolve in a matter of hours. Spinal paralytic polio originally presents with the same symptoms as abortive polio, followed by a symptom-free interval of several days. Afterward, the fever recurs along with meningeal irritation causing headache, vomiting, and stiff neck, as well as muscle pains. A characteristic feature of paralytic polio is development of asymmetric paralysis with involvement of different muscle groups. Legs are usually more affected than arms. A paralysis or loss of muscle control in polio is described as flaccid (floppy) and can range from the involvement of some muscle groups to the involvement of trunk and both arms and legs (quadriplegia). Involvement of the chest wall muscles and diaphragm results in compromised breathing, which frequently necessitates mechanical support. Additional symptoms include muscle twitching and muscle spasms. The development of paralysis usually stops when the fever resolves. Some factors were found to be associated with a higher chance of paralysis, such as pregnancy, strenuous exercise, tonsillectomy, and intramuscular injection. Up to one-third of paralytic polio cases could evolve into a form called bulbar polio, in which the virus invades the brain stem and involves cranial nerves that control muscles responsible for swallowing and breathing.

Bulbar polio is associated with the highest mortality compared to the other forms of polio. Overall mortality from paralytic polio is 5 to 10 percent and is commonly a result of respiratory suppression.

Encephalitis is a rare and uncommon form of poliomyelitis that presents with confusion, altered consciousness, and seizures.

Subclinical and abortive polio resolve without any sequelae. Up to two-thirds of patients with paralytic polio continue to have residual weakness for the rest of their lives, resulting in disability. Infection with poliovirus results in a serotype-specific antibody development. This is not necessarily protective against infection with other polioviruses.

A condition called postpoliomyelitis syndrome is described in up to 40 percent of survivors of paralytic polio; it develops 20 to 30 years after the original infection. This condition is not well understood, but it is believed that new onset muscle weakness is a result of a premature death of the nerve cells.

Diagnosis and treatments

Polioviruses can be commonly recovered by viral culture from throat secretions or feces, and on some occasions from the cerebrospinal fluid. Virus isolation is important when the differentiation of the wild (found in nature) type virus from the vaccine-associated virus is necessary. Cerebrospinal fluid is often analyzed to check the number of cells and the protein content. A blood test detecting the antibody response to this virus is also available; for confirmation, the blood tests are performed in the acute and recovery phase. The diagnosis of poliomyelitis is confirmed if there is a fourfold increase in two antibody measurements.

There is no specific treatment for poliomyelitis. Treatment is typically aimed toward relief of symptoms. Bed rest is especially important in paralytic illness. In cases in which muscles of respiration are involved, mechanical ventilation is sometimes necessary.

Prevention

The best way to prevent poliomyelitis is vaccination, which induces antibody production and subsequent protection from the infection. Two vaccines have been widely used in the world. The first licensed vaccine was the inactivated poliovirus vaccine (IPV) developed by Jonas Salk. IPV is an injectable vaccine and is given at 2, 4, and 6 to 18 months, and at the age of 4 to 6 years. After improving the vaccine's ability to induce antibody responses, it is now exclusively used in the United States. IPV does not induce local immuni-

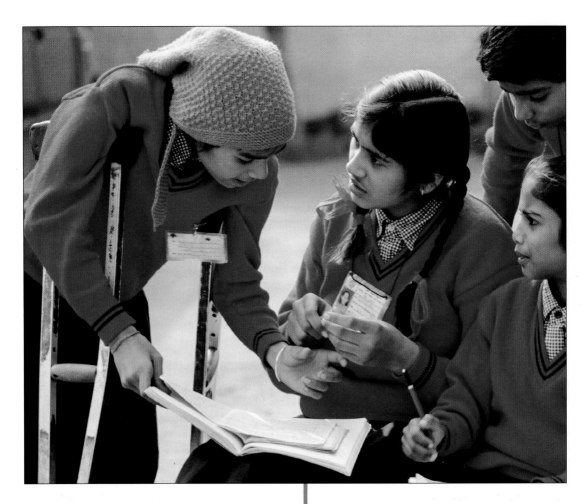

An Indian schoolgirl disabled by polio confers with her classmates. Although a global initiative to eradicate the disease is underway, setbacks in parts of India have been encountered. Overall the number of cases has decreased worldwide.

ty (antibody production) in the gastrointestinal tract; therefore IPV vaccinated individuals could theoretically shed the virus with feces and become a source of the infection.

Another vaccine that was introduced in the 1960s is a live oral poliovirus vaccine (OPV) developed by Albert Sabin. Due to ease of administration and cost effectiveness, it is widely used in most of the developing world. The advantage of this vaccine is development of local antibody response in the gastrointestinal tract and shedding of the vaccine-associated virus in the stool. In this situation the virus could be passively spread to nonimmune individuals and result in the development of protective antibody.

The oral vaccine is given at two, four, and six months of age with a booster dose at the age of four. The use of this vaccine is responsible for a significant worldwide decrease in cases of poliomyelitis. OPV is also available in a monovalent serotype specific formulation (mOPV). As part of the Global Polio Eradication Initiative, mOPV1 is now being increasingly used.

In contrast to the inactivated poliovirus vaccination, on rare occasions OPV is a cause of vaccine-associated paralytic poliomyelitis (VAPP). Around 93 cases of VAPP were reported per 291.4 million doses of vaccine that were distributed in 1969 to 1980 in the United States. The disorder occurs in recipients of the vaccine, in a close family member, or in caregivers. Clinical features of the VAPP are similar to naturally occurring paralytic polio.

Diana Nurutdinova

See also
• Paralysis

Post-traumatic stress disorder

Post-traumatic stress disorder (PTSD) is an anxiety disorder in which psychological and physiological symptoms follow an exposure or confrontation with life-threatening traumatic experiences. These may be military combat, hostage situations, rape, torture, or natural and man-made disasters. The intensity of this trauma relates to the severity of symptoms of PTSD. PTSD patients can be effectively treated with different pharmacological agents and psychotherapy.

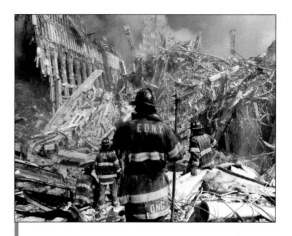

Firefighters clear debris after the devastation of the twin towers tragedy in 2001 in New York. Many people, including rescue workers, suffered from PTSD following the attack.

PTSD is a psychiatric disorder that historically has been studied in the context of combat experience. However, it has been recognized that other types of trauma, such as child abuse, torture, hostage situations, or violent crimes can also be associated with the development of PTSD. *The Diagnostic and Statistical Manual of Mental Disorders,* fourth edition (DSM-IV), specifies that a life-threatening traumatic event must be witnessed or experienced by the individual, and the response to this event must involve intense fear or horror. Based on currently available data, it is evident that the proximity to and the intensity of the traumatic event are related to the probability of developing the disorder and the severity of its symptoms.

Causes and risk factors

The development of PTSD reflects an interaction of constitutional and environmental factors. Research indicates that a smaller hippocampus, a part of the brain that is actively involved in the processes of fear and memory, may be associated in PTSD patients with specific risk and resilience factors. Experiencing a traumatic event increases plasma and brain concentrations of corticosteroids and neuroactive steroids, which increases responsiveness to glucocorticoids or other neuroendocrine measures, or both, that have been observed in combat-related PTSD. It has been also shown that a person's coping strategies could play a critical role in the development of the disorder. Specifically, avoidant coping strategies have been associated with greater PTSD symptoms, while more problem-focused cognitive style applied to reinterpretation and adaptation to the traumatic experience has been associated with fewer symptoms.

A growing body of evidence indicates that individuals who have a history of childhood trauma are more likely to develop PTSD later in life. The severity and duration of this initial traumatic experience are associated with increased severity of PTSD symptoms later in life. Also, a history of depression in first-degree relatives increases someone's vulnerability to PTSD.

Diagnosis and symptoms

In PTSD, people primarily develop three domains of symptoms: reexperiencing the traumatic event, avoiding stimuli associated with the trauma, and experiencing an increase in autonomic arousal. Symptoms of reexperiencing the trauma include recurrent and intrusive recollections of events, distressing dreams, acting or feeling as if the traumatic events are recurring, and physiological and psychological distress following exposure to the internal or external cues related to the trauma. Symptoms of avoidance include an effort to avoid recurrent thoughts or activities associated with the trauma, inability to recall an important aspect of the traumatic event, decreased interest and participation in significant activities, feelings of being numb or detached from reality, restricted affect, and a sense of a foreshortened future. Symptoms of increased arousal include irritability, insomnia, hypervigilance, difficulty concentrating, and enhanced startle response. The diagnosis of PTSD is only made when symptoms persist for at least one month. According to the DSM-IV, there are three subtypes of PTSD, based on the time course. Acute PTSD refers to an episode that lasts less than three months. Chronic PTSD refers to an episode lasting three months or longer. Delayed-onset PTSD refers to an episode that develops six months or more after exposure to the trauma.

Treatments

Pharmacotherapy is effective in the treatment of PTSD, acting to reduce its core symptoms and commonly associated symptoms of depression. Selective serotonin reuptake inhibitors, or SSRIs (citalopram, escitalopram, fluvoxatine, fluvoxetine, paroxetine, and sertraline), along with venlafaxine, a serotonin-norepinephrine reuptake inhibitor, have become first-line treatments of PTSD based on their overall efficacy and tolerability. Sexual dysfunction, weight gain, and sleep disturbance are common adverse effects associated with SSRI treatment. In the case of PTSD, benzodiazepines, such as alprazolam, diazepam, and clonazepam, have been also shown to be effective, well tolerated, and safe, in the absence of comorbid substance- and alcohol-abuse disorders. However, in the long term, antidepressants may may help target depressive symptoms. In addition, discontinuing long-term therapy with benzodiazepines can be difficult because, in some patients, anxiety symptoms could be exacerbated. Side effects of benzodiazepines include general sedation, slurred speech, memory impairment, and ataxia.

There is a growing body of data that indicates that a course of propranolol started shortly after an acute traumatic event helps reduce PTSD symptoms one month later. However, larger studies are needed for propranolol. Psychotherapeutic interventions include supportive techniques, cognitive-behavioral therapy, psychodynamic therapy, and group therapy. The most common therapeutic targets include dealing with intense emotional content, recovering a sense of self, new coping strategies, and reestablishing connections with the outside world. A combination of psychotherapy and medications is the most effective therapeutic option for PTSD.

Prevention

Individuals whose professional responsibilities expose them to possibilities of experiencing or witnessing traumatic events may benefit from additional education about the signs and features of PTSD. Treatment such as a critical incident stress debriefing is a proven therapeutic modality intended to prevent the development of full-blown PTSD following trauma. In addition, administration of propranolol shortly after traumatic exposure may be useful to mitigate PTSD symptoms or perhaps even prevent its development.

Epidemiology

In the United States, lifetime prevalence of PTSD in the adult community population is around 8 percent. However, in specific populations, such as military personnel, firefighters, police officers, search-and-rescue personnel, refugees, and victims of natural and man-made disasters, prevalence of PTSD is higher.

Oleg Tcheremissine and Lori Lieving

KEY FACTS

Description
An anxiety disorder with psychological and physiological symptoms after experiencing or witnessing a life-threatening trauma.

Causes
Changes in neural system in response to a life-threatening traumatic event.

Risk factors
Childhood trauma and family history of depression.

Symptoms
Reexperiencing the trauma; avoiding emotional experiences related to the trauma; sleep disturbances, and feeling increased arousal.

Diagnosis
If the symptoms last at least one month.

Treatments
Antidepressants, anxiolytics, adrenergic agents, and psychotherapy.

Pathogenesis
PTSD can occur at any age, including childhood.

Prevention
Educating people whose professions expose them to traumatic experiences.

Epidemiology
The lifetime prevalence among adults in the United States is around 8 percent. Women are twice as likely as men to be diagnosed with PTSD; in specific populations of patients, these figures are higher.

See also
• Anxiety disorders • Depressive disorders

Prostate disorders

Several disorders may affect the prostate, including benign prostatic hyperplasia (enlarged prostate), prostatitis (inflammation of prostate), and prostate cancer.

The prostate is part of the male reproductive system. It is a walnut-sized gland that produces fluid that mixes with sperm to form semen. The prostate lies below the bladder and surrounds the upper part of the urethra, the tube that carries urine from the bladder through the penis to the exterior. Because of this proximity to the urinary system, prostate disorders often affect urination.

Benign prostatic hyperplasia

Benign prostatic hyperplasia (BPH) is a noncancerous enlargement of the prostate gland. Because the prostate continues to grow during a man's lifetime, BPH becomes increasingly common with older age, affecting around half of men aged 50 years and 90 percent of men aged 80 years. BPH is not linked to prostate cancer. Other terms for BPH include benign prostatic hypertrophy, lower urinary tract symptoms (LUTS), prostatism, or bladder outflow obstruction.

Causes and risk factors

The precise cause of BPH is not known. Some studies suggest that BPH is associated with hormones that regulate prostate growth, such as testosterone, estrogen, and dihydrotestosterone. Other evidence suggests BPH is linked with aging and the testes, since the disorder is more common in older men and does not develop in men whose testes were removed before puberty. The major risk factors for BPH are older age and a family history of BPH.

Symptoms, signs, and diagnosis

As the prostate enlarges, it compresses the urethra, obstructing the passage of urine; the bladder cannot produce enough force to empty itself, hence urine is left in the bladder. The symptoms of BPH vary from person to person and do not necessarily indicate the size of the prostate or the severity of disease. It is also possible to have BPH without suffering any symptoms.

Common symptoms include difficulty or pain when passing urine, frequent or urgent need to urinate (especially at night), a weak stream of urine, inability to

KEY FACTS: BPH

Description

Benign prostatic hyperplasia (BPH) is a non-cancerous enlargement of the prostate gland. The prostate gland is part of the male reproductive system and produces fluid that mixes with sperm during ejaculation.

Causes

The cause of BPH is not known. Contributing factors are likely to include advancing age and male hormones. Prostate enlargement is a normal part of aging, and most men have enlarged prostates by the age of 80 years.

Risk factors

The main risk factors for BPH are older age and a family history of the disorder. The only men not at risk of developing BPH are those whose testes were removed before puberty.

Symptoms

BPH puts pressure on the urethra, causing problems with urination. Common symptoms are pain or difficulty urinating; a frequent or urgent need to urinate, or both; difficulty starting to urinate; a weak urine stream; leaking or dribbling; and feeling that the bladder is still full despite urinating.

Diagnosis

BPH is diagnosed from symptoms, examination of the prostate, and the results of blood, urine, and imaging tests. The symptoms of BPH are similar to other prostate disorders, so tests may be done to exclude prostatitis and prostate cancer.

Treatments

Some cases improve without treatment. Mild BPH may simply require regular monitoring. Severe or persistent BPH is treated with drugs or surgery to remove excess prostatic tissue that is compressing the urethra, or shrink the prostate.

Pathogenesis

Without treatment, symptoms may improve, stay the same, or increase in frequency or severity, or both. BPH may also recur after successful treatment. Long-standing BPH can cause serious complications, such as inability to urinate, urinary tract infections, and kidney damage.

Prevention

BPH cannot be prevented.

Epidemiology

BPH becomes more common after the age of 40 and affects most men after 80, although not all will have symptoms. After adjusting for age, there is very little geographic or racial variation in the prevalence of BPH around the world.

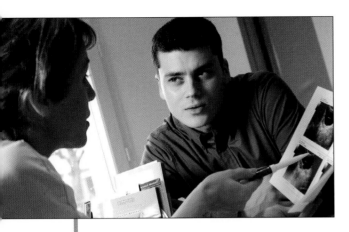

A consultant discusses the findings on a prostate ultrasound scan with a patient. Ultrasound scanning may be done to confirm that there is prostate enlargement.

begin urinating, leaking or dribbling, and the feeling of incomplete bladder emptying.

BPH is diagnosed on the basis of symptoms and investigations. The main test is a digital rectal examination (DRE), during which the doctor inserts a gloved and lubricated finger into the rectum to feel the size and condition of the prostate. A blood test called prostate-specific antigen (PSA) may be performed to help rule out prostate cancer, which has similar symptoms to BPH. Other tests include analysis of urine samples for glucose, blood, or signs of infection; urinary flow studies to measure the strength and volume of urine flow; imaging tests or cystoscopy to view the prostate; and urodynamic studies to determine bladder function.

Treatments and prevention

Many cases of BPH do not require treatment. If the prostate is only slightly enlarged or the symptoms are mild, the patient may simply be monitored with regular checkups. This is known as "watchful waiting."

For more severe or persistent symptoms, several treatments are used. Drugs can help relax the muscles around the prostate or shrink the prostate gland itself; ultrasound waves, microwaves, or radiofrequency energy may be used to destroy excess prostate tissue; or part of the prostate may be removed surgically. Surgery for BPH is usually performed via the urethra so that no external incision is needed. At present there is no way of preventing BPH.

Prostatitis

Prostatitis means inflammation of the prostate gland. It is the most common prostate disorder in men under 50 years of age. There are different types of prostatitis. It may develop suddenly (acute prostatitis) or gradually (chronic prostatitis) and may be caused by infection (bacterial prostatitis) or have no known cause (nonbacterial prostatitis). Other terms for prostatitis include *prostatodynia* and *pelvic pain syndrome*.

Bacterial prostatitis is an infection of the prostate gland caused by bacteria spreading from the urethra, bladder, large intestine, or other part of the body. Nonbacterial prostatitis is not due to bacteria, but the precise cause is unknown. Potential causes include other infectious agents, structural abnormalities of the urinary tract, or pelvic muscle spasm.

Risk factors for prostatitis include urinary tract infection, a urinary catheter, rectal or perineal injury, structural abnormalities of the urinary tract, and occupations or activities that subject the prostate to vibration.

In acute prostatitis the symptoms typically arise suddenly and are severe, whereas chronic prostatitis may be asymptomatic or cause symptoms that are mild or variable in severity.

All forms of prostatitis can cause problems with urination similar to those for BPH. Additionally, prostatitis can cause symptoms of infection, such as fever, chills, nausea, and vomiting; pain in the lower back, pelvis, and genital area; pain when urinating; blood in the urine; pain with ejaculation; painful bowel movements; and blood in the semen or urine.

Prostatitis is diagnosed based on symptoms, physical examination (often including DRE), and analysis of urine for bacteria and white blood cells. Samples of prostatic fluid and semen may also be tested for bacteria.

Treatments and prevention of prostatitis

Bacterial prostatitis is treated with antibiotics, sometimes with muscle-relaxant, analgesic, and anti-inflammatory drugs. If treatment is not successful, part of the prostate may be removed surgically via the urethra. Nonbacterial prostatitis may also be treated with antibiotics. Other treatments include exercises, relaxation techniques, and lifestyle changes to relieve symptoms. Some cases of prostatitis can be prevented by avoiding infection of the urinary and reproductive tracts.

Joanna Lyford

See also
• Cancer, bladder • Cancer, prostate

Psoriasis

Psoriasis is a chronic inflammatory disease that results from a genetic predisposition to the disease and from environmental factors. The genetic basis is evident because it is seen more often in some families and there is a high rate of concordance among twins. Triggering factors include skin trauma, infection, psychological stress, certain medications, alcohol consumption, and pregnancy. Patients with a family history of psoriasis are at increased risk for developing the disease.

Psoriasis is typically diagnosed by its characteristic clinical appearance. Classically patients develop sharply demarcated red plaques (raised plateaulike lesions) with silvery white scale distributed about the scalp, trunk, and limbs, with a predilection for extensor surfaces such as the elbows and knees.

The second most common form of psoriasis is called guttate psoriasis and is typified by red droplike lesions that classically appear on younger patients after streptococcal sore throat.

Other forms include pustular (small blisters containing sterile pus on a red base) and erythrodermic (redness of more than 90 percent of the body surface area due to persistent and severe inflammation). Psoriasis frequently affects the nails, causing small pits, discoloration, and lifting of the nail plate. Of particular importance, up to one-third of patients with psoriasis can have an associated arthritis called psoriatic arthritis.

Treatments and prevention

There are many topical and systemic therapies for psoriasis. Management of this chronic disease requires recognizing the extent of the disease, as well as the possible side effects of treatment. In general, limited skin disease can be managed with topical corticosteroids in combination with other steroid-free agents such as vitamin D_3 analogues, retinoids (vitamin A–type molecules), salicylic acid, and coal tar.

More widespread disease may be treated by exposure to ultraviolet light (phototherapy), without additional medications (psoralens) to increase light sensitivity. Additional therapies include oral vitamin A–type drugs (retinoids), chemotherapy agents such as methotrexate, or immunosuppressive agents such as cyclosporine. A group of medications known as biologics has become available for the treatment of extensive psoriasis. Biologics are proteins produced by molecular biology techniques and include antibodies that bind molecules involved in causing psoriasis. Often topical therapies are combined with light therapy or nontopical medications for adequate relief. There are no known preventive measures at this time.

Adam Korzenko
and Richard Kalish

KEY FACTS

Description

Psoriasis is a chronic inflammatory disease of the skin.

Causes

Both genetic and environmental factors contribute to psoriasis.

Risk factors

The most important risk factor is a family history of psoriasis.

Symptoms

Red patches and plaques with silvery white scale over extensor surfaces. Psoriasis may also affect scalp, nails, palms and soles, and joints.

Diagnosis

Clinical grounds and skin biopsy.

Treatment

Topical corticosteroids, vitamin D_3 analogues, coal tar, salicylic acid, topical and oral retinoids, phototherapy without additional psoralens, methotrexate, cyclosporine, and biologics.

Pathogenesis

The exact mechanism remains unclear. Several lines of evidence suggest that psoriasis is an autoimmune disease mediated by T-lymphocytes.

Prevention

There are no known preventive measures at this time.

Epidemiology

The prevalence of psoriasis has been estimated at 2 percent of the world's population. There is a bimodal incidence with peaks at 20 to 30 years and 50 to 60 years. Psoriasis affects males and females equally.

See also
• Arthritis

Psychotic disorders

Psychosis is a general term that refers to distortions or alteration in a person's thoughts or perceptions. The person loses touch with reality and has frightening thoughts, for example that someone is trying to kill him or her. The person's thoughts and perceptions have changed or distorted. This is one of many examples of the symptoms that may be experienced by someone with a psychotic disorder.

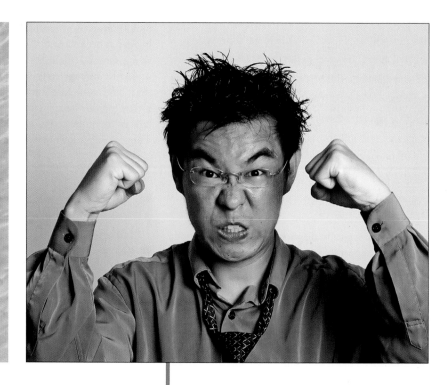

Auditory hallucinations, in which the individual hears one or two voices talking, can be distressing for the person involved. Usually, but not in every case, these voices make very negative comments about the person.

Everyone continually takes in information from their environment, information that is received through the senses, including visual (sight), auditory (sound), gustatory (taste), olfactory (smell), and tactile (touch). Each of these five important sensory functions, functions that are taken for granted each day, become distorted in psychosis and result in people viewing things or people around them that are not present. Individuals with psychosis may also experience delusions, which are fixed beliefs that are not based in reality, or they have difficulties in organizing or generating their thoughts.

Psychotic disorders are illnesses in which psychosis is the primary symptom. It is important to keep in mind that many disorders, including nonpsychiatric medical illnesses, may have psychosis as a symptom. For example, individuals with epilepsy, brain tumors, or those who have suffered a severe head injury may develop psychosis.

Another common cause of psychosis is drugs of abuse, such as amphetamines, PCP, or cocaine. In addition, drugs such as LSD are in a class of drugs called hallucinogens, which bring about changes in beliefs and perceptions. Although these drugs of abuse can induce psychosis, drug abuse and dependence are not considered psychotic disorders. Psychotic disorders include several psychiatric illnesses that are associated with psychosis (see box, page 352). Since how people perceive the world around them is essential to ground them in reality, it can easily be seen how psychotic disorders, which alter the perception of reality, can be such devastating illnesses.

Causes

More is known about the cause of psychosis than the cause of psychotic disorders. The symptom of psychosis is nonspecific, being present not only in psychotic disorders but also in a number of nonpsychiatric medical disorders and substance abuse disorders.

Psychosis is a symptom, whereas psychotic disorders are illnesses. The development of psychosis appears to be related to an overabundance of the neurochemical dopamine. Drugs that increase dopamine, such as amphetamines or cocaine, or medications used to treat Parkinson's disease, can result in psychosis.

Both genetic and environmental factors are associated with psychotic disorders. For example, if an identical twin develops schizophrenia, the other twin has a 50 percent chance of also developing the illness. This decreases to a 15 percent chance in fraternal twins. Since identical twins have identical genes, but fraternal twins, like siblings, share only 50 percent of their genes, genetic factors play a large role in the development of schizophrenia. However, 50 percent of identical twins who have a co-twin with schizophrenia do not develop the illness.

Thus it can be reasoned that environmental factors also play a role in the development of schizophrenia, as well as the other psychotic disorders.

Environmental factors

There have been numerous environmental factors that have been implicated in psychotic disorders. Many of the factors that have been investigated include events that occur very early in life, such as an infection during pregnancy or complications during birth. The current thinking about the cause of psychotic disorders is that there are individuals born who are genetically predisposed toward illness but only develop the illness in the context of specific environmental stressors.

Symptoms

Psychotic disorders have psychosis as their common feature. Psychosis can come in a number of different forms, but the characteristic features include hallucinations, delusions, or disordered thought. Auditory hallucinations are the most common type of hallucination and can vary from indistinct noises (for example, mumblings, people shouting in the distance, or the wind blowing) to one or more distinct voices. The voices most often make negative and degrading comments about or directed toward the person, and at times two voices may converse among themselves. Command hallucinations, or voices that make demands, are not uncommon and are often very upsetting. Not all auditory hallucinations are negative, and some individuals have voices telling them that they are wonderful, gifted, or that they have special powers or abilities.

Visual hallucinations have similar characteristics. They can be either nondescript (for example, flashing lights or moving shapes) or apparent real images of faces, animals, or monsters. Visual hallucinations are more common in children and become less common in later adolescence and adulthood. Feeling insects crawling on the skin is a common tactile hallucination, and olfactory hallucinations are typically foul smelling. Gustatory hallucinations, or hallucinations of taste, are rare in individuals with psychotic disorders.

Delusions are false beliefs that remain fixed despite being far-fetched or having considerable evidence to the contrary. Delusions can only be understood within their cultural and ethnic context. Thus certain religious or ethnic beliefs, although they may appear odd to those outside that culture, would not be considered delusions.

Interestingly, individuals within the cultural or ethnic group are often able to readily identify delusional beliefs when someone within that same group deviates from the cultural norms. Psychosis is a worldwide phenomonen that crosses all ethnic and religious

KEY FACTS

Description

Psychotic disorders are those disorders that are associated with psychosis, or an alteration of a person's thoughts and perceptions.

Causes

Although the underlying cause of psychotic disorders are as yet unknown, there are both genetic and environmental factors associated with these illnesses.

Symptoms

An alteration in someone's thoughts and perceptions, causing hallucinations, delusions, and disorders of thought and speech.

Diagnosis

The diagnosis of the psychotic disorder will require a thorough history, physical and neurological examination, laboratory studies, and often imaging studies of the brain.

Treatments

The treatment of psychotic disorders often includes antipsychotic medications. Supportive or cognitive behavioral therapy is also important.

Pathogenesis

Psychotic symptoms are related to the brain chemical known as dopamine.

Prevention

Little is known about the prevention of psychotic disorders, although there is emerging evidence that avoiding marijuana will reduce the chance of developing schizophrenia.

Epidemiology

Rare during childhood, and the primary age of onset is late adolescence and early adulthood. Males tend to present with symptoms earlier than females.

lines and can be found equally on all continents. Delusions can be divided into those that are false but yet fall within the realm of possibility (for example, "the government is plotting to kill me"), and those that are unrealistic ("the government has implanted chips in the brains of everyone at birth so that they can know and manipulate our thoughts").

The most common types of delusions that people have are paranoid delusions, such as the feeling that others want to cause harm. Other types of delusions include grandiose delusions (having special powers or abilities), somatic delusions (feeling that the body has some disease or illness), or religious delusions (having a special relationship with God that others do not have). Most individuals who suffer with delusions do not have insight into the possibility that their belief system is distorted. Thus, their actions will reflect their beliefs. For instance, an individual who fears that his food is poisoned may avoid eating certain types of food. Although delusions can alter one's beliefs, most individuals with psychosis are not aggressive.

An additional symptom that may or may not be present in individuals with a psychotic disorder is called a formal thought disorder. This refers to the disruption in the flow or processing of a person's thoughts and becomes apparent during normal conversation. The severity of the thought disorder can be quite variable, ranging from rather mild disruptions in thought, such as a long latency between asking a question and obtaining a response, to a complete lack of communication or speaking gibberish ("word salad").

Additional symptoms of a thought disorder include moving rapidly between one topic and another (flight of ideas), rapid or pressured speech, creating new words (neologisms), or suddenly switching to a completely unrelated topic during conversation (tangentiality).

Diagnosis

When individuals develop obvious symptoms of psychosis, it is first very important for physicians to correctly determine if there is an underlying medical or substance use disorder.

Psychosis can have many causes, and the treatments differ, depending on the diagnosis. In order to obtain an accurate diagnosis, the physician will perform a thorough history and physical examination, laboratory tests, and often brain imaging studies. Although nonpsychiatric medical illnesses that cause psychosis are quite rare, they will only worsen if not identified and treated.

In addition, psychiatric disorders such as bipolar disorder, major depressive disorder, substance abuse, post-traumatic stress disorder, or borderline personality disorder may have psychosis as a secondary symptom. Substance abuse is one of the most common causes of psychosis and can be identified either through the history or by laboratory studies.

Once it is determined that the psychosis is a part of a psychotic disorder, there are differences between the psychotic disorders (see box, below) that help solidify the diagnosis.

PSYCHOTIC DISORDERS

Brief psychotic disorder is a condition in which the psychotic symptoms develop suddenly, usually within a day or two. The psychosis may follow some tragic event or a period of considerable stress and disappear as quickly as it came. The psychosis must come and go within a month for it to be considered a brief psychotic disorder.

Schizophrenia is a devastating illness that affects approximately 0.5 to 1 percent of the world's population. Along with psychotic symptoms, schizophrenia is also associated with a lack of motivation, withdrawal from social interactions, a flattening of facial expressions, and greater difficulties performing cognitive tasks.

Schizoaffective disorder is similar to schizophrenia and is a hybrid of schizophrenia and a mood disorder. It is defined by the presence of both psychosis and a mood disorder in the same individual, but at different times.

Schizophreniform disorder is similar to schizophrenia, except that the symptoms are present for less than six months.

Delusional disorder is a condition in which an individual experiences only nonbizarre delusions, without hallucinations or a thought disorder.

Shared psychotic disorder is an illness in which delusional beliefs are transferred to another. It usually involves two family members or a married couple. The person who first develops the delusion is typically more dominant; the person who adopts the delusions tends to be more suggestible.

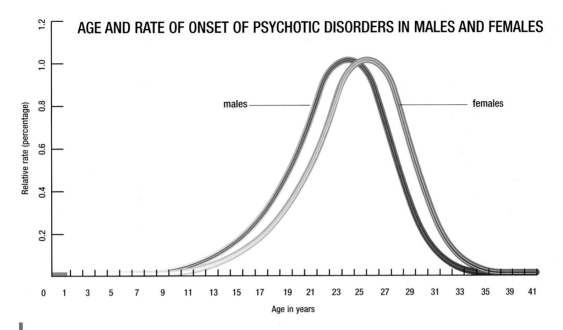

AGE AND RATE OF ONSET OF PSYCHOTIC DISORDERS IN MALES AND FEMALES

The graph shows that the incidence of psychotic disorders peaks between age twenty and thirty.

Treatments

The treatment will be dependent on the diagnosis. Psychotic symptoms that are a result of nonpsychiatric medical disorders should resolve when the medical illness is treated. For psychotic disorders, the mainstay of treatment is an antipsychotic medication. Antipsychotic medications were first used during the 1950s and dramatically altered the lives of many individuals with psychotic disorders.

Since the 1980s, newer medications have been developed with fewer side effects. These antipsychotic medications are also used for psychosis in the presence of mood disorders. Treatment of shared psychotic disorder requires the separation of the two or more individuals who adhere to the delusion. This may result in rapid improvement in the individual who adopted the delusion.

Cognitive behavioral therapy

There is emerging evidence that people with a psychotic disorder may benefit from a specific type of therapy called cognitive behavioral therapy (CBT). The goal of CBT is to assist patients to recognize when they are experiencing hallucinations and delusions and to help them learn that it is a part of their illness. The support and encouragement of parents and friends is also very important to help a person suffering from a psychotic disorder.

Pathogenesis

Long-term treatment is usually needed, and recurrence is likely. Individual outcomes vary but seem worse if the person is young when the disorder begins.

Prevention

There is emerging evidence that individuals who are genetically predisposed to develop a psychotic disorder increase their risk with the use of marijuana during early and middle adolescence. Being familiar with the symptoms of psychosis may promote early identification and treatment.

Epidemiology

The most common age to develop psychotic disorders is during late adolescence and early adulthood. Psychotic disorders are rare during childhood. Males tend to have an earlier age of onset than females, although the rates are equal in delusional disorders.

Finally, it is important to note that upward of 15 percent of children and adolescents may experience mild hallucinations, such as hearing their name called. These events are considered to be normal developmental events and are not psychosis.

Tonya White

See also
- Anxiety disorders • Bipolar disorder
- Depressive disorders • Mood disorders
- Personality disorders • Schizophrenia

Rabies

Rabies is a life-threatening viral disease that mainly involves the central nervous system. The illness is usually transmitted to humans from the bite of a rabid animal. Rabies is a rare but feared disease that has been documented in every country except Australia and Antarctica and in all U.S. states except Hawaii.

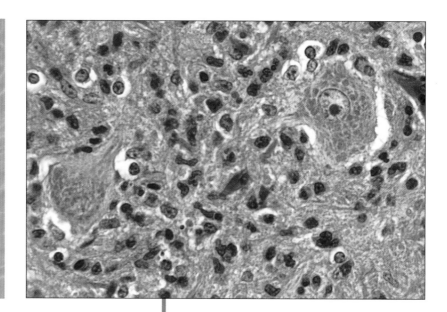

This magnified and colored microscopic image of cerebellar tissue from someone who died of rabies shows characteristic negri bodies, which are found in the brain in cases of rabies. The negri bodies are the dark round structures with basophilic granules at the center.

Rabies can be contracted through contact with animals infected with rabies virus or by contact with the virus in a research laboratory. Rabid animals usually spread the illness to humans through a bite wound. In some cases, the bite goes unnoticed, particularly instances involving bat bites. It is thought that such bite injuries can go undetected because of the small teeth of a bat. There is a possibility of aerosol transmission of the virus from bats to humans.

Nonbite transmission can occur through scratches made by a rabid animal, by the animal licking over an open wound or mucous membrane, or by exposure to brain fluid or tissue that is infected with the rabies virus. Rabies is not transmitted by simply petting a rabid animal or by contact with blood, urine, or feces of a rabid animal; nor is it transmitted from person to person. In a few cases, rabies has been transmitted by corneal transplantation.

The type of rabies virus (varies by species), the body site where the virus enters, and the dose of virus introduced at the entry site are all factors in risk of infection and progression of illness. The immune status of the host also plays a role.

Animal control and vaccination programs account for the low rates of rabies in the United States compared to developing countries. Most animal rabies cases in the United States are identified in raccoons, skunks, foxes, and bats. Except for the woodchuck, rodents and lagomorphs (hares) usually do not transmit rabies.

Symptoms and signs

Rabies starts out as a nonspecific, flulike illness. Symptoms usually begin within 20 to 90 days after exposure to the virus, but can occur within only a few days or up to one year or more after this exposure. Fever, headache, and malaise are common symptoms. Pain, numbness, and tingling may occur at the injury site. As the illness progresses, the person develops changes in behavior, hallucinations, and agitation. Difficulty in swallowing develops from neurological dysfunction, leading to fear of water. Excessive salivation, convulsions, cardiac arrhythmias, respiratory failure, and death usually follow. In almost all cases, once classic symptoms appear, death results.

Diagnosis

Early symptoms of rabies are nonspecific and difficult to distinguish from common, benign illnesses, making diagnosis difficult and often untimely. In animals, diagnosis of rabies is made by examining postmortem brain tissue. In humans, multiple specimen sources are examined, including serum and spinal fluid for antibody to the virus. The virus may be grown in culture in a laboratory. Saliva specimens may be analyzed for the presence of rabies viral genetic material.

Treatments

There is no effective treatment once symptoms appear. Wounds inflicted by a potentially rabid animal should be washed with soap and water. Immediate medical attention should be sought. The geographical location of the incident, the animal involved and its vaccination status, and whether or not provocation was involved is important. Capture of the animal and testing of postmortem tissue, or, in the case of a domesticated animal that has documented up-to-date rabies vaccine status, confinement and observation for a specified period of time are needed. In the latter case, the animal is watched for any signs of rabies.

For potential exposures to rabies, immune globulin and five doses of rabies vaccine are administered. This is referred to as post-exposure prophylaxis. Immune globulin provides antibody to the virus and is administered around the site of the wound. The vaccine induces the body to produce antibody to rabies virus, a situation that takes some time. The vaccine is administered in the upper arm and is given over a period of 4 weeks.

Pre-exposure prophylaxis, used by those at high risk of exposures, such as veterinarians, field biologists, and laboratory personnel working with rabies virus, involves the administration of three doses of rabies vaccine given over three to four weeks. The recipient's antibody levels are monitored periodically, with boosters administered as needed to maintain adequate antirabies antibody levels in the blood.

Pathogenesis

Once rabies virus enters the body through a bite or mucous membrane contact, the virus multiplies in the muscle cells. No symptoms appear during this time. The virus spreads along nerves, traveling to the spinal cord. At this time, the person may have numbness, tingling, and discomfort along the path of the nerve. The virus eventually infects the central nervous system. Since salivary glands are supplied with a dense amount of nerve tissue, excessive salivation may be seen. Inflammation of the brain, or encephalitis, and cardiopulmonary failure follow. Death usually occurs within one week after the onset of signs and symptoms.

Prevention and epidemiology

No vaccine is available. Every year, about 40,000 people in the United States receive rabies pre-exposure

prophylaxis and about 18,000 people receive post-exposure prophylaxis. The best way to avoid rabies is to avoid contact with wild animals and with unknown animals. Those who are planning travel to a country where rabies is a problem should visit their physician in the event that rabies pre-exposure prophylaxis is required. Pet owners should keep their pets' vaccines up to date. Any openings in the home through which animals could enter should be sealed. If someone is bitten or exposed to an animal that could potentially be infected with rabies, immediate medical attention should be sought.

Rita Washko

KEY FACTS

Description
Viral infectious disease of mammals.

Cause
Rabies virus.

Risk factors
Contact with animals infected with the virus, or with rabies virus in a laboratory setting.

Symptoms
Nonspecific, flulike initially, then hallucinations, excessive salivation, convulsions, and death.

Diagnosis
In animals, postmortem brain tissue is examined for presence of the virus. In humans, blood and cerebrospinal fluid are examined.

Treatments
Rabies vaccine for those at risk of exposure to rabies; vaccine plus immunoglobulin (preformed antibodies) for someone exposed to rabies.

Pathogenesis
The virus enters at the site of injury, or perhaps via mucous membrane inoculation, and travels to the central nervous system. Inflammation of the brain and death usually follow.

Prevention
Avoid contact with unknown or wild animals, keep pets' vaccines up to date. Seek immediate medical attention for exposures to potentially rabid animals.

Epidemiology
In the United States, rabies causes only 1–2 deaths yearly; worldwide, the virus causes more than 35,000 human deaths every year.

See also
• Arrhythmia

Radiation sickness

Radiation sickness, also known as acute radiation syndrome (ARS), is caused by exposure to an excessive amount of radiation. The exposure may be in a series of doses over time (chronic) or in a single large dose (acute). The larger the dose, the greater the risk of developing radiation sickness. The effects are felt first in each cell. With very high doses of radiation, many cells are affected, and the tissues cease to function. Eventually the body is unable to repair itself, and if the damage is great enough, the person will die.

Radiation is the process of emitting energy in the form of waves or particles. There are various types of radiation, which are distinguished according to their properties of emitted energy and matter. Radiation occurs naturally in the environment, so everyone is exposed to some daily radiation without harmful consequences. For example, routine cases of exposure to artificial radiation are living near a nuclear power plant or undergoing a medical test, such as an X-ray. This kind of radiation occurs in amounts too small to cause any damage.

Radiation is normally classified into ionizing and nonionizing types. Nonionizing radiation comes in the form of light, radio waves, microwaves and radar, which are relatively harmless. These types of radiation generally do not cause tissue damage. On the other hand, ionizing radiation is radiation that produces immediate chemical effects (ionization) on human tissue. X-rays, gamma rays, and particle bombardment (neutron beam, electron beam, protons, and mesons) emit ionizing radiation. This type of radiation is used for medical testing and treatment, industrial testing, manufacturing, sterilization, weapons and weapons development, and many other uses.

Too much exposure to excessive ionizing radiation can cause serious health problems. Any living tissue in the human body can be damaged by radiation, but some body parts are more sensitive to radiation than others. These are the breasts, thyroid gland, reproductive organs, and bone marrow. The body's cells attempt to repair the damage, but if the damage is too severe, radiation sickness will result.

The major factors that determine the severity of radiation injury are the amount and length of time of radiation received and the length of exposure time. For example, a person exposed to ionizing radiation in a focused medical procedure such as a knee X-ray will usually not suffer any symptoms of radiation sickness since the procedure is short, localized, and radiation exposure is minimal. However, a person can be exposed to radiation anywhere radioactive materials are used. Someone exposed to a large nuclear plant leak such as the Chernobyl nuclear reactor accident is likely to suffer from severe radiation sickness if the radiation was in the atmosphere for long periods of time and exposure occurred to the whole body. Thus, the larger and longer the dose, the greater the risk for radiation sickness.

Causes and risk factors

Ionizing radiation causes cells to die by damaging DNA, which becomes so impaired that it can no longer function and support the biochemical processes that keep the cells alive. Children and fetuses are more sensitive to radiation because they are growing more rapidly, and there are more cells dividing and a greater opportunity for radiation to disrupt the process. Anyone can be exposed to radiation if radiation sources or radioactive materials are used, such as in nuclear power plants, medical centers, research laboratories, or if radioactive material is removed from mines.

The degree of radiation sickness depends on the dose and the rate of exposure. Exposure from X-rays or gamma rays is measured in units of roentgens. For example, a total body exposure of 100 roentgens causes radiation sickness. A person with a total body exposure of 400 roentgens will get radiation sickness; death occurs in half of these individuals. A dose of 100,000 rads (radiation absorbed dose) causes almost immediate unconsciousness and death within an hour. The severity of symptoms and sickness depends on the type and amount of radiation, the duration of the exposure, and the body areas exposed. Symptoms of radiation sickness usually do not occur immediately following exposure.

A person who is contaminated with radioactive materials will expose others. Contaminated materials must be handled by specially trained people. Once the radioactive material has been removed, the person cannot spread radiation.

Signs and symptoms

Cell death is manifested in the body through the symptoms of radiation sickness. Symptoms of radiation sickness usually do not occur immediately following exposure but over the course of a few days or months. These symptoms appear gradually and include nausea and vomiting; diarrhea; skin burns (radiodermatitis); weakness; fatigue; loss of appetite; fainting; dehydration; inflammation (swelling, redness or tenderness) of tissues; bleeding from the nose, mouth, gums, or rectum; low red blood cell count (anemia); and hair loss.

Because it is difficult to determine the amount of radiation exposure from accidents, the best indications of the severity of the exposure are the length of time between the exposure and the onset of symptoms, the severity of symptoms, and severity of changes in white blood cells. Generally, the higher the amount of radiation, the greater the severity of early effects and greater possibility of later effects, such as cancer. The effects of radiation exposure on the body vary according to the circumstances in which they occur. Radiation sickness can be acute or chronic. The acute form of the disease can develop quickly, within a few hours or days of exposure. A set of symptoms appear in an orderly fashion. A person with acute radiation sickness has usually been exposed to large amounts of radiation over a very brief period of time. This happens in the case of a nuclear plant accident or a nuclear bomb explosion. It may take several days or weeks to develop the chronic form of the disease. A person with chronic radiation sickness has usually been exposed to lower doses over a longer period of time, as in the case of radioactive outcome from a nuclear explosion or accident. It may also be caused by long-term exposure to radiation in the workplace. Chronic sickness is usually associated with delayed medical problems such as cancer and premature aging, which may happen over a long period of time.

The main phase of the intestinal form of the sickness typically begins two to three days after radiation exposure with abdominal pain, fever, and diarrhea, which progress rapidly in severity for several days to dehydration, total exhaustion or weakness, and a fatal, shocklike state. The main phase of the hematopoietic (production of blood cells) form of the illness usually begins in the second or third week after radiation exposure with fever, weakness, infection, and hemorrhage. If damage to the bone marrow is severe, death from infection or hemorrhage may follow four to six weeks after exposure unless corrected by transplantation of unexposed bone marrow cells.

The diagnosis is based on the symptoms and a person's report of radiation exposure. There is no effective treatment cure for radiation sickness after exposure. Only supportive treatments to alleviate symptoms can be offered; there is no medication that can prevent or reverse the damage caused by radiation.

Recovery from radiation injuries may take months or years. Chronic problems, such as damage to the chromosomes, may be permanent and can last a lifetime. A person who has been exposed to radiation will be monitored closely. Laboratory studies of blood samples, including a complete blood count, will reveal how well the body is working to recover. Physical exams will also be done to check for the development of late effects from the radiation poisoning.

Rashmi Nemade

KEY FACTS

Description
Damage to living tissue as a result of excessive exposure to ionizing radiation.

Causes
Accidental or intentional exposure to radiation.

Risk factors
Working with or around radioactive materials and equipment, as well as receiving medical treatments that require radiation. Children and fetuses and people who work with radiation and radiation equipment are at risk.

Symptoms
Nausea, vomiting, diarrhea, hair loss, weakness, bleeding, swelling of mouth or throat, or both, fatigue, skin ulcers, and low blood count.

Diagnosis
History of exposure to radiation, physical signs and symptoms, and a complete blood count.

Treatments
No effective treatment for reversing the effects. Treatment is aimed at relieving symptoms.

Prevention
Avoiding unnecessary exposure to radiation.

Epidemiology
A person is exposed to about 0.002 grays of radiation from natural, medical, and work-related sources per year. One gray is the absorption of 1 joule of radiation energy by 1 kilogram of matter.

See also
• Burns

Repetitive strain injury

Repetitive strain injury (RSI) describes a spectrum of musculoskeletal pain disorders as a result of occupational overuse or repetitive motion. Such overuse injuries can occur in people who do repetitive movements over a long time, for example, when using a computer, handheld instrument, or tool. RSI may also occur in occupations that require a person to maintain a fixed position for long periods of time. RSI can eventually become a chronic condition, in which the person suffers pain even when he or she is not carrying out the repetitive action that originally caused the pain.

RSI is also known as repetitive stress injury, repetitive strain injury, work-related upper limb disorder (WRULD), and occupational overuse syndrome. Specific disorders that may fall under the classification of RSI include adhesive capsulitis, bursitis, carpal tunnel syndrome, cervical spondylosis, writer's cramp, cubital tunnel syndrome (ulnar nerve entrapment), De Quervain's syndrome, Dupuytren's contracture, epicondylitis, ganglion cyst, peritendonitis, rotator cuff syndrome, tendonitis, tenosynovitis, trigger finger or thumb, and thoracic outlet syndrome.

Nonspecific disorders may affect muscles, tendons, bursae, or joints of the neck, shoulders, upper back, elbows, wrists, or hands, or all of them. "Diffuse RSI" refers to a nonspecific pain syndrome in which pain is present in several areas, attributed to underlying nerve damage as a result of repetitive motions. Occupations commonly associated with RSI disorders include working for long periods of time without rest breaks at a computer, desk, or assembly line.

Causes

Repetitive motion and prolonged tension in muscles that are held in a continuous position are believed to cause microtrauma to underlying tissues, which injures muscles, tendon sheaths, ligaments, nerve sheaths, or other structures, resulting in swelling and pain.

Swelling of muscles or tendon sheaths is believed to reduce blood flow to the affected tissues and the surrounding area, exacerbating the symptoms. Repetitive motions aggravate the underlying microtrauma to tissues and prevent healing.

KEY FACTS

Description

Spectrum of soft tissue injury disorders of the neck, shoulders, upper back, arms, wrists, or hands.

Causes

Occupations or activities that require prolonged repetitive motion or a prolonged fixed position, such as work with a computer, a handheld instrument, or a tool.

Risk factors

An ergonomically unsound work station, poor posture, excessive workload, prolonged periods of work without rest, repetitive movements with work (such as typing), repetitive forceful hand motions (such as twisting or gripping), prolonged body vibrations (such as from power tools), fatigue, cold work environments, and psychosocial stressors.

Symptoms

Sharp or dull pain, soreness, stiffness, tingling and numbness, loss of sensation, limited range of motion, weakness, fatigue, or persistent tension in the neck, shoulders, upper back, elbows, wrists, or hands. Pain may develop in the back or lower extremities or be referred from one area to another.

Diagnosis

Thorough history and physical exam.

Treatment

Depends on the specific underlying syndrome and its cause. Options include rest, anti-inflammatory medications, anti-convulsant medications for neuropathic pain, deep tissue massage for acute pain and trigger points, stretching or strengthening exercises, specialized orthopedic braces for immobilization, or surgery.

Pathogenesis

Repetitive microtrauma to muscles, tendon sheaths, and nerve sheaths of the neck, upper back or upper extremities, causing swelling and pain. Reduced blood circulation after soft tissue swelling exacerbates symptoms.

Prevention

Good posture, frequent breaks from prolonged fixed positions, adaptive technology in the workplace, and maintenance of general good health through physical activity.

Epidemiology

Exact prevalence and incidence is unknown because of underreporting and misdiagnosis. Reporting varies by industry.

Risk factors

Risk factors include an ergonomically unsound work station, poor posture, and excessive workload. Working for long periods without rest and using repetitive movements or repetitive forceful hand motions (twisting or gripping) are also contributing factors, as are prolonged body vibrations (such as from power tools), fatigue, cold work environments, and psychosocial stressors.

Symptoms

Symptoms may accumulate over long periods of time and include recurring sharp or dull pain, soreness, stiffness, tingling and numbness, loss of sensation, limited range of motion, weakness, fatigue, or persistent tension in the neck, shoulders, upper back, elbows, wrists, or hands. Pain may be referred from one area to another, such as when nerve impingement in the neck or shoulder causes pain in the forearm or hand. Less commonly, pain may also be referred to the back or lower extremities.

Symptoms in the arms or hands may worsen when lying in bed. Routine daily activities such as driving, carrying groceries, housework, or gardening may worsen symptoms. Without treatment, symptoms may become continuous and progress to long-term injury and disability.

Diagnosis

Diagnosis is often difficult and is based upon a thorough history and physical examination by a physician familiar with RSI syndromes. Injuries are not identifiable with X-rays or other radiological studies since the injuries involve soft tissues. Several different specialists may be involved with the diagnosis and treatment plan, such as occupational therapists, physical therapists, physiatrists, surgeons, massage therapists, and alternative medicine practitioners.

Treatments and prevention

Treatment of RSI will vary and will depend on the specific underlying syndrome and its cause. Possible treatment options include rest, anti-inflammatory medications, anti-convulsant medications for neuropathic pain, deep tissue massage for acute pain and trigger points, stretching or strengthening exercises (or both), biofeedback techniques, or specialized orthopedic braces for immobilization. Surgery is considered a last resort. Cessation of hand activity both at work and in routine daily activities may be required for a period of time to prevent worsening of symptoms and to promote healing of affected tissues.

Adaptive technology such as specialized keyboards, computer mouse replacements, and speech recognition software may be considered for certain work environments. Computer users are encouraged to decrease the risk of RSI by adjusting their work stations so that the top of their computer screen is at eye level, to keep their arms at a 90-degree angle to the computer keyboard, to use a chair back that supports the spine and tilts the pelvis forward, and to keep feet flat on the floor. People who type for prolonged periods are encouraged to avoid bending their wrists or resting their hands on the keyboard. People in occupations at risk for RSI are encouraged to take frequent breaks to stretch and increase blood circulation to muscles. General physical activity to maintain flexibility is encouraged, as is a healthy diet, as well as smoking cessation to promote general health.

Epidemiology

RSI has a significant economic impact; research in the United States reveals that in Washington State alone, compensation for workers affected by RSI was in the region of $20 billion, and one-third of worker's compensation costs in the United States are directly related to RSI. Added to that is the burden of the cost of lost revenue and the cost to employers when workers take sick leave.

Although statistics regarding RSI are controversial, it seems clear that RSI is almost always occupational in nature, and the huge increase in the use of computers in the workplace and computers at home puts people at risk for the condition. In the United States, around 50 percent of injury claims for upper limb disorders involve a computer. A European survey showed that 30 percent of workers suffered from backache and 17 percent, about 25 million people, complained of muscular pain in the arms and legs. The British Health and Safety Executive reported that around half a million workers complained of some type of neck or limb disorder. In 2002 in the United Kingdom, 5.4 million working days were lost in sick leave as a result of RSI.

Ergonomically designed workstations, combined with appropriate strategies in the workplace, are essential in order to combat RSI.

Joanne L. Oakes

See also
• Sports injury

Retinal disorders

Retinal disorders are caused by injury, genetic mutations, hypertension, vessel occlusion, premature birth, glaucoma, diabetes, cancer, or unknown causes. Several disorders involve retinal cell degeneration due to retinal detachment or damaged blood supply and induced growth of abnormal, leaky vessels. Treatment of underlying disease and surgery to keep the retina attached to its source of oxygen and nutrients may slow vision loss.

The retina has connections to the brain. Adjacent to the whitish sclera of the eye is a vascular tissue layer known as the choroid, which feeds and supports the innermost lining of the eye, the retina. The retina is made up of the retinal pigment epithelium (RPE) layer, located next to the choroid, and the sub-adjacent multilayered neural retina. Photoreceptors (rods and cones) transform light energy into electrical impulses. Rods are motion-sensitive and work best in dim light, whereas cones respond optimally in bright light and are highly concentrated in the macula, the small portion of central retina necessary for seeing fine details and color.

Electrical signals from photoreceptors travel through other retinal layers to the innermost sheet of retinal ganglion cells. Axons of these cells collect together at the back of the eyeball and exit as the optic nerve, which transmits impulses from the retina to the brain, where they are interpreted. Thus, "seeing" an image involves collaboration between the outer layers of the eye (serving to focus the light): the retina, optic nerve, and brain. Vision may be affected if one or more of these components is compromised, or if information transfer from eye to brain is disrupted.

Retinal detachment occurs when the retina pulls away from its position against the choroid, causing the cells to degenerate due to lack of oxygen and nutrients. This can result from age-related shrinking of the vitreous, causing the layers to pull apart, or an injury that tears the retina, allowing fluid to pass through the tear under the retina, detaching it from the rest of the eye. A macular (central retina) pucker may also follow trauma, inflammation, or vitreous shrinking. Symptoms include blurry vision, seeing flashes, new floaters, or a shadow across the visual field. Retinal tears or detachments require immediate attention to prevent permanent vision loss, since the cells cannot survive away from the choroid.

Retinoschisis. Although sharing symptoms of retinal detachment, retinoschisis involves splitting of the retina into two layers. It is usually diagnosed after age 50 and frequently affects both eyes. If the affected area is stable, small, and peripheral, no treatment is recommended; larger, progressive, central conditions require treatment. A juvenile, congenital, X-linked form is less prevalent but affects the central retina.

Retinal cancers

Retinoblastoma is a rare retinal cancer detected in young children. Common symptoms are redness of the eye, irritation, pain, and loss of vision in the affected eye. It may be associated with mental retardation and slow growth. Mutations in *RB1*, a tumor suppressor gene (normally prevents uncontrolled cell growth) is associated with retinoblastoma; mutated genes are inherited (autosomal dominant) or occur spontaneously during embryonic life or later.

Choroidal melanomas originate in pigment-producing choroids cells; metastases originate elsewhere and spread to the choroid via its rich blood supply. The condition may be asymptomatic initially, then cause floaters, flashes, and retinal detachment.

Degenerative changes

Many changes affect the retina, including different types of macular degeneration and various syndromes.

Macular degeneration (MD). Age-related MD (ARMD), the leading cause of impaired vision in the elderly, involves a progressive degeneration of the central retina. Dry MD (90 percent of ARMD patients) is caused by damage to macular photoreceptors and retinal thinning. Wet MD is more severe, though less common. It occurs when new, leaky blood vessels form around a damaged macula, fluid leaks under the macula, and the retina may scar and detach. Blurry vision and a central blind spot develop in both forms of ARMD; straight lines appear wavy in wet MD. The vascular endothelial growth factor (VEGF) is required for growth of the vessels; when anti-VEGF antibody is administered as an intravitreous injection, it is effective in reducing leakage from blood from the abnormal vessels and slowing further loss of vision. Age, race (white, blue eyes), gender (female), smoking, high cholesterol, and family history are predisposing factors.

Stargardt disease (fundus flavimaculatus). This disorder is an inherited (autosomal recessive; also dominant), gradually progressive MD affecting both eyes, usually before age 20. Mutations in the *ABCR* gene cause degeneration of cones, blurry vision, deterioration of central vision (acuity stabilizes at 20/200), and reduced color vision, but peripheral vision is spared.

Best's disease (vitelliform macular dystrophy). This rare inherited disorder involves damage to the macula; it may be asymptomatic until the age of about 50. Mutations in the *RDS* or *VMD2* genes cause Best's MD.

Retinitis pigmentosa (RP), or retrolental fibroplasia, is a group of inherited disorders, detected before age 30, that is linked with progressive photoreceptor degeneration. Symptoms of rod-cone dystrophy (more common) are an inability to adapt to dim light due to degeneration of rods with progressive peripheral vision loss. Less frequently, cones are affected first in cone-rod dystrophy; central vision and color perception are impaired, with later rod loss, sometimes accompanied by cataracts. More than 100 gene mutations cause RP, with differing inheritance patterns.

Usher syndrome. RP and severe hearing loss are both present, often at birth, in this inherited condition (autosomal recessive) associated with mutations in at least 10 genes related to balance, hearing, and vision. Peripheral vision deteriorates first, then central vision becomes blurred; cataracts may develop. Incidence is higher in Ashkenazi Jews and the Louisiana Acadian population.

Bardet-Biedl syndrome. Symptoms of this inherited disorder (autosomal recessive) include rapidly progressing RP in childhood, obesity, polydactyly (extra digits), short stature, broad feet, small genitalia (males); approximately 50 percent of affected individuals are mildly retarded and may exhibit kidney disease.

Choroideremia (tapetochoroidal dystrophy). This is a rare, inherited (X-linked) disorder associated with loss of *REP-1* gene, degeneration of choroid and retinal pigmented epithelial (RPE) cells, and photoreceptor loss. Choroideremia is diagnosed almost exclusively in male children, with initial peripheral vision loss, sometimes followed by central vision; degeneration continues throughout life.

Leber congenital amaurosis (LCA). This is an inherited (autosomal recessive) disorder, which is characterized by abnormal, prematurely degenerating photoreceptors and severe visual impairment in infancy. Keratoconus, cataracts, and retardation may also be present.

Retinal vessel occlusion

Blockage of the retinal artery, retinal vein, or their branches compromises the supply of blood, oxygen, and nutrients to and from the retina. Artery occlusion leads to sudden loss of vision in part of the visual field, then an irreversible death of retinal cells; blocked retinal veins cause backed-up blood flow, swelling, hemorrhaging of tiny vessels, and a gradual effect on vision. Occlusion results from a thrombus (blood clot) buildup, or an embolus (blood-borne floating clot or debris) lodging in vessel walls that may already be damaged from hypertension, diabetes, atherosclerosis, glaucoma, inflammation, malignancies, sickle-cell disease, medications, trauma, or radiation treatment.

KEY FACTS

Description
Disorders of the light-sensitive, inner layer of the eye.

Causes
Most unknown; some disorders are inherited; few contributing genes identified.

Risk factors
Diabetes, hypertension, family history, injury, premature birth, and age.

Symptoms
Blurry vision, flashes, new floaters, shadow across visual field, night blindness, tunnel vision.

Diagnosis
Eye exams with pupil dilation, imaging with fluorescent dye, tonometry, electroretinogram, electro-oculogram, family history.

Treatments
Laser microsurgery, cryotherapy, laser photocoagulation to reattach the retina or arrest vessel leaking; vitreous removal; medically or surgically treating intraocular pressure (IOP), hypertension. Gene or stem cell therapies are in development.

Pathogenesis
Retinal cells or axons, or both, degenerate as a result of vitreous shrinkage, injury to eye, vessel damage or blockage, IOP, cancers originating in or metastasizing to retina. Visual impairments are sudden or progressive, permanent or resolvable.

Prevention
Regular eye exams, control of blood pressure, immediate attention to alterations in vision.

Epidemiology
1.8 million (0.66 percent) Americans have severe visual impairment stemming from retinal disorder.

Diabetic retinopathy

Retinopathy refers to a disease of the retina; many retinopathies are caused by retinal vessel abnormalities. Problems with glucose metabolism as a result of diabetes may damage blood vessels. Three stages of diabetic retinopathy are: nonproliferative, with damaged vessels and retinal swelling; macular edema, with leaky vessels and fluid collecting in the retina; proliferative, characterized by growth of abnormal vessels that bleed into the retina, damage cells, and lead to scar formation and retinal detachment. Symptoms, initially detectable in the second stage, include blurry vision, progressing to vision loss. Maintaining blood sugar levels may slow deterioration.

Hypertensive retinopathy. Hypertensive retinal atherosclerosis may result from chronic hypertension. At first, arterioles look constricted, then they hemorrhage. "Cotton wool" spots (retina deprived of blood) and yellowish lipid deposits (exudates) are visible on eye exam. Symptoms are managed by controlling blood pressure.

Familial exudative vitreoretinopathy (FEVR). Peripheral retinal vessels are not fully formed; the resulting oxygen loss (ischemia) induces formation of new vessels that are leaky, may cause retinal tears, fluid collection (exudates), and detachment. The condition may be congenital (present from birth). Mutations in the *FZD*4 and *LRP*5 genes are associated with 20 percent of the autosomal dominant inheritance of FEVR and in the *NDP* gene with the X-linked form.

Retinopathy of prematurity (ROP). A sporadic disorder, ROP resembles FEVR in that peripheral vessels have not fully developed by the time of the premature birth.

Other retinal disorders

Several other various conditions affect the retina. Some of them are inherited disorders.

Coat's disease (exudative retinitis). Typically diagnosed before age 10, Coat's disease primarily affects males. Retinal capillaries dilate and leak fluid that may collect under the retina, leading to detachment, usually in the central retina. Spontaneous arrest of disease progress is not uncommon.

Cystoid macular edema (CME). This disorder presents with swelling of the central retina, with fluid collecting in layers of the macula, which leads to distorted vision. CME is difficult to diagnose, but fluorescein angiography may allow detection. Anti-inflammatory medications applied directly to the eye are effective in reducing swelling.

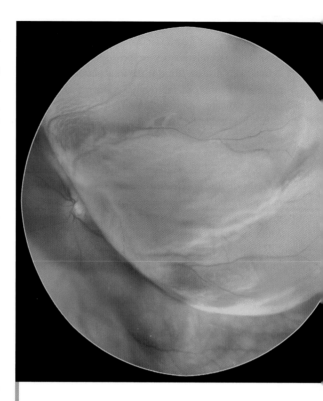

This retinal photomontage shows a retinal detachment, which is the separation of the sensory retina from the underlying pigment epithelium. The condition disturbs vision and usually requires immediate surgery to correct.

Central serous chorioretinopathy (CSC). CSC is characterized by a breakdown of RPE cells or choroidal vessels that supply the RPE, and fluid collection under the retina; vessel leaks may seal spontaneously. In the chronic condition, the retina thins, and may detach. CSC occurs mostly in males of 20 to 50 years and can be associated with stress.

Bieti's crystalline dystrophy (BCD). This is a rare autosomal recessive inherited disorder in which crystal deposits form on the cornea and retina, and the retinal layers and choroid progressively atrophy.

Color blindness is an inherited impairment in perceiving certain colors. It is much more common in males than females. Mostly, there is a loss of one or two types of cones (red-green color blindness is most common); fully color-blind individuals are rare. Occasionally, color blindness results from brain damage.

Coloboma. This is a rare birth defect in which the individual has a congenital gap (malformation) in the retina, optic nerve, iris, or lens.

Night blindness. Although people with this condition cannot see well in poor light, there may be no ob-

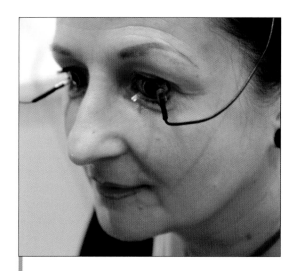

A patient with anomalies of the visual field undergoes electroretinography, an eye electrophysiology examination. Electrodes are placed on the cornea to allow measurement of the electrical response of the retina to light stimulation.

vious eye defect. Night blindness can be a result of vitamin A deficiency and may be a precursor to retinitis pigmentosa.

Glaucoma. This incurable disease is caused by degeneration of optic nerve axons, severing connections between eye and brain; retinal ganglion cells are secondarily damaged. Glaucoma may be caused by high intraocular pressure (IOP) but also occurs without it. Medication and surgery can relieve IOP.

Optic nerve atrophy (hypoplasia, optic nerve neuritis). The nerve is abnormal, due to a congenital degenerative condition (atrophy), underdevelopment (hypoplasia), or inflammation (neuritis). Retinal signals cannot be interpreted, leading to loss of vision.

Uveitis. In this condition there is an inflammation inside the eye, which affects the blood supply to the retina, often in otherwise healthy people. Symptoms include pain, itching, redness, floaters, and light sensitivity. Eye drops and anti-inflammatory medications are prescribed at once to prevent vision loss and scarring.

Diagnostic tests

These include tests of visual acuity and perimetry (to establish the extent of the visual field). Cat's eye reflex or whiteness in pupil, gonioscopy, ophthalmic examination with pupil dilation, and fluorescein angiography (injecting a fluorescent dye) are tests done to assess blood flow in the eye, as well as tonometry for IOP and blood tests for inflammation and cholesterol levels.

The Ambler grid is used for testing blurriness. Electroretinogram (ERG) measures the electrical response of retinal cells to a light stimulus; this is useful in differentiating between disorders such as RP and cone dystrophy. Electro-oculogram (EOG) is useful for evaluating disorders such as RP.

Treatments

A paramount concern is to treat conditions prior to the death of retinal cells. Regular eye exams, eye protection, and early detection are essential. For retinal detachment or vessel proliferation, treatments are laser microsurgery, laser photocoagulation, cryotherapy, or vitrectomy. If there is vessel occlusion, treatments include eye massage, breathing carbogen and rebreathing carbon dioxide to widen arteries, anterior chamber paracentesis (removing fluid), injecting clot-dissolving medications into the eye, and laser coagulation. Low vision aids are useful when peripheral vision is minimally affected. To slow RP progression, high doses of vitamin A are given (these are anecdotal reports). Many inherited disorders are not treatable; genetic counseling is recommended for these cases.

Preliminary experimental treatments are microretinal implants to replace photoreceptors; gene therapy for replacing or blocking defective gene action; neuroprotective proteins, survival factors, or stem cells to protect blood vessels and rescue photoreceptors.

Epidemiology

In the United States, 1.75 million people over age 40 have ARMD-related reduced vision; this may reach 3 million by 2020. The prevalence of retinitis pigmentosa is 100,000. Each year, 30,000 people (1 in 10,000) are diagnosed with retinal detachment; it is most common in severely myopic individuals. Around 10,000 to 15,000 people have Usher syndrome. An estimated 4 to 5.6 million (40 percent of diabetics) have at least some form of diabetic retinopathy; 65,000 per year develop stage 3 retinopathy. About 14,000 to 16,000 infants per year are affected with ROP; 400 to 600 infants become legally blind each year. Retinoblastoma (eye cancer) affects 1 in 15,000 to 20,000 live births (about 250 diagnoses yearly); around 1,300 retinal melanomas are diagnosed each year. One in 10 males is color-blind; it is rare in females.

Sonal Jhaveri

See also
• Cataract • Diabetes • Macular degeneration

Rheumatic fever

Rheumatic fever is a disease of the joints and heart. It occurs as a result of an immune reaction following infection with specific types of streptococcal bacteria. It is acute but may become chronic and progressive.

After an episode of pharyngitis (painful inflammation of the throat) caused by streptococcal bacteria and commonly called "strep throat," acute rheumatic fever occurs in 0.4 to 3 percent of untreated people. The disease usually begins one to five weeks after the sore throat. Affected people develop fever, along with painful swelling of the large joints (such as knee, elbow, and hip). Some people may have a heart murmur, along with chest pain and shortness of breath. In some cases there may even be small, firm swellings under the skin, and a typical rash called erythema marginatum. The disease usually lasts 3 months and can be serious and life threatening. It may also be recurrent.

Diagnosis and treatment

Diagnosis of rheumatic fever is based on signs and symptoms and laboratory evidence of prior streptococcal infection, such as culture or detection of antibodies to the streptococcal bacteria. The disease is treated with high dose aspirin and sometimes steroid drugs. Aspirin should not be given to young children because of the risk of Reye's syndrome.

The long-term consequence of acute rheumatic fever is rheumatic heart disease, which is a disorder of the heart valves, or sometimes the outer lining of the heart. It occurs in 30 to 40 percent of patients if they had carditis and in 6 percent if they did not have carditis (inflammation of the heart or its linings). It is chronic and progressive. The most common abnormality in rheumatic heart disease is mitral stenosis, a tightening of the mitral valve of the heart. A rare complication of acute rheumatic fever is chorea, which is abnormal movements of the face, hands, and feet.

Individuals who develop chronic rheumatic heart disease need lifelong treatment with heart medications and may need surgical repair or replacement of the heart valves. Acute rheumatic fever may be prevented by prompt treatment of strep throat. Once acute rheumatic fever has occurred, chronic heart disease may be prevented by prolonged therapy with penicillin for 5 to 10 years or until adulthood. Efforts are ongoing to develop a safe and effective vaccine to prevent streptococcal infection and acute rheumatic fever.

Epidemiology

Acute rheumatic fever is most common in children between 5 and 15 years of age. Some complications of rheumatic fever such as mitral stenosis and chorea are more common in women. The disease is more common in African Americans compared to Caucasians. Although rare in the United States, rheumatic fever is widespread in the Middle East, India, selected areas of Africa, and South America, and in the aboriginal populations in Australia and New Zealand.

Pranavi Sreeramoju

KEY FACTS

Description

An acute disease affecting joints and sometimes the heart. It may become chronic and progressive.

Causes

An immune reaction following infection with streptococcal bacteria.

Risk factors

Crowded living conditions in a low-income country.

Symptoms and signs

Fever, rash, nodules under the skin, pain and swelling of the large joints, shortness of breath, chest pain, and heart murmur.

Diagnosis

From symptoms and signs, along with laboratory evidence for streptococcal infection.

Treatments

No specific treatments; rest, aspirin, and steroids depending on the severity of the illness.

Pathogenesis

Unknown.

Prevention

Treatment of streptococcal pharyngitis; once rheumatic fever occurs, prolonged treatment with penicillin for years to prevent heart disease.

Epidemiology

Rare in the United States, with incidence less than 1 per 200,000 people per year. Widespread in some low-income countries.

See also
• Influenza

Rickettsial infections

The term *rickettsiae* embraces a broad group of potentially lethal microorganisms that have caused devastating epidemics among the world's population. Dr. Howard Ricketts, for whom the bacteria are named, died from epidemic typhus, a type of rickettsial infection that he was researching. Rickettsiae are small bacteria associated with arthropods. Rickettsial infections vary in severity but can be life threatening.

Most rickettsia are carried by arthropod vectors, with the exception of Q fever (caused by *Coxiella burnetti*), which is transmitted through exposure to body fluids of infected animals. *Ehrlichia chaffeensis* and *Anaplasma phagocytophilum* cause human monocytic ehrlichiosis and human granulocytic anaplasmosis, respectively, and are transmitted by ticks during ticks' blood meals. Epidemic typhus is a louse-borne disease caused by *Rickettsia prowazekii*, while scrub typhus is caused by *Orienta tsutsugamishi* and is transmitted by mites. Rickettsialpox is a mite-borne illness caused by *Rickettsia akari*.

Risk factors

Most rickettsial diseases are transmitted to humans by bacteria-harboring arthropod vectors (ticks, mites, fleas, and lice) during feeding, and the greatest risk of acquiring these infections occurs with exposure to these vectors. Animals and humans can be infested with these arthropods and transmit them to others. Areas of poor sanitation, such as impoverished or rural communities, have higher infestation levels and higher rates of infection among the inhabitants.

Symptoms and signs

Symptoms vary depending on the specific infection. The incubation period varies from one to three weeks. Patients often do not recall exposure to an insect vector. High fever, headache, muscle aches, and lymphadenopathy are often seen. Rash may be prominent (vesicular in rickettsialpox, macular in epidemic and scrub typhus and monocytic ehrlichiosis) or absent (granulocytic anaplasmosis). Patients may also develop a localized area of dead tissue, often black in color, at the site of an arthropod bite, also called an "eschar." An eschar is prominent in rickettsialpox and scrub typhus. Pneumonia can occur in Q fever. As the bacteria replicate, patients may develop inflammation in the blood vessels, heart muscle, lungs, liver, and central nervous system, leading to widespread organ dysfunction.

KEY FACTS

Description
A group of bacterial infections distributed worldwide that range in severity from a mild flulike illness to multi-organ failure and death.

Causes
Bacteria that are usually transmitted to humans through the bite of an infected arthropod. Common pathogens include *Ehrlichia chaffeensis*, *Anaplasma phagocytophilum*, *Coxiella burnetti*, *Rickettsia prowazekii*, and *Rickettsia akari*.

Risk factors
Exposure to bacteria in lice, fleas, and mites poses the greatest risk. Infestation levels are likely to be higher in areas of poor sanitation.

Symptoms
Vary widely depending on the specific infection. A lesion or ulcer may develop at the site of the bite. Fevers, muscle aches, and diffuse rash may also occur. In very severe cases, patients can develop pneumonia and organ failure.

Diagnosis
Blood tests measuring antibody; skin biopsies. Treatment should not be delayed while these tests are in progress.

Treatments
Antibiotics; doxycycline and tetracycline are most effective. Chloramphenicol is a second choice.

Pathogenesis
The infecting organisms target the inner lining of blood vessels or blood leukocytes (white blood cells). Inflammation develops, leading to leakage of fluid into surrounding tissues and possible damage to various organs.

Prevention
Avoidance of arthropod vectors and appropriate hygiene and sanitation practices. There is no vaccine available.

Epidemiology
Worldwide distribution, determined by their vectors. Often occur as outbreaks due to poverty, overcrowding, or animal exposure.

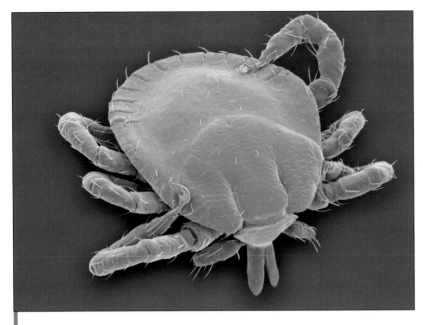

This brown dog tick larva (Rhipicephalus sanguineus) *has mouthparts adapted to suck blood. Although it prefers dogs, it will feed on many mammals. It can transmit Rocky Mountain spotted fever and tularemia to humans.*

Thrombocytopenia, leukopenia, and hepatitis can be seen in most rickettsial infections. Because of the potential lethality, *Rickettsia prowazekii* (epidemic typhus) is listed as a potential agent of bioterrorism.

Diagnosis and treatments

Rickettsiae are difficult to culture. Rickettsial infections can be diagnosed with various blood tests that detect components of the host immune response, specifically antibody levels that fight the infection. Testing for antibodies to rickettsial antigens provides a retrospective diagnosis. Polymerase chain reaction assays on blood are useful in diagnosing ehrlichiosis. Biopsies of skin lesions are helpful in rickettsialpox and scrub typhus, but these tests are time consuming, labor intensive, and not available at all medical institutions.

Treatment should be started immediately if rickettsial infection is suspected. Irreversible complications and death may result when therapy is delayed. The treatment of choice is doxycycline or tetracycline.

Pathogenesis

Most rickettsiae target the vascular endothelium in the wall of blood vessels and cause a vasculitis (inflammation of blood vessels). *Orienta*, *Ehrlichia* and *R. akari* multiply in blood monocytes, and *Anaplasma* targets neutrophils. All induce inflammation and clotting abnormalities, leading to fluid discharge into tissues. Severe infection can damage multiple organs. Without treatment, complications like pneumonia, central nervous system damage, and gangrene of the extremities can occur.

Prevention

Avoidance of insect vectors that carry the bacteria is the best method of prevention. In wooded areas, protective clothing and insect repellant should be applied to skin and clothing. The body should be carefully inspected for ticks. If found, these should be removed immediately using tweezers. Good hygiene and sanitation help eradicate carriers in areas of high infestation. Control programs for animals, both wild and domestic, may be necessary. Avoiding contact with fluids from potentially infected animals helps prevent Q fever.

Epidemiology

Rickettsial infections can be found all over the world. Their geographic distribution is determined by their vectors, and specific infections are limited to certain areas. Ehrlichiosis and anaplasmosis are predominantly found in the United States in the southeastern, south central, and mid-Atlantic regions, with an annual incidence of two to three cases in 1 million. Q fever occurs worldwide wherever there is animal exposure (for example, farmers and slaughterhouse workers are at risk). Epidemic typhus has killed millions of people since the Middle Ages but is now limited to a few locations in Africa, Asia, and Central and South America. Rickettsialpox has been reported in the United States, South Africa, and eastern Europe.

Joseph M. Fritz and Nigar Kirmani

See also
• Rocky Mountain spotted fever • Typhus

River blindness

River blindness, or onchocerciasis, is a chronic parasitic illness found mainly in tropical Africa that causes intense suffering and can lead to visual impairment and blindness. The disease is found only in humans and has been the focus of control and eradication efforts by international health and aid agencies.

River blindness gets its name from the fact that the disease is transmitted along fertile river areas, mainly in Africa but also in several Latin American countries and Yemen, and can lead to blindness. About 123 million people live in areas where the disease is endemic. It is the second leading infectious cause of blindness and thus is a preventable cause of blindness. The illness has been blamed for adversely affecting the socioeconomic status of people living in endemic regions, because populations may abandon areas where the blackfly lives and breeds. In the United States the disease is rare; it has been diagnosed only in immigrants or travelers who spent time in endemic areas.

Causes and risk factors

The parasitic worm *Onchocerca volvulus* causes the debilitating illness river blindness. It is transmitted by the bite of an infected *Simulium* blackfly, found mainly in tropical Africa near fast-flowing waters. Humans are the only known host. Risk of contracting the illness is only in areas where the blackfly lives.

When an infected blackfly bites a human, usually only one to two of the larval forms of the parasite are injected into the skin. Multiple bites can occur and are common in regions endemic for this illness. In humans who contract this disease, the intensity of their illness (number of the parasitic worms) is related to the number of such bites.

Symptoms and signs

The earliest symptom is severe itching, or pruritis. The itching can become so severe that it interferes with sleep and results in social isolation. Scratching can produce skin trauma such as excoriations and can result in thickened, dry skin. Skin nodules are common, especially overlying bony prominences, as are skin rashes and depigmentation. Skin color changes resulting from depigmentation in some areas and normal-looking skin in others has been referred to as "leopard skin." Lymphadenoapthy (enlargement of lymph nodes) in the groin and femoral areas may become quite pronounced, resulting in elephantiasis of the genitalia. General debilitation can occur. The most feared outcome is blindness. Because the probability of blindness is related to the length of illness, the peak age when affected is 40 to 50. Even though the illness

---

KEY FACTS

Description
Chronic parasitic illness involving mainly the skin, lymph nodes, and eyes.

Cause
Onchocerca volvulus, a parasite transmitted by the bite of infected blackflies.

Risk factors
Risk increases with time spent in areas where the disease is endemic.

Symptoms
Severe itching, skin nodules, swelling of the groin lymph nodes, possible blindness.

Diagnosis
Identification of larvae in skin snips or of adult parasitic forms from the deeper skin nodules. In some cases, examination of the eye with a special lamp allows identification of the parasite.

Treatments
Ivermectin, an oral medicine, for 10 years or more.

Pathogenesis
Infected blackflies deposit larval forms of the parasite into human skin. There, the parasites mature and produce offspring (microfilariae) that then migrate to other tissues. Microfilariae live up to 30 months; an inflammatory response to dying microfilariae is responsible for the human tissue damage, including blindness. The life cycle is completed when an infected human is bitten by a blackfly, which takes up the parasite and thus can continue the cycle.

Prevention
Avoidance of areas where the vector blackflies live; insecticides to control blackfly populations.

Epidemiology
More than 18 million people are currently infected; up to 1 to 2 million have been blinded by the disease.

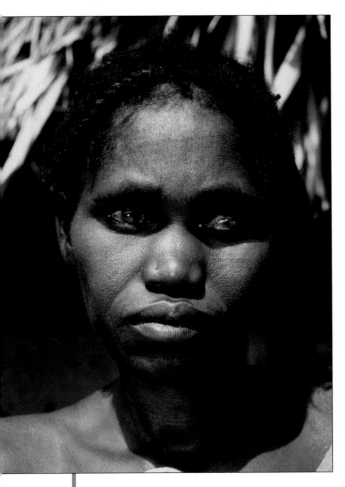

This young woman in Sudan has been blinded by onchocerciasis (river blindness). The blindness in this condition is caused by the death of the worms in or near to tissues of the eye. It can be effectively treated if caught in time.

tense involvement of the eye by the infecting parasite, pretreatment with prednisone (an anti-inflammatory medication similar to cortisone) may be required to protect the eye from the inflammatory effects of the dying parasites.

Since the adult forms may live in the human for up to 14 years, treatment must be continued for as long as 15 years. Treatment is well tolerated. Excision of accessible subcutaneous nodules may help some patients.

Pathogenesis

Once an infected blackfly bites a human and deposits the infective larval forms of the worm in the skin, the parasites mature over a 6 to 12 month period. Female adults grow to a size of 8 to 31½ inches (20 to 80 cm) and are surrounded by a fibrous capsule. They are fertilized by the smaller, adult males, which are 1 to 2 inches (3 to 5 cm) long. The males travel from capsule to capsule. About one year after the initial infection, females produce new larvae, called microfilariae. Each female can produce 1,000 to 3,000 microfilariae per day. These microfilariae migrate through the human body, remain alive for 6 to 30 months, and subsequently incite an inflammatory response by the host's tissues as they are dying. It is this inflammatory response that causes tissue damage, particularly when the eye is involved, leading to visual impairment and possible blindness.

The life cycle is completed when a human infected with this illness is bitten by a blackfly that ingests the microfilariae; these larvae go on to mature within the blackfly into larvae that can infect humans.

Prevention and epidemiology

No vaccine is available. Arrest of the disease rests on controlling blackfly with insecticide programs. Mass treatment programs have been implemented that consist of once or twice yearly ivermectin treatment of people in endemic regions. Travelers to areas where the disease is endemic are advised to use insecticide repellants and to wear long sleeves and pants to reduce the risk of bites. It is felt, though, that short-term travelers to these endemic regions are at low risk of contracting the illness since a minimum of several months in these areas is required before infection occurs.

Rita Washko

is not life threatening, the overall life expectancy among those who are affected by river blindness is only about one-third of that found in uninfected people.

Diagnosis and treatments

Diagnosis is made by identification of larvae in skin snips or adult worms in deeper tissue specimens. In some cases, examination of the eye using a special lamp called a slit lamp may reveal the parasite. Once to twice a year, ivermectin, an oral medication developed initially for use in veterinary medicine, is effective against the larval forms but ineffective against adult worms. This antiparasitic medication reduces further transmission of the disease, improves symptoms such as pruritis, and reduces the possibility of blindness. When there is in-

See also
• Giardiasis • Malaria

Rocky Mountain spotted fever

First described in the late 1800s, Rocky Mountain spotted fever is caused by the bacterium *Rickettsia rickettsii*. It is transmitted to humans by tick bites and is the most lethal tick-borne illness in the United States.

Ticks acquire the bacterium *Rickettsia rickettsii* after feeding on infected animals, then transmit the organism to humans during feeding. There are no specific risk factors for this disease, but heavy tick exposure increases the risk of acquiring the infection.

Symptoms and signs

Patients typically develop symptoms 2 to 14 days after the tick bite. Initial symptoms may include fever, headache, nausea, muscle aches, joint pain, and diarrhea. A rash is common and typically develops between the third and fifth day of the illness. It usually first appears over the ankles and wrists as flat areas of red discoloration but later spreads to the trunk, palms, and soles. Patients may develop inflammation in the blood vessels, heart wall, lungs, and central nervous system, leading to widespread organ dysfunction. Gangrene of the extremities and seizures are possible late complications of this disease.

Diagnosis and treatments

There is no reliable diagnostic test in the early stages of illness. Blood tests can be obtained to confirm the diagnosis, but they are highly specialized and time-consuming. Treatment should not be delayed while blood tests are in progress. Typically, the diagnosis is made based on detailed history (especially with history of tick exposure) and clinical presentation.

Antibiotics should be started as soon as this condition is suspected; doxycycline is the drug of choice. Other antibiotics may be effective, although there is less experience in the clinical setting.

Pathogenesis

Once in the bloodstream, the bacteria replicate in the cells lining the blood vessels. Focal areas of bacterial and cellular infiltration within the blood vessels lead to damage of the vessel wall and surrounding tissue.

Prevention and epidemiology

Avoidance of ticks is the most effective prevention. In a tick-infested area, protective clothing and tick repellents should be used. If a tick is found, it should be removed as soon as possible under the guidance of a physician. Currently there is no available vaccine.

Despite its name, most cases of the disease are reported from the southern Atlantic region. Two-thirds of cases occur in children younger than 15. From 1994 to 2003, the average number of cases reported to the Centers for Disease Control and Prevention was 585 per year. The mortality rate is 2 to 4 percent.

Joseph M. Fritz and Bernard C. Camins

KEY FACTS

Description

Acute bacterial infection transmitted to humans through tick bites.

Causes

Rickettsia rickettsii carried by tick vectors.

Risk factors

Heavy tick exposure.

Symptoms

Fever, headaches, muscle and joint pain, vomiting, diarrhea. Rash on extremities, then spreads.

Diagnosis

Based on clinic presentation.

Treatments

Antibiotics.

Pathogenesis

Organism gains access to the bloodstream via tick bite. It creates inflammation within blood vessel wall and damages surrounding tissues.

Prevention

Avoidance of tick exposure, tick repellent, protective clothing, and careful inspection for potential tick bites. No available vaccine.

Epidemiology

Several hundred cases per year in the United States.

See also

- Lice infestation • Rickettsial infections
- Toxoplasmosis

Rubella

Rubella is also known as German measles. However, it is not caused by the same virus that causes measles. Rubella is highly contagious; it is transmitted through the air or by close contact with an infected person. Children and adults who contract this viral infection will usually experience mild symptoms and a rash. A rubella virus vaccine helps prevent the spread of this infection.

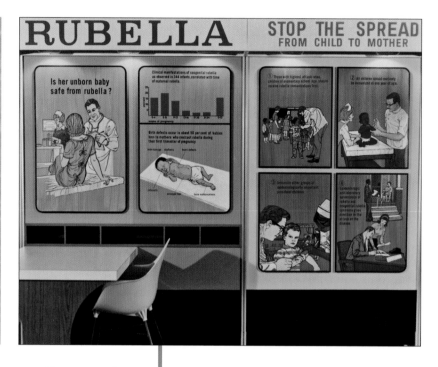

Posters in a clinic highlight the dangers of rubella. If a woman who has not previously had rubella contracts the disease during the first few months of pregnancy, the rubella virus can cause severe birth defects in the unborn child.

Rubella, commonly known as German measles or three-day measles, is a viral infection that mainly causes a skin rash and fever. It is caused by an RNA rubella virus, not the same virus that causes measles. *Rubella* is a name derived from the Latin and means "little red." It became known as "German measles" ever since it was first described in the German medical literature.

Causes and risk factors

Rubella is a viral illness mainly spread through the air by droplets of fluid from the infected person. The fluid contains the virus; coughing, talking, sneezing, hugging, and sharing food and drinks with an infected person can spread the virus. Also, if someone touches a surface contaminated with viral droplets and then touches the nose, face, eyes, or mouth afterward, they can become infected. From the time of exposure to an outbreak with the infection is usually 13 to 20 days. Rubella usually causes a mild infection in children and adults. If contracted in the first months of pregnancy, it can lead to severe abnormalities in the unborn child. Rubella vaccine is used in over one-half of all countries worldwide. It remains a common viral infection, and the risk of exposure to rubella outside the United Kingdom and United States can be high.

Symptoms and signs

A person infected with the rubella virus may have one or more symptoms. They may have rash with skin redness or inflammation, fever, headache, general discomfort (malaise), bruising, runny nose, loss of appetite, and swollen lymph nodes. Many infected people have few or no symptoms at all. The rash usually appears on the second day of infection; it begins on the face and spreads downward on the body. The rash can itch and may last up to three days. Complications can occur, usually more often in adults than children. Over one-half of adult females who contract rubella develop a type of arthritis that mainly affects the fingers, wrists, and knees. These joint symptoms may last up to one month after the infection. Hemorrhaging is a rare complication that occurs more often in children with the rubella infection. Most patients do recover.

If a pregnant woman becomes infected with the rubella virus, it may cause congenital rubella syndrome, with potentially severe birth defects for the unborn child. The infection may lead to premature delivery or death, or both, to the child. Children who are infected with the rubella virus before birth may be born with abnormalities of the heart and eyes; deafness; mental retardation; and growth retardation. Deafness is the most common abnormality of congenital rubella infection. Cataracts and glaucoma can result from congenital rubella syndrome. Diabetes mellitus often occurs in affected children.

Diagnosis

A blood test for rubella antibodies is usually performed on a woman who is or wants to become pregnant to determine whether she is at risk for a rubella infection. Several laboratory methods are available to detect the rubella antibodies. The most common test is the enzyme-linked immunosorbent assay (ELISA).

KEY FACTS

Description
A contagious viral infection with mild symptoms and a skin rash.

Causes
A virus spread through the air or by close contact.

Risk factors
Contact with infected people. It can be transmitted to an unborn child by a mother with a rubella infection, causing severe disease in the unborn child (fetus).

Symptoms
There may be fever, headache, runny nose, general discomfort, and a skin rash. When rubella occurs in a pregnant woman, it can cause congenital rubella syndrome with mental and growth retardation in the newborn, as well as other abnormalities.

Diagnosis
Laboratory blood test for rubella antibodies; a nasal or throat swab for viral culture.

Treatments
There is no treatment. Medication may be given to reduce fever. Congenital rubella syndrome requires treatments for any abnormalities.

Pathogenesis
This viral infection usually has mild symptoms that occur over a three-day period. When rubella occurs in a pregnant woman, it may cause severe abnormalities in the infant, such as deafness and mental retardation.

Prevention
Vaccination; isolation of infected people.

Epidemiology
Rubella occurs worldwide.

Prevention and treatments

When a person has a rubella infection, antibodies are made by the body's immune system to fight and kill the rubella virus. These antibodies remain in the blood for years. In the clinical laboratory, testing is available to detect the presence of rubella antibodies in a person's blood, verifying that the person either had been infected with the rubella virus or had received the vaccination available for rubella. If the rubella blood test is negative for antibodies in a woman who wants to become pregnant, she can receive the rubella vaccination to help protect her against contracting the rubella infection. However, she needs to wait one month after she receives the rubella vaccination before becoming pregnant to provide full protection for her baby against the rubella virus. A pregnant woman cannot receive a rubella vaccination during her pregnancy, since it may be harmful to the unborn child. If a pregnant woman has not had a rubella infection or received the rubella vaccination, she must avoid anyone who has or may have rubella.

The rubella vaccination is given as a single preparation, combined with the measles and mumps vaccine. It is referred to as the measles, mumps, and rubella (MMR) vaccine. In some countries, it is a measles, mumps, rubella, and varicella combination vaccine called the MMRV. At least one dose of rubella vaccine, as the combination MMR or MMRV, is usually recommended for all children. The first dose of MMR or MMRV is usually given on or after the first birthday, followed with an additional dose given at age 4 to 6 years, before a child enters school.

A woman of childbearing age who is not pregnant should be immunized with MMR if she has not been immunized previously or had a rubella infection. Rubella is a very safe vaccine. A mild fever or joint pains, or both, are the most common complaints that follow rubella vaccination.

Rubella infection does not require any special treatment. The infected person usually needs a few days of rest at home. Since it is highly contagious, the infected person needs to avoid public places until one week after the rash has disappeared.

Kathleen Becan-McBride

See also
• Chicken pox and shingles • Diphtheria
• Measles • Mumps • Scarlet fever
• Whooping cough

SARS

Severe acute respiratory syndrome, or SARS, is an acute viral infection of the respiratory tract marked by a high fever of more than 100.4°F (38°C). Other symptoms include chills, headache, body aches, dry cough, an overall feeling of discomfort, and diarrhea. Most people infected with the virus develop pneumonia. Some people with SARS will have difficulty breathing and will not be able to get enough oxygen into the blood. About 10 percent of people infected with SARS may die.

A coronavirus called SARS-associated coronavirus (SARS-CoV) is the cause of SARS. This disease was unknown before the first outbreak began in southern China in 2002. It was, however, not reported in the world press until 2003. It developed into the first new serious contagious illness of the twenty-first century. SARS was notable because it spread so rapidly and unexpectedly. Public health efforts contained the disease, and the first epidemic ended in 2003. SARS seems to spread in several different ways. It can spread in the respiratory droplets produced when an infected person sneezes. Like the common cold, it can spread when a person touches an object like a telephone or a doorknob that a person with SARS contaminated from a touch or a sneeze. There is also some suggestion that the virus may travel in the air. This may explain how some buildings seem to be at risk if they have poorly designed sewer systems—air coming from the sewer pipes may carry the virus through the building. People are not at risk to get SARS unless there is an outbreak. If this occurs, then people who have close contact with infected people are at risk. Close contact is defined as being near someone or having direct physical contact.

A diagnosis of SARS is made if the patient has a temperature of more than 100.4°F (38°C), cough, difficulty breathing, pneumonialike symptoms, body aches, and a feeling of general discomfort.

Treatment and prevention

Treatment for SARS is similar to that for viral pneumonia, but people with SARS are treated in isolation. Health care workers have to wear protective equipment, including filter masks. Although antiviral medications and antibiotics have been tried, there is currently no known effective treatment for the infection. SARS is only a concern when an outbreak occurs, when people can take simple steps to reduce the chance of infection. The most important thing is to wash the hands frequently and avoid touching the eyes, nose, or mouth with hands. A disposable tissue should be used to cover the mouth and nose when sneezing.

Pathogenesis and epidemiology

Because people have no immunity to the SARS virus, unless they are treated promptly there is a risk of death, particularly in groups such as the elderly or those who have a compromised immune system.

The cumulative number of cases worldwide from the start of the outbreak in China in November 2002 until December 2003 was just more than 8,000.

Richard Bradley

KEY FACTS

Description
Viral infection of the human respiratory tract.

Causes
Infection by SARS-associated coronavirus.

Risk factors
Direct, close contact with an infected person.

Symptoms
Fever over 100.4°F (38°C), headache, body aches, dry cough, a feeling of discomfort, and pneumonia.

Diagnosis
Lab tests of blood, nasal secretions, or feces.

Treatments
Experimental use of antiviral treatments. No approved treatments are available yet.

Pathogenesis
Humans lack immunity to SARS-CoV, and severe symptoms develop quickly.

Prevention
Hygienic practices such as frequent hand washing and covering one's mouth when sneezing.

Epidemiology
Around 8,000 cases occurred worldwide between November 2002 and December 2003.

See also
- Pneumonia

Scarlet fever

Scarlet fever is an infectious disease caused by streptococcal bacteria. Usually, this infection involves the throat, in which case it is called pharyngitis. In some cases it involves the skin; then it is called impetigo. Symptoms are fever and rash.

Scarlet fever is an illness affecting young persons, mainly children. Cases of this illness have declined over time, even though cases of strep pharyngitis have not undergone similar decreases. Reasons for this are unknown.

Causes and risk factors

Infection of the throat with toxin-producing group A *Streptococcus* (strep) precedes scarlet fever. In some cases, strep infection of the skin leads to scarlet fever. Not everyone who becomes infected with group A *Streptococcus* develops scarlet fever, however. The disease is transmitted through contact with the secretions of someone infected, including respiratory droplets produced by coughing or sneezing. Touching something that has been contaminated with such infectious secretions, followed by touching one's mouth, eyes, or nose, can also cause this illness.

Symptoms and signs

Sore throat, fever, and a bright red, finely textured, and raised rash (sandpaper rash) are most common. With impetigo, the skin sores are red and weeping and then crust over (honey-crusted lesions). On examination, a strep throat infection appears as red, swollen tissue in the back of the throat. White or yellow patches called exudates may be present. The normal bumps on the tongue may become exaggerated (strawberry tongue), and the area surrounding the mouth may appear pale. The creases of the skin may look darker than usual, referred to as Pastia's lines. Other common symptoms include chills, body aches, and headache. Nausea and vomiting may occur. The rash usually starts in the central areas of the body, then spreads over the rest of the body, and persists for several days. Afterward, the skin of the fingertips and toes may peel.

Diagnosis is made by physical exam and a throat culture that tests positive for group A *Streptococcus* or, in the case of impetigo, a culture of skin lesions that tests positive for this organism. Antibiotics such as penicillin are used as treatment. Fever can be treated with acetaminophen. Bed rest and increased fluid intake are recommended. With appropriate treatment, persons are usually cured within about one week.

Pathogenesis, prevention, and epidemiology

For scarlet fever to develop, the strep bacteria must be a strain that produces toxin and the person must be sensitive to this toxin. In a few cases, infection with the bacteria staphylococci can cause scarlet fever. If treated appropriately, complications are rare. Otherwise, complications may include pneumonia, sinusitis, ear infections, inflammation of the kidneys, or rheumatic fever.

Hand washing, avoiding contact with people who have the illness, and avoiding the sharing of drinking cups and eating utensils can prevent this illness. Group A *Streptococcus* infections are very common in the United States; there are about 10 million cases yearly.

Rita Washko

KEY FACTS

Description
Illness consisting of rash and fever.

Cause
Group A *Streptococcus* bacteria.

Risk factors
Contact with infected persons or their airborne droplets created by coughs, sneezes, exhalations.

Symptoms
Fever, sore throat, or skin infection and rash.

Diagnosis
Physical exam and a throat or skin culture that is positive for Group A *Streptococcus*.

Treatments
Antibiotics.

Pathogenesis
If treated appropriately, complications are rare.

Prevention
Frequent hand washing; avoid sharing utensils.

Epidemiology
Once considered a serious threat, the frequency has dropped over time.

See also
• Pneumonia • Throat infections

Schizophrenia

Schizophrenia is one of the most devastating of all the mental illnesses. It is the most common of the psychotic disorders, affecting about 0.5 to 1 percent of the population in the United States. It also presents during late adolescence and early adulthood, a time when individuals are making the transition from adolescence to adulthood. Schizophrenia affects all cultures around the globe equally. As such, it is an illness that can be found described in various writings in many countries throughout history.

The term *schizophrenia* was first coined by Eugen Bleuler in the early 1900s and was not meant to describe a splitting of personalities, which is a common misperception, but rather a splitting of psychic processes. Individuals who are psychotic have a distortion, or a split from reality. This typically takes the form of hallucinations or delusions, which are two of the primary symptoms in schizophrenia.

However, individuals may have no delusions or hallucinations and still receive a diagnosis of schizophrenia. In these cases, other symptoms of schizophrenia predominate, such as a reduction of the emotions seen in facial expressions (affective flattening), withdrawing socially from others, a loss of interest in activities (anhedonia), disorganized or catatonic behavior, and a disruption in the thought processes (thought disorder). This wide diversity of symptoms may be the result of several different causes.

Schizophrenia is an illness that is surrounded by many misconceptions. These misconceptions may have arisen through television shows and movies that have depicted individuals with schizophrenia as having either multiple personalities or psychopathic traits. Individuals with personality or trait disorders have very different symptoms from those with psychotic disorders. There is also a misconception that individuals with schizophrenia are overly aggressive. Although individuals with schizophrenia have engaged in horrible crimes, as is true of individuals without schizophrenia, people tend to perceive them as more aggressive than they really are. This is perhaps due to attempts by some people to avoid prosecution for their crimes by attempting to obtain a diagnosis of schizophrenia in order to plead not guilty by reason of insanity.

Causes and risk factors

Although the actual cause of schizophrenia is not known, it involves both genetic and environmental factors. People are born with certain genes that may put them at risk for developing schizophrenia, but they do not develop the illness without specific environmental influences. It is likely not just one gene or one environmental factor that places an individual at risk, but rather a number of different factors that all contribute in some way to the development of the illness. These differences in the genes and environmental factors account for the variability in the types of symptoms that people experience.

As an example, consider an individual who has a grandmother with schizophrenia and whose mother developed influenza infection while he was developing inside her womb. He had no other difficulties during early childhood and seemed to be no different from any other child. As a teenager he used marijuana and cocaine. Finally, when he was 18 years old, he began to exhibit psychotic symptoms that became worse over eight months until he was brought to the hospital for an evaluation. Both influenza during pregnancy and the use of marijuana in early to mid-adolescence have been shown to increase the risk of schizophrenia. Thus, it is possible that this individual would have never developed schizophrenia if the influenza infection and drug use had never taken place.

To simplify a complex situation, both genes and environmental factors could be considered as a dose. If someone gets a high dose of genes that lead to schizophrenia, then it takes fewer environmental factors to develop the illness. On the other hand, certain genes may be protective; that is, they are protective in spite of the dose of environmental factors. There is still a considerable amount of research to be done to understand the cause of the disorder, and many questions remain unanswered.

Symptoms

The symptoms of schizophrenia have been categorized as either positive and negative symptoms.

Positive symptoms are those symptoms that are expressed outwardly by the individual. These include delusions and hallucinations and disorganized thoughts. Hallucinations commonly include hearing voices, feeling odd sensations, and smelling foul odors. Delusions are exaggerated or distorted beliefs, such as the idea that one is being conspired against or a belief that one has special powers. These can range from the plausible ("The police are trying to kill me") to the

completely implausible ("My parents are aliens who abandoned me on earth when I was a child"). Positive symptoms are more likely to improve with medication, and thus individuals with only positive symptoms do better than those with negative symptoms.

Unlike positive symptoms, which come and go throughout the course of the disease, negative symptoms are often always present. They are also less responsive to medications and are linked to how well one functions in one's environment (for example, greater negative symptoms are associated with greater difficulties in areas such as work and social relationships). Negative symptoms include apathy, a lack of motivation, poverty of speech, inability to experience pleasure, and flattened affect (lack of emotional expressions or response).

Cognitive deficits are also prevalent in people with schizophrenia and are closely tied to the negative symptoms. These deficits include impaired memory and attention and greater difficulty with what are termed *higher order brain functions*. These higher order brain functions include the ability to solve problems and to use abstract reasoning. Since memory, attention, and problem-solving skills are all important for both school and vocation, and since cognitive symptoms are linked to negative symptoms, it is not surprising that individuals with greater negative symptoms tend to have greater difficulties with vocational issues.

Finally, individuals with schizophrenia may have difficulties ordering their thoughts. This is known as a formal thought disorder.

Course of schizophrenia

There are four phases of schizophrenia. These include the pre-illness, the prodromal, the active, and the residual phase. Although individuals will experience all of these phases, the duration in each phase can vary significantly from individual to individual.

Pre-illness phase. During the pre-illness phase, some individuals, but not all, may exhibit minor difficulties with memory, attention, and their motor skills. These symptoms are common in the population, and so most people with deficits in these areas will not go on to develop schizophrenia.

Prodromal phase. *Prodrome* is a term to describe an early symptom of illness that heralds what is yet to come. Symptoms in the prodromal phase are variable and nonspecific. The phase includes symptoms such as worsening academic performance, social withdrawal, attention problems, conduct problems, and difficulties

KEY FACTS

Description
Schizophrenia is a disorder that includes a combination of hallucinations, delusions, disordered thought, lack of motivation, flattening of affect, and disruptions in social functioning. Not all of these symptoms are present in everyone with schizophrenia, and there is considerable variability in the severity of the symptoms.

Causes
The cause of schizophrenia is not yet known. Evidence shows that both genetic and environmental factors play a role in who will get the illness and who will not.

Symptoms
An alteration in a person's thoughts and perceptions, including hallucinations, delusions, and disorders of thought and speech. Cognitive deficits are also commonly associated with schizophrenia.

Diagnosis
The diagnosis of schizophrenia requires a thorough history, physical and neurological examination, laboratory studies, and often imaging studies of the brain.

Treatments
Antipsychotic medications are the mainstay for treating schizophrenia. Supportive therapy and sometimes cognitive behavioral therapy are also important.

Pathogenesis
Psychotic symptoms are related to the brain chemical known as dopamine.

Prevention
There is no direct evidence that schizophrenia can be prevented. Evidence is emerging that avoiding marijuana will reduce the chance of developing schizophrenia.

Epidemiology
Affects 0.5 to 1 percent of the population worldwide. It affects males and females equally, although females have a slightly later age of onset.

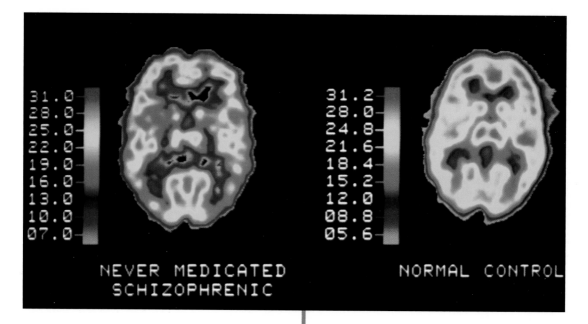

NEVER MEDICATED SCHIZOPHRENIC

NORMAL CONTROL

A positron emission tomography scan shows a horizontal slice of the brain from a normal person (right) and a schizophrenic (left) after a radioactively labeled substance was introduced into the body. In this scan, red shows a high level of activity; blue or purple indicates low levels of activity. The scan reflects the function of tissues rather than the structure.

with hygiene. What is meant by nonspecific is that these symptoms could also be seen in someone who has other illnesses, such as major depression, bipolar affective disorder, or in someone who is actively using drugs. The duration of the prodrome varies from several days to several years.

Active phase. The active phase is the time period when the diagnosis of schizophrenia is made. During the active phase, individuals meet the criteria that are shown in the box on page 758. Normally, an individual with schizophrenia experiences several active stages over the course of his or her life, with periods of relative remission, or a residual period, in between.

Residual phase. The time between active stages is called the residual phase. Although a person may experience low-grade hallucinations and delusions during the residual stage, they often display negative symptoms and cognitive deficits.

Diagnosis

An accurate diagnosis is obtained through a similar approach to that used for psychotic disorders. It is first important to eliminate any nonpsychiatric medical conditions that would have symptoms similar to those seen in schizophrenia. There are several rare conditions that do this, and since the treatments are often quite different from those for schizophrenia, it is important to make sure that tests are done to ensure that these do not account for the symptoms.

Once a nonpsychiatric medical condition is ruled out, schizophrenia is diagnosed by a careful psychiatric

history and examination of the patient's mental status. The criteria that are used during the examination are the same for any age and are shown on page 758. Diagnosis during the prodromal period is very difficult, since the symptoms overlap with other psychiatric disorders.

Once a patient is in the active stage of the illness and it has been determined that the symptoms are not a result of a nonpsychiatric illnesses, the diagnosis is often readily made.

Treatments

The mainstays of treatment for individuals with schizophrenia are the antipsychotic medications. These medications have been widely studied in adults and have been shown to work well in controlling the positive symptoms and thought disorder.

The negative symptoms are more difficult to treat, being less responsive to medications. As individuals are different, not everybody responds equally to the same medication and dose.

Sometimes an individual takes several medications before they find one that works. However, it will soon be possible to test a person's genes and be able to

DIAGNOSTIC CRITERIA FOR SCHIZOPHRENIA FROM THE DSM-IV

There are several characteristic symptoms of schizophrenia, and to make a definitive diagnosis, two or more of the symptoms must each be present for a significant portion of time during a one-month period, or less if the condition has been successfully treated.

Symptoms

Typical symptoms of schizophrenia are: delusions; hallucinations; disorganized speech; grossly disorganized or catatonic behavior; negative symptoms such as affective flattening (lack of emotional response), alogia (lack of speech), or avolition (lack of any motivation).

Making a diagnosis

Only one of the above symptoms is required if the person has delusions that are bizarre or hallucinations that consist of a voice keeping up a running commentary on the person's behavior or thoughts, or two or more voices conversing with each other.

In addition, there must be social or occupational dysfunction, or both; continuous signs of the disturbance persisting for at least 6 months; and evidence to show that the disturbance is not due to the direct physiological effects of a substance, such as a drug of abuse or a medication, or a general medical condition.

determine which medications will be most efficacious. Two different types of therapies have been shown to be helpful in individuals with schizophrenia.

The first therapy, which should be provided to all patients, is supportive psychotherapy. This therapy works to support the patient and often the family in all facets of dealing with the illness and its effects. It involves educating the patient and family early on about the illness and getting them connected to any support systems in the community. It is often helpful for those diagnosed with schizophrenia to meet regularly with their psychiatrist or therapist to discuss the issues and problem solve.

The second type of therapy is called cognitive behavioral therapy. This therapy, which also is useful for those with anxiety and mood disorders, helps the patient understand the distortions in how they perceive things. For example, it will work so that the patient understands that when he hears voices, they are a result of his illness and he should try to ignore them. Since not all patients have insight into their illness, this tends to work best with those who understand that they are ill.

Finally, it is very important that physicians ask whether or not their patients with schizophrenia are having thoughts of harming themselves. Approximately 5 percent of individuals with schizophrenia commit suicide, and those who do are more likely to do so during the first six months of the illness. Those who have insight into their illness seem to be at a greater risk. Also, some individuals with schizophrenia experience auditory hallucinations that tell them to kill themselves. It is important to understand the devastating effects of the perceived stigma of hav-

ing schizophrenia. Such stigma can result from unfair reporting in the media of incidents involving schizophrenic patients. An isolated occurrence may be described as if it were common, which can foster attitudes of intolerance toward, and rejection of, people with mental problems. Because people with schizophrenia find it difficult to find employment or housing, they become socially isolated. Studies in 2005 show that stigma in developed countries is universal, that stigma is attached to mental illness in many different socio-cultural communities worldwide, and that the negative consequences of stigma are increasing.

Epidemiology

Schizophrenia affects approximately 0.5 to 1 percent of the population. If this statistic is extrapolated in a school of 1,000 people, 5 to 10 people in that school will one day develop schizophrenia. The prevalence of schizophrenia is the same in all countries across the globe. Thus, schizophrenia affects an extremely large number of people worldwide.

Males and females are affected equally, although females tend to develop the illness at older ages than males. The disease generally develops in the late teens or early twenties. Onset of schizophrenia prior to the age of 12 is rare, and the incidence increases afterward.

Tonya White

See also

• Bipolar disorder • Depressive disorders
• Personality disorders • Psychotic disorders

SCID

SCID (severe combined immunodeficiency) is a rare disorder in which the immune system's two major weapons against disease—antibodies and T cells—are genetically missing or disabled. Babies born with SCID usually experience multiple and persistent infections, such as pneumonia and oral thrush, and may fail to develop physically at a normal rate.

SCID is a group of inherited disorders distinguished by a lack of immune response. It is the most serious of the primary immunodeficiencies. It occurs when a child lacks lymphocytes (B and T lymphocytes), which are the specialized white blood cells that the body uses to fight infection. During fetal development, lymphocytes are made in the bone marrow. Some lymphocytes move to the thymus gland behind the breastbone, where they become T cells; others remain in the bone marrow to become B cells. Each specialized type of cell is responsible for a particular immune response: T cells attack antigens (microorganisms and foreign substances) and help the body reject unfamiliar tissue. T cells are also needed to trigger the B cells that produce antibodies to fight specific invaders.

There are many causes of SCID. The most common type is that in which the X chromosome harbors a genetic defect; the mechanism that allows T and B cells to receive signals from growth factors is flawed. Since a male child has only one X chromosome inherited from his mother, SCID is more common in males. In females, typically there is one normal X chromosome that compensates for the defective one.

Symptoms of the disorder can vary from mild to life threatening. Typical signs of SCID are an increased vulnerability to infection and failure to grow and gain weight. A baby with SCID may have persistent bacterial, viral, or fungal infections—such as ear infections, sinus infections, mouth thrush, and pneumonia—that may not respond well to treatment. Infants with SCID may also have persistent diarrhea.

Early diagnosis of SCID is uncommon because routine white blood cells counts are not performed on newborns. After multiple infections, if SCID is suspected, T- and B-cell counts are done. SCID can be successfully treated if it is identified early; otherwise, the disease is often fatal within the first year of life. Patients with SCID can be treated with antibiotics and immune serum to protect them from infections, but these treatments cannot cure the disorder. Until recently, SCID eventually ended in death; now, with advances in biomedical research, SCID patients have hopes of surviving much longer. Bone marrow transplantation, if performed early, is an effective treatment for SCID, and it will help rebuild a defective immune system.

Another treatment for SCID is a hematopoietic stem cell transplant. This is a procedure in which blood-forming stem cells (early cells found in the bone marrow where blood cells develop) are placed into the body in the hope that these new cells will help rebuild the immune system.

Rashmi Nemade

KEY FACTS

Description

A rare disorder in which the immune system components are genetically missing or disabled.

Causes

Genetic defects.

Risk factors

Children with a family history of SCID.

Symptoms

Many infections in first few months of life, and persistent diarrhea.

Diagnosis

Positive family history of SCID and blood tests.

Treatments

Bone marrow transplant, special diet, and stem-cell transplantation.

Pathogenesis

Until recently, SCID was always fatal.

Prevention

None, since it is an inherited disease.

Epidemiology

Occurs in approximately 1 in 5,100,000 births and is most common in boys; 50 percent of all cases are linked with the X chromosome.

See also
• Pneumonia

Sexual and gender identity disorders

A sexual dysfunction or disorder can be defined as a problem in someone's desire to engage in sexual activity, or an inability to experience the natural unfolding of the sexual response cycle. Such disorders can cause personal distress or relationship problems. Gender identity disorder is a condition that is characterized by two components. First, the person has a persistent belief that he or she should be, or actually is, a member of the opposite sex. Second, there is a feeling of distress or inappropriateness that the person has about her or his birth sex and the accompanying role, body characteristics, and appearance. Both criteria must be present to establish the diagnosis.

Media bombardment of erotic images and frank discussion of previously taboo topics create the impression that sexual activity in modern society is a well-understood, uncomplicated endeavor. In reality, many people, including those who display no other physical or psychological problems, have distressing sexual dysfunctions. It is very difficult to know precisely how widespread these difficulties are, and estimates vary considerably.

One large survey revealed that 43 percent of women and 31 percent of men reported some form of sexual disturbance in a previous one-year period. Sexual dysfunctions include disorders of desire and disorders of arousal.

Disorders of desire

There are two disorders of desire. The first is hypoactive sexual disorder, a condition that is diagnosed in individuals with little or no interest in sexual activity. It affects approximately 20 percent of women and 10 percent of men.

If a hormone deficiency is thought to be a causative factor, testosterone may be used in treatment. However, the disorder is more often a result of depression, stress, or relationship problems. These disorders require psychotherapeutic treatment.

The other disorder of desire, sexual aversion disorder, is diagnosed in individuals who avoid sexual contact or become anxious when confronted with a

KEY FACTS: GENDER IDENTITY DISORDERS

Description
A disorder in which someone feels that they are, or should be, a member of the opposite sex.

Causes
Thought to be a neurodevelopmental condition in the prenatal brain.

Risk factors
Unknown.

Symptoms
A wish or a belief expressed by a child, at between two and four years of age, that he or she belongs to the other sex. Boys may prefer female role playing and dressing in girls' clothes. Girls may refuse to wear feminine clothes, such as dresses, and reject stereotypical norms, such as playing with dolls or playing house. Adults want to change their appearance to fit in with the other gender.

Diagnosis
Evaluation of symptoms by a psychiatrist.

Treatments
Treatment is largely psycho-educational and focuses on combating the ostracism that is experienced by children who have an identity disorder. Separation anxiety is also a problem that is addressed through treatment.

Pathogenesis
The disorder can emerge when the person is a child or it may not present itself until the person is adult.

Prevention
There is no known way of preventing gender identity disorders.

Epidemiology
Because many cases are not reported, in the mistaken belief that a child will grow out of wanting to change gender, it is not known how many people have this condition. It is estimated that transsexualism occurs in 1 in 30,000 genetic males and 1 in 100,000 females.

sexual situation. This dysfunction is usually caused by emotional problems. In women it can result from a previous traumatic incident such as rape or incest. In men it may reflect guilt about sexuality if the individual has a family background in which sexual behavior was considered shameful.

The disorder ranges in intensity from mild to severe. Therapy is aimed at unmasking the cause of the disorder and tailoring therapeutic interventions to extinguish conditioned responses. Without treatment, disorders of desire may persist for a lifetime.

Disorders of arousal

This class of disorders is characterized by an inability to attain the pleasurable sensation and accompanying physiological accommodation that is required for sexual activity. Female sexual arousal disorder is characterized by a lack of adequate vaginal lubrication. Male erectile disorder is the inability to maintain an erection to complete sexual activity. These disorders, which often result from fears about sexual performance or depression, need to be distinguished from those caused by medical problems.

Treatment for arousal disorders begins with a complete sexual history to determine the cause of the disorder. Many cases of infertility occur in marriages where disorders of arousal prevent insemination.

Following normal arousal, some women may be persistently unable to reach orgasm. If this causes personal distress or relationship problems, female orgasmic disorder is diagnosed. This appears to be more prevalent in younger women and may be lifelong. For men, an inability or recurrent delay in reaching orgasm may be situational.

Premature ejaculation refers to orgasm and ejaculation in men that occurs with little sexual stimulation and before the person is ready. It is thought to be caused by both psychological and physiological factors. Some men have this problem early in life but then learn to delay orgasm. Good therapeutic outcomes for premature ejaculation have been reported with certain types of antidepressant medications that target serotonin receptors.

Another category of sexual dysfunction, sexual pain disorder, is characterized by pain that occurs during sexual intercourse. Dyspareunia refers to genital pain, ranging from mild to severe. Little is known about sexual pain disorder or its cause. In men, the cause is usually a physical one, although in rare cases, there can be a psychological cause. If no physical problem can be discovered, such as prostate infection,

then it is presumed to be a symptom of guilt about sexual behavior.

Vaginismus is a condition in which females involuntarily contract the muscles surrounding the vagina, so that they go into painful spasms. This can happen before or after penetration, which, in mild cases, causes tightness and discomfort, and, in severe cases, prevents penetration. The disorder usually has a sudden onset and may follow a sexual trauma (such as abuse or rape) or a first gynecological exam. Vaginal inflammation can lead to vaginismus because intercourse is painful. If not treated by teaching the patient techniques to relax the paravagina muscles, the disorder can persist for a lifetime.

Disorders of sexual desire or sexual arousal can also result from medical conditions, certain prescription drugs, intoxication, or substance abuse.

Paraphilias

Paraphilias are conditions in which a person fantasizes or acts out a sexual desire that is atypical, extreme, or inappropriate. The focus of the paraphilia can be an object, children, or other nonconsenting participants, or the suffering or humiliation of oneself or a partner. The paraphilias cause personal distress, relationship problems, or constitute criminal activity. For some, images of the arousing topic are necessary for sexual activity. Others with paraphilias can sometimes function sexually without the paraphiliac stimulation. The object or stimulus may be very specific. Some people hire prostitutes to act out fantasies, or own collections of objects that they find sexually arousing.

As people generally do not admit to having paraphilias, the disorders are much more prevalent than can be deduced from estimates taken from medical or legal settings. It is not known what causes paraphilias to develop, but they usually begin in early adolescence and tend to be lifelong. Stress may increase the intensity of the paraphilia. These disorders are almost never diagnosed in women. The most common of the paraphilias are listed here.

Exhibitionism describes the exposure of the genitals to an unwitting stranger, typically a female or a child, although no attempt at sexual activity with the stranger is involved. For the exhibitionist, the thought of startling or shocking the observer is sexually arousing. This behavior usually begins in the mid-twenties. Exhibitionists comprise about 30 percent of criminal sex offenders. The behavior is chronic, and many exhibitionists have been arrested multiple times.

Fetishism is a disorder in which a person focuses on

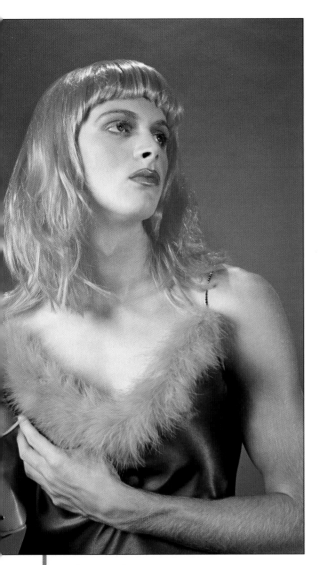

A young man is made up as a woman and dressed in a woman's clothes for his performance on stage as a transvestite artist. Men who entertain in this way at cabarets and discotheques are often called drag queens.

ed places, such as a subway or theater, where a quick escape is possible. This paraphilia typically develops at puberty and wanes in adulthood.

Pedophilia refers to the desire to engage in sexual activity with a child. The pedophile can be attracted to boys or girls, or both, and usually prefers preteens. The range of activities in which the pedophile engages or fantasizes about varies. For some, it may consist of looking at naked children, or exposing themselves, or both, to a child while masturbating. Other pedophiles use force to engage in sexual acts with children. Treatment for this disorder is multifaceted and may involve court-mandated administration of anti-androgenic substances to reduce sexual arousal patterns.

Sexual masochism is a paraphilia in which pain or humiliation and the psychological or physical suffering that ensues create sexual excitement. For some, this may only involve fantasizing about being overpowered during sex. Such fantasies develop early, often in childhood.

However, for others, sexual masochism involves aggressive acts undertaken alone or with a partner. These can include enlisting someone to shock them, whip them, clothe them in diapers, urinate on them, or perform other demeaning or abusive acts. Individuals with this disorder repeat the same masochistic act. Injuries and deaths have occurred as a result of acting out such urges.

Sexual sadism is a chronic disorder that usually begins in early adulthood. With this disorder, a person derives sexual pleasure from inflicting abuse or pain on someone else. In some cases, the partner may be a sexual masochist who consents to the abuse. However, if the partner is nonconsenting, he or she may be injured or killed as a result of the attack. Individuals who attack nonconsenting victims tend to escalate the intensity of the pain they inflict over time, until they are apprehended.

Transvestic fetishism is an urge by a heterosexual male to wear women's clothing and fantasize that he is a female during a sex act. Some men have a cache of clothes that they keep for this purpose; others may use a single item of clothing, such as female undergarments. The behavior usually first appears at puberty and may vary in intensity throughout a lifetime.

For some men, the condition becomes less erotic after puberty, but still creates the desired feeling of tension reduction. Men who cross-dress do not necessarily have other psychiatric problems or seek treatment; they may have spouses who are comfortable with the behavior. For others, however, the feeling may

an object in order to generate sexual arousal. The object or "fetish" is typically an item of women's clothing, such as an apron, underpants, shoes, or boots. Men with such fetishes often need a partner to wear the garment in order to engage in sexual activity. Fetishism is chronic, and the object that is the focus has a special meaning to the individual, perhaps dating back to early childhood.

Frotteurism is a paraphilia wherein an individual derives sexual gratification from rubbing against or fondling a stranger. These acts usually occur in crowd-

escalate into gender identity disorder, a desire to be a member of the opposite sex.

Voyeurism, often referred to as "peeping," is diagnosed when, in order to create sexual arousal, a man must engage in spying on unsuspecting persons who are either undressing or having sex. Voyeurism usually begins in adolescence or early adulthood. It often results in arrest.

Gender identity disorder

The condition of gender identity disorder is differentiated from gender issues that arise in intersexed persons (who are born with some aspects of both sexes, anatomically or hormonally). Cultures differ in what they deem as appropriate for males and females. Persons who stray from the cultural guidelines are considered gender nonconforming. But gender nonconformity does not constitute gender dysphoria, that is, the belief that one would be better suited as a member of the opposite sex or the feeling that one is "trapped in the wrong body."

Gender identity disorder in children

Children who show distress about being a boy or a girl usually alarm their parents. The first evidence of their gender-variant behavior usually appears between two and four years of age. These children state a wish to be a member of, or the belief that they belong to, the other sex.

For boys, female role-playing and dressing up in girls' clothing is a preferred activity. They avoid rough-and-tumble play, and choose girls as playmates.

Girls with the disorder may state that they will grow a penis. They refuse to wear dresses or engage in any gender-stereotypical activities, such as playing with dolls or playing house.

Gender identity disorder in childhood is rare, and experts do not know how frequently it occurs. Since many parents think the behavior is just a "phase" that the child will outgrow, and few clinics treat this condition, many children with the disorder never come to the attention of professionals. About 75 percent will grow up to have a homosexual orientation but will not have gender identity disorder in adulthood.

Treatment for children who do present to professionals is largely psycho-educational and involves the parents, who can help the child counteract the ostracism that inevitably accompanies this disorder. These children often have other problems, such as separation anxiety. This manifests as feelings of great distress when a child is separated from his or her parents for any reason. The symptoms are holding onto the parent and crying. This behavior is common until the age of about four years, but it diminishes after that. In separation anxiety disorder, the child exhibits clinging behavior that is not usual for the age of the child. Physical symptoms can ensue, such as problems sleeping and headaches. Separation anxiety is addressed during treatment.

Gender identity disorder in adults

With adults, gender identity disorder may have started in childhood. These individuals are preoccupied with changing their appearance to reduce the incongruence between the gender with which they identify and aspire to and the body and sexual gender into which they were born.

Men who want to be women and women who want to be men have existed throughout history and are often referred to as transsexuals. It is estimated that transsexualism occurs in 1 in 30,000 genetic males and 1 in 100,000 females. Some experts believe that the disorder is caused, at least in part, by a neurodevelopmental condition in the prenatal brain.

Psychotherapy alone is not effective in reversing a cross-gender identity. In severe cases of gender identity disorder, a person may be eligible for a program of hormones and genital surgery to reassign the gender.

Some men have a less severe degree of the disorder, wishing to remain male while they occasionally appear as female. These individuals may not be interested in genital surgery, but may desire some feminizing procedures, such as beard removal, to eliminate secondary sex characteristics and avoid detection when appearing in public. Cross-dressers, as such men are called, tend to experience an intensification of the cross-gender longings when they are under stress, or following a major loss or trauma in life. If such urges are accompanied by erotic arousal and masturbation, then a diagnosis of transvestic fetishism is made. If the motive for appearing feminine comes from a desire to express one's sense of a female identity and is not erotically focused, then a diagnosis of gender identity disorder is appropriate.

Randi Ettner

See also
• Prostate disorders • Sleep disorders

Shock

Shock is a life-threatening state of an inadequate volume of blood circulating around the body. There is insufficient delivery of oxygen and nutrients to body tissues. There are four major categories of shock: cardiogenic, hypovolemic, distributive, and obstructive.

Cardiogenic shock is caused by the failure of the heart to pump effectively. Hypovolemic shock involves loss of fluid, usually blood. Septic, anaphylactic, and neurogenic shock are types of distributive shock, characterized by insufficient circulating volume due to vasodilation and leaky capillaries. Obstructive shock is caused by conditions that prevent blood flow to or from the heart. Sepsis is caused by overwhelming infection. Anaphylaxis results from severe allergic reactions; neurogenic shock is a consequence of spinal cord damage. In cardiac tamponade, fluid fills the sac around the heart. In tension pneumothorax, air progressively accumulates between the lung and chest wall. A blood clot obstructs lung vessels in pulmonary embolism. Hardening and narrowing of the aortic valve leads to aortic stenosis. Endocrine shock can result from thyroid dysfunction or adrenal insufficiency.

All forms of shock can result in dry mouth, rapid respiration, restlessness, hypothermia, hypotension, unconsciousness, and low urine output. In hypovolemic shock there is a faint, rapid pulse with cool, clammy skin. In cardiogenic and obstructive shock there may be distended neck veins from fluid backup. In septic shock there may be fever and warm extremities. In neurogenic shock there may be a normal or low heart rate and paralysis. In anaphylactic shock there may be rash, breathlessness, and airway swelling.

A careful history and physical exam are essential to recognize the type of shock. Ancillary testing and treatment depend on the causes of shock. Most forms of shock require intravenous fluids, then medications to support blood pressure. A breathing tube may be needed to support respiration. Chest pain, palpitations, and shortness of breath suggest cardiogenic shock. A myocardial infarction needs clot-breaking medication or angioplasty. A cardiac valve may need surgical repair. Profuse bleeding and major trauma suggest hypovolemic shock; blood replacement and surgery are indicated to stop the bleeding. Fever and infection suggest septic shock, requiring antibiotics. An insect sting or allergen exposure with airway swelling indicates anaphylactic shock, calling for antihistamines, steroids, and epinephrine. Paralysis after trauma suggests neurogenic shock. Tension pneumothorax requires needle decompression, then a chest tube. Cardiac tamponade necessitates fluid drainage from the pericardium by a needle or catheter. Massive pulmonary embolism may require clot-breaking medications or surgical clot removal.

There are four stages of shock: initial, compensatory, progressive, and refractory. Initially the lack of oxygen leads to anaerobic metabolism and metabolic acidosis, then hyperventilation and adrenaline release attempt to compensate for the hypoxia and hypotension. Elevated heart rate, low urine output, and cool extremities ensue as the body struggles to maintain blood flow to critical organs. In progressive shock, there is inadequate blood flow to vital organs, acid-base balance is disturbed, and fluid accumulates peripherally. In refractory shock, vital organs fail, and shock is no longer reversible. Brain damage will be present, and death is imminent. The outcome of shock depends on the cause and concurrent problems. Hypovolemic, anaphylactic, neurogenic, obstructive, and endocrine shock respond to treatment in their early stages. Septic shock has a mortality rate of 30 to 50 percent. The prognosis of cardiogenic shock is worse.

Medley O'Keefe Gatewood

KEY FACTS

Description
Hypoperfusion of bodily tissues and organs.

Causes
Cardiogenic, hypovolemic, distributive, obstructive, and endocrine.

Signs
Hypotension, hyperventilation, altered consciousness, low urine output.

Diagnosis
History and clinical exam.

Treatment
Varies with the type of shock.

Pathogenesis
All are treatable early, except for cardiogenic and septic shock, which carry a grave prognosis.

See also
• Allergy and sensitivity

Sick building syndrome

Sick building syndrome describes a disorder in which individuals experience acute problems with their health or well-being that are associated with the amount of time spent in a particular building, but no specific illness or cause can be identified.

Sick building syndrome is characterized by symptoms that affects clusters of people from the same building. The symptoms will improve or disappear once the affected individuals leave the building. Investigators often believe that inadequate ventilation is the cause of sick building syndrome. This may occur when HVAC (heating, ventilation, and air conditioning) systems do not bring enough fresh air into the building. Designed to conserve energy, some buildings have HVAC systems that introduce only one-third of the recommended amount of fresh air. Another possible cause may be chemical contaminants that come from either indoor or outdoor sources. These may come from adhesives, carpets, furniture, copy machines, pesticides, cleaning agents, and volatile organic compounds. Environmental tobacco smoke and products of combustion (usually from furnaces) may also be part of the problem. Other sources may include motor vehicle exhaust, plumbing vents, and smells from kitchens or shops in the building.

Biological contaminants such as bacteria, mold, pollen, and viruses may also be factors. In many cases, sick building syndrome affects the entire building, but in other locations, it will affect only certain parts of the building.

The World Health Organization states that up to 30 percent of new and remodeled buildings around the world may cause occupants to complain of sick building syndrome. Some studies suggest that psychosocial factors may be equally or more important than the physical factors present in the building. For example, one study showed a relationship between the presence of sick building symptoms and both psychosocial stress at work and the amount of control over one's work environment. This study suggested that such factors as the inability to open the windows or control humidity or temperature lead to an increased incidence of symptoms. There was also a direct correlation between the amount of on-the-job stress and the prevalence of symptoms.

The symptoms of sick building syndrome include: headaches; eye, nose, and throat irritation; dry cough; dry or itchy skin; dizziness; nausea; difficulty in concentrating; fatigue; and sensitivity to odors. These problems usually improve when the person leaves the building. Sick building syndrome can be difficult to resolve, since engineers and building managers must focus on the building and not on the patient. Managers may replace water-damaged carpet and ceilings or eliminate any mold. They may prohibit smoking and improve ventilation where there are adhesives, paint, or solvents. Repairing HVAC systems or increasing ventilation rates will help. Some building owners have added high-performance air cleaners to their HVAC systems. Open communications with the building occupants are needed to educate them about efforts to resolve the situation.

Richard N. Bradley

KEY FACTS

Description
People in buildings are sick for no known reason.

Causes
Unclear, but it may be poor building ventilation, contaminants, or workplace stress.

Risk Factors
Working in large, energy-efficient buildings.

Symptoms
Headache, eye, nose, or throat irritation, cough, dry or itchy skin, dizziness, nausea, difficulty concentrating, fatigue, and sensitivity to odors.

Diagnosis
Elimination of other possible causes of symptoms.

Treatments
Increased ventilation, air cleaning, removal of pollutant source, education, and communication.

Pathogenesis
Unknown.

Prevention
Careful construction of new buildings.

Epidemiology
One in five workers may have some symptoms.

See also
• Allergy and sensitivity • Throat infections

Sickle-cell anemia

Sickle-cell anemia (SCA) is a severe genetic illness characterized by the production of sickle-shaped blood cells because of an abnormality of hemoglobin (HbS), leading to chronic anemia and vaso-occlusive crises.

SCA follows an autosomal-recessive mode of inheritance. The parents are usually unaffected carriers of the abnormal gene. Couples in which both partners carry the sickle-cell trait have a 25 percent probability of conceiving a child (heterozygote) with SCA.

Risk factors and symptoms

Certain risk factors for SCA have been identified; most important is the percentage contribution of sickle-cell hemoglobin (HbS) in the blood.

Patients with SCA have moderate to severe anemia, although red cell volume is generally normal. Many SCA patients suffer from chronic bone pain. The most common clinical presentation of SCA is a sickle-cell crisis: the blocking of small blood vessels, caused by sickle-shaped red cells clumping together. Occlusion of capillaries leads to painful microinfarcts (obstructions). Common sites include bone, spleen, and lung, the latter resulting in a dramatic acute chest crisis. There is another possible complication in younger children, in which the spleen acutely pools large volumes of blood (splenic sequestration syndrome), causing a drop in hemoglobin levels and circulatory failure. A feared sequel of SCA is stroke, which can occur at any age. Severe systemic infections with encapsulated bacteria, as a result of impaired function of the spleen and salmonella osteomyelitis (favored by dead areas in bone), are a significant problem.

Diagnosis and treatments

The diagnosis is made from a blood sample by hemoglobin (Hb) electrophoresis. In this assay, the different Hb species are separated in a gel based on their electrical charge. Instead of the normal HbA band, SCA patients have HbS. Bone marrow studies show increased erythropoiesis (production of red blood cells).

The mainstay of SCA treatment is pain control and prevention of sickle cell crises and other severe aftereffects of SCA. Behavioral recommendations aim at prevention of hypoxia (lack of oxygen to the body's tissues) by avoidance of cold environments, high altitude and overexertion, and prevention of dehydration, by maintaining high fluid intake, particularly during febrile illnesses, hot weather, or exercise. Parents are taught to check the spleen in their young children for enlargement. Daily folate is recommended for all patients. All patients should receive immunizations against encapsulated bacteria (*Streptococcus pneumoniae*, *Hemophilus influenzae* type B, and *Neisseria meningitides*). Children up to 5 years of age also receive daily

KEY FACTS

Description
Chronic anemia and recurrent painful crises due to inborn defect of hemoglobin.

Causes
Inheritance as an autosomal recessive trait.

Risk factors
The sickle cell mutation is prevalent in equatorial Africa, the Mediterranean, the Middle East, and India. In the United States, 95 percent of sickle-cell anemia patients are African American.

Symptoms
Chronic anemia and pain, acute painful "sickle cell crises," splenic sequestration syndrome, bacterial sepsis, chronic organ damage (spleen, kidney, heart, eye), leg ulcers, stroke.

Diagnosis
Blood test; hemoglobin electrophoresis.

Treatments
Folate, pain medication, hydroxyurea, prevention of infections and sickle-cell crises, erythrocyte transfusion, bone marrow transplantation, induction of fetal hemoglobin, experimental therapies.

Pathogenesis
Anemia results from decreased life span of sickle-shaped red blood cells, which occlude capillaries and block oxygen and nutrient supply. The result is pain and tissue infarction.

Prevention
Neonatal screening for hemoglobin diseases is performed in most federal states. Prenatal diagnosis is possible. Prevention of crises uses behavioral and pharmacological measures.

Epidemiology
In African Americans in the United States, the frequency is approximately 1 in 600 newborns. More than 70,000 people in the United States are afflicted with sickle-cell disease.

prophylactic penicillin. Low doses of the cancer drug hydroxyurea halve the amount of pain and the frequency of hospitalizations, reduce the number of blood transfusions, and elevate the amount of hemoglobin in the blood, with generally few adverse effects. The mechanism of action is not clear, but induction of fetal hemoglobin may play a role. Sickle-cell clinics address the specific medical needs of these patients.

Acute pain crises require treatment with strong analgesics, generally morphine or derivatives, alone or with anti-inflammatory agents. Oxygen is administered to patients with compromised respiratory function. Bacterial infections can take a more severe course in SCA patients and require aggressive treatment. Antibiotics and intravenous fluids are often required. Patients with severe anemia, with aplastic crises (lack of development of blood cells), and with splenic sequestration syndrome require red blood cell transfusions. Regular transfusions are indicated for individuals at high risk for cerebral stroke.

Bone marrow transplantation is the only cure for SCA. Because of its toxicity, transplantation is currently reserved for high-risk people who have an optimal donor, usually a matched but healthy sibling. Gene therapy is considered a potential emerging cure for SCA; studies are ongoing.

Pathogenesis

Normal hemoglobin is a molecule made up of four protein subunits, two alpha chains and two beta chains. A mutation of the beta globin gene leads to replacement of the amino acid glutamine for valine. This forms hemoglobin S, called HbS rather than the normal HbA. HbS is principally functional, in that it is stable and can carry oxygen. However, HbS molecules form large homopolymers in red cells, and cells containing such HbS aggregates are misshapen. Instead of the normal donut shape, they assume a sickle shape. Some sickle cells are present at all times and are removed by the spleen, leading to decreased erythrocyte survival (10 to 20 days, as opposed to 120 days for normal cells) and anemia. Under conditions of decreased oxygen tension (high altitude, cold, increased oxygen consumption due to exercise or fever) or dehydration, critical numbers of sickle erythrocytes form at the same time, resulting in vaso-occlusive pain crises: the abnormally shaped erythrocytes cannot squeeze through capillary blood vessels. Instead, they clog the capillaries or damage the vessel lining, or both, leading to sticking of inflammatory cells, which contributes to blockage of capillaries. Areas of tissue behind the oc-

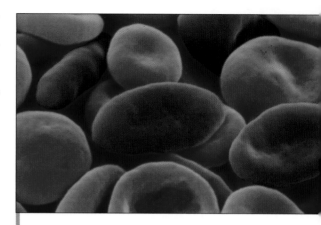

The shape of red blood cells in sickle-cell anemia changes; the normal cells are red and the distorted cells are shown in green. They become fragile and take on a sickle shape.

clusion are deprived of oxygen and nutrients, resulting in tissue death (infarct) and pain. Sickle cells chronically damage kidneys, heart, spleen, bone, skin, eyes, brain, and essentially any other organ in the body.

Prevention and epidemiology

All individuals should be informed about their carrier status prior to making reproductive choices. Genetic counseling is advised for couples in which both partners carry pathological hemoglobin genes. Prenatal diagnostic is possible.

In the United States, 95 percent of SCA patients are African American. In this population, the heterozygote frequency is approximately 1 in 12, and 1 in 600 children is born with SCA. Thus over 70,000 people in the United States are affected by SCA and other, rarer sickle-cell diseases. In some West African countries, more than 1 in 50 children are born with SCA. The high frequency of the mutation may be due to the fact that erythrocytes containing HbS are resistant to malaria. The survival advantage from malaria resistance must have been enormous, since endemic malaria drove Darwinian selection of HbS carriers despite the fact that HbS homozygotes used to die early in infancy. In the United States, which has no malaria, sickle-cell trait is not advantageous, and HbS heterozygote frequency in the United States is decreasing.

Halvard Boenig

See also
• Anemia • Malaria • Stroke and related disorders

SIDS

Sudden infant death syndrome (SIDS) is the abrupt and unexpected death of an infant less than one year of age that remains unexplained after a thorough investigation, including performance of a complete autopsy, review of the circumstances of death, and the clinical history. SIDS (also called crib death) is the leading cause of infant mortality between one month and one year of age in the United States. Many factors have been associated with an increased risk of SIDS, including the infant's sleeping position and exposure to tobacco smoke.

Each year, more than 4,500 infants in the United States die suddenly with no evidence of an obvious cause. This sudden and apparently unexplained loss of life in a normal-appearing infant can be difficult for the baby's parents and family to deal with. A great amount of emotional energy is spent trying to find any clue that would suggest a reason for this loss of life, with parents blaming themselves, their partners, or other caregivers, such as baby sitters. Fortunately, the rate of fatal child abuse (filicide) represents only a minority of these cases when fully evaluated.

The current rate of SIDS in the United States is less than 1 in 1,000 live births. This rate represents a significant decrease in the rate of SIDS and is related to lower rates of maternal smoking during pregnancy, but it is mainly a result of the Back-to-Sleep program. In 1992 the American Academy of Pediatrics issued a recommendation that infants always be placed on their back for sleeping. This measure, along with increasing public awareness campaigns, has minimized the incidence of this devastating problem for families.

About 90 percent of SIDS cases occur before 6 months of age. The median age at death is 11 weeks, with a peak incidence between 2 to 4 months. Interestingly, in premature infants, the median age is 4 to 6 weeks sooner than in full-term infants, using postconception dating criteria. This unique distribution suggests that critical stages of development or maturation after birth are more likely to lead to SIDS. A recent multicenter study by National Institute of Child Health and Human Development concluded that there are no strong predictors that would permit screening for infants at high-risk for SIDS. But numerous similarities between infants succumbing to SIDS have been noted.

Causes and risk factors

The association between exposure to tobacco smoke and SIDS has been known since the 1950s. But public awareness campaigns of this fact have been slow until recently. Maternal smoking during pregnancy and tobacco smoke exposure in the home or day care environment increase the risk of SIDS two- to four-fold. This risk of SIDS appears to increase with the amount of tobacco smoke to which the child is exposed. This finding has led many researchers and educators to label tobacco use one of the most current preventable risk factors for SIDS.

Many infants dying of SIDS have been found when they did not wake up, leading researchers to investigate napping and nighttime rest for possible causes. Co-sleeping, the bed and bedding, and clothing have been implicated in numerous studies. Prone (sleeping on the stomach) or side sleeping (particularly in an infant unaccustomed to sleeping on his or her side or stomach) has an increased risk of SIDS. Although babies need to lie on their stomach to strengthen the shoulder girdle, this position should only be allowed when the child is awake and someone is available to watch the baby.

Co-sleeping involves parents or other siblings sleeping in the same space as the infant. The concern is that the larger person would roll on top of or pull bedding over an infant who could not pull them out of the way, leading to suffocation of the infant. Conflicting studies have been noted between parents co-sleeping with the infant in bed, although the risk appears greatest while co-sleeping on a couch or sofa. The risk of SIDS is lower when the infant sleeps in a separate bed in the parent's room, but this reduced risk is not seen when sharing another sibling's room in different beds.

Likewise, the surface the infant sleeps on or clothing has been implicated in SIDS deaths. Soft sleep surfaces, such as soft mattresses, sheepskin, or polystyrene-filled cushions, have all been associated with a twofold increased risk of SIDS. The crib, or cradle, should always be kept clear of soft objects such as pillows and stuffed toys. Overheating the room in which the infant sleeps should be avoided by maintaining the room temperature at a comfortable level for a lightly clothed infant (65°F–68°F; 18.3°C–20°C). Infants should not sleep in the direct sunlight or near a source of heat such as a heater or radiator. A sixfold increased rate of SIDS has been reported in certain Northern Plains Native American communities when two or more layers of clothing are used on sleeping infants.

Other factors that have been associated with SIDS include gestational age, birth weight, and ethnicity. Preterm infants have a three- to fourfold increased risk of SIDS compared to infants born at term. Low birth weight or growth-restricted infants also are noted to have a higher risk of SIDS. African Americans and Native Americans have a two- to threefold higher rate of SIDS compared to Caucasian people in the United States.

The role of genetics in the cause of SIDS is unclear. The risk of SIDS in fellow siblings is noted to represent a five to six times increased incidence (this still totals less than 1 percent using current prevention strategies). The identification of certain gene polymorphisms (different types of the same gene) in certain SIDS cases would suggest a possible genetic role, but the low incidence of SIDS in both twins and the lack of difference in the rate of SIDS between same sex and different sex twins suggest that genetics may play a lesser role as a cause of these unexplained deaths.

Many other factors have been evaluated as risk factors or causes of SIDS. Maternal drug abuse during and after pregnancy has been associated with a fivefold increase in the risk. Sleep apnea—a sleeping disorder in which a person transiently stops breathing—is more commonly seen in premature infants. The Collaborative study from the National Institutes of Health (NIH) on SIDS showed a slightly higher percentage of mothers with infants that died from SIDS recalling an episode of the baby turning blue compared to control infants. Immunizations and pacifier use have not been associated with an increased risk of SIDS and may actually decrease the risks in infants during the first year of life.

Symptoms and diagnosis

SIDS cases need to be differentiated from other causes of infant death that can mimic or are similar to unexpected demise in an otherwise normal and healthy appearing baby. Other causes of death that need to be

KEY FACTS

Description

Sudden infant death syndrome (SIDS) is defined as the sudden, unexpected death of an infant less than one year of age, with onset of a fatal episode apparently occurring during sleep that remains unexplained after a thorough investigation, including a complete autopsy and review of the circumstances of death and the clinical history.

Causes

The current "triple-risk hypothesis" states that SIDS occurs when three events happen in an infant simultaneously: 1) an underlying vulnerability in control (most likely the central nervous system); 2) a critical developmental period (maturation of the nervous system); and 3) a stressor (such as infection or tobacco smoke).

Risk factors

While many factors have been identified as associated with SIDS, common factors including young maternal age, ethnicity (less common in Caucasians), minimal or no prenatal care, preterm birth or low birth weight, and male gender have all been associated with an increased risk of SIDS. Other factors associated with SIDS include tobacco use during pregnancy or after birth around the child, sleeping position (prone), overheating, and sleeping on a soft surface.

Diagnosis

By definition, SIDS can only be diagnosed after no apparent cause of death is found after thorough evaluation of the death scene, review of the clinical history, and careful autopsy in infants less than one year of age.

Treatments

As no treatment is available after infant death, current strategies focus on prevention of SIDS.

Pathogenesis

SIDS occurs in otherwise normal-appearing infants. Delayed maturation of the central nervous system and abnormal development of the arcuate nucleus have been used in the triple-risk hypothesis to help explain why certain infants die of SIDS.

Prevention

Current strategies to prevent SIDS have successfully focused on modifiable risks, including sleeping position (Back-to-Sleep), smoking cessation during pregnancy and around the infant, avoiding overheating, and attention to providing a safe sleeping environment. There is no evidence that the use of home monitors to prevent SIDS in infants with apnea decreases the risk.

Epidemiology

The rate of SIDS in the United States is about 0.56 in 1,000 live births, with a median age at death of 11 weeks.

PREVENTING SIDS

To prevent or minimize the risk of SIDS, the following measures should always be applied. Infants should always be placed on their back (face up) when resting, sleeping, or left alone. Infants who are used to sleeping on their back are more susceptible to SIDS when sleeping on their stomachs for the first or occasional times. Everyone who cares for the child should be aware of the best position, including babysitters, friends, and grandparents. The baby should sleep on a firm surface or on a mattress that fits snugly in the crib's frame. Do not allow soft (pillows, stuffed toys such as teddy bears, or bumpers) or loose bedding in the same area that the baby is sleeping in and do not allow him or her to sleep on chairs, sofas, or waterbeds. Dress the infant in clothes appropriate for the room temperature instead of covering with a blanket. Never smoke or allow others to smoke in a room in which the infant plays, eats, or sleeps. A clean, dry pacifier may be used when placing the infant to sleep.

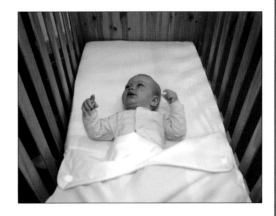

The safest position for a baby in a crib is to lie on his or her back with the feet at the end of the crib so that it is impossible for him or her to move downward and get under the bedcovers.

evaluated include infection, congenital birth defects, congenital metabolic disorders, accidental or intentional suffocation or strangulation, poisoning, obstruction of the respiratory tract, accidental falls, neglect, abandonment, and other maltreatment syndromes, assault and homicide, and other symptoms, signs, and abnormal clinical and laboratory findings. Essential components of this evaluation would include a complete autopsy, assessment of the area of death, and review of the infant and family history. Adjuncts to this evaluation could include a full skeletal survey, assessment of the infant's blood and body fluids for possible infection, metabolic derangement, genetic studies, and toxicology screen. Careful evaluation in the case of apparent SIDS can identify a cause of death in 15 to 20 percent of cases after autopsy in an otherwise normal-appearing but dead infant.

Pathogenesis

The autopsy findings noted in SIDS cases have several common features. None of these features would be considered significant enough by themselves to provide a plausible explanation for the demise of the infant. Infants that die from SIDS are typically normal appearing in size and weight. There is also typically blood-tinged frothy fluid around the child's nostrils. Examination of the internal body on autopsy include congestion of the lungs and small focal areas of bleeding on the inside of the chest.

The triple-risk hypothesis has been proposed to explain the susceptibility of certain infants to SIDS. This triple-risk hypothesis suggests that infants can have a predisposing condition (genetic predisposition or development of the brain tissue), which is triggered by an inciting event such as caused by tobacco-smoke exposure or an infection at a vulnerable time in the development of the infant. Researchers have noted a delay in the maturation of certain portions of the brain, along with a specific change in a portion of the brain called the arcuate nucleus, in infants who have died from SIDS. This area of the brain appears to help in the regulation of the respiratory system. Certain receptors in the ventral portion of the arcuate nucleus are markedly reduced in greater than 50 percent of the SIDS infants.

Interestingly, the peak incidence of SIDS occurs during a period of time when the significant changes are happening in infants' sleeping patterns and the controlling mechanisms for the heart and the lungs. Several recent reports have suggested that cardiac dysfunction or mutations in cardiac channels, a condition called long QT syndrome, may also be seen more frequently in infants who have died from SIDS.

Brian Brost

See also
• Sleep disorders

Sinusitis

Sinusitis is an infection or inflammation of the paranasal sinuses. Viral, bacterial, and fungal infections, as well as allergic reactions, can cause sinusitis. Conditions that obstruct the sinuses, including infections, allergies, and nasogastric tubes, predispose patients to sinusitis.

Sinuses are hollow air cavities located in the skull or bones surrounding the nose. All the sinuses have an opening into the nose for the free exchange of air and mucus and are lined by a continuous mucous membrane. Acute sinusitis lasts for four weeks or less; chronic sinusitis usually last up to eight weeks, but can continue for months or even years.

Acute sinusitis is caused by *Streptococcus pneumoniae*, *Hemophilus influenzae*, and other organisms and is often precipitated by a common cold or other viral respiratory infection that causes swollen mucous membranes to obstruct the sinuses. Sometimes fungal infection can cause acute sinusitis in people whose immune system is not functioning properly. Allergic rhinitis is another common cause of sinusitis.

Chronic sinusitis is usually caused by inflammation, not infection, although colonizing bacteria can make it worse. Typically, a prolonged inflammatory process such as nasal polyps, thick mucus, allergies, tumor, trauma, or viral upper respiratory infections cause thickened mucous membranes and inflammation and obstruction of the sinuses.

Allergic conditions, a deviated septum, nasal polyps, and immunosuppression increase the risk of contracting sinusitis. People with nasogastric tubes used for feeding, people who are sedated, and patients unable to protect their airways are at extra risk of sinusitis. Drinking alcohol, cocaine abuse, swimming in chlorinated pools, and diving into water all increase the risk. Certain cancers, diabetes, cirrhosis, smoking, kidney failure, and severe burns increase the risk of contracting sinusitis.

Acute and chronic sinusitis have similar signs and symptoms. The area over the sinus is tender and may be swollen. Malaise is frequently present. Other symptoms are fever, fatigue, weakness, running nose, purulent nasal discharge, halitosis, congestion, a cough that is more severe at night, and postnasal drip. Acute sinusitis can last longer than two weeks and causes more symptoms than a cold. Diagnosis is often based on the history of symptoms and physical examination findings. X-ray signs of sinusitis are cloudy (opacified) sinuses, fluid in the sinuses, and thickened mucosa.

Treatment of sinusitis involves antibiotics, decongestants, and pain relievers. Nonprescription decongestants and nose drops or sprays are used for up to 7 days. Antibiotics should be given for 10 to 12 days. Sinusitis that is unresponsive to antibiotics and other measures may require surgery to improve drainage and to remove impacted debris. Some chronic sinusitis may require treatment with oral or topical steroids, or both.

Preventive measures include the early treatment of respiratory infections and avoiding conditions or practices that may increase the risk of sinusitis.

The average adult has two to three colds and influenzalike illnesses yearly; 20 million Americans are affected by sinusitis each year; and 0.5 to 2 percent of colds and flulike illnesses are complicated by acute sinusitis.

Isaac Grate

KEY FACTS

Description

Sinusitis is an infection or inflammation of the paranasal sinuses.

Causes

Streptococcus, hemophilus, and moraxella infections.

Risk factors

Allergic conditions, deviated septum, nasal polyps, immunosuppression, nasogastric tubes for feeding, sedation, alcohol and cocaine abuse.

Symptoms and signs

Tenderness over sinuses, fever, headache, malaise, runny nose, congestion, purulent nasal discharge, cough, and halitosis.

Diagnosis

Symptoms, physical exam. X-rays and CT scans.

Treatments

Decongestants, antibiotics, and pain relievers.

Epidemiology

20 million Americans are affected by sinusitis each year. About 0.5 to 2 percent of colds and flulike illnesses are complicated by acute sinusitis.

See also
- Allergy and sensitivity • Cold, common
- Influenza

Sleep disorders

Disruptive patterns of sleep, sleeping too long, difficulty falling and staying asleep, and any unusual associated behavior indicate a sleep disorder. Sleep disorders are classified as primary (disturbances in the amount, quality, or timing of sleep, abnormal events in behavior or physiology during sleep) and secondary (due to general medical condition or substance abuse). There are two stages of sleep: non–rapid eye movement (NREM) and rapid eye movement (REM). Sleep disorders are related to alterations in the sleep-wake cycle of NREM and REM.

Good sleep quality is essential for overall physical and mental health. Inadequate sleep may cause fatigue, changes in mood, impaired performance, and can also negatively affect quality of life, safety, and productivity.

Causes

Certain medical conditions such as pain, metabolic disorders, endocrine disorders, and physical conditions (obesity) may cause sleep disorders. Other causes include: use of stimulants such as caffeine, amphetamines, and cocaine; sedative withdrawal; psychiatric conditions (for example, major depression, bipolar disorders, and anxiety disorders); and neurotransmitters (brain chemicals), for example, elevated levels of dopamine, norepinephrine, acetylcholine, and serotonin. Genetic and environmental factors are also associated with sleep disorders.

Although insomnia is not a disease, it is a chronic problem for about 25 percent of the population. A person with this disorder has difficulty in falling asleep and staying asleep, or they may get no benefit from sleep, resulting in daytime drowsiness and decreased energy and motivation. The condition is diagnosed if disturbance of sleep occurs three or more times per week for at least 1 month. This should not be associated with general medical conditions, substance abuse, or other sleep disorders. For treatment, medications are recommended for short-term use. They include sleeping drugs, antidepressants, and antihistamines. Insomnia can become chronic if untreated; it is exacerbated by stress and other environmental factors. Stress management and sleep hygiene (regular bed-

time, no alcohol or caffeine) are forms of prevention. This disorder affects approximately 30 percent of the general population. It is more common in women.

Primary hypersomnia

A person with this disorder experiences excessive or persistent daytime sleepiness that is not relieved by napping. To diagnose the condition, at least one month of the described symptoms should be present. Medications such as stimulants (amphetamines) are first-line treatments. Selective serotonin reuptake inhibitors (SSRIs) may be useful in some patients. Without treatment, hypersomnia may interfere with social and occupational functioning. Environmental stimulation could be helpful as a form of prevention. The course the disorder will take is unknown.

Narcolepsy

A person with this disorder has repeated, sudden attacks of sleep during the daytime with loss of muscle tone (cataplexy), which occurs in 70 percent of patients. Frequent REM sleep with brief paralysis occurs upon awakening (sleep paralysis) in 50 percent of patients. To confirm the diagnosis, the above symptoms must exist for at least 3 months. Treatment involves scheduled daily naps and stimulant drugs (amphetamines and ritalin). In case of sudden loss of muscle power, adjunctive antidepressants may be useful. If untreated, narcolepsy may cause serious occupational and social impairment. Most cases are treated successfully. There is no known prevention for the disorder. The exact prevalence in the population is unknown. Both males and females are equally affected. The onset is usually during adolescence or young adulthood. There may be a genetic predisposition.

Breathing-related disorders

Sleep disruption and daytime sleepiness can be caused by abnormal sleep ventilation from either obstructive or central sleep apnea. Sleep apnea is associated with headaches, depression, and pulmonary hypertension (respiratory problems). These symptoms should be enough to form a diagnosis. Treatment for the condition is nasal continuous positive airway pressure (nCPAP), and weight loss. Nasal surgery or uvuloplasty may treat obstructive sleep apnea. For central sleep apnea, mechanical ventilation (nCPAP) is helpful. These disorders take a chronic course if untreated and cause significant impairment in daily functioning and medical complications. Prevention includes weight reduction by diet and exercise. Approximately 10 percent of adults suffer from this type of sleep disorder. It is more common in men and obese individuals.

Circadian rhythm sleep disorder

This type of sleep disturbance is associated with a mismatch between a person's intrinsic circadian rhythm and external sleep-wake demands. Some of the conditions associated with this disorder include jet lag, shift work, and delayed sleep phase. These symptoms should be enough to make a diagnosis. Jet lag usually resolves spontaneously after 2 to 7 days. Light therapy may be useful for shift workers. The likely progression of the disease is not known. The only way to prevent this disorder is to avoid long travel time and to rearrange shift work schedules. It is not known how many people suffer from this sleep disorder.

Nightmare disorder

A person may experience repeated episodes of scary dreams with recall during REM sleep causing signifi-

cant distress. The disorder is diagnosed by these symptoms. There is no specific treatment for this type of sleep disorder. Occasionally, tricyclic antidepressants (TCAs) could be used to suppress total REM sleep. The likely outcome of this disorder is also unknown. Stress management is helpful in some cases as a preventive. The onset of this disorder is most often in childhood. It may occur more frequently during stress and illness.

Sleep terror disorder

Repeated episodes of apparent fearfulness during sleep (non-REM stages 3 or 4) with a scream appear. The individual may sit up or cry out and be extremely frightened or anxious. He or she will not awaken and not remember the episode. These symptoms allow diagnosis. There is usually no treatment, but some patients may benefit from small doses of benzodiazepine (valium) or other types of antianxiety medications at bedtime. The likely progression of the disorder is unknown, and there is no known prevention. This disorder usually occurs in children and is more common in boys. Prevalence of the disorder is 1 to 6 percent of children, and it has a familial tendency.

Sleepwalking disorder

Also known as somnambulism, a person with this disorder has repeated episodes of getting out of bed, walking with a blank stare, and is awakened only with difficulty. Other activities during such episodes include getting dressed, talking, or screaming. This behavior usually remits when the patient returns to bed. Some patients appear to be confused for several minutes and are unable to remember the event. It occurs during the non-REM sleep at stages 3 or 4. These symptoms are enough to diagnose the disorder.

Treatment is to provide a safe environment to prevent injury. Sometimes medications such as tricyclic antidepressants can help suppress non-REM sleep at stages 3 or 4. The likely outcome is unknown, and there are no known preventive measures. The onset of the disorder is usually between ages 4 and 8; peak prevalence is at age 12. This disorder is more common in boys and has a familial tendency.

Nurun Shah

KEY FACTS

Description

Disorders associated with disturbances in the amount, quality, and time of sleep, or abnormal events in behavior or physiology during sleep.

Causes and risk factors

Genetic, biochemical, and environmental factors. Secondary sleep disorders are associated with general medical conditions and substance abuse.

Symptoms

Difficulty in falling or staying asleep, excessive sleepiness, sleep attacks during the day with sudden loss of muscle tone, abnormal breathing, sleep disturbances, repeated episodes of frightening dreams, and sleepwalking.

Diagnosis

Evaluation and interview by a psychiatrist.

Treatment

Sleep hygiene, stress management, short-term medications, and breathing treatment.

Pathogenesis

Chronic course.

Epidemiology

10 percent of adults with breathing-related disorder; 1–6 percent have sleep terror disorder. Insomnia is more common in women; breathing-related sleep disorder is more common in men.

See also

- Anxiety disorders • Bipolar disorder
- Depressive disorders • Obesity
- Sleeping sickness

Sleeping sickness

Sleeping sickness, or African trypanosomiasis, is a parasitic illness caused by one of the *Trypanosoma* species. The parasite is a single-cell organism with a flagellum, which is a tail-like structure that helps the organism to move. This parasite exists outside the human cells in the body fluids and multiplies by division. Sleeping sickness is transmitted through a tsetse fly bite; in addition, it can be transmitted from mother to child during pregnancy.

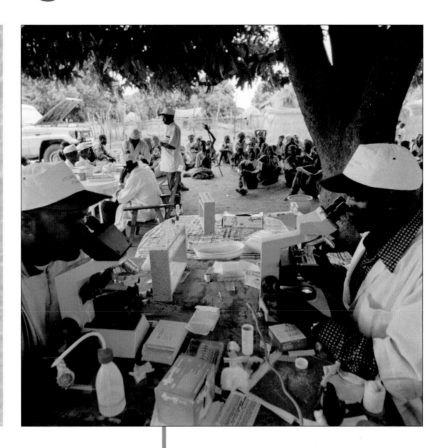

The parasite that causes sleeping sickness has two distinct life-cycle forms called epimastigote and trypomastigote. Tsetse flies feed on an infected human or another mammalian; the trypomastigotes multiply in the fly's gut and transform into epimastogotes. The parasites then travel to the fly's salivary glands so they can be injected by the fly into another human during the bite, so the transmission cycle continues. Once the parasite enters the human body, it transforms again and starts to multiply. Inside the body, the parasite exists in a trypomastigote form, which is distinguished into a long and a short one. Only the short trypomastigote will continue the parasite's life cycle in the fly's body and maintain the transmission.

Causes and epidemiology

The two parasite subtypes have similar structure but cause quite distinct clinical diseases and are transmitted by different species of tsetse fly. They also have a different geographic distribution. *Trypanosoma brucei gambiense*, which causes West African trypanosomiasis

As part of a World Health Organization (WHO) initiative, in 2002 screenings for sleeping sickness were set up in 15 African countries. Around 5 to 9 percent of the population tested during the campaign were infected.

(or gambiense trypanosomiasis), is common in West and Central Africa. *Trypanosoma brucei rhodesiense*, which causes East African trypanosomiasis (or rhodesiense trypanosomiasis), is common in Central and East Africa. Because this disease is transmitted only by a tsetse fly, it is prevalent only on the African continent, where tsetse flies are common. Infection among travelers is rare, unless they travel into rural areas. The actual number of people with sleeping sickness is difficult to establish; this disease is more common in the rural setting, where health resources are frequently scarce. The infection is found in 36 countries of sub-Saharan Africa. According to the World Health Organization (WHO), this infection became very uncommon on the African continent by the 1960s as a result of an aggressive surveillance campaign, but about a decade later the disease reappeared and continues to be a public health issue. West African trypanosomiasis is less commonly reported, while the majority of cases of sleeping sickness are due to East African trypanosomiasis.

Risk factors and pathogenesis

A major risk factor for the illness is contact with the tsetse fly and the presence of environmental factors to support the existence of this vector. Tsetse flies inhabit woody areas along rivers and lakes. People involved in activities such as fishing or hunting in infested areas are at risk for the infection. The parasite causing East African trypanosomiasis can also infect other mammals like cattle and antelopes. Persons traveling to or working at the game parks in East Africa may also be at risk for acquiring this infection.

Pathogenesis of sleeping sickness is defined by the dissemination of the parasite into the blood and lymphatic system. A unique feature of this parasite is the ability to escape the body's immune response. The immune response is determined by the production of antibodies against the antigens contained in the infecting organism. In the case of African trypanosomiasis, the parasite continues to change its antigenic structure, so the antibody response does not become sufficient, and the parasite continues to multiply and spread. Untreated infection will lead to death.

After the tsetse fly bite, a primary skin lesion called chancre can sometimes develop. From the bite area the parasite enters the human body and travels until it reaches the central nervous system. The process of dissemination takes weeks to months. The disease is usually described in two stages. During the first stage, multiplication of the parasite in blood and lymph occurs, followed by a second stage when the parasite enters the central nervous system.

Symptoms

West African (gambiense) trypanosomiasis is comparatively less severe and has a more chronic course. Infection can present as a local skin lesion at the site of a tsetse fly bite one to two weeks later. The first stage of the disease can develop weeks to months after the bite with systemic symptoms such as fever and prominent lymph node enlargement, as well as liver and spleen enlargement. Lymph node enlargement is especially prominent on the back of the neck. The lymph nodes can eventually become firm. Other findings include rash, weight loss, and generalized weakness. During the second stage of the illness, a progressive impairment in the central nervous system would even-

tually lead to coma and death. A major finding in this stage is daytime sleepiness, hence the name of the disease. It is accompanied by insomnia, as well as headache and personality and mood changes. Other impairments, such as loss of speech, movement disorders, or disturbances in coordination, can develop.

East African (rhodesiense) trypanosomiasis frequently presents itself as the more acute illness. Symptoms can develop days after the bite. During the first stage of the East African trypanosomiasis, the swelling of the lymph nodes is much less prominent, but rash and fever are common. Invasion of the heart by the parasite is more common with East African trypanosomiasis and leads to elevated heartbeat (tachycardia) and the development of heart failure. In weeks to months, the infection progresses to the second stage

KEY FACTS

Description
Sleeping sickness (or African trypanosomiasis) is a parasitic disease caused by a protozoan.

Causes
Sleeping sickness is caused by *Trypanosoma brucei*, which has two subtypes (subspecies).

Risk factors
The bite of a tsetse fly (vector) that lives only in sub-Saharan Africa. The flies are common in rural areas of tropical Africa.

Symptoms
Tend to develop in two stages: in the first stage, fever, malaise and lymph node enlargement; in the second stage, the organism invades the central nervous system, causing changes in behavior, sleepiness, and weight loss.

Diagnosis
Diagnosis is made by demonstration of a parasite in the body fluids, such as blood or spinal fluid.

Treatments
The disease is fatal if not treated. Treatment is given based on the type and stage of the illness.

Pathogenesis
The organism enters the body through a tsetse fly bite and eventually reaches the central nervous system, where it causes coma and death.

Prevention
The best way to prevent trypanosomiasis is to avoid areas infested with tsetse flies.

Epidemiology
It is estimated that the total number of people with sleeping sickness is somewhere between 50,000 to 70,000, but actual estimates are hard to predict.

LIFE CYCLE OF TRYPANOSOMES

A A tsetse fly feeds on an infected human or other mammal and ingests *Trypanosoma* parasites.

B The parasites reproduce in the fly's gut.

C The parasites travel to the fly's salivary glands; it is there that the parasites become infective.

D A fly with infective parasites in its saliva bites a human, transferring the parasites; the person will then develop sleeping sickness.

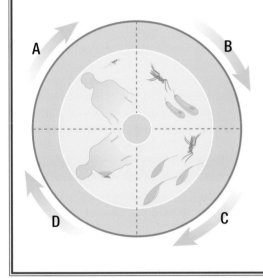

and invades the central nervous system with features similar to West African trypanosomiasis. Persons with East African trypanosomiasis commonly have low blood counts and wasting; coma and death develops in the late stage of the disease if no treatment is given.

Diagnosis and treatments

Demonstration of a parasite in the body fluids or tissue such as the bone marrow or lymph nodes is necessary for definitive diagnosis. The organisms can be found in fluid from chancre, blood, or a small sample of lymph node tissue. These tests may have to be repeated several times to increase the chance of detection. History of tsetse fly exposure in the endemic area of sub-Saharan Africa is also helpful in suspecting this disease. Tests that look for specific antibody response in the blood are available, although they are used for population screening only. If the serological screening is positive, further confirmatory diagnostic tests

should be done. It is important to examine the cerebrospinal fluid in all patients with African trypanosomiasis because it determines the specific treatment course. The typical cerebrospinal fluid abnormalities include elevated amounts of cells and protein.

It is imperative to timely treat the sleeping sickness to avoid progressive damage to the central nervous system. The treatment course is specific to the trypanosome subspecies and the clinical disease stage. The medications for trypanosomiasis are pentamidine, suramin, eflornithine, and melarsoprol. They are effective in clearing the infection but are sometimes not readily available in resource-limited settings. In addition, these medications are difficult to administer (most of them need to be given intravenously) and require monitoring due to toxicities and side effects. For West African trypanosomiasis, pentamidine is used for the first stage and eflornithine is used for the second-stage disease. For East African trypanosomiasis, suramin is used for the first stage and melarsoprol is used for the second-stage disease. The specific suggestions for disease stage and subtype were developed based on the side effect profile, toxicity, and penetration to the central nervous system. Suramin can cause fatal intolerance and kidney damage. Melarsoprol, which is an organic arsenical compound, is associated with a spectrum of side effects and toxicities, including central nervous system damage. It is always given in combination with steroid medication that reduces the inflammation and potential damage.

Prevention

There is no vaccine for this infection. None of the preventive medicines for African trypanosomiasis can be used because of the high risk of toxicity.

The WHO has established a surveillance team to try to eliminate this disease and assist with treatment to those infected. The best prevention method is to avoid areas of heavy tsetse fly infestation or wear neutral colored protective clothing (the flies are attracted to some bright colors). The flies can bite through light fabric, and insect repellants are not usually effective.

Other ways to stop the spread of the infection are tsetse fly control. Fly traps, insecticide use, elimination of breeding sites, or irradiation of the male flies to make them sterile are examples of vector control measures.

Diana Nurutdinova

See also
• Sleep disorders

Smallpox

Smallpox first appeared more than three thousand years ago. The first cases probably occurred in India or Egypt. Smallpox eventually spread worldwide and became one of the most devastating diseases known to humanity. For centuries, repeated epidemics swept across continents, wiping out populations and changing the course of history. As early as the 1700s, smallpox killed 1 in 10 children born in Sweden and France and 1 in 7 children born in Russia.

In 1798 an English physician named Edward Jenner showed that inoculation with a cowpox virus, which is similar to the smallpox virus, could protect a person against the smallpox virus. The development of the vaccine led to a global eradication program. This effort was completely successful; vaccination eliminated naturally occurring smallpox from the world. The last case was in Somalia in 1977.

Several laboratories maintained stocks of the virus in storage after the eradication of the disease. Eventually, these storage sites consolidated, and by 1984 they had centralized the remaining stocks at the Centers for Disease Control and Prevention (CDC), in Atlanta, and the Research Institute of Viral Preparations, in Moscow. In 1994 the storage site in the Soviet Union was moved to the State Research Center of Virology and Biotechnology (the Vektor Institute), in Novosibirsk, Russia. This center may have been vulnerable when the Soviet Union collapsed in the early 1990s, and many experts are concerned that someone may have misappropriated some of the virus that causes smallpox during this time.

If this happened, smallpox could pose a significant bioterrorism threat. The virus is easy to grow, and experts could probably modify it in a way that protects it from heat. It can survive in aerosol form and thus someone could load it into weapons or deliver it from a spray device. Today many countries are preparing to deal with a potential attack that uses smallpox.

Causes and risk factors

The variola virus causes smallpox. It affects only humans and is very contagious. It usually spreads from person to person by tiny droplets created when an infected person coughs. Contaminated clothes and bedding can also spread the disease, but the risk of infection from these sources is much lower. Although direct face-to-face contact is usually required for smallpox to spread from person to person, the disease does spread relatively easily.

Before 1970 almost everyone in the world had some immunity against smallpox. Either they had been infected and survived, which gave them natural immunity, or they had received a vaccination that gave them artificial immunity. These people may have some protection in the event of a future smallpox outbreak, but no one knows how long protection lasts after a smallpox vaccination. Some experts recommended revaccination every ten years. Health officials, however, discontinued all of the routine vaccination programs after they eradicated the disease. Only a very few people have received a vaccination against smallpox since 1980. Therefore, almost no one in the world has any immunity that would provide protection in a

KEY FACTS

Description
Viral infection of the human respiratory tract.

Causes
Infection by variola virus.

Risk factors
Contact with an infected person; exposure to a biological weapon.

Symptoms
Fever, cough, and body aches, followed by a spotted, bumpy rash.

Diagnosis
Confirmed by testing blood or the fluid from the blisters.

Treatments
None currently approved, but experts are testing some medications.

Pathogenesis
The virus enters and multiplies in the respiratory passages.

Prevention
Avoiding those with the disease. During an outbreak, a vaccine is available that will prevent the disease or lessen its severity.

Epidemiology
Completely eradicated from nature but could be a potential biological weapon.

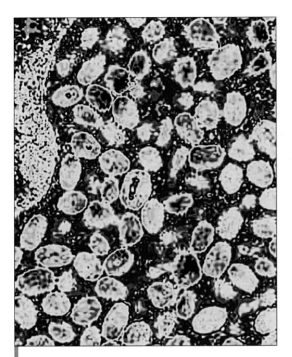

In this colored and magnified photomicrograph, the variola virus can be seen (yellow) against a blue background. The virus causes smallpox, but the disease has been eradicated since the late 1970s.

appears, first on the face, hands, and forearms, and then after a few days moving to the chest, abdomen, and back. The rash starts as pink bumps. The name *smallpox* comes from the Latin word for "spotted" and refers to these bumps. The bumps eventually become blisters and then fill with pus. After several days, they dry up and form scabs.

Complications of smallpox

Smallpox can lead to blindness, and brain inflammation has also been reported. Other disorders are eye infections, bacterial skin infections at the site of the lesions, pneumonia, arthritis, and bone infections. People who have recovered from the disease usually have severe scars on the face, legs, and arms.

Treatment

There is no effective treatment for smallpox, although many different medications are under investigation. Since there is no cure for smallpox, medical treatment is limited to caring for complications of the disease, such as shock or respiratory failure.

Prevention

People who have been around smallpox but have not yet started to have any symptoms can receive the smallpox vaccination. If it is given early enough, it can prevent the disease or reduce its severity.

In the event of an outbreak, many governments have stockpiles of the smallpox vaccine that they could use in an emergency. The governments of both the United Kingdom and the United States, for example, have enough to vaccinate the entire population of their countries, if necessary.

Another important step to stop the spread of a future outbreak will be to ensure that healthy people stay away from those who are sick. Those with smallpox must be isolated until the last scab comes off the body. In a large outbreak, infected individuals would be encouraged to stay at home to help reduce the spread of the disease. Public health authorities may recommend "social distancing," which involves requesting people to avoid crowded places, in order to reduce the spread of smallpox. In the event of a smallpox outbreak, it is important that the public stays informed.

Richard N. Bradley

future smallpox outbreak. During previous decades when smallpox was occurring, about 3 in 10 cases of smallpox among individuals without immunity were fatal. Even though most people in the world probably do not have any immunity today, advances in modern health care might moderate the relatively high fatality rate.

Symptoms and signs

Smallpox, like many infectious diseases, has an incubation period. During this time, the virus is multiplying in the person's body, but he or she looks and feels healthy and cannot infect others. The incubation period for smallpox is from seven to seventeen days, but for most people, it will be between 12 and 14 days.

After the incubation period, the infected person will quickly become very ill with flulike symptoms. The symptoms include fever, weakness, headache, and muscle and joint pain. Two to three days later, the fever improves and the patient feels somewhat better. At this point, sores develop in the person's nose and mouth. These become raw and release large amounts of virus. Each cough propels large numbers of these virus particles into the air. Next, the characteristic rash

See also
• Influenza • Pneumonia

Spina bifida

Spina bifida is one of the most common birth defects in the world, and it is also one of the easiest to prevent. Simply adding folic acid to a mother's diet before pregnancy can dramatically reduce the number of cases of spina bifida each year, though the actual cause remains a mystery.

Spina bifida is a birth defect that can occur before a woman even knows she is pregnant. Preventive measures therefore focus on the general population. In the United States, breads, cereals, and other grain products have been fortified with extra folic acid, a nutrient that appears essential to normal embryonic development. In this way, most women of childbearing age will have sufficient folic acid in their diets well before a pregnancy begins.

Causes

Just 18 days after a sperm fertilizes an egg, a critical developmental milestone occurs. The neural tube begins to close up around the developing brain and spinal cord. By the fourth week of pregnancy, the process is complete. If the mother is at risk or suffers from a nutritional deficiency, the neural tube may not close properly. When the gap occurs along the spine, the result is spina bifida, which means "split spine."

Different forms and different outcomes

There are multiple forms of spina bifida. The two major forms are spina bifida occulta, which means "hidden," and spina bifida manifesta, in which the spinal defects are obvious. Spina bifida manifesta can be subdivided into two types: meningocele and myelomeningocele. These names describe the specific type of damage caused by the disorder.

Spina bifida occulta is a common condition, and some health professionals estimate that it may occur in up to 20 percent of apparently healthy people. There might be a slight dimple along the spine, unusual pigmentation, or a hairy patch over the area. This disorder rarely causes symptoms or problems for the patient unless there is an associated fatty deposit that can press on the spinal cord and spinal nerves.

The meningocele form of spina bifida is the least common form. In this disorder, only the meninges, which are the protective membranes around the spinal cord, extrude from the spinal column. Nerve damage can result, and these patients might suffer minor disabilities or neurological problems later in life.

The most severe form of spina bifida is myelomeningocele, and this is the form most people recognize as spina bifida. In this case, the opening extends along several vertebrae, and both the meninges and spinal cord itself are pushed out of the opening. It is quite common for these patients to experience some degree of paralysis or weakness in their legs and lower back. Nerve damage can affect both bladder and bowel functions. In addition, 70 to 90 percent of patients with this form of spina bifida will also have hydrocephalus, or "water on the brain." This condition can lead to problems with learning and memory, behavior, and decision making.

One of the most important factors in determining how severe the damage will be is the actual location of the lesion. Lesions higher on the spinal column are more likely to result in paralysis and severe disabilities. Patients with lower lesions can often lead normal lives and even raise families of their own.

Risk factors

The cause of spina bifida remains unknown, but several risk factors have been identified. The most important risk factor is insufficient folic acid in the diet before and during early pregnancy. Other risk factors include certain drugs used to treat epilepsy, kidney dialysis, alcohol abuse, obesity, diabetes, and fevers or high temperatures during early pregnancy. Although whites and Hispanics are at higher risk overall, socioeconomic factors that lead to poor nutrition can raise the risk for other racial groups. Parents who have had one child with spina bifida are at higher risk of having a second child with the disease. Spina bifida patients also have a higher risk. However, scientists have not located a specific gene associated with the disorder.

Since 1997, the U.S. government has officially recognized exposure to Agent Orange as an additional risk factor for spina bifida. Agent Orange was a defoliant used during the Vietnam War, and many veterans were exposed. Veterans who have children with spina bifida can receive up to $1,200 a month in disability payments and assistance with vocational training and rehabilitation. No benefits are provided to patients with spina bifida occulta.

Symptoms and diagnosis

Most cases of spina bifida can be identified by routine prenatal blood tests during the second trimester of pregnancy. A triple screen test looks for the presence of alpha-fetoprotein (AFP) and measures levels of two important hormones. If the AFP levels are abnormally high, an ultrasound scan will be used to look for defects along the spinal column. The test is not definitive, because not all cases of spina bifida will produce high levels of AFP.

In the more severe forms of spina bifida, the physical defects are obvious at birth. A fluid-filled sac protrudes from the back, and there may be an opening in the skin around the lesion. In less severe cases, symptoms such as weakness in the legs and lower back pain may develop later in life. Spina bifida occulta may never be diagnosed unless the patient happens to need a spinal X-ray at some point.

Treatments

There is no cure for spina bifida. Damaged nerves can never be repaired or replaced. Therefore, the most important treatment for spina bifida is surgery to prevent additional nerve damage by repairing the hole in the spinal column. This surgery is normally performed within the first 24 hours of life, although some doctors are experimenting with prenatal surgery. For patients with hydrocephalus, a shunt is normally implanted to help drain cerebrospinal fluid. Without the shunt, pressure can build up and damage the brain and central nervous system. Patients need additional surgery later in life. A common complication is a condition called "tethered spinal cord." As the patient grows, the spinal cord becomes stuck and must be surgically freed to allow proper movement and fluid flow around the cord. If the spinal cord remains tethered and stretched, additional nerve damage can occur.

Other treatments focus on keeping a patient active, healthy, and mentally fit. Even patients confined to wheelchairs will get special exercise programs to keep their weight under control, to prevent pressure sores, and to maximize their fitness. Good hygiene is also important to avoid infections and skin sores. Many patients have very poor sensation in their lower limbs, so it is important to check frequently for skin damage and bruises. Patients are also more likely to have latex allergies, so it is important to avoid all latex products, such as balloons.

Social impact

It is estimated that 70,000 people in the United States are living with spina bifida. The highest rates of the disease are in the southeastern part of the country. Worldwide, the highest rates are found in China. Differences in nutritional status and the availability of medical care can greatly affect the quality of life for these patients.

Patients with myleomeningocele spina bifida are often confined to wheelchairs or require braces to walk. Problems with learning and memory are common; however, most patients will have average IQs. Advocacy groups have been established to help patients with spina bifida lead normal productive lives. Special training or educational programs can help patients cope with learning disabilities, poor hand-eye

---

KEY FACTS

Description
A developmental disorder that can lead to paralysis in severe cases.

Cause
Unknown, but both genetics and environmental factors probably play a role.

Risk factors
Insufficient folic acid in the mother's diet before and during pregnancy; anti-epileptic medicines; obesity; and diabetes.

Symptoms
Congenital deformities of the spine, lower back pain, and weakness in the back or legs.

Diagnosis
Prenatal blood tests and ultrasound can be used to diagnose most cases in utero. Spinal deformities are obvious at birth.

Treatments
Severe cases require surgery in the first days of life. Mild cases may need no treatment at all.

Pathogenesis
The course of the disease varies considerably and depends on both the location and severity of the malformation. About 90 percent of babies born with spina bifida will survive to adulthood.

Prevention
Adequate consumption of folic acid before and during pregnancy.

Epidemiology
Hispanics and whites of European descent are at highest risk. In the United States, the current rate is about 1 in 5,000 live births.

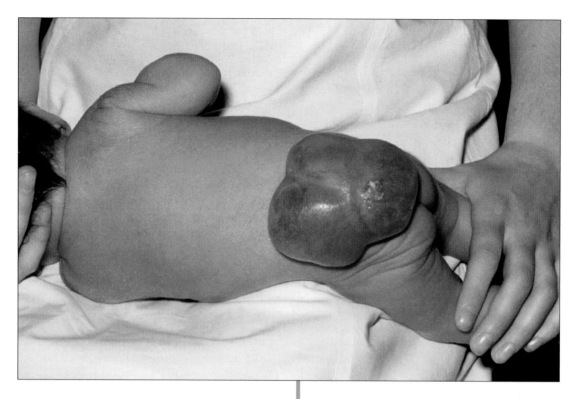

A newborn baby has spina bifida, in which part of the spinal cord and its coverings are exposed through a gap in the backbone. Symptoms can include paralysis, incontinence, and mental retardation.

coordination, and behavioral disorders associated with spina bifida and hydrocephalus. Mental health professionals can help patients deal with the stress and depression that often occur in people who have chronic illnesses.

Pathogenesis

Comprehensive care is required throughout life, which makes spina bifida a very expensive disorder. The lifetime cost can be as high as $1 million per patient in the United States. With proper care, however, the majority of patients will survive to adulthood and some are able to raise families of their own. These patients do face an increased risk of having a child with the disorder, however.

Patients with spina bifida occulta may not experience serious health problems, but they might discover they have difficulty getting health insurance or getting hired. To avoid these potential difficulties, many health professionals do not use the term *spina bifida occulta*. They will report the defect as a "vertebral fusion defect" instead.

Prevention and epidemiology

Spina bifida cases dropped 28 percent from 1995 to 2003 after the U.S. government mandated the addition of folic acid to grain products such as bread and cereal. Studies indicate that one-half to three-quarters of all cases of spina bifida can be prevented by folic acid supplementation.

However, scientists still cannot determine exactly how folic acid prevents birth defects. They do know that it is essential for cells to make RNA and DNA, for the production of new red blood cells, and for the breakdown of homocysteine, a metabolite that can damage tissue when present in high concentrations. Foods high in folic acid include leafy green vegetables, orange juice, eggs, and enriched grain products.

According to the Centers for Disease Control and Prevention (CDC), approximately 20 cases of spina bifida occur in every 100,000 live births in the United States.

Chris Curran

See also
- Alcohol-related disorders • Diabetes
- Obesity • Vitamin deficiency

Spinal curvature

The human spine, or backbone, has natural gentle curves. However, poor posture or inheritance can result in misaligned curves, pain, and impaired respiration.

The normal vertebral column forms a straight line down the center of the back. Viewed from the side, the vertebral column displays a curvature that develops with growth and age. The infant spine is flexible and forms a C curve (viewed from the side) as infants curl their head toward the center of their body. This early curve is a kyophotic curvature because the spinal convexity is directed backward. As infants grow and develop muscle control, they begin to lift their heads against gravity when they are lying on their stomachs. The neck muscles bring the cervical spine into a reverse curvature, with the convexity directed toward the body's front. A curvature with an forward-directed convexity is called a lordotic curvature. When a baby learns to sit up, a second lordotic curvature forms in the lumbar region of the lower back. The result is alternating curvatures: lordotic curvatures in the cervical and lumbar regions and kyphotic curvatures in the thoracic and sacrococcygeal regions. The spine continues to change throughout adolescence until growth is completed.

Types of spinal curvatures

The vertebrae are connected individually and as segments by an intricate array of muscles and ligaments. Column segments are so interdependent that shifting or injury associated with any vertebra can alter the alignment of articulating vertebrae. It is inevitable that a cascade effect will alter the mechanics and alignment of the vertebral column as a whole. An idiopathic curvature is inherited. A postural curvature is due to poor posture. Individuals may choose to sit or stand with a postural curvature to protect themselves from pain.

Kyphosis

Kyphosis is a posterior curvature normal to the thoracic and sacrococcygeal areas. Excessive thoracic kyphosis appears as a "humped" area in the shoulders and midback. Postural kyphosis is flexible and is the result of poor posture. Individuals with a "flat" lower back often slump in the shoulders to optimize their center of gravity, resulting in a kyphotic stance. The hump ofidiopathic kyphosis is called a "gibbus" and is often the result of a fracture, tumor, or bone disease that altered the shape of some thoracic vertebrae. Postmenopausal women may have a so-called dowager's hump as a result of osteoporosis of the upper and mid-thoracic vertebrae. Severe and persistent kyphosis related to changes in the vertebral column can lead to painful nerve root impingements and muscle discomfort.

Lordosis

Lordosis is a forward-directed convexity. Excessive lordosis is a condition of the lumbar spine and often

---

KEY FACTS: SCOLIOSIS

Description

A lateral shift and rotation of the spinal vertebrae. The spine forms an S or a C shape.

Causes

Postural or idiopathic, which may be due to vertebral abnormalities or abnormal muscle control in the trunk.

Risk factors

A strong genetic component to idiopathic scoliosis.

Symptoms

Usually asymptomatic at adolescence. Severe curve progression and rib cage rotation can lead to impaired respiration. Large lumbar deviations may lead to painful osteoarthritis.

Diagnosis

Physical examination and X-ray.

Treatments

A mild scoliotic curvature (less than 30 degrees deviation) is generally monitored. Moderate curvatures (30–45 degrees deviation) may need bracing; severe curvatures may require surgery.

Pathogenesis

Predispositions include heredity, connective tissue disorders, and neuromuscular disorders. Progression of scoliotic curve can lead to pain, restricted movement in the trunk and arms, and impaired respiration.

Prevention

Bracing may prevent curve progression, but there is disagreement about the success of bracing. Early intervention offers best results.

Epidemiology

Thoracic curvatures of greater than 60 degrees deviation are associated with reduced life span. Adolescent girls are affected by scoliosis at least five times more often than boys.

accompanies scoliosis. Lordosis is often the result of an anteriorly tilted pelvis and shortened hip flexor muscles. Individuals with weak trunk and hip muscles, such as those with muscular dystrophy, often compensate for their weakness by assuming a lordotic stance.

Scoliosis

Lateral shifting occurs when the spinal column does not form a straight line or deviates from the vertical center of the back. Lateral spinal column deviation is referred to as scoliosis. These lateral deformities usually occur in either the thoracic or lumbar spine, or both coincidentally. The spinal column shifts laterally as a result of rotational forces on the vertebrae. Because the vertebrae articulate directly with the rib cage, severe scoliosis alters the rib cage and impairs the lungs' ability to expand. Impaired respiratory function is a very serious consequence of severe scoliosis. A rib hump is often apparent at the most severe rotational point.

A scoliotic curvature may form a C curve, with one lateral convexity (to the left or to the right), or an S curve, with two convexities directed in opposite directions. Scoliosis can be mild and nearly unidentifiable, or severe. Postural scoliosis is flexible and often the result of body posturing. It can be corrected by pressure at the lateral convexities or with conscientious effort to improve posture. Often, postural scoliosis is the result of a posture that protects a painful back.

Individuals with one leg longer than the other may also display postural scoliosis as they shift their posture in standing to keep their field of vision level and centered.

Girls are at least five times more likely than boys to be affected by idiopathic scoliosis. It is usually painless and asymptomatic; however, severe curvatures may cause respiratory limitations and pain in adult years. Idiopathic scoliosis is often the result of a vertebral abnormality that changes the structural alignment of the spinal column.

Scoliosis is common in individuals with neuromuscular disorders such as cerebral palsy and poliomyelitis. An imbalance in muscle "pull" on either side of the spinal column results in a lateral shift and vertebral rotation toward the stronger side of the back. Neuromuscular disorders that result in weakness and poor trunk control, such as muscular dystrophy, spina bifida, or spinal cord injury are also at risk for scoliosis. Since trunk muscles help enhance breathing, individuals with weak trunk muscles due to neuromuscular disorders may be at higher risk of respiratory compromise if they also have severe scoliosis.

Diagnosis

A diagnosis of kyphosis or lordosis is generally made through observation and measurement. Idiopathic causes of these spinal curvatures, such as vertebral wedging or other abnormalities, can be confirmed through X-ray. Osteoporosis, a potential cause of kyphosis, can be confirmed with a bone density scan.

A plumb line centered at vertical midline of the back can help identify both subtle and obvious scoliosis. Idiopathic scoliosis may also be detected when an individual with scoliosis bends forward with hands joined and arms hanging down. Individuals with scoliosis show asymmetries in the two sides of the back when bending forward. An X-ray can confirm scoliosis and help monitor its progression. An MRI may be necessary if the individual presents with neurological signs.

Practicing good posture is the best way to prevent postural disorders of the spinal column. Postural scoliosis related to back pain is best resolved by treating the source of back pain, possibly nerve root impingement or other inflammatory conditions. Postural thoracic kyphosis can often be treated with posture reeducation and focused strengthening exercises.

Idiopathic thoracic kyphosis due to vertebral wedging, fractures, or vertebral abnormalities is more difficult to manage, since assuming a correct posture may not be possible with structural changes in the vertebrae. Children who have not completed their growth may show long-lasting improvements with bracing. Exercises may be prescribed to alleviate discomfort associated with overstretched back muscles. A variety of gravity-assisted positions or gentle traction can minimize pain associated with nerve root impingement. Surgery may be recommended for severe idiopathic kyphosis.

Treatment for idiopathic scoliosis depends upon the severity of the curvature, the spine's potential for further growth, and the risk that the curvature will progress. Mild scoliosis (less than 30 degrees deviation) may simply be monitored and treated with exercise. Moderately severe scoliosis (30–45 degrees) in a child who is still growing may require bracing. Severe curvatures that rapidly progress may be treated surgically with spinal rod placement. Bracing may prevent a progressive curvature, but evidence is not strong in favor of correction with brace wear. In all cases, early intervention offers the best results.

Patti Berg

See also
• Osteoporosis

402

Sports injury

All bones, joints, muscles, and tissues are susceptible to injury, which can occur in both athletes and non-athletes. The most common injuries are caused by carelessness, lack of training, biomechanical factors, accident, and overuse of muscles. More than 10 million sports injuries are treated each year in the United States; just under half of these are in children under 15.

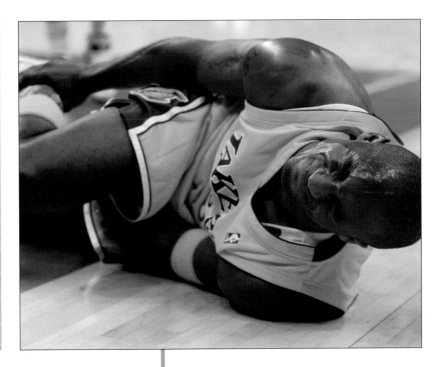

Improving physical performance was essential for ancient man to stay alive to fight. Egyptian hieroglyphics depict running, swimming, rowing, archery, and wrestling competitions. The first sports-related medical text was the Kahun Papyrus, dated around 1700 B.C.E. For the Olympic Games in 776 B.C.E., Greek athletes were given specialized training under the supervision of specialists in the gymnasium. Sports medicine developed early in history and has become a major specialty within orthopedic surgery during the twenty-first century.

With the increase in physical activity as a remedy for the problem of obesity, more sports-related injuries are being reported, primarily related to carelessness, poor training, and the improper use of equipment. Everyone has tissues that are susceptible to injury because of inherent body weakness or biomechanical factors. For example, people who have a deep curvature of the spine (lumbar lordosis) are at risk for back pain when they swing a baseball bat; people with flat feet whose feet turn out (pronation) are at risk for knee pain when they run long distances. In all sports, specific motions must be repeated. When the activity is stopped, pain usually stops until the activity is tried again.

Whether an athlete experiences the thrill of success or the distress of defeat, physical pain may occur, in-

Athletes are prone to muscle and tendon injuries. They can be caused by insufficient warm-up, tiredness, and using excessive force, such as pushing or pulling, during games. Ligament sprains and strains are also common sports injuries.

juring bones, joints, ligaments, or muscles. Some injuries require no treatment other than rest; others require immediate attention.

Sports injuries to bone

The thrills of the school playground come with a price: fractures. A fracture is a broken bone. Bones are hard because they contain mineral, notably calcium, but surrounding the calcium are living bone cells and blood vessels. Usually bones absorb shocks by bending, then returning to their normal rigid position, but if bones are weakened or if the force is too great, bones will break.

There are four types of fractures that are more common in sports injuries. For a simple fracture, a clean break occurs, but the skin is not broken. Surrounding muscle and blood vessels are not damaged. In a compound fracture, broken bone penetrates the skin and is visible; considerable damage may occur to surrounding tissue. Greenstick fractures are usually seen in children; bone cracks and bends as if it were a green stick.

A comminuted fracture is when the bone is broken in two or more places or is crushed.

Children with broken bones heal much faster than adults. However, injuries to children are so common that most children have seen an orthopedic surgeon (a doctor who specializes in bone repair) before they reach the age of five.

Recognizing an open or compound fracture is obvious when a piece of the bone is visible, but the following symptoms indicate a closed or simple fracture: a break or snap is heard; a grating sensation is felt with movement; swelling, bruising, or reddening may occur; limbs may look deformed with different lengths, sizes, or shapes; an improper angle may be noted; when the person moves, there is intense pain; numbness or tingling may occur in the extremities; or unusual pain in the rib cage occurs when one breathes or coughs. Breaking a bone is a shock to the entire body. Some people may feel sick or dizzy, and others feel no pain because of shock.

A concussion is a hairline fracture to the skull. It is the most common head injury and results in temporary brain disturbance due to trauma. Concussion may be caused by a sudden or violent movement of the head, which may occur in a tackle or collision, or spinning of the head caused by a blow to the side of the head. The player may have a concussion and be conscious or may have a vacant stare with slow responses, slurred or incoherent speech, or may forget events after the impact. The following signs indicate a concussion: bruising around the eye or ear; bleeding from the nose; pupils unequal in size; and swelling of the skull.

If there is any risk of neck or head injury, the player should be stabilized and taken from the field on a stretcher. No player with a concussion should return to the sport unless checked by a medical practitioner.

Metatarsals are the long bones of the foot. A march fracture is a type of injury usually found in walkers or runners, resulting from repeated periods of excessive stress on the metatarsals. Runners often push off from their toes and place great stress on the first two metatarsal heads. There, the bones are thin, and a fracture may occur. Resting and strapping the foot with adhesive plaster for a few weeks helps healing.

KEY FACTS

Description
Injuries that occur when participating in a variety of sports activities; injuries can involve bone, cartilage, joints and ligaments, tendons, and muscles.

Causes
Carelessness, lack of training, overuse of muscles, improper use of equipment; intrinsic factors, or the way the body is constructed, and extrinsic factors, may cause injuries.

Symptoms
Pain; severity depends on the injury.

Diagnosis
After physical examination and taking of medical history, the person may be referred to specialists for carefully selected tests such as X-rays, computed tomography scans, bone scans, and magnetic resonance imaging scans.

Treatments
First aid treatment includes rest, ice, compression, elevation (RICE); depending on the injury, the person may be recommended to a specialist in sports medicine.

Pathogenesis
If treatment is followed, recovery is usually good.

Prevention
Warming up, stretching, cooling down; focusing or paying attention.

Epidemiology
More than 10 million sports injuries are treated each year in the United States; around 3.5 million of these are in children under the age of 15.

Ligaments and sprains

Although the word *sprain* is used to describe a variety of medical conditions, a true sprain is an injury to a ligament, the tough elastic band that connects bone to bone at a joint. A violent twist can damage any ligament. Following are three types of sprains:

In a simple stretch (grade I sprain), ligament fibers are overstretched with minor pain and some tenderness and swelling. X-rays are normal and the person can put weight on the area without too much pain.

In a partial tear (grade II sprain), a ligament tears but does not rupture. Movement is moderately painful with some swelling and discoloration.

A complete tear (grade III sprain) is a severe injury because the joint is completely misaligned. The whole area is swollen and discolored.

Sports injuries to the ankle and knee joints are the most common. An ankle sprain results in overstretching or tearing of one or more ankle ligaments. Sprains usually occur on the outside, making the foot turn inward and causing excess tension on the outer ankle ligaments. When a sprain occurs the "RICED" procedure can be used (see box, page 405). Rehabilitation and exercise are necessary to restore function.

Sprained knees occur when a tear or complete rupture occurs of one or more of the knee ligaments, most commonly the anterior cruciate ligament (ACL). When a runner makes a sudden movement (for example, when tackling or twisting in football or rugby), the knee is suddenly rotated. A blow to the outer knee when the leg or foot is firmly planted damages the medial collateral ligament (MCL), the large ligament supporting the inside of the knee. Posterior cruciate ligament (PCL) injuries occur when a force hits the front of a bent knee. Using the RICED procedure is important to lessen the impact of such injuries. Some charts add "P" in front of "RICED" for "protect." Prevention involves two important factors: warm-up and cool-down exercise. Many amateur participants are eager to jump into the activity and forget important procedures, such as use of devices that tape, brace, or wrap knees, ankles, wrists, and elbows. "Train, don't sprain" should be the motto of all athletes.

Dislocations occur when a bone is moved out of place at the joint. Usually a blow has enough force to tear the ligaments, and in addition, damage may occur to the surrounding muscles, blood vessels, and bone. Shoulder dislocations happen when a force moves the ball-and-socket joint in one of four directions: forward, backward, up, or down. Dislocations are common in sports that use a large range of motion of the shoulder, such as swimming, gymnastics, or collision sports. The recommended procedure here is "RICD"; elevation is left out because of the normal position of the shoulder. If someone has a dislocation, it is difficult to move the joint; medical help should be sought as soon as possible.

Tendons and tendonitis

Tendons are strong fibrous bands that attach muscle to bones. Sports injuries of tearing and inflammation of tendons are common in the shoulder, elbow, wrist, and lower leg or ankle.

The rotator cuff holds the head of the humerus, or bone of the upper arm, into the scapula or shoulder blade. Certain sports that require the arm to be moved over the head repeatedly often tear or inflame tendons in this area. Examples are baseball, swimming freestyle, backstroke, butterfly, weight lifting, and racket sports. Chronic irritation can cause bursitis or inflammation of the bursae, small fluid-filled sacs that cushion areas where muscles cross bones or other muscles. The sacs lubricate the area for smooth movement of muscle.

RICED

For sports injuries, follow this procedure:
REST No weight should be put on the injured part.
ICE Applied as packs, massage, or immersion. Ice cools the tissue and reduces pain, swelling, and bleeding, by slowing metabolism in the cells and allowing tissue to survive a temporary lack of oxygen. The ice must not be applied directly to the skin; it should be first wrapped in a cloth.
COMPRESSION Firm bandaging helps to reduce bleeding and swelling.
ELEVATION This helps to stop bleeding and reduce swelling.
DIAGNOSIS A medical professional should be consulted if pain or swelling does not go down within 48 hours.

Many repetitive movement disorders are common in sports. Tennis elbow is known also as lateral humerus tendonitis epicondylitis and is caused by repetitive strenuous pushing of the wrist against resistance when hitting a ball. A tear or inflammation of the tendon that links muscle to bone may become a chronic condition if the area is not rested. Tennis elbow can also be caused by frisbee throwing and other activities that tighten the muscles in the hand or forearm. Often reconstructive surgery is necessary.

When running, the calf muscles lower the forefoot to the ground after the heels strikes the ground and raise the heel when the toe lifts off. Although most tendons have a sheath that surrounds them, the Achilles tendon located at the back of the lower leg has only the lining or fatty tissue that separates the tendon from the sheath. Early pain of Achilles tendonitis is due to injury to this covering; if the pain is ignored, inflammation spreads to the tendon and causes degeneration. The athlete must stop running and reduce tension on the area by placing a heel lift in the shoes and stretching the hamstring muscles.

Muscles and strain

Pulled muscles can occur anywhere, but certain muscles appear more at risk in sports injuries. The hamstrings are a group of three muscles at the back of the thigh. A strain is caused when an overstretch results in a tear or complete rupture of one or more of these muscles. Hamstring strains are common in sports that require explosive stop-start running motions, such as football or rugby, volleyball, and athletic sprinting events. The injuries often occur at the beginning of a game or training session due to inadequate warm-up or

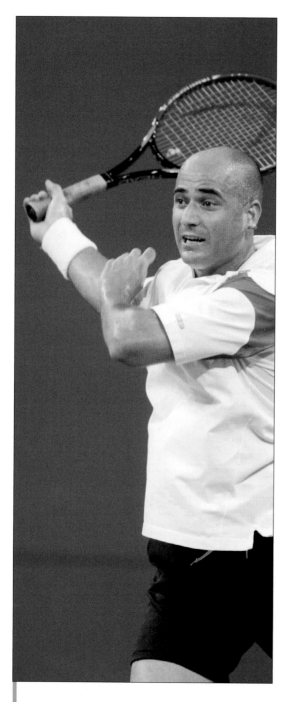

Tennis players, such as U.S. player Andre Agassi, are vulnerable to many muscle, bone, and joint injuries because playing in one tournament after another often does not give them time to recover fully from injuries. Tennis elbow is a common injury in tennis players.

near the end of a game when fatigue becomes a factor. For hamstring injuries, the RICED procedure is used.

Any great force can tear the muscles and tendons of the lower back. Lumbar strain occurs in sports that require pushing or pulling against great resistance, such as weight lifting, football, basketball, baseball, or golf. The person should be treated with RICD (because elevation is not essential); once healing has begun, the person can benefit from exercises that strengthen the abdominal muscles and stretch the back muscles to restore flexibility.

Shin splints, known as anterior compartment syndrome, are probably the most common overuse problem. Resulting from the repeated straining of muscles between the shinbones, shin splints cause pain in the lower leg between the ankle and knee. The swollen muscles press on blood vessels, thus transferring stress to the bones, causing tiny cracks. Shin splints may occur, for example, when a tennis player shifts from a soft to a hard surface, or a basketball player suddenly has to play extra time. These microfractures are so fine that they do not show up in X-rays. Treatments include rest, proper diet rich in calcium, and training in the proper use of equipment.

Drug abuse in sports

When an athlete exercises, the nervous system produces hormones, such as adrenaline, that in turn increase the amount of blood for muscles and glucose to provide muscle energy. Some athletes illegally take drugs that will give them an unfair advantage over other athletes. The problem is international; it involves both amateur and professional athletes in a wide range of sports and includes the use of anabolic steroids, ephedrine and its derivatives, stimulant drugs, painkillers, nerve relaxants, growth hormone, diuretics to lose weight quickly, and corticosteroids. The U.S. Olympic Committee and the International Olympic Committee bans the use of these enhancers and stimulants.

Anabolic steroids are chemically related to natural hormones and mimic the effects of the male hormone testosterone. The athlete gains weight, muscle mass, and strength. However, use of these steroids has been linked to liver failure, heart damage, reproductive system damage, and extreme aggressiveness.

Evelyn B. Kelly

See also
• Backache • Dislocation • Fracture
• Head injury • Repetitive strain injury

Stomach ulcer

Stomach ulcers are small holes or sores in the lining of either the stomach or the duodenum. Most often the result of a bacterial infection, ulcers cause a burning feeling in the upper abdomen, and in severe cases may cause bleeding, vomiting, or weight loss. Every year, more than 500,000 new cases of peptic ulcer disease are diagnosed in the United States.

Stomach ulcers, more accurately called peptic ulcers, are small, painful sores that can develop in the lining of the stomach or the duodenum, the upper part of the small intestine. Long ascribed to stress and dietary factors, most ulcers are now believed to be caused by infection with *Helicobacter pylori*, a common bacterium that weakens the protective mucous coating of the stomach and duodenum, allowing acid to penetrate to the sensitive lining beneath. Left untreated, severe ulcers may eventually eat a hole through the wall of the stomach and cause infection of the abdominal cavity.

Causes and risk factors

A definitive link between ulcers and the *Helicobacter pylori* bacterium was established only in 1982. Though acceptance of this connection has been slow to spread, the majority of peptic ulcers are now treated as bacterial infections, spread from person to person primarily via the gastro-oral route, or through contaminated water sources. Long-term use of anti-inflammatory drugs such as aspirin or ibuprofen may also irritate the lining of the stomach, while stress and the use of tobacco and alcohol can worsen the symptoms.

Signs and symptoms

Symptoms are a burning sensation in the abdomen, which is worse when the stomach is empty and may last several hours. Less common symptoms include nausea, vomiting, or loss of appetite. Blood from severe ulcers may appear in vomit or bowel movements.

Diagnosis and treatments

Ulcers may be seen directly through endoscopy, in which a tiny camera is threaded down the esophagus into the stomach. If an ulcer is seen, a tissue sample may be taken to identify the presence of *H. pylori*, which may also be detected by blood, breath, or stool tests.

Treatment for *H. pylori*–related ulcers typically involves a short course of antibiotics, combined with the use of drugs that reduce or neutralize acid production in the stomach. Ulcers that fail to respond to such treatment may be due to antibiotic-resistant *H. pylori*, or, in rare cases, to diseases and syndromes that affect the digestive system. Surgery is necessary only when the ulcer does not respond to aggressive drug treatment.

Prevention

Recommendations for avoiding *H. pylori* infection involve washing hands thoroughly, eating food that has been properly prepared, and drinking water from a clean source.

Jonathon Cross

KEY FACTS

Description
Sores or holes in the lining of the stomach or duodenum.

Causes
Infection by *Helicobacter pylori* bacterium.

Risk factors
Use of nonsteroidal anti-inflammatories, smoking, and alcohol use.

Symptoms
Burning sensation in the upper abdomen.

Diagnosis
By endoscopy, biopsy, breath, blood, or stool tests.

Treatments
Antibiotics in combination with acid-reducing drugs.

Pathogenesis
Left untreated, ulcers may eventually penetrate the stomach or intestinal wall.

Prevention
Basic hygiene methods to prevent oral-oral or fecal-oral transmission.

Epidemiology
H. pylori affects up to 70 percent of people worldwide. Up to 15 percent of these will develop peptic ulcers.

See also
• Alcohol-related disorders

Stroke and related disorders

Strokes occur when the blood supply to part of the brain is suddenly stopped or when a blood vessel bursts, spilling blood into the area vessels surrounding the brain cells. A stroke is often referred to as a "brain attack." Strokes are the leading cause of adult disability. Each year about 760,000 people have symptomatic strokes; more than 11 million suffer silent strokes.

The Greek physician Hippocrates (460–377 B.C.E.) observed a condition in which people suddenly became unable to speak or walk. The Roman physician Galen (129–216) continued these studies and called the condition *apoplexy*. He theorized that women had these attacks because of the female menstrual cycle. Centuries later, a Swiss doctor Johann Wepfer (b. 1620) performed autopsies of humans and connected the postmortem signs of bleeding in the brain with persons who died from apoplexy. He also observed the blockage of the carotid and vertebral arteries that supply blood to the brain.

Like Galen and Wepfer, physicians throughout the centuries had no power over the condition. However, stroke medicine is changing rapidly, and scientists of the twenty-first century are garnering better therapies each day.

Description of stroke

The medical term for stroke is *cerebrovascular disease*, and it is sometimes referred to as a cerebrovascular accident, or CVA. The word *cerebrovascular* comes from the Latin word *cerebro*, which means "brain," and *vasa*, which means "vessel."

The brain requires about 20 percent of the heart's output of fresh blood to supply its requirements for oxygen and glucose. Two artery systems, the carotid arteries, carry blood through the neck to the brain.

Anything that disturbs the blood flow, even for a few seconds, affects the brain's function. Depending on the area of the brain, a variety of following symptoms may occur: sudden numbness, weakness, or paralysis on one side of the body, such as the face, arm, or leg; sudden nausea, fever, or vomiting; sudden difficulty speaking or understanding speech (aphasia); sudden blurred vision, double vision, or decreased vision in one or both eyes; sudden dizziness, loss of balance, or loss of coordination; sudden loss of consciousness; sudden confu-

sion or memory problems, loss of spatial orientation or perception; sudden headache, as a bolt out of the blue. The key word for each of these symptoms is sudden. There will frequently be more than one sign. Any of these symptoms signal a medical emergency. Every minute the brain cells are deprived of oxygen increases the risk of damage. Chances for recovery are much better when the right treatment is begun within the first few hours of noticing stroke symptoms.

Two major types of cerebrovascular events are ischemic stroke, in which blood does not get to part of the brain due to a disturbance in blood flow; and cerebral hemorrhage, during which blood vessels in the brain bleed and the released (hemorrhagic) blood damages brain tissue. The term *stroke* is commonly applied to the clinical symptoms and not to a specific condition.

Ischemic stroke

The word *ischemia* literally means "to hold back blood." This type of stroke occurs when an artery suddenly becomes blocked and decreases or stops the flow of blood to the brain. Cells may begin to die within minutes. This type is responsible for 80 percent of all strokes. There are two conditions that cause this type of stroke. The first is embolic stroke, which is a type of ischemia, in which a clot forms in another part of the body, travels through blood vessels, and becomes wedged in a brain artery. The free-roaming clot or embolus often forms in the heart. The type of clot is often caused by irregular beating in the two upper chambers of the heart. This irregular beating is called atrial fibrillation, which leads to poor blood flow and the formation of a clot.

The second type is thrombotic stroke, in which a blood clot forms in one of the cerebral arteries and grows until it is large enough to block the blood flow. Buildup of plaques (a mixture of fatty substances including cholesterol and other lipids) causes stenosis or narrowing of the artery as a result of these fatty deposits in the artery wall. When a stroke occurs as a result of small vessel disease, an infarction occurs. An infarction is the deprivation of blood supply of part of a tissue or organ in which an area of dead tissue (infarct) forms. Infarcted tissue swells and becomes firm, blood vessels around the infarct widen, and plasma and blood may flow into the infarct, thus increasing the swelling. The infarct then shrinks and is replaced by fibrous scar tissue, and function is lost.

Transient ischemic attacks (TIAs) may indicate that a stroke is coming. These are minor attacks in which the person may have a sudden onset of weakness, vertigo, or imbalance that lasts only a few minutes. These attacks have the same origin as ischemic stroke. Attacks are probably due to atherosclerosis, when plaque fragments break off and travel to a site in the brain. Major risk factors are high blood pressure, smoking, diabetes, and advanced age. The most significant factor is that the symptoms and signs last no more than 24 hours. If the symptom recurs, it often is a warning that a stroke may follow. One of the most common treatments for this condition is aspirin. Aspirin inhibits the way in which platelets clump together. Too many platelets gathered in a constricted area may block the flow to the brain.

Hemorrhagic stroke

Hemorrhage is the medical word for bleeding. A hemorrhagic stroke occurs when an artery in the brain bursts, sending blood into surrounding tissue. Symptoms include severe headache, drowsiness, seizures, or confusion after a head injury, paralysis on one side of the body, or changes in personality. This type of stroke accounts for about 20 percent of all strokes and happens in two ways. First, it can happen as an aneurysm; a thin or weak spot on the artery wall balloons out and ruptures, spilling blood into spaces surrounding the brain tissue. The ruptured brain arteries bleed into the brain itself or into spaces surrounding the brain.

Second, the stroke can occur as an intracerebral hemorrhage, when the vessel in the brain leaks blood into the brain itself. In this case, brain cells beyond the leak are deprived of blood and are also damaged.

High blood pressure is the most common cause of hemorrhagic stroke. High blood pressure causes small arteries in the brain to become stiff and subject to cracking or rupture. A subarachnoid hemorrhage is bleeding under the meninges into the outer covering

of the brain, which contaminates the cerebrospinal fluid (CSF). Because the CSF circulates through the cranium, this type of stroke can lead to extensive damage and is the most deadly of all strokes.

A head injury or blow to the head, such as a car accident or simply bumping the head, may cause a hemorrhage (this type of hemorrhage is never classified as a stroke). Subdural hemorrhages occur when an injury results in bleeding between the brain and the dura matter (the outer covering of the spinal cord and brain). Blood accumulates and produces a mass called a hematoma, which is literally a blood tumor. If the hematoma forms between the skull and the brain, it is called an extradural hematoma. Both these conditions put pressure on the brain and require immediate

KEY FACTS

Description
A stroke is a condition that occurs when the blood supply to part of the brain is suddenly stopped or when a blood vessel bursts, then spills blood into the vessels surrounding the brain cells.

Risk factors
Family history, hypertension (high blood pressure), atherosclerosis (hardening of the arteries), high levels of lipids or fat in bloodstream, sleep disorders, high homocysteine levels, age, and certain lifestyle behaviors.

Symptoms
Sudden numbness, weakness or paralysis on one side of the body, loss of speech, sudden nausea, dizziness, blurred vision, loss of balance, sudden headache, person has difficulty swallowing and talking.

Diagnosis
Suddenness of the attack and symptoms; physician will study blood vessels using a variety of imaging techniques.

Treatments
Drugs to improve blood flow and also neuroprotective agents.

Pathogenesis
Getting the victim to a physician who can quickly treat and determine the type of stroke. The stroke may be disabling or lethal.

Prevention
Lifestyle changes in eating and exercise, drugs to keep channels open, and neuroprotective agents

Epidemiology
The leading cause of adult disability; each year about 760,000 people have symptomatic strokes; more than 11 million suffer silent strokes.

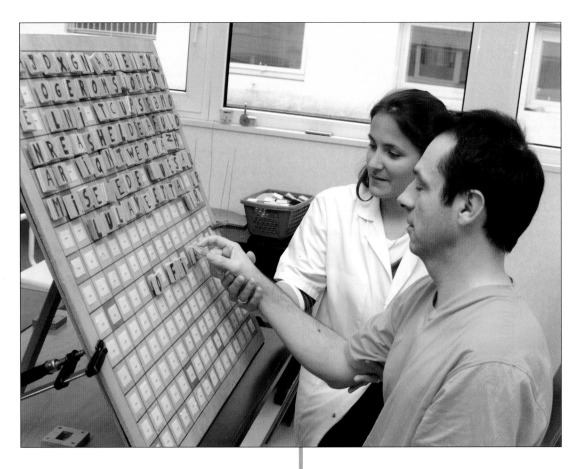

attention. The risk of dying is substantial with this type of injury and hemorrhage.

Risk factors

Several red flags for stroke include hypertension, hyperlipidemia, obesity, sleep disorders, homocysteine levels, and certain lifestyle behaviors. The chance of risk is slightly higher if one of the parents or brother or sister has had a stroke or TIA; age is also a risk factor. High blood pressure (HBP), also called hypertension, is highly correlated to stroke. Blood pressure is measured on a device called a sphygmomanometer, which reads the pressure during the relaxing phase (diastolic pressure) and also the peak pressure reached during the pumping contraction (systolic pressure). People who have abdominal fat (apple shapes) tend to have elevated blood pressure. For example, obese adults ages 20 to 45 are six times more likely to have high blood pressure than normal adults of the same age. Obese people who are 20 percent above standard weight show a 10 percent risk of stroke. A 2001 study by the North Manhattan Group found that doctors were prescribing few medications for

An occupational therapist helps a patient who is recovering from a stroke to construct words on a board. This exercise is part of a rehabilitation program designed to improve the patient's coordination and help with muscle control.

hypertension but were encouraging more attention to blood pressure control.

Hyperlipidemia or elevated levels of serum triglycerides (fats) are linked to stroke. Healthy arteries have a thin and smooth inner surface that allows blood to flow freely to deliver oxygen to the cells, including the 20 percent payload that the brain demands. In a diseased artery, the inner layer consists of a pool of fat that becomes covered with a hard crust called plaque, which forms inside the artery. Smooth muscle cells migrate to the built-up area, and a small crack appears in the lining, where a blood clot forms.

The buildup can be in any artery in the body, including the carotid artery in the neck that leads to the brain. As the abnormal deposits of fats and cholesterol grow and develop, the internal bore (lumen) of the artery gets narrower and narrower. Also, some of the plaque may break away and circulate in the bloodstream to the brain. According to several studies, TIA strokes appear closely related to hyperlipidemia.

People who sleep more than eight hours a night, who snore, or who experience daytime drowsiness have increased risk for stroke. Obstructive sleep apnea (OSA) is a sleep disorder characterized by episodes of not breathing, called apnea. This condition results from a collapse of the upper airway at the area of the back of the throat called the pharnyx. During an episode of apnea, the person tries to breathe against the closed airway, but he or she is not getting oxygen, and a condition called hypoxia occurs. The brain senses the lack of oxygen, and the person wakes up briefly to restore the upper-airway passage. The cycle may be repeated a hundred times during the night, disrupting normal sleep. The person rarely remembers. OSA can lead to stroke by reducing the amount of oxygen that reaches the brain.

Several lifestyle behavioral factors correlate with stroke. One study found that 28 percent of strokes follow alcohol use and 8 percent after heavy exertion. Other examples were lifting more than 50 pounds, 10 percent; straining during urination or defecation, 4 percent; anger outbursts, 4 percent; and sexual intercourse, 2 percent. Another lifestyle condition is metabolic syndrome, or Syndrome X, in which a cluster of major risk factors of life habits such as alcohol abuse, improper nutrition, inadequate physical activity, and increased body weight all converge to create cardiovascular problems and risk of stroke. Other factors include gender (women tend to die more with strokes), cigarette smoking, diabetes, and use of birth control bills, and hormone therapy.

Certain medications have been related to stroke. In October 2000 the U.S. Food and Drug Administration (FDA) removed phenylpropanolamine (PPA) from over 400 over-the-counter cold, cough, and some diet medications. The FDA found PPA caused 200 to 500 strokes in people under 50, who were mostly women.

Epidemiology

Accurate reporting techniques are being developed and refined. A 2001 study reported that rates of the first ischemic stroke, intracerebral hemorrhage, and subarachnoid hemorrhage were 25 to 50 percent higher among people of African American descent than among Caucasians. The study found that the general U.S. population will suffer 760,000 strokes each year, and more than 11 million suffer silent strokes or TIAs. Historically, the Southeast, especially Alabama and Mississippi, has been referred to as the stroke belt because the area had more strokes than other sections of the country. However, there are indications that the western states of Oregon, Washington, and Arizona may, in the future, have the highest incidence of strokes.

Figures from the National Stroke Foundation have revealed a startling number of young adults who have had strokes. About 225,000 Americans under the age of 45, including young and middle-aged women, have had strokes. One stroke victim of a brain aneurysm was 13; she was fortunate the aneurysm had only ballooned out, and it was caught before it burst. Drug abuse has led to 85 to 90 percent of hemorrhagic strokes occurring in people in their 20s and 30s. In 2002 around 275,000 people in the United States died after having a stroke; stroke accounted for 1 in 15 deaths in the United States. Stroke is the third leading cause of death after heart disease and cancer.

Diagnosis and treatments

When the rapid development of symptoms of stroke occur, emergency facilities should be contacted immediately, but first aid care must be taken in the meantime. Timely first aid is of vital importance for the patient. If breathing stops, cardiopulmonary resuscitation (CPR) should be administered. For minor breathing difficulties, the head should be elevated by positioning the head and shoulders on a pillow. The affected person should not be given anything to eat or drink, and the paralyzed parts must be protected. Depending on circumstances, emergency personnel may begin to administer anti-clotting medications, such as aspirin and ticlopidine, and anticoagulants, such as heparin or warfarin.

In order for the doctor to pinpoint treatments, an image of the brain is necessary. One type of image is called cerebral arteriography or angiography, which is an X-ray that shows the fluid in the arteries to the brain. This image allows the physician to see blood circulating through the brain and to note exactly where there are abnormalities, such as narrowing of the arteries or escape of blood from an artery. The patient is conscious during the procedure. A long flexible catheter is inserted through an artery in the groin, then is passed through the trunk and into the carotid artery or vertebral artery. Dye is injected through the catheter to reveal abnormalities or obstructions. This type of procedure lasts from one to three hours and can be very tiring for the patient.

Many advances in imaging have occurred in the past

few years. Computerized tomography (CT) scans image brain anatomy and blood movement in a series of scans. A new generation of CT scanner applies noncontrast CT, perfusion (the way in which the blood passes through the brain), and CT angiography, all in a scanning time of 23 minutes. Magnetic resonance imaging (MRI) uses a strong magnetic field to generate a three-dimensional view of the brain. This test is sensitive for detecting brain tissue damaged by ischemic stroke. Also, MRI techniques have improved. A technique called fluid-attenuated inversion recovery, or FLAIR, suppresses bright signal images from the cerebrospinal fluid that interfere with reading. Echocardiography is an ultrasound technology that creates images of the heart. A new procedure called neurosonology applies transcranial Doppler (TCD) ultrasound to monitor therapy.

Drugs for acute therapy treatment fall into two categories: medication to improve blood flow and neuroprotective agents.

Improving blood flow. At present, treatment with intravenous thrombolytic tissue plasminogen activator (t-PA) continues to be the first choice for acute stroke within the first three hours. Genetech, a biotechnology firm, developed the clot dissolving Activase (r), a genetically engineered version of naturally occurring t-PA. Since approval in 1996, more than one million people have benefited from the drug.

Other anti-thrombotic drugs include heparin, aspirin, and abciximab. A seven-year study of 2,206 patients at 48 centers compared aspirin to warfarin for recurrent stroke prevention and found that aspirin works as well as warfarin in helping to prevent strokes in most patients. Aspirin affects blood platelets and clotting and has been used for over one hundred years. However, its beneficial effects to prevent stroke and heart attack were only recognized in the 1970s. A large group of new thrombolytics is being investigated. Another new strategy is the use of the laser-based endovascular photo acoustic recanalization (EPAR) system, which combines laser "clotbusters" with pharmaceuticals.

Neuroprotective agents. It is now known that substantial amounts of neuronal tissue damage may be reversible. These strategies consider how to preserve or even reverse neuronal areas. Many of these drugs are in trials. Hypothermia or reducing body temperature as a neuroprotective in animal models continues to be explored in adults. An experiment compared patients who had been wrapped in cooling blankets with water baths at 90°F (32°C) to those without the blankets. The study found that the patients treated with hypothermia had less disability three months after the stroke.

Surgical procedures are sometimes necessary to remove blood that has been leaking into the tissue from a cerebral hemorrhage. An operation called a carotid endarectomy may be used to clean arterial plaque deposits as a preventive measure. Sometimes this is used to prevent a minor stroke from recurring. If there has been a subarachnoid hemorrhage, surgical treatment of the aneurysm is often needed.

Rehabilitation

Over 500,000 people survive strokes each year. Half of these patients live over five years, and 10 to 13 percent live ten years. There are an estimated 2.5 million disabled stroke survivors in the United States. Some have only minor disabilities. It is hopeful that many of these patients will walk again and be able to care for themselves. However, about two out of ten will require extended care in a long-term care facility.

Rehabilitation for people who have had strokes is very important for their livelihood and morale. Living at home, if possible, is a great booster. Ingenious adaptive devices and modifications can help the person at home, to allow them to be more independent and to remain a useful part of society. In 1990 the Americans with Disabilities Act (ADA) prohibits discrimination on the basis of disability. Public facilities must accommodate those who have some type of disability to enable them to do things that other people can do. Ramps, special chairs, and bathroom accommodations must be available. Recovery and rehabilitation depend on the area of the brain involved and the amount of tissue damaged. If the speech area is affected, the person may need speech therapy.

Prevention

Prevention of stroke by a healthy lifestyle and avoiding risk factors makes good common sense. A number of strategies include taking preventive drugs that keep open channels and act as neuroprotective agents. Some doctors recommend routinely taking a low-level dose of aspirin (75 mg) as a routine protective against heart disease and stroke. The aspirin keeps the blood flowing and attacks the clotting mechanism of the blood platelets. Other anti-platelet agents are estradiol and vitamins.

For those who have had strokes or TIAs, one of the most hopeful areas of research is that of stem cell

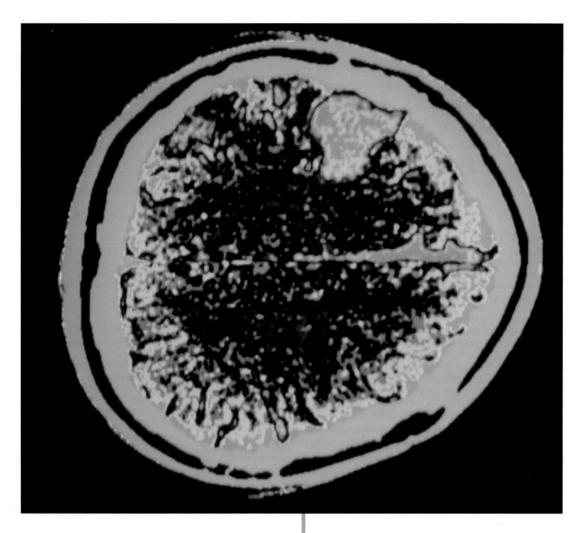

This computed tomography scan is a transverse cross section of the brain of a person after a vascular accident. A cerebrovascular accident or stroke is caused by hemorrhage and results in the destruction of brain tissue (green patch at top center right of picture).

transplants to enhance recovery from cerebrovascular damage. Adult stem cells found in the bone marrow or embryonic tissue can develop into brain cells. In rat models of stroke, stem cells have grown in the area of the damage and formed connections with adjacent cells. A study showed that human umbilical cord blood cells injected into rat's tails migrated to the brain within hours and began repairing damage. The umbilical cord is a rich source of immature stem and progenitor cells.

Other new medical procedures are currently under investigation. Putting stroke victims in a hyperbaric oxygen chamber, in which oxygen is at greater pressure than in the normal atmosphere, has proved helpful to some stroke victims.

Stroke may have a genetic element. A 2001 study found a genetic link to hemorrhagic strokes in young white women. The investigators focused on genetic variations in factor XIII, a protein involved in blood clotting. Although few data exist, gene therapy may offer promise for stroke recovery.

Research has come a long way in offering hope to stroke victims. Studies have shown that brain injury occurs within minutes and can continue for days afterward. Timing is critical; educating the public for the signs, symptoms, and necessary action is essential.

Evelyn B. Kelly

See also
• Alcohol-related disorders • Head injury
• Heart attack • Paralysis • Thrombosis
and embolism

Sunburn and sunstroke

Sunburn is the skin's reaction to too much exposure to the ultraviolet radiation of the sun. A person's skin type may determine how quickly the burn occurs. Extreme exposure to sun may cause sunstroke, a life-threatening condition in which the body's heat-regulating mechanism shuts down.

From the time of the ancient Egyptians, who worshipped the sun god Ra, the sun has been recognized as an essential for life. But the sun can also be a source of great agony if precautions are not taken. In addition to heat and light, the sun gives off invisible ultraviolet radiation in three types: UVA, which penetrates into deeper skin layers and damages the production of new skin cells and causes tanning and wrinkling; UVB, which is even more damaging because it affects the surface of the skin by releasing chemicals that dilate the blood vessels; and UVC rays, which are absorbed by Earth's atmosphere before they strike earth. Sunburn results from too much sun on the skin; sunstroke occurs when the body's mechanisms are overwhelmed by a very hot and humid environment or by strenuous physical activity.

Causes, risk factors, and symptoms

Unlike a thermal burn, sunburn is not immediately apparent. Once the skin appears painful and red, the damage has been done. The skin turns red about 2 to 6 hours after exposure, and peak effects are noted at 12 to 24 hours.

Melanocytes in skin produce melanin for protection from UV rays. However, if the UV rays exceed the blocking power of melanin, sunburn occurs. Because their level of melanin (skin pigment) is sparse, certain light-skinned and fair-haired people are at greater risk for sunburn.

Symptoms of severe sunburn include chills, fever, nausea, vomiting, flulike symptoms, and blisters, which may vary from very fine to large water-filled blisters that have red, raw skin underneath. Medical care should be sought if pain is severe.

Sunstroke is a type of heatstroke that occurs when the body's thermostat cannot keep it cool. When temperature rises, evaporation of perspiration cools the body. In humid air, sweat does not evaporate, causing the body temperature to rise rapidly. If not treated, heatstroke can cause organ shutdowns, brain damage, and death. Treatment includes cooling the body core and giving intravenous injections to restore lost fluid.

Prevention

The best prevention is to avoid the sun. Other strategies include covering up with wide-brimmed hats, long-sleeved shirts, and long pants; wearing a sunscreen with a sun protection factor (SPF) of at least 15; and drinking plenty of water but avoiding alcohol and caffeine. Chronic sun exposure may lead to premature aging, severe wrinkling, and various cancerous skin tumors. Premature cataract formation may also occur.

Evelyn B. Kelly

KEY FACTS

Description
Sunburn is the skin's reaction to the sun; sunstroke occurs when the body's heat-regulating system shuts down.

Risk factors
Sunlight and humid temperatures.

Symptoms
Red, tender, blistered, and swollen skin; sunstroke includes elevated body temperature, hot dry skin, and often unconsciousness.

Diagnosis
Severe burn and blisters; hot dry skin, fainting, confusion, and dizziness are all indications.

Treatments
Home treatments for mild sunburn include medication for pain, cool compresses, or cool baths; for severe cases or stroke, IV fluids may be given upon admission to a hospital.

Pathogenesis
Untreated severe sunburn can lead to complications; repeated sunburns precede premature wrinkling, sunspots, and skin cancer.

Prevention
Sunscreen, wide brim hats, covering, and avoiding sun in the hottest part of the day.

Epidemiology
Sunstroke kills 10 percent of its victims.

See also
- Burns • Cancer, skin • Cataract
- Melanoma

Syphilis

Syphilis is a sexually transmitted disease (STD) that can cause chronic infection and irreversible health problems if left untreated. It can be transmitted during pregnancy from mother to infant, causing a serious and sometimes fatal condition called congenital syphilis. In other parts of the world where there are crowded and poor hygienic conditions, syphilis may also be transmitted though close nonsexual contact.

Syphilis has been known as a disease for thousands of years and is still a prominent STD. Syphilis is caused by *Treponema pallidum*, a motile corkscrew-shaped bacterium known for its undulating behavior, which belongs to the order Spirochaeta, commonly called spirochetes. *T. pallidum* enters the body through a break in the skin or mucous membranes of the reproductive tract or mouth after sexual contact (oral, anal, or vaginal) with an infected person.

Syphilis goes through four stages of infection that sometimes overlap. In the first stage, primary syphilis, a small, round, painless sore called a chancre (pronounced "shanker") generally develops 10 to 90 days after exposure at the entry point of *T. pallidum*, usually on the penis, vulva, or cervix, or in the vagina or rectum, on the mouth, tongue or lips after oral sex, or other parts of the body. The sore contains *T. pallidum*, so it is highly contagious. Since the sore is painless, if it is on the cervix, inside the vagina, or inside the rectum, a woman may not even know she has been infected. Because the sore heals on its own, men and women may not seek treatment, and the disease progresses. The open sore increases the risk of HIV transmission.

The secondary stage begins about two to ten weeks after the sore appears, as *T. pallidum* spreads through the bloodstream. The result is a non-itchy rash, usually on the palms of the hands and soles of the feet, but also in the mouth, other areas, or the entire body. Symptoms can include fever, swollen glands, fatigue, headache, muscle aches, or hair loss. Because many of these symptoms can be found in many other diseases, syphilis is called "the great imitator." The rash contains the bacterium *T. pallidum*, so the secondary stage is also highly contagious. Despite being able to provoke an immune response in the body, untreated *T. pallidum* can last in the body for decades.

The third stage is called latent (hidden) syphilis. There can be few or no symptoms, and this stage can last for years. The early part of this stage is still infectious, the later part much less so, and risk of transmission is low. If not treated, some people progress to tertiary, or late syphilis. During this stage *T. pallidum* can damage the heart, blood vessels, brain, nervous system, bones, liver, and joints. Some of the results are blindness, mental illness, memory loss, heart disease, stroke or even death.

KEY FACTS

Description

Sexually transmitted disease; untreated can lead to serious health problems; can be passed from mothers to babies at any stage of pregnancy.

Causes

The bacterium *Treponema pallidum*.

Risk factors

Sexual activity; multiple sex partners; living in area with high rates; inconsistent use of condoms.

Symptoms and signs

Painless sore, then may have skin rash, general flulike symptoms, mouth sores, swollen glands, headache, muscle aches, weight loss, hair loss. Symptoms may cease. Final stage: neurological, cardiovascular, and musculoskeletal damage.

Diagnosis

Detecting *T. pallidum* from sore using darkfield microscopic exam; blood tests.

Treatments

Antibiotics, usually penicillin; in later stage damage cannot be reversed. Partner notification.

Pathogenesis

T. pallidum penetrates broken skin or mucous membranes and progresses in stages. First stage: sore at site of infection. Second stage: spreads through blood, damaging organs. Increases likelihood of HIV transmission.

Prevention

Sexual abstinence. Avoiding contact with infected people; monogamous relationship with uninfected person; consistent and correct use of condoms.

Epidemiology

Lowest rate of highly infectious forms, primary and secondary syphilis, in 2000 (less than 6,000 reported cases) since reporting began in 1941 (600,000 cases). Rates from 2000 to 2004 have increased (almost 8,000) mostly due to infection of men who have sex with men.

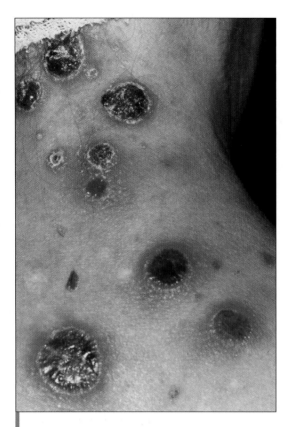

This inflamed rash on the neck is a secondary syphilis rash, which occurs about 6 to 12 weeks after infection with Treponema pallidum. *The rash is accompanied by headache, fatigue, and fever. Treatment is with antibiotics.*

Pregnant women with untreated syphilis can pass the infection to their unborn babies, resulting in miscarriages, premature births, or stillbirths. Newborns can have deformities, seizures, liver problems, anemia, and developmental delays, and as many as 40 percent of babies will die. Blood tests for syphilis are recommended routinely in pregnant women.

Diagnosis

Darkfield examination of a sample from the sore or skin rash uses a special lighting technique that makes *T. pallidum* easier to see than with standard microscope lighting. The VDRL (Venereal Disease Research Laboratory) blood test measures antibodies to the bacterium. This test may be positive when syphilis is really not present, so a more specific blood test, the FTA-ABS (fluorescent treponemal antibody absorption), can confirm the infection. If advanced syphilis involving the brain, called neurosyphilis, is suspected, a spinal tap is done to test the cerebrospinal fluid.

Because many people who have the infection may have no symptoms, many states still require a blood test for syphilis before marriage. Syphilis remains an important public health problem in poor and urban areas. The Centers for Disease Control has launched a program to eliminate syphilis in the United States, focusing on high risk populations.

Treatments

In the early stages, syphilis is easily curable with antibiotics, usually penicillin. *T. pallidum* divides slowly, so the long-acting forms of penicillin are used. During the later stages, *T. pallidum* divides even more slowly, and this requires a longer course of antibiotics. Damage from late syphilis cannot be reversed. Neurosyphilis is treated with daily intravenous (in the vein) penicillin.

Partner notification identifies sex partners of those people with HIV and other STDs so that they can be tested, evaluated, and treated for STDs.

Prevention

Prevention includes abstaining from sexual contact. Condoms used consistently and correctly and a monogamous sexual relationship with an uninfected person can reduce risk. Infection does not make a person immune; reinfection can occur.

Epidemiology

In the United States, rates of reported cases of the early infectious forms of syphilis, called primary and secondary syphilis, decreased during the 1990s, to an all-time low in 2000 of less than 6,000 since reporting began in 1941, when there were almost 600,000 cases. Reported cases increased in 2004 to almost 8,000, with rates higher in African Americans and Hispanics than in whites.

Rates in women remained stable but increased in men who have sex with men. The increase is thought to be due to an increase in high-risk sexual behavior (multiple sex partners, not using condoms consistently). Syphilis is known as a genital ulcer disease because during the early stage of infection an ulcer, or deep sore, appears at the site of infection.

Ramona Jenkin

See also
• AIDS • Cancer, cervical • Chlamydial infections • Gonorrhea • Hepatitis infections • HPV infection • Pelvic inflammatory disease

Tapeworm infestation

Tapeworms are long, segmented worms of the class Cestoda (cestodes). Infestation occurs either as fully developed (mature) tapeworms in the intestinal lumen or as fluid-filled masses (cysts) in the liver, lung, muscle, brain, eye, or other organs.

Cestodes that can infest humans include the intestinal tapeworms *Diphyllobothrium latum* (fish tapeworm), *Hymenolepis nana* (dwarf tapeworm), *Taenia saginata* (beef tapeworm), and *T. solium* (pork tapeworm) and the invasive tapeworms *Echinococcus spp.* and pork tapeworm. Tapeworms divide their life cycle between two animal hosts (intermediate and definitive), vary in size from several millimeters to 82 feet (25 m), lack an intestine, and absorb nutrients through their external surface.

The mature worm consists of a head (scolex) that attaches to the lining of the intestine, a neck, and a segmented body that contains both male and female sex organs (proglottids) and produces the parasite's eggs. Proglottids become gravid (full of eggs), break free from the tapeworm, degenerate in the stool, and release thousands of eggs per day into the feces.

Life cycle of tapeworms

The eggs of *Echinococcus spp.*, and pork and dwarf tapeworms infest an intermediate host (such as cattle and pigs) through ingestion of contaminated food. Once ingested, the egg hatches in the intestine and releases a larval form (oncosphere). The oncosphere penetrates the intestinal wall, reaches the circulation, and migrates to different organs to form a cyst. When a definitive host (such as a human) eats the cyst-containing tissues of the intermediate host, the cyst develops into a mature tapeworm in the intestinal lumen. Fish tapeworm eggs hatch in the water, and if the larval form is eaten by a small crustacean called a copepod, the larvae develops in the copepod's tissues. After the copepod is eaten by a fish (intermediate host), the larva migrates to its muscles and encysts. When an uncooked cyst is eaten by a human (definitive host), it develops into a mature tapeworm in the intestine.

Humans are solely definitive hosts for fish tapeworm and beef tapeworm and are solely intermediate hosts for *Echinococcus spp.*, which are located as mature tapeworms in the intestine of canines such as dogs and

KEY FACTS

Description

Parasitic infestation leading to the development of mature tapeworms in the intestine or to the development of cysts in different organs.

Causes

Long segmented worms of the class Cestoda.

Risk factors

Ingestion of cyst-containing tissues (meat) or of food contaminated with tapeworm eggs.

Symptoms

Intestinal infestation is often symptomless but can lead to nutrient malabsorption. Invasive infestation in the brain can cause seizures.

Diagnosis

Examination of stool samples for eggs or proglottids for intestine worms. Imaging techniques and antibody tests for invasive infestation.

Treatments

Antiparasitic drugs for intestinal infestations. Drugs and surgery for invasive infestations.

Pathogenesis

Intestinal tapeworms compete for nutrients with the host, and may lead to nutrient deficiencies in infested people. *Echinococcus* cysts may compress other organs, develop into abscesses, and rupture, causing seeding of new cysts and an allergic reaction. When pork tapeworm cysts die, they release parts of the parasite in the surrounding tissues, causing local inflammation and damage.

Prevention

Intestinal tapeworm infestations can be prevented by careful disposal of human sewage; using uncontaminated food for animals that serve as intermediate hosts; inspecting meat before marketing; and freezing or cooking meat.

Epidemiology

There is great geographic variability in the incidence and prevalence of tapeworm infestations, depending on the types of intermediate and definitive hosts involved in the tapeworm's life cycle.

foxes. However, humans serve both as intermediate and definitive hosts for pork and dwarf tapeworms.

The immune response to intestinal infestations leads to an increase in eosinophil white blood cells and immunoglobulin E (IgE) levels in the blood, but it is not known whether this alters the course of the infestation. The immune response to a cyst often does not lead to its eradication but to its encapsulation with fibrous tissue, thus limiting damage to nearby organs.

Risk factors and epidemiology

Fish tapeworm infestation is acquired by eating un-cooked freshwater fish that contain cysts. It is common in Siberia, northern Europe, Canada, Japan, Chile, and now also in the United States partly because of the increasing popularity of ceviche, sushi, and sashimi. Mature tapeworms reach up to 82 feet (25 m) long.

Dwarf tapeworm is acquired by ingestion of the eggs on fecally contaminated food and is the only tapeworm with direct human-to-human transmission. The mature tapeworm releases eggs that infest direct-ly the mucosal lining and increase the number of ma-ture tapeworms in the intestine of the infested host in the absence of further ingestion of eggs from the envi-ronment. It is very common in Asia, southern and eastern Europe, Central and South America, and Africa, whereas in North America it is found principally in people who are institutionalized, malnourished, or have a poorly functioning immune system. Mature tapeworms are small 0.6 to 2 inches (15–50 mm) long.

Beef tapeworm is acquired by eating uncooked beef containing the cysts. It is common in cattle-breeding areas of the world such as central Asia, the Near East, and Central and East Africa, and South America. Mature tapeworms reach up to 33 feet (10 m) long.

Pork tapeworm is acquired either by ingestion of eggs on fecally contaminated food, leading to the de-velopment of cysts in organs (cysticercosis) or by in-gestion of uncooked pork containing the cysts, leading to the development of a mature tapeworm living the intestine. In 25 percent of cases, both forms are pres-ent simultaneously. It is common in Mexico, Central America, South America, Africa, Southeast Asia, India, the Philippines, and southern Europe. Mature tapeworms reach up to 6.5 to 26 feet (2–8 m) long.

In people with cysticercosis, the cysts are located in different organs, and involvement of the brain (neuro-cysticercosis) or of the heart can be life threatening. Echinococcosis results from the ingestion of eggs on food contaminated by canine feces. There are two forms of echinococcosis: hydatid disease, caused by *E. granulosus* or *E. vogeli*, and alveolar cyst disease, caused by *E. multilocularis*. *E. granulosus* is transmitted by do-mestic dogs and is common worldwide, whereas *E. multilocularis* and *E. vogeli* are transmitted by wild ca-nines and are common in the northern regions of Europe, Asia, and North America, and in the Arctic regions of South America, respectively. Hydatid cysts of *E. granulosus* most commonly form in the liver or lungs and reach up to 2 to 4 inches (5–10 cm) in size. Cysts of *E. multilocularis*, which infest the lungs, tend to be smaller but invade surrounding tissues very aggressively and can spread to distant organs via the bloodstream.

Symptoms and diagnosis

Mature tapeworms in the intestine cause few symp-toms, although nutrient malabsorption and a change in intestinal motility may occur. Fish tapeworm infes-tation may result in vitamin B_{12} deficiency and mega-loblastic anemia. Patients with neurocysticercosis have few symptoms while the cysts are alive but can devel-op epilepsy and other neurological symptoms when the cysts die, swell, and release parts of the dead para-site in the surrounding tissues, causing local inflam-mation and brain damage. Symptoms of echinococcosis occur as a result of compression of other organs by an enlarging cyst, bacterial superinfection of a cyst, and rupture, causing release of offspring cysts or an allergic reaction to the dead parasite.

Diagnosis of intestinal infestation is made by exam-ination under a microscope of stool samples for eggs or proglottids, but multiple stool samples are often need-ed because of the irregular rate of proglottid detach-ment. Invasive infestation is suspected on the basis of imaging techniques such as computed tomography (CT) or magnetic resonance imaging (MRI) and is confirmed by tests for specific antibodies in the blood or cerebrospinal fluid (in neurocysticercosis).

Treatment and prevention

Intestinal tapeworm infestation should be treated with the drugs praziquantel or niclosamide. Pork tapeworm cysts outside the brain can be surgically removed. For neurocysticercosis, surgery is often too dangerous, al-though treatment with drugs such as praziquantel and albendazole together with corticosteroid drugs may be beneficial. For *Echinococcus spp.* cysts, treatment is sur-gical removal after killing of cysts with ethanol injec-tions or drugs such as albendazole and melbendazole.

Intestinal infestation can be prevented by careful disposal of human sewage; using uncontaminated food for animals that can be intermediate hosts; inspecting the meat before marketing to rule out cyst infestation; and freezing or cooking meat to kill cysts. Invasive in-festations are more difficult to prevent because infec-tious eggs are widespread in the environment.

Corrado Cancedda

See also
• Anemia • Vitamin deficiency

Tay-Sachs disease

First described in the late 1800s by physicians Warren Tay and Bernard Sachs, Tay-Sachs disease is an inherited and lethal disorder that affects the central nervous system. Though found predominantly in Jewish families of eastern European origin, Tay-Sachs disease also affects other ethnic groups. A mutation in the gene that makes the enzyme hexoaminidase A is responsible for causing central nervous system deterioration. Although it is not currently possible to treat Tay-Sachs disease, public education, genetic counseling, and genetic testing help reduce the incidence of this devastating metabolic disorder.

Tay-Sachs disease is named after the two clinicians who separately described this inherited condition. In 1881 the British ophthalmologist Warren Tay (1843–1927) linked the presence of a cherry-red spot located in the retina to symptoms of physical and mental decline—symptoms later observed in children. Several years later, Bernard Sachs (1858–1944), a New York neurologist, described this condition at the cellular level. He also discovered its genetic causes by noticing that most families who had babies with what he called "amaurotic familial idiocy" were Jews of eastern European origin.

Causes

Tay-Sachs is caused by an autosomal recessive disorder in which a faulty gene is inherited from both parents. People who have this inherited metabolic disorder either lack the enzyme hexosaminidase A (Hex A) or make Hex A enzyme molecules that do not work properly. Normally this enzyme breaks down the fatty substance GM2 ganglioside into materials needed to make nerve cell membranes. Without Hex A, GM2 ganglioside accumulates in nerve cells thus causing them to swell and die.

Symptoms and signs

Tay-Sachs babies appear normal at birth. By about three to six months, because of the effects of enzyme deficiency and nerve-cell damage, parents notice their baby startles easily in response to any noise, appears unaware of his or her surroundings, and has poor vision and muscle weakness, with floppy arms and legs. The baby will also show other developmental and behavioral abnormalities. By two years, most Tay-Sachs children experience uncontrollable seizures, diminishing mental capacity, and loss of physical skills, such as sitting and crawling. Eventually, the child becomes blind, paralyzed and nonresponsive. Most Tay-Sachs children die before their fifth birthday.

Risk factors

Medical researchers have known for more than 40 years that Hex A is absent in Tay-Sachs patients. Inherited in an autosomal recessive manner, people who have one Tay-Sachs gene make enough Hex A enzyme molecules to prevent damage. However, those who inherit two Tay-Sachs genes are completely deficient in this vital enzyme and do not survive.

The Hex A gene that causes Tay-Sachs disease is located on chromosome 15. Recent advances in DNA sequencing technology reveals nearly one hundred Hex A mutations that cause Tay-Sachs disease. Some

KEY FACTS

Description

A fatal genetic disorder in children that destroys the central nervous system.

Causes and risk factors

Absence of the enzyme hexoaminidase A causes Tay-Sachs disease. Inheriting two copies of the Tay-Sachs gene is the risk factor.

Symptoms

Vision loss, an abnormal startle response, developmental regression, seizures, diminishing mental function.

Diagnosis

DNA testing for the presence of Tay-Sachs mutations and the absence of hexoaminidase A in blood.

Treatments

Supportive care. There is no cure for Tay-Sachs disease.

Pathogenesis

The absence of hexoaminidase A causes accumulations of a lipid, GM2 ganglioside, in the brain.

Epidemiology

Primarily affects Jews of eastern European origin.

mutations prevent Hex A synthesis and others produce Hex A molecules that do not efficiently break down GM2 ganglioside. Infantile Tay-Sachs, the condition marked by Hex A enzyme deficiency, is the most severe and rapidly progressing form.

People who have late-onset Tay-Sachs disease (LOTS) make Hex A molecules that do not work properly. In this situation, the disease progresses slowly, and people usually experience poor coordinations, tremor, and slurred speech—symptoms of neurological degeneration—by the time they reach adolescence. Over time, LOTS patients develop other neurologic symptoms that may include unsteady gait, muscle weakness, and mental and behavioral changes.

Genetic testing and prevention

At the present time, there is no cure for Tay-Sachs disease, although the disease is lessening as a result of more available information. Public education, carrier screening, and prenatal diagnosis are effective preventive measures. Testing blood and DNA identifies people who carry Tay-Sachs mutations.

Blood testing identifies carriers because their single Hex A gene produces smaller amounts of enzyme than people who have two functional genes. DNA testing identifies many Hex A mutations, including those which cause LOTS.

Preimplantation genetic diagnosis (PGD) may be considered for couples when there is a known mutation. The technique identifies defects in embryos created through in vitro fertilization before transferring them to the uterus.

Genetic counseling and treatment

If the woman is already pregnant, genetic counselors can offer referrals for diagnostic tests to determine if the baby is unaffected, is a carrier, or has Tay-Sachs disease. Amniocentesis involves testing the fetal cells contained in the surrounding amniotic fluid for Hex A. Doctors perform this test between the fifteenth and eighteenth week of pregnancy.

Testing placental tissue, or chorionic villus sampling, provides similar diagnostic information. Doctors perform this test between the tenth and twelfth week of pregnancy. Overall, the incidence of Tay-Sachs disease in Ashkenazi Jews was 1 in every 3,600 births; as a result of extensive genetic counseling of carriers the incidence has been reduced by more than 90 percent. In Sephardic Jews and non-Jews, the incidence of Tay-Sachs disease is 1 in 250,000 people.

Genetic counselors, professionals who receive extensive education and training in genetics and psychology, believe that it is better if the family receives some genetic counseling information before testing. During the initial session, the genetic counselor explains the purpose of testing, how to prepare for the test procedure, and how to understand the range of possible test results. Often families see the counselor after having already received a positive Tay-Sachs report. In either situation, the genetic counselor helps the couple understand and interpret their test results and explains the range of available options.

The baby does not have Tay-Sachs disease if neither family member carries the Tay-Sachs gene. If either the mother or the father is a Tay-Sachs carrier, the baby has a 50 percent chance of also receiving a single copy of the Tay-Sachs gene. There are several possible outcomes if both parents are Tay-Sachs carriers. For each pregnancy, there is a 1 in 4 chance that the baby will not inherit the Tay-Sachs gene. There is also a 50 percent chance that the baby will be a carrier and a 25 percent chance that the baby will have Tay-Sachs disease. The genetic counselor, rather than telling the family what they should do, helps them make decisions that are compatible with their personal beliefs.

Options range from giving birth to having a therapeutic abortion. It is very important that counselors present information in a way that supports family discussion and does not stigmatize individuals.

There is currently no treatment for Tay-Sachs disease. All that is possible is to treat any symptoms when they occur, and to keep the child as comfortable as possible.

Pathogenesis and epidemiology

Tay-Sachs is a fatal disease for children who have inherited two Tay-Sachs genes. They rarely live beyond the age of five.

Medical geneticists estimate that everybody carries six to eight disease-causing genes. According to the Chicago Center for Jewish Genetic Disorders, nearly 1 in 30 Jewish people of eastern European or Ashkenazi descent carry a Tay-Sachs gene. By comparison, in the general population that also includes Mediterranean or Sephardic Jews, about 1 in 250 people have this mutation.

Janet Yagoda Shagam

See also
• Paralysis

Tetanus

Tetanus is a disorder of the nervous system caused by the bacterium *Clostridium tetani*. It typically occurs when traumatic injuries and wounds are contaminated by this toxin-producing organism. The disease is characterized by intense muscle spasms and is often fatal. With the advent of vaccination, the incidence of tetanus has decreased among the developed world. However, it is still very prevalent in developing nations.

The bacterium *Clostridium tetani* commonly exists in the environment, especially in soil. The organism produces spores that can gain access to the host through penetrating trauma or wounds. Once inside host tissue, the organism germinates into the bacterium and produces harmful toxins. Injury and wounds, including those seen in postsurgical patients, are the main predisposing factors for the development of tetanus.

Symptoms and signs

In its most classic form, symptoms include painful, involuntary muscular contractions that can involve the entire body. Muscles of the jaw may be affected, referred to as "trismus" or "lockjaw." In addition to muscle spasms, patients may experience fever, sweating, irritability, and restlessness. As spasms progress, airway obstruction and respiratory failure may ensue necessitating the use of a mechanical ventilator.

Diagnosis and treatments

The diagnosis is typically made based on the presentation of the patient, especially if any history of an injury or wound is reported. The bacteria do not grow well in the laboratory; therefore culture and other blood tests are rarely helpful in the diagnosis.

Several different treatment modalities should be implemented to treat tetanus. Antibiotics are universally recommended, and acceptable agents include penicillins or metronidazole. Antibodies to the toxin, also known as tetanus immune globulin (TIG), should be administered with the hope of neutralizing its effects. The vaccination series should also be started to confer long-term immunity. Surgical removal of devitalized tissue or wounds may be necessary. Finally, measures to decrease muscle spasms and support the respiratory system, possibly with a mechanical ventilator, are often required.

Once in host tissue, the organism produces its primary toxin, called tetanospasmin, which travels through neurons to the spinal cord and brain stem. The toxin then interferes with normal neuronal activity to induce muscular rigidity and other symptoms.

Vaccination with tetanus toxoid is recommended. In the United States, it is given as a series of five shots. Booster injections should be given every ten years to ensure lifelong immunity.

The annual incidence of tetanus in the United States is 0.16 cases per million people, or 35 to 70 cases per year. Worldwide incidence is higher, with roughly 18 cases per 100,000 people, about 1 million cases per year.

Joseph M. Fritz and Bernard C. Camins

KEY FACTS

Description
A disease of the nervous system caused by toxin-producing bacteria.

Causes
Clostridium tetani.

Risk factors
Deep injuries or wounds, postsurgical patients, drug users, neonates.

Symptoms and signs
Muscular rigidity and pain, often of the jaw; fever, sweating, and mental changes. Spasms lead to airway obstruction and respiratory compromise.

Diagnosis
Based on clinical presentation of the patient.

Treatments
Antibiotics, tetanus immune globulin to neutralize the toxin, and vaccination to confer immunity after treatment. Surgical debridement, muscle relaxants, and respiratory support.

Pathogenesis
Bacteria produce tetanospasmin toxin. Affects spinal cord and brain stem, causing muscle spasms.

Prevention
Vaccination series through childhood, followed by booster injections every ten years.

Epidemiology
35 to 70 cases per year in United States and about 1 million cases per year worldwide.

See also
• Diphtheria

Throat infections

A painful infection of the throat caused by viruses, bacteria, or fungi. Usually these infections are limited and cause no lasting effects. The incidence of throat infections is unknown but presumed to be very high.

Throat infections are usually caused by bacteria, viruses, or fungi. They produce a painful swelling of the throat, and the throat becomes red and sore. Sometimes, when the infection is isolated to a specific portion of the throat, it takes on the name of that part. For example, tonsillitis is an infection in the tonsils only. It is possible to have some of the symptoms of a throat infection without really having an infection. We call these conditions sore throats. They are often caused by irritants and pollutants in the air, such as cigarette smoke and chemicals.

Nearly 90 percent of all throat infections are caused by viruses. The remainder are due to bacteria and fungi. Although any virus can cause a throat infection, the most common causes are rhinoviruses, which are the same viruses that cause the common cold. Many other well-known infections are caused by viruses, including mononucleosis, influenza, measles, and herpes.

A strep throat infection is caused by bacteria. Other types of bacteria, such as *Corynebacterium diphtheriae*, which at one time caused plaguelike illnesses, have been largely eradicated by vaccination programs around the world. However, they still exist in some developing nations and in parts of eastern Europe.

A third type of throat infection, called thrush, is caused by fungi and is usually only seen in people with weakened immune systems due to diabetes, AIDS, medications, or chronic illness.

Risk factors

In a generally healthy population, people are not at a high risk for getting a throat infection. They become sick only when they are exposed to the virus, bacteria, or fungi that causes the illness. However, throat infections seem to be more common among certain groups. For instance, children in day care or school pass the illness to each other and to their teachers easily. Additionally, hospital workers who are exposed to infected people frequently also become sick.

Some people seem to be more prone to throat infections because they have pockets in their tonsils (called crypts), which store bacteria. The bacteria make thick impenetrable films inside these crypts, making it difficult to eliminate them. Since they are always present, they often cause throat infections.

Unlike healthy people, those with weak immune systems do not have the ability to fight off infections. Therefore, this group is at greater risk than all others because there are viruses and bacteria all around us.

Symptoms and signs

Throat infections usually begin almost unnoticed, but the common symptoms that develop quickly are unmistakable. The throat pain becomes sharp and more intense over a few days. The infected person cannot eat or drink comfortably because it hurts too much when he or she swallows. Sometimes, when the pain is very severe, the person becomes dehydrated and requires emergency intravenous fluids. Also, if the pain

KEY FACTS

Description
A painful infection of the throat.

Causes
Viruses, bacteria, and occasionally fungi create inflammation in the throat.

Risk factors
People with weakened immune systems are at increased risk. In healthy people the highest risk is among children and young adults.

Symptoms
Painful swallowing and sore throat. Drooling and difficulty breathing are occasional danger signs. Associated fever and muscle and joint aches.

Diagnosis
Patient history and findings of inflamed throat. Bacterial cultures and X-rays may be helpful.

Treatments
Generally, symptomatic treatment and hydration are adequate. If bacterial infection is present, antibiotics are used.

Pathogenesis
Develops from local throat infection by viruses, bacteria, or fungi.

Prevention
Hand washing is the best. Maintaining a healthy immune system is also important.

Epidemiology
Unknown, but believed to be very high.

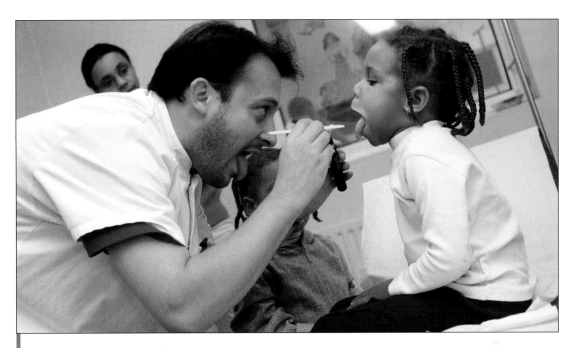

A doctor examines a child's throat. One of the most common bacteria that affects throats is Streptococcus faecalis, *hence the term* strep throat. *Left untreated, it can result in kidney problems or rheumatic fever.*

is very severe, the person may start to drool because it is too painful to swallow his or her own saliva. Lastly, a throat infection almost always causes a sore throat that changes the sound of a person's voice.

The most dangerous symptom of a throat infection is severe swelling that narrows a person's airway and results in difficulty breathing. Other significant symptoms and signs of throat infections include high fevers, rashes, headaches, aching muscles and joints, eye irritation, and general exhaustion.

Diagnosis and treatments

Doctors can diagnose a throat infection by listening to the patient's symptoms and by a routine physical examination. Sometimes it is not so obvious and the doctor has to order tests, blood sample analyses, and X-rays.

Most of the time, throat infections can be cured without long-term problems or complications. The treatment for a throat infection will depend upon the cause. The body cures most viral infections with its own disease-fighting mechanisms. Throat infections caused by bacteria are treated with antibiotics. Since strep bacteria can also cause complications such as kidney failure and heart disease, the infection must be treated aggressively and the patient must be monitored

carefully. Gargling with salty water is a popular home remedy, but there is little scientific evidence to show its effectiveness. In those people who have repeated throat infections from bacteria hiding in tonsillar crypts, the surgical removal of the tonsils may be recommended.

Prevention

The best cure for a throat infection is to prevent it before it happens. Hand washing is the most effective way of avoiding an infection. Some people recommend taking extra doses of vitamin C, vitamin E, and beta carotene. Most scientific studies have shown that these are not effective. A sufficient supply of these substances is found in a well-balanced diet, and the human body cannot use or store these extra vitamins taken as supplements.

About 15,000 cases of invasive strep infections occur each year in the United States. It is not known how many people have throat infections every year because most people do not visit the doctor with every sore throat. However, the number of missed days of work and the economic impact from throat infections is very significant, costing society millions of dollars annually.

Y. Etan Weinstock
and Kevin D. Pereira

See also
• Cold, common • Croup • Rheumatic fever

Thrombosis and embolism

Thrombosis and embolism are disorders of blood clotting and circulation. Thrombosis means the development of a clot in a blood vessel; embolism means the obstruction of a blood vessel by a mass (usually a clot) that has traveled through the circulation. The most common forms are deep vein thrombosis and pulmonary embolism.

The body's ability to control the flow of blood through the arteries, veins, and capillaries is critical to survival. In normal conditions, when blood vessels remain intact (non-injured), blood flows smoothly through the vessels but quickly forms a clot at the site of any vascular injury (coagulation). Once the injury has been repaired, there is a reversible process of repair, in which the clot dissolves (fibrinolysis). The mechanisms that control the delicate balance between coagulation and fibrinolysis are known as hemostasis (arrest of bleeding).

Thrombosis and embolism are disorders in which hemostasis is unbalanced, leading to clots in arteries that obstruct blood flow to different parts of the body. Without adequate blood supply, the affected tissue or organ is damaged and ultimately loses its ability to function normally.

Depending on the location of the blood clot, thrombosis and embolism may be termed *arterial* (occurring in the arteries) or *venous* (occurring in the veins).

The most common forms are deep vein thrombosis (DVT), in which a clot forms within a vein (usually in the leg), and pulmonary embolism (PE), in which there is a blockage in the artery supplying the lungs, usually caused by a clot that developed in the leg veins and traveled to the lungs.

Causes and risk factors

Three risk factors influence the blood's tendency to clot (Virchow's Triad): the constituents of the blood itself; the vessel wall; and the flow of blood. Problems in any of these areas can lead to an increased tendency to clotting, also known as a prothrombotic or hypercoagulable state.

KEY FACTS: DVT

Description

DVT is the formation of a blood clot within a deep vein, usually in the leg. The clot may obstruct the flow of blood, causing swelling, pain, and damage to the tissues; or the clot may break free and travel to the lungs, causing pulmonary embolism, a potentially fatal complication.

Causes

Derangement in the blood's ability to flow smoothly through the vessels. Three main factors encourage the formation of blood clots: constituents in blood promoting coagulation, damage to the vessel wall, and stagnant flow through the vessels (stasis).

Risk factors

Prolonged immobility, surgery (particularly orthopedic surgery), older age, cancer, varicose veins, smoking, obesity, pregnancy, estrogen therapy, and thrombophilia (excessive clotting).

Symptoms

Many cases of DVT are asymptomatic. Common symptoms include swelling, pain, cramp, redness, and changes in the temperature and appearance of the skin of the affected limb.

Diagnosis

By ultrasound, venography, and other imaging tests to visualize blood vessels and locate the clot.

Treatments

Anticoagulant drugs to thin the blood. Less often, thrombolytic drugs are used to dissolve the clot. Compression stockings may be worn to help reduce swelling in the legs. In rare cases, a filtering device is placed in the vein to catch clots before they reach the lungs.

Pathogenesis

Without treatment, DVT can cause pain, difficulty with walking, and damage to the valves in the blood vessels, leading to venous hypertension and pulmonary embolism.

Prevention

Avoiding risk factors and prophylactic measures. For example, people who need orthopedic surgery often take anticoagulant drugs, wear compression stockings, and are mobilized one day after surgery.

Epidemiology

DVT affects around 1 person in 1,000 and is fatal in around 5 percent of cases.

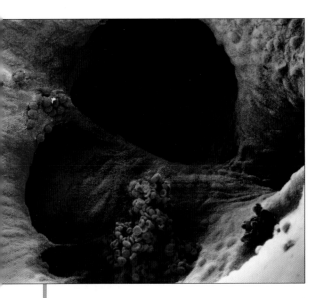

This false-color scanning electron micrograph shows a thrombus (blood clot) protruding from an arterial entrance in a chamber of the heart. This type of thrombus is called a coronary thrombosis.

Common causes of thrombosis include prolonged immobility, for example, during air travel; cancer; pregnancy; surgery, especially orthopedic surgery; oral contraceptives and hormone replacement therapy; and central venous catheters (medical devices used to deliver drugs and fluids to the body over a long period of time).

Other risk factors for thrombosis are older age, obesity, smoking, a family history of thrombosis, varicose veins, and thrombophilias (conditions in which there is an increased tendency for excessive blood clotting). The risk of thrombosis increases with the number of risk factors present.

Common thrombophilias are factor V Leiden (activated protein C resistance); deficiency of protein C, protein S, or antithrombin III; prothrombin mutation (G20210A); antiphospholipid syndrome (due to lupus anticoagulant or anticardiolipin antibodies); and high homocysteine levels (due to a genetic mutation or vitamin deficiency). Thrombophilias may be inherited (caused by genetic mutations) or acquired (caused by other medical conditions).

Symptoms, signs, and diagnosis

The symptoms of thrombosis and embolism depend on the location of the blood clot. DVT typically affects the legs (usually the thigh and calf) and may cause swelling, pain, tenderness, cramp, or changes in the color or temperature of the affected limb. DVT in the upper body may cause swelling of the arm or neck. However, many cases of DVT are asymptomatic.

The symptoms of PE are often vague or resemble other diseases. The most common symptoms of PE are sudden shortness of breath, chest pain, cough, rapid heart rate, and dizziness or fainting.

Both DVT and PE are diagnosed using tests such as ultrasound, venography (X-ray of the veins), and computed tomography to visualize the blood flow and locate the clot. A blood test may be performed to rule out thrombophilias, and other investigations may be needed to explore the underlying causes and to see how much damage the clot has caused.

Treatments and prevention

Thrombosis and embolism are serious disorders that are usually treated in a hospital. Urgent treatment is needed to reduce the risk of serious complications and death. The goals of treating thrombosis and embolism are to stop the blood clot from growing, prevent the clot from breaking off and traveling elsewhere, and to reduce the likelihood of another clot forming.

Treatment usually involves drugs to thin the blood (anticoagulants) or dissolve the clot (thrombolytics, thrombin inhibitors). Patients who cannot take these drugs may have a filtering device implanted in the large vein below the heart to stop blood clots from reaching the lungs. Patients with DVT often wear compression stockings to help reduce swelling in their legs.

Many cases of thrombosis and embolism can be prevented. Some risk factors, such as obesity and cigarette smoking, can be avoided through lifestyle changes. Other risk factors, such as being immobilized following surgery, can be modified with blood-thinning drugs, compression devices, and early rehabilitation. Preventive measures are particularly important in people with thrombophilias, who may take blood-thinning drugs on a routine basis.

DVT becomes more common with increasing age. DVT is believed to affect up to 25 percent of all hospitalized patients, although many will not have any symptoms. There is no obvious cause in 25 to 50 percent of people with DVT. Around 7 percent of people with DVT suffer a recurrence within six months.

Joanna Lyford

See also
• Heart attack • Obesity
• Stroke and related disorders

Thyroid disorders

The thyroid gland is an endocrine gland that makes and releases thyroid hormones T3 and T4 into the blood. These hormones are responsible for regulating the body's metabolism and the way that the body uses fats and carbohydrates, affecting the tissues of every organ.

About 15 million people in the United States have been diagnosed with some form of thyroid disease. Because many people have mild forms of thyroid disease, there may be an equal number undiagnosed. The two main types of thyroid disease are hypothyroidism, an underactive thyroid gland; and hyperthyroidism, an overactive thyroid gland. More than 75 percent of people with thyroid disease are women. Symptoms of thyroid disease can be nonspecific, sometimes making diagnosis difficult. There are about 20,000 new cases of thyroid cancer each year; it is more common in men.

The thyroid gland is a two-lobed butterfly-shaped gland sitting in the front of the neck just below the Adam's apple. It produces and secretes the iodine-containing thyroid hormones T4 (thyroxine) and T3 (triiodothyronine). As part of a feedback loop to keep the body's metabolism in check, the thyroid gland works with the hypothalamus and pituitary gland, located at the base of the brain. Circulating thyroid hormones in the blood signal the hypothalamus to release TRH (thyroid-releasing hormone). TRH signals the pituitary gland to secrete TSH (thyroid stimulating hormone), and TSH signals the thyroid to produce T3 and T4. A shift in any of these hormones can cause an alteration in the feedback loop.

Causes

In hypothyroidism too little circulating thyroid hormone is present. If the hypothalamus and pituitary glands are normal, TRH and TSH levels are elevated because of lack of negative feedback by thyroid hormones. In hyperthyroidism, too much thyroid hormone signals the hypothalamus to reduce the amount of TRH secreted; this decreases the amount of TSH secreted. Because of this feedback loop, blood tests for T3, T4, and TSH are used routinely to diagnose thyroid disease. Since iodine plays a key role in thyroid hormone production and is pulled from the blood to manufacture T3 and T4, special scans of the thyroid can be made after small amounts of the harmless radioactive iodine (I-123) are swallowed or injected in a vein; the concentration in the thyroid gland indicates how much hormone the thyroid is making. Another isotope, I-131, is used to destroy normal and cancerous thyroid tissue.

Hypothyroidism

As people age, the thyroid gland may produce less thyroid hormone, more commonly in women over age 50. But the most common cause of hypothyroidism in the United States is Hashimoto's thyroiditis, an autoimmune disorder that attacks and destroys the thyroid gland. Other causes include: pituitary failure; surgical removal of the thyroid gland, or radioactive iodine or anti-thyroid medication for treatment for thyroid cancer or hyperthyroidism; previous head and neck exposure to radiation as cancer treatment; and medications, like lithium, used to treat psychiatric dis-

KEY FACTS

Description

Too or much or too little thyroid hormone.

Causes and risk factors

Increasing age, female gender, iodine deficiency, family history, autoimmune disorder, radiation treatment of head or neck cancers.

Symptoms

Many people have mild or no symptoms. Hypothyroidism: sluggish, weight gain, pale dry skin, fatigue. Hyperthyroidism: nervousness, sweating, tremors, weight loss, hair loss, increased heart rate.

Diagnosis

Thyroid function blood tests T3, T4, and TSH; thyroid scans; ultrasound; biopsy.

Treatments

Hypothyroidism: replacement medication for life; Hyperthyroidism: destroy thyroid tissue, thyroid replacement medication.

Prevention

Adequate iodine in the diet.

Epidemiology

About 15 million people in United States with thyroid disease; many more undiagnosed. Iodine deficiency throughout the world causes 100 million cases of hypothyroidism.

orders. Hypothyroidism due to iodine deficiency is uncommon in the United States, where iodine is added to some table salt. In other parts of the world where dietary iodine is insufficient, 100 million people suffer from iodine-deficiency hypothyroidism.

Symptoms include sensitivity to cold, slow speech, constipation, coarse hair, hoarse voice, heavy menstrual periods, pale dry skin, cold skin, weight gain, puffy face, and depression. In some cases there may be heart problems, goiter, birth defects, and myxedema, a life threatening condition due to long-standing undiagnosed hypothyroidism that can result in coma. Hypothyroidism is particularly dangerous in newborn infants (congenital hypothyroidism). Diagnosis is made by blood tests T3 and T4 (low), TSH (high), and TSAb, thyroid stimulating antibodies (high).

Hyperthyroidism

Hyperthyroidism occurs in about 1 percent of people in the United States and is at least five times more common in women, especially between the age of 20 and 60. Excess thyroid hormone causes nervousness, sweating, tremors, change in appetite, weight loss, sleep disturbances, increased heart rate, and vision changes. About 85 percent of cases are caused by Graves' disease, an autoimmune disorder that increases the size and activity of the thyroid. Graves' disease can cause inflammation of the tissues around the eyes, so they appear to bulge. Thyroid nodules can produce too much thyroid hormone and are another cause of hyperthyroidism. In thyroiditis, a general inflammation of the gland, sometimes caused by infection or unknown mechanisms, excess thyroid hormones leak into the blood. Diagnosis is made by T3 and T4 (usually high), TSH (low), and TSAb, and increased uptake on thyroid scan. Biopsy can be done for nodules. Graves' disease can be treated with radioactive iodine to destroy thyroid tissue, surgery, or both. Drugs that block production of thyroid hormone may be used. Beta blockers can treat blood pressure and heart rate. After treatment, many people become hypothyroid and need thyroid replacement medication for life.

Goiters

A goiter is a general enlargement of the thyroid gland. Causes include inadequate iodine or autoimmune disorder, such as Hashimoto's thyroiditis, and can take months or years to develop. Goiters are treated if there is trouble swallowing or breathing, from compression of the esophagus or windpipe behind the thyroid gland. Blood tests include TSH, and T3 and T4

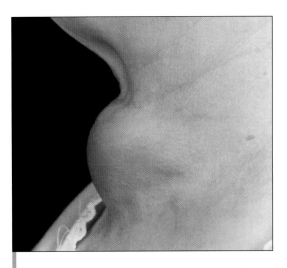

The swelling in this woman's neck is caused by carcinoma of the thyroid. Cancer of the thyroid is fairly rare and the causes are generally unknown.

(low or normal), thyroid scans, and ultrasound. Once treated, the thyroid gland shrinks back to a normal size.

Pregnancy

About 2 percent of pregnant women in the United States are diagnosed with hypothyroidism, which can lead to miscarriages, preeclampsia, bleeding after birth, and low birth-weight babies. The most common cause is Hashimoto's thyroiditis. Iodine deficiency can cause hypothyroidism during pregnancy. The most common cause of hyperthyroidism during pregnancy in the United States is Graves' disease, which occurs in 1 in 1,500 pregnancies.

Congenital hypothyroidism

Also called cretinism, hypothyroidism in a newborn occurs in about 1 in 3,000 births, twice as often in girls. It can be due to abnormal development of the thyroid or pituitary gland, or abnormal formation of thyroid hormones. The child requires rapid treatment with thyroid replacement hormone to prevent developmental problems; untreated, an infant can become mentally and physically retarded. Lifelong treatment is needed to avoid chronic symptoms. Most states require newborns to be screened for hypothyroidism.

Ramona Jenkin

See also
• Cancer, thyroid

Tooth decay

Tooth decay, also known as caries, is a disorder in which a hole or defect forms in the outer mineral layer of a tooth. The normal tooth is made of a hard mineral layer, which surrounds a softer layer. The outer layer or enamel is above the gum line; underneath is dentin, which is a softer mineral layer in which the nerves and pulp of a tooth lie. When a cavity forms, the outer enamel layer has a hole, which, if deep enough, exposes the layer containing the pulp. This can lead to nerve damage, tooth loss, and even death from infection spreading past the tooth to the jaw.

Each person has numerous bacteria naturally living in the mouth, which can form plaques. When a person eats, the food meets the bacteria in the mouth, and sugars and starches are digested, leaving behind acid. This acid can then demineralize and erode the protective enamel of the teeth.

Risk factors

One of the risks for developing tooth decay is poor oral hygiene. Not brushing or flossing properly or often enough can allow plaques to develop. Not seeing a dentist can also allow early signs of decay to progress. Because the other component leading to cavities is food, a diet high in sugar and refined starch is a risk factor for decay. This includes foods such as candy, honey, sweetened snacks, and even juice. For tooth decay, how often these foods are eaten determines the risk of developing decay—that is, if a person eats these foods three separate times a day, he or she would have more risk than someone who eats them just once a day. Other risk factors include not having access to fluoride, either in the water or in items such as toothpaste or mouthwash.

Babies are at risk of developing "baby bottle caries" when they are allowed to fall asleep with sweetened liquids in their bottles or if they receive multiple feedings of sweetened liquids.

Symptoms and signs

Early tooth decay has no signs or symptoms. If the cavity enlarges, there can be increased sensitivity to cold and cold drinks or pain after having sweet drinks or food. There can also be softening of the teeth around the decay. There have also been associations with foul odors or bad breath in progressed decay.

Diagnosis and treatments

Most cavities are diagnosed by X-ray on a routine dental visit, before symptoms and signs have developed. In a dental X-ray, tooth caries can show up as darkened areas. Dentists can also find larger cavities by looking or probing with dental instruments.

There is a wide range of treatments that dentists can offer for cavities. The most important thing to re-

KEY FACTS

Description

A defect or hole in the enamel of a tooth. Also known as "cavities" or "caries."

Causes

Bacteria on teeth digest sugars from eaten food, leaving behind acid, which dissolves the outer layer of teeth.

Risk factors

Inadequate brushing, flossing, and dental care. A diet high in refined starches and sugar. Lack of preventive measures such as fluoride.

Symptoms

There are often no signs or symptoms of early decay. If the decay progresses, there can be tooth pain worsened by heat, cold, or sweet food and drinks.

Diagnosis

Dentists can find cavities on dental X-rays.

Treatments

Range from fluoride treatments, dental fillings, or root canal, depending on the extent of decay.

Pathogenesis

Can lead to tooth loss. If severe, can lead to infection of the surrounding tissues of the face and neck, and even death.

Prevention

Good oral care, diet low in refined sugars, fluoride in water, and toothpaste. Dental sealants are an option in some cases.

Epidemiology

The most common chronic disease of children. About 90 percent of schoolchildren and most adults have been affected.

member is that the earlier the cavity is found, the easier the treatment. One of the simplest treatments is topical fluoride. This treatment can be used if the cavity is very small and dental hygiene is good. Fluoride affects the enamel part of the tooth. It binds to the minerals in the enamel area, making it harder for the bacteria to stick there, and therefore harder for cavities to form. Fluoride is also used as a preventive measure in water and toothpaste.

If the decay has progressed enough into the enamel layer of the tooth, the treatment includes removing the decayed enamel by drilling it out and then replacing it with a dental filling. Many materials can be used for filling a cavity, such as gold, amalgam, resin, and porcelain. The material chosen for the filling depends on where the tooth is, what role it plays in chewing food, and how noticeable the filling will be. For example, resin and porcelain can be colored to match the color of teeth and would be used in areas where the filling would be noticeable. However, these materials are not as strong as amalgam and gold, and so may not be used in teeth that are used for chewing food.

Pathogenesis

If a cavity is not treated, it can reach the pulp of a tooth and cause the nerve to die from infection or from being exposed. For these cases, root canal treatment is necessary. In this procedure, the nerve and blood supply of a tooth are removed in addition to the decayed enamel. The tooth is filled with a rubberlike filling, and a crown is then placed over the tooth. If tooth decay progresses, the entire tooth may need to be removed, which is called dental extraction. An extraction can be necessary if the tooth is destroyed beyond an ability to repair it, or if the cost to fix it is too high. There are also severe cases of tooth decay in which an infection can spread past the tooth to include the jaw and the tissues in the mouth and neck, a condition known as Ludwig's angina. Very rarely, this condition can progress to death.

Prevention

One key way to prevent cavities is to routinely and properly brush and floss. This action prevents plaque, a pale yellow-to-white coating of bacteria on the teeth. Routine visits to the dentist to look for early signs of decay, as well as for dental cleanings, are also important. Dentists use X-rays to detect early signs of cavities.

A diet low in refined sugars and starches is key to minimizing bacteria's ability to produce decay-causing

TOOTH DECAY

Decay can penetrate the enamel and dentin of a tooth and the affected tooth will have to be filled. If decay reaches the pulp, which contains the nerves and blood vessels, root canal treatment is carried out.

The decay in the tooth has spread from the outer layer of the tooth (enamel) to the dentin. The area around the decay will be removed then filled.

acids. In fact, tooth decay only became a worldwide problem after sugar cane plantations were developed in the 1700s, which made sugar easily available worldwide. Before sugar was commonly available, cavities were less frequently encountered. Fluoridation of both water supply and toothpaste has reduced the incidence of tooth decay. Dentists may also use dental sealant on developing teeth in children to prevent cavities.

Epidemiology

By World Health Organization (WHO) estimates, nearly 90 percent of all schoolchildren and young adults have tooth decay. It is the most common chronic disease of children and is at least five times more common than asthma.

Nisha Bhatt

See also
• Gum disease

Toxic shock syndrome

Toxic shock syndrome is a bacterial disease caused by *Staphylococcus aureus* and *Streptococcus pyogenes*.

Toxic shock syndrome (TSS) is caused by *Staphylococcus aureus* and *Streptococcus pyogenes*. *S. aureus* is present in the nose of about 50 percent of humans; and it can affect other people. Many types of *S. aureus* exist; only some have the ability to cause TSS. *S. pyogenes*, the other cause of TSS, more commonly causes strep throat (pharyngitis). Streptococci are contracted from other humans, usually by coughing. Only certain types of streptococci can cause TSS, via breaks in the skin. TSS, whether staphylococcal or streptococcal, is caused by toxins called superantigens that are produced and released by both bacteria.

Risk factors include infections as a result of surgery, trauma, drug use, and infection with the influenza or chickenpox virus. The viruses damage both skin and mucous membranes, allowing subsequent infection by streptococci and staphylococci. Tampon usage during menstruation can create conditions favorable for staphylococcal toxin production; thus menstruating women are at greater risk of developing menstrual TSS.

The signs of TSS include flulike symptoms, vomiting and diarrhea, then a drop in blood pressure and multiple organ involvement. Other signs may include a sunburn-like rash. Streptococcal TSS is often complicated by a deep soft-tissue infection known as necrotizing fasciitis (flesh-eating disease), which causes severe pain, usually around bruised areas. Diagnosis requires drop in blood pressure or dizziness on standing, multiple organ involvement (such as vomiting, diarrhea, and confusion or combativeness), and fever. Diagnosis of TSS should include the isolation of *S. aureus* or *S. pyogenes* from mucosal surfaces or from normally sterile sites on the body. Septicemia is far more common in streptococcal TSS than in staphylococcal TSS.

The risk of menstrual staphylococcal TSS can be reduced by not using tampons or alternating with pads, and using tampons of the lowest absorbency. Nonsteroidal anti-inflammatory drugs may mask the pain of streptococcal TSS, so use of these drugs may be risk factors. Treatment options for both types of TSS are available. *S. pyogenes* responds to antibiotics such as penicillin and clindamycin; however, the selection of antibiotics can be challenging for *S. aureus*, because of

prevalent antibiotic resistance. Treatment of TSS also should include intravenous immunoglobulin (IVIG), a mixture of antibodies that neutralizes the superantigens. TSS treatment can include drainage of wounds, removal of the tampon, and surgery to remove gangrenous limbs. In the case of streptococcal TSS with necrotizing fasciitis, surgical removal of dead tissue is often required, or possible amputation of the limb.

Kristi L. Strandberg, Amanda J. Brosnahan,
and Patrick M. Schlievert

KEY FACTS

Description
Uncommon illness caused by bacterial toxins.

Causes
Staphylococcus aureus (tampon disease) or *Streptococcus pyogenes* (flesh-eating disease).

Risk factors
Tampon use and vaginal barrier contraception, viruses, surgery, burns, skin trauma, and use of nonsteroidal anti-inflammatory agents.

Symptoms
Flulike symptoms, then dizziness upon standing. Symptoms of streptococcal TSS may include pain in areas of bruising that have become infected.

Diagnosis
Based on signs, changes in liver and kidney function, high fever, rash, and isolation of the organism from infection site.

Treatments
In the case of antibiotic resistance, the antibiotic vancomycin is used. Intravenous immunoglobulin to neutralize toxins, removal of tampons, and surgery.

Pathogenesis
Without treatment, multiple organ failure and death.

Prevention
Not using tampons. No preventive measures exist for streptococcal TSS.

Epidemiology
The annual incidence of staphylococcal TSS is about 3 in 100,000, affecting males and females equally. Worldwide, 5 in 100,000 are affected by streptococcal TSS; males and females and all ages affected about equally.

See also
• Antibiotic-resistant infections

Toxoplasmosis

Toxoplasmosis is an infection caused by *Toxoplasma gondii*, a parasite that infects birds and mammals, including humans. Very few infected people show symptoms, since a healthy person's immune system usually keeps the parasite from causing illness. However, toxoplasmosis in pregnant women and people with weak immune systems can cause serious health problems.

Toxoplasmosis is an infection caused by *Toxoplasma gondii*, a parasite found in most warm-blooded animals and birds. Domestic cats can contract the parasite by eating infected birds or rodents. They shed the parasites in their feces, and infection can spread to people through direct contact with the cat's feces or with soil that has been in contact with it. People can also get toxoplasmosis from eating undercooked infected meat. Less commonly, a pregnant woman may pass the infection to her unborn baby. Though toxoplasmosis is generally asymptomatic, infection in unborn children and individuals with a weak immune system can cause serious health problems.

Causes and risk factors

Humans may contract toxoplasmosis by touching the mouth after gardening or cleaning a cat's litter box; by eating or handling undercooked infected meat; by drinking contaminated water; or, in rare cases, by receiving an infected organ transplant or blood transfusion. If a pregnant woman contracts toxoplasmosis, there is a 40 percent chance that her unborn child will also become infected. Toxoplasmosis is most dangerous for babies born to mothers who became infected during or just before pregnancy, and for people with severely weakened immune systems, such as those with HIV/AIDS, or chemotherapy or transplant patients.

Signs and symptoms

A minority of healthy individuals may develop mild, flulike symptoms that typically resolve within a few months. However, toxoplasmosis in those with weakened immune systems may damage the brain, eyes, or other organs. Unborn children infected in early pregnancy may later suffer blindness, deafness, seizures, and mental retardation, though only about 1 in 10 infected babies show signs of infection at birth.

Diagnosis and treatments

Blood testing is the routine method of diagnosis. In a pregnant woman with an active infection, amniocentesis or ultrasound may help determine if the fetus is also infected. Medical treatment is generally needed only for pregnant women and people with weak immune systems, who are given pyrimethamine (an antimalarial), sulfadiazine (an antibiotic), and folic acid. The antibiotic spiramycin can halve the chance of an infected woman passing the infection to her unborn child.

Jonathon Cross

KEY FACTS

Description
An infection caused by *Toxoplasma gondii*, a common parasite.

Causes
Contact with infected cat feces or soil; infection of fetus by pregnant mother; eating infected meat.

Risk factors
Infected soil, cat litter, and blood transfusion.

Symptoms
Usually none, though may cause flulike symptoms. Severe toxoplasmosis may damage the brain, eyes, or other organs.

Diagnosis
Blood testing. Amniocentesis and ultrasound may determine infection in a fetus.

Treatments
Generally not needed, though pregnant women and immunodeficient individuals may be treated with antibiotics and other drugs.

Pathogenesis
Symptoms in healthy people usually resolve in a few months. Severe health problems in babies infected in early pregnancy may be apparent at birth but usually appear months or years later.

Prevention
Avoiding contact with cat feces, soil, or raw meat.

Epidemiology
It is estimated that more than 60 million people in the United States have toxoplasmosis. One to two in 1,000 infected babies are born each year.

See also
• Food poisoning

Tuberculosis

Tuberculosis (TB) is a life threatening infection that worldwide kills nearly 2 million people per year. The World Health Organization has predicted that this number will increase. Presently, one new TB infection occurs every second. The bacterium *Mycobacterium tuberculosis* causes most cases of tuberculosis infections. It usually affects the lungs but can result in a localized lesion or lesions throughout the body.

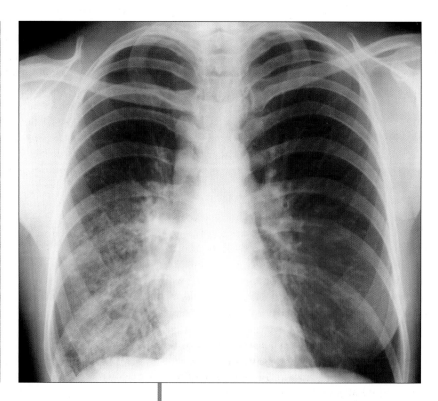

This colored chest X-ray of a woman with pulmonary tuberculosis shows black areas, which are the lungs; the areas affected by tuberculosis are red.

Tuberculosis has been known to cause disease from ancient times to the present. Egyptian mummies have been found with tubercles, which are tuberculous lesions. The most common form of TB is tuberculosis of the lungs. The bacteria are spread in the air and enter the body through the respiratory tract. General symptoms include fever and weight loss. The symptoms of tuberculosis depend upon the area of infiltration of the microorganisms. For example, Pott's disease is a presentation of TB that affects the spine. Tuberculosis is the most common major communicable disease today, infecting 2 billion people, equating to one-third of the world's population. Some famous people who had or are believed to have had TB include Jane Austen, Robert Burns, Edgar Allan Poe, Fredric Chopin, and Stephen Foster.

Causes and risk factors

Tuberculosis is a bacterial infection which may or may not cause disease. *Mycobacterium tuberculosis* is the bacterium responsible for most cases of tuberculosis as a respiratory disease. This disease, also known as consumption, has occurred in all eras and worldwide climates. In 1882 Robert Koch discovered a stain that he used to microscopically identify *Mycobacterium tuberculosis*. His accomplishment provided a new approach to fighting this deadly disease. *Mycobacterium bovis*, *Mycobacterium bovis BCG*, and *Mycobacterium africanum* are other species that cause tuberculosis. *Mycobacterium tuberculosis* and *Mycobacterium bovis* cause infections worldwide. The organism *Mycobacterium africanum* causes human infections mainly in East and West Africa. *Mycobacterium bovis* can cause respiratory or intestinal tuberculosis and is contracted by drinking contaminated milk or through airborne transmission. Humans and a wide host range of animals, including cattle, goats, cats, dogs, and pigs, can be infected with *Mycobacterium bovis*. This species of mycobacterium is mainly seen in countries that have tuberculous dairy cows and unpasteurized milk.

After human immunodeficiency virus (HIV), tuberculosis is the leading infectious cause of death in the world. Individuals with HIV are highly susceptible to rapidly active tuberculosis because their bodies are being immunosuppressed by the virus. Studies have shown there is a connection between the rise in HIV infections and the increasing rate of TB infections. Mycobacterial organisms can live for a considerable period of time in dust or air. Tuberculosis is most commonly acquired by person-to-person transmission of airborne droplets of mycobacterial organisms from a person with active disease to a susceptible person, the host. When a person with infectious (active) tuberculosis coughs or sneezes without covering the mouth, the tubercle droplets are expelled into the air. Other people may inhale the air containing these airborne droplets of mycobacteria and become infected.

Some populations are at higher risk for the active (infectious) TB disease because they are more likely to be exposed or infected. Tuberculosis thrives wherever there is poverty, crowded living conditions, and chronic illness (for example, HIV, diabetes mellitus, and alcoholism). In jails and homeless shelters, the crowded conditions and inadequate testing and treatment also lead to extremely high TB infection rates. Also, people born in regions of the world where tuberculosis is highly prevalent, elderly people, people who inject illegal drugs, and health care workers are all at a much higher risk of becoming infected with TB.

In 1993 the World Health Organization (WHO) declared TB a global health emergency since one-third of the world's population is infected. Regions and countries afflicted by wars, poverty, and natural disasters are seriously affected. The highest incidences are seen in countries with the lowest gross national products, in Africa, Asia, and Latin America. As the HIV and AIDS epidemic spreads in Africa, TB rates are increasing, not only in those afflicted with AIDS, but also in the general population.

Symptoms and signs

The tuberculosis infection begins when the bacterial organisms enter the lungs and multiply in the small air sacs of the lungs. Some of these tubercle microorganisms enter the bloodstream and spread throughout the body, but the body's immune system usually keeps the bacterial organisms under control. The primary infection is contained and, in many cases, the infection is permanently stopped. Thus, the infection does not cause any symptoms. This controlled disease is referred to as latent TB infection (LTBI). If the body's immune defenses decrease, the tuberculosis disease may break out again and become active. It is highly probable for a person infected with HIV to have LTBI progress to active TB disease. Most people who have latent TB infection never develop the active TB disease, and they cannot spread the infection to others. Latent TB infection is detected through a positive reaction to the tuberculin skin test or the QuantiFERON TB Gold blood test, used to diagnose both latent and active TB infections.

Patients with a tuberculosis infection may or may not have symptoms. Common presenting symptoms include fever, cough, loss of appetite, night sweats, weight loss, weakness, or chills, or all the symptoms. Also, the person may cough a small amount of yellow, green, or bloody sputum (saliva, pus, blood, and other matter discharged from diseased lungs). These symptoms are seen in those people with mainly tuberculosis of the lungs. Other regions of the body that can become infected with the mycobacterial organisms include the bones, lymph nodes, joints, abdominal cavity, pericardium (membrane around the heart), kidneys, reproductive organs, and central nervous system.

KEY FACTS

Description
A life-threatening infection that usually affects the lungs. Commonly called TB.

Cause
Bacteria in the genus *Mycobacterium*, particulary *M. tuberculosis*.

Risk factors
Contact with infected people or animals or contaminated food; chronic illness such as HIV infection; poor and unsanitary living conditions.

Symptoms
In latent TB, no symptoms; in active TB of the lungs, there may be fever, cough, loss of appetite, night sweats, weight loss, and chills; coughing up yellow, green, or bloody sputum.

Diagnosis
Tuberculin skin test; QuantiFERON TB Gold blood test; chest X-ray; sputum smear and culture.

Treatments
Antibiotics such as isoniazid, rifampicin, pyrazinamide, and pyridoxine.

Pathogenesis
Mycobacterium causes lesions called tubercles in the lungs. Without treatment the infection can spread to other body organs.

Prevention
Vaccination; isolation of infected people.

Epidemiology
Affects one-third of the world's population. Most common in Africa, Asia, and Central America.

Many people with untreated TB develop shortness of breath as the infection spreads in the lungs. The kidneys and lymph nodes are the most common sites of the body affected by TB outside the lungs (extrapulmonary tuberculosis). Tuberculosis that infects the central nervous system tissues covering the brain is called tubercular meningitis.

Diagnosis

When a person has symptoms that suggest tuberculosis, a tuberculin skin test (PPD-purified protein derivative test) or QuantiFERON TB blood test, a chest X-ray, a sputum smear, and a culture are normally ordered by the physician. A person who has contracted the type of tuberculosis that affects the lungs will have tubercules (lesions) that will appear on a chest X-ray. The tuberculin skin test is performed by injecting a small amount of protein derived from TB bacteria between the layers of skin on the forearm of the patient. Two days later, the injection site is checked and measured. A positive test result is indicated by swelling that feels firm to the touch and is larger than the specified normal size. The tuberculin skin test may show false-positive results due to a recent vaccination against tuberculosis. The QuantiFERON TB blood test requires that a sample of blood be taken from the patient and tested in a clinical laboratory with special chemical reagents that identify if a person has a TB infection.

The patient's sputum is examined in the clinical laboratory by smearing some of the sputum on a glass slide, staining the smear, and looking at this stained smear using a microscope. When the stained smear is viewed microscopically, the tuberculosis bacteria will appear as red rods. Also, some of the sputum is placed on culture media and in an incubator to see which microorganisms grow. Cultures do not provide results for several days because mycobacteria organisms grow slowly. A positive culture for *Mycobacterium tuberculosis* confirms that the patient has TB disease. After the culture has identified the TB bacteria, a drug susceptibility test is performed, which will help the physician choose the correct medication for use in the patient's treatment.

It is extremely important that TB disease be diagnosed as early as possible since pulmonary tuberculosis can cause permanent lung damage if not treated early.

Prevention and treatments

The infectiousness of a patient with TB disease is directly related to the number of tubercle bacteria that he or she expels into the air from the lungs. Patients who expel many mycobacteria are more infectious than patients who expel few bacteria. Patients who have signs and symptoms of tuberculosis must be placed in an area separated from other people, promptly evaluated, then given treatment to avoid spreading the disease. Infectiousness decreases very rapidly after treatment is started. Patients who have been receiving appropriate medication for TB for two to three weeks, whose symptoms have improved, and who have three consecutive negative sputum smears collected on different days can usually be considered noninfectious.

Latent tuberculosis infection in a patient must be treated with antibiotics so that the patient does not contract active TB disease. The usual medication for latent tuberculosis infection, isoniazid, abbreviated as INH, is given daily for nine months to the patient. The patient must be checked by a physician monthly since this TB medication and others may cause side effects such as skin rashes, upset stomach, or liver damage. Taking the medication rifampin for four months is an alternative treatment for latent tuberculosis infection. The patient must not miss taking the daily medication and must take all of it to avoid the possibility of TB disease.

TB disease in the lungs must be treated much more rigorously than latent TB infection. The disease is usually treated with daily doses of rifampin, isoniazid, pyrazinamide, and pyridoxine over a six-month period. All of the medications are given since resistance to one or more of these drugs occurs in many patients. Because it is so important to take all of these medications on a daily basis, the patient may be required to see a nurse who will administer the medications every day.

Treatment of tuberculosis in other parts of the body, such as the bones or central nervous system, must occur over nine months to one year for full effective recovery from the disease.

Prevention of TB infection and disease has occurred through vaccination with BCG (bacilli Calmette–Guerin). It is given to school children in some countries in an attempt to decrease the risk of developing tuberculosis.

Kathleen Becan-McBride

See also
• AIDS • Antibiotic-resistant infections
• Diabetes

Typhoid and paratyphoid

Typhoid is a life-threatening, feverish disease caused by the bacterium *Salmonella typhi*, which seriously affects the digestive system. Paratyphoid is a less severe disease caused by *Salmonella paratyphi*. Most cases of both diseases are reported in developing countries where hygiene is poor.

Salmonella typhi is a bacterium that is exclusive to humans. While other animals, such as birds, cows, and turtles, may pass other types of *Salmonella*, this hardy bacterium has a protective coat that helps it hide from the human immune system. The bacterium is transmitted with water and foods and can withstand drying and freezing. Also, certain humans may carry the disease without being ill themselves. *Salmonella paratyphi* causes paratyphoid fever, a condition that is similar in the way it is spread but that has milder symptoms than typhoid.

Signs and symptoms

Typhoid fever makes its victims feel very ill. Classic typhoid goes through two phases. In the first phase, the bacterium gets into the intestine from water or food that has been contaminated by the feces or urine of people who have the disease or are carriers of the disease. The bacterium penetrates the intestinal lining, or mucosa, to the underlying tissue. If the immune system does not stop the infection there, the bacteria multiply and spread to the bloodstream, causing the first observable symptoms of fever and sweating. The patient will have loss of appetite and may have a fever pattern of as high as 105°F (40.6°C), which may gradually rise and fall and last for weeks at a time. Then the bacteria penetrate the bone marrow, liver, and bile ducts, and are excreted into the bowel contents. Rose spots on the trunk appear in about 25 percent of Caucasians.

The second phase of the disease occurs when the bacteria penetrate the immune tissue of the small intestine, causing violent and prolonged diarrhea, interspersed with constipation. Usually this happens in the second or third week. Severe abdominal pain and blinding headache with a continued cough and slow heart rate begin within one to two weeks after exposure, but this period can be from three days to three months. In the third week, severe diarrhea resembling pea soup may also contain blood. In severe cases, the person may lie motionless, appearing as dead, with eyes half open, a state referred to as "typhoid state."

Around the fifth week, the fever may drop and the condition may slowly improve.

Left untreated, complications such as potentially fatal intestinal bleeding can occur. Other complications include pneumonia, psychosis, meningitis, bladder and kidney infection, a condition known as typhoid spine, and coma.

Diagnosis

It took several years for people to connect unsanitary conditions with disease, especially with typhoid. During the early decades of the nineteenth century, physicians proposed the "filth" theory of disease. As the industrial revolution brought people into crowded cities, diseases like typhoid and typhus, a disease carried by lice, became endemic. Some speculated that conditions spontaneously generated from the bad air and open sewage.

In 1839 Englishman William Budd argued that typhoid did not arise from filth but that it was a contagious disease. After investigating several epidemics, he found that some students became ill from using a common well and concluded that the well water was poisoned. By the 1870s it was accepted that the poison of typhoid was from sewage-contaminated water. With the advance of microbiology, the organism was finally grown in culture, and by 1896 physicians had tools for diagnosing the bacteria.

Because early symptoms resemble other conditions, such as malaria, the doctor's clinical picture must include information on travel and which countries have been visited. The final diagnosis should include analysis of stool, blood, and tissue samples. Stool samples are teeming with *S. typhi*. Food and water contaminated by feces and urine transmit typhoid fever. In some countries, shellfish taken from sewage-contaminated beds, particularly oyster beds, may transmit the organism. Fruit and vegetables that are fertilized by "night soil" (human feces) can be sources of typhoid infection. Other sources include contaminated milk and milk products. Flies may infect foods in which the organism can multiply to an infective dose.

Epidemiology

Typhoid fever is common in certain parts of Asia, Africa, and Latin America. With the development of sanitary facilities, the disease has been eliminated in many areas, with most cases occurring in endemic areas. Six countries—India, Pakistan, Mexico, Bangladesh, the Philippines, and Haiti—accounted for 76 percent of the cases. Strains resistant to chloramphenicol and other antibiotics have been recently reported.

Treatments

Treatment requires admission to a hospital, where antibiotics and in some cases steroid medicines are administered. In addition, treatment for dehydration (loss of fluids and electrolytes) demands a high-calorie, nonbulky diet and possibly intravenous feeding. In the hospital, infected people are isolated, and the staff must be vigilant to avoid unprotected contact with contaminated clothing or bedding.

If the appropriate antibiotics are administered, the prospects of cure are very good, and the person may be discharged when the condition is stable. Choice of antibiotic depends upon the strain of *S. typhi*.

At present 107 types of typhoid can be distinguished by a technique called phage typing; three types of *S. paratyphi* are recognized. However, care must be taken because the bacteria may be excreted for several more weeks.

Paratyphoid fever is caused by a different bacterium called *Salmonella paratyphi*. The incubation is shorter, and although there may be carriers, they are not as likely to transmit the disease in the way that typhoid carriers do.

Paratyphoid has a similar clinical picture to typhoid but is much milder, and the fatality rate is much lower. No generalized symptoms occur; rather, the patient suffers an acute bout of gastroenteritis. The ratio of disease caused by *S. typhi* to *S. paratyphi* is about 10 to 1. Some experts believe paratyphoid occurs more frequently than reports suggest and may be infrequently identified in Canada and the United States.

If a traveler is in a developing country and becomes very ill, there is reason to suspect typhoid fever. The U.S. consulate is the source for a list of recommended doctors. Immediately, the physician will start the patient on the most common antibiotics to treat the disease: ampicillin, ciprofloxacin, and trimethoprim-sulfamethoxazole. As soon as the antibiotics are in the system, the person begins to feel better in a few days, and deaths rarely occur.

Although the symptoms go away, a person may be carrying *S. typhi*, so the illness could return or be passed on to other people. If the person works in food service, he or she may be legally barred from going back to work until it is proven that he or she no longer harbors the bacteria.

A person being treated for typhoid should take the prescribed antibiotics until the whole course is finished. Good hygiene practices should be observed, such as washing hands carefully with soap and water after each bathroom use. Someone with typhoid should not prepare or serve food to other people, and the doctor should arrange for a series of stool cultures to be performed until it can be demonstrated that no *S. typhi* remain in the body.

KEY FACTS

Description

Bacterial diseases that affect the digestive system; typhoid is the most serious, paratyphoid has milder symptoms.

Causes

The bacteria *Salmonella typhi* causes typhoid; *Salmonella paratyphi* causes paratyphoid.

Risk factors

Unsanitary food and drinking water.

Symptoms

Typhoid: fever, headache, weakness, sore throat, cough, diarrhea. Paratyphoid: acute gastroenteritis, but without the general malaise.

Diagnosis

A physician takes a blood or stool sample to identify the bacteria.

Treatments

Antibiotics.

Pathogenesis

Without treatment for typhoid, mortality is high; as many as 20 percent die from complications of the infection. Only rarely is paratyphoid fatal.

Prevention

Vaccination, care in eating food and drinking water. Rigorous hygiene such as washing hands after bathroom use, peeling fruit and vegetables, and drinking bottled water.

Epidemiology

Worldwide the annual incidence of typhoid is estimated at about 17 million cases with about 600,000 deaths. Only about 400 cases occur in the United States each year, and these are related to travel to developing countries. The global annual incidence of paratyphoid fever is estimated to be 5.4 million people.

TYPHOID MARY

Mary Mellon, an Irish immigrant, was the first person to be identified as a carrier of typhoid in the United States. She was the picture of health when the New York health inspector knocked on her door in 1907. She was informed that although healthy and immune to the disease, she spread disease while working as a cook in the New York City area. Charles Henry Warren, a wealthy banker, hired Mary to be the cook at their summer home in 1906. Soon, 6 out of 11 people in the household came down with typhoid. George Soper, a sanitary engineer, found that Mary had worked at several jobs where 22 people had become ill. When he asked Mary for stool samples to test for typhoid, she refused and ran away. Soper found her and obtained a court order incarcerating her for examination, but she was freed after three years on the condition that she would never take a job as a cook. Mary disappeared, but five years later, Soper found her working as a cook in a hospital under another name. In 1914 she was confined in a former isolation hospital, Riverside Hospital, on North Brother Island (an island in the East River), where she was institutionalized for more than two decades until she died in 1938. Mary, who became known as "Typhoid Mary," had unwittingly caused three typhoid deaths and 47 cases of typhoid. She died showing complete unwillingness to admit there was a problem or to comply with restrictions.

Typhoid is a very serious disease when untreated. Even when treated, a small number of people may not survive. Elderly people or those with disabilities may be vulnerable; however, in children the disease is usually milder. Typhoid can adversely affect many organs of the body, and when complications develop, the outlook is poor.

This light micrograph shows gram negative, rod-shaped bacteria called Salmonella typhi. *They are magnified 500 times.* Salmonella typhi *are the causative agent of typhoid fever in humans, and they are transmitted through contaminated food or drinking water.*

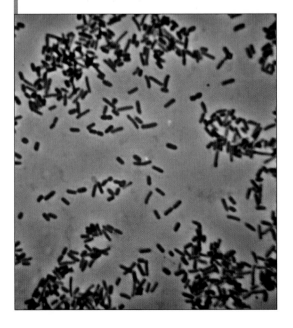

Prevention

Travelers to areas where the disease is common are recommended to visit a doctor or a travel clinic to get vaccinated. TY21a is an oral vaccine; four doses are necessary and last about six years. A booster is needed every five years. VICPS is an injectable vaccine in which one dose is given; a booster is needed every two years. Vaccines are not completely effective, so it is wise to continue to take food and drink precautions. There is no effective immunization for paratyphoid.

Other preventive measures include carefully selecting food and drink while visiting a developing country. This measure will also protect from cholera, dysentery, and hepatitis A. Drinking water should be bottled or boiled. Bottled carbonated water is safer than noncarbonated drinks. Drinks should be taken without ice; when brushing teeth, bottled water should be used rather than tap water. Foods should have been thoroughly cooked, and hands washed with soap and water after bathroom use. When eating raw fruits or vegetables that can be peeled, a good procedure is "boil it, cook it, peel it, or forget it." It is best to avoid foods and beverages from street vendors, which are a common source of illness for travelers.

Pathogenesis

With prompt treatment, typhoid usually clears up, but if not treated, the consequences can be fatal.

Evelyn B. Kelly

See also
• Meningitis • Pneumonia

Typhus

Typhus is a group of infectious diseases transmitted to humans by lice or fleas. It is characterized by high fever, a transient rash, and intractable headache.

Typhus is prevalent worldwide and is transmitted to humans in the feces of body lice, which contaminate wounds on human skin. There are three kinds of typhus: murine, epidemic, and scrub typhus. They are caused by different rickettsial bacteria.

Murine typhus occurs in the southeastern region of the United States, mainly southern Texas and southern California. It is primarily transmitted by the rat flea *Xeonpsylla cheopis*. Murine typhus is mild and is seldom fatal; less than 100 cases are reported annually. This disease is often seen in the summer and fall and lasts for two to three weeks.

Epidemic typhus may have caused more deaths in the twentieth century than any other infectious disease. Epidemic typhus occurs in conditions of war, poverty, famine, crowding, and poor hygiene (called "jail fever") when the temperature is cold. The disease spreads by lice, although it is rare in the United States. Outbreaks of the disease occur in Ethiopia, Uganda, Rwanda, and Peru. Brill-Zinsser disease is a reoccurrance of epidemic typhus, years after the initial attack. This is more common in the elderly when the host defense mechanism falters. Acute sporadic infections occur during the winter months in the eastern and southern United States. It appears to be associated with contact with the parasites of flying squirrels.

Symptoms

Murine (endemic) typhus is an uncommon flea-borne infectious disease caused by *Rickettsia typhi*. After an incubation period of 7 to 14 days, headaches, fever, backache, and arthralgia (joint pain) occurs. Temperatures of 105°F–106°F (40.5°C–41°C) may last two weeks with slight remission in the morning. A rash begins on the trunk and spreads to the periphery, sparing the face, palms, and soles. Nausea, vomiting, dry cough, and abdominal pain are common symptoms.

In contrast, epidemic typhus is characterized by shaking chills, headaches, and fever lasting 12 days, then returning to normal. Rash and other symptoms are similar to murine typhus but are not as severe. Hypotension and stupor or delirium, or both, occurs in the more seriously ill patients. Without treatment, death occurs in 10 to 60 percent of patients with epidemic typhus. Less than 2 percent of untreated patients with murine typhus may die; however, appropriate antibiotics will cure virtually all patients.

Diagnosis and treatments

Blood tests may show anemia and low platelets; liver function enzymes are mildly elevated. Antibody test to typhus should be elevated. Definitive diagnosis is best made by analysis of typhus group antigens. Because these tests take time, many physicians begin treatment based solely on a patient's symptoms.

Symptoms and signs are alleviated if an effective antibiotic, such as tetracycline, is given when the rash first begins. Intravenous fluids and oxygen may be required to stabilize patients with epidemic typhus.

Immunization and lice control are highly effective. Dusting infected persons with DDT, malathion, or lindane may eliminate lice. However, no effective vaccine exists. Keeping out rats and rat fleas from food depots and granaries is a preventive measure.

Isaac Grate

KEY FACTS

Description
Infectious diseases transmitted by fleas or lice.

Causes
Typhus is a rickettsial disease caused by *R. prowazekii* and *R. typhi*.

Risk factors
War, poverty, overcrowding, poor hygiene, cold temperature, rat fleas, rat feces, or fleas.

Symptoms
Headache, myalgias, arthralgia, backache, high fevers, a rash, nausea, vomiting, dry cough, gut pain. Other symptoms include low blood pressure, delirium or stupor, and photophobia.

Diagnosis
By analysis of acute and convalescent phase sera for typhus antibodies.

Treatments
Antibiotics.

See also
• Lice infestation • Lyme disease • Malaria

Vitamin deficiency

Vitamins are small noncaloric, carbon-containing organic compounds that are essential for normal physiological functions, such as growth and development, maintenance, and reproduction. Vitamins are required in minute amounts, but they are either not synthesized by the body, or they are produced in insufficient quantities to meet the requirements for the normal functioning of the body.

Vitamins are classified as either fat- or water-soluble. The fat-soluble vitamins include Vitamin A, Vitamin D, Vitamin E, and Vitamin K. They are absorbed along with dietary fat. After being transported to the liver, they are either used immediately or stored there or in fatty tissues for future use.

The water-soluble vitamins include the vitamin B complex group comprising thiamine (vitamin B_1), riboflavin (vitamin B_2), niacin (vitamin B_3), biotin, pantothenic acid, pyridoxine (vitamin B_6), folic acid, and vitamin B_{12}. Vitamin C (ascorbic acid) is also water soluble. Water-soluble vitamins are absorbed from the intestine into the bloodstream and are transported to various cells to be used as needed. Since these vitamins are not stored in large amounts, any excess will be excreted by the kidneys in the urine, so water-soluble vitamins need to be consumed at least weekly, if not daily. If not consumed on a regular basis, deficiency symptoms or, in some cases, disease may develop fairly quickly.

Although vitamins are sometimes grouped in terms of general function, ultimately each has a specific purpose in the body and, when deficiencies develop, they are specific to the vitamin or vitamins that are lacking. Vitamin deficiencies may come about due to inadequate intake, poor absorption as a result of various medical conditions, or even the use of medication (drug-nutrient interaction). Although a deficiency of the fat-soluble vitamins or vitamin C may occur singly, deficiencies of B vitamins usually appear together. Deficiency symptoms will be addressed individually for each vitamin.

Treatment and prevention of deficiencies are similar for all vitamins. They include a diet high in foods rich in the missing nutrient, and if necessary, use of a high-dose vitamin supplement. If a medical condition causes malabsorption, it must be treated and corrected. If the deficiency is caused by a drug-nutrient interaction, physicians often consider changing the medication or utilizing large doses of a supplement to overcome the effects of the drug.

The following discussion will focus on each of the above-named vitamins, first detailing functions of the vitamin, and then concentrating on the deficiency of each, including the causes and risk factors, symptoms, and diagnosis. Treatment and prevention will not be discussed unless it differs from that stated above. Vitamin A will be discussed in the Key Facts Box.

Fat-soluble vitamins

Vitamin A (retinol) is involved in a number of functions in the human body. These functions include roles in night and color vision; cell differentiation of epithelial cells (the cells that line the body surfaces, including the skin mucous membranes, mouth, stomach and intestines, lungs, urinary tract, uterus, vagina, cornea, and sinus passageways); sperm production in men and fertilization in women; maintaining healthy bones; and contributing to a healthy immune system. Beta-carotene, a precursor (provitamin) of Vitamin A acts as an antioxidant.

Vitamin A deficiency is most common in individuals who do not consume dark-green, orange, and deep-yellow fruits and vegetables (excellent sources of beta-carotene) or animal foods such as liver, eggs, or dairy products. Disorders of the intestine can also impair absorption, and liver disorders negatively impact storage of the vitamin.

Night blindness, the inability to see in dim light, is the earliest symptom of a deficiency. If left untreated, it may progress to xerophthalmia, which is irreversible total blindness as a result of hardening of the cornea. Other deficiency symptoms include impairment of growth, immunity, and reproductive function. Vitamin A deficiency affects as many as 5 million people, mainly infants and children in developing countries. Diagnosis of vitamin A deficiency is based on symptoms and a low level of the vitamin in the blood.

Vitamin D promotes the absorption of calcium and phosphorus from the small intestine; regulates blood calcium levels; is required for bone mineralization, growth and repair; and is important in cell differentiation (maturation). Interestingly, the body can actually synthesize vitamin D when sunlight strikes the skin. Thus it is not considered an essential nutrient if individuals spend enough time in the sun.

Vitamin D deficiency is more common in people who are not exposed very often to the sun (10 or 15 minutes of exposure on hands, face, and arms on a summer day appears to be all that is needed) or have dark skin (less vitamin D is made by these individuals), in infants who are breastfed without any supplementation, and in those who do not use fortified milk or fortified margarine (major sources of vitamin D).

The classical vitamin D deficiency is known as rickets in children and osteomalacia in adults. Children develop bowed legs because the leg bones cannot support their body weight and a protruding abdomen due to weakened musculature. Rickets is still a problem in many less developed nations. Adults who develop osteomalacia exhibit softened bones of the legs and spine, causing some individuals to become bowlegged and bent. Diagnosis of rickets or osteomalacia is based on symptoms, the appearance of abnormal bones on X-rays, and a low level of vitamin D metabolites in the blood.

Vitamin E functions as an antioxidant, protecting the cells against oxidative damage by free radicals (unstable, highly reactive products of normal cellular activity). It is especially important in stabilizing cell membranes and protecting polyunsaturated fatty acids and vitamin A.

A deficiency of vitamin E from a poor intake is rare, since the vitamin is so widespread in foods. However, newborn premature infants who are not supplemented are at risk for a deficiency. They may develop a hemolytic anemia, causing red blood cells to rupture. Disorders that impair fat absorption, such as liver, gall bladder, or pancreatic disease, can also reduce vitamin E absorption and may cause a deficiency. Symptoms of deficiency include difficulty walking, loss of coordination, and muscle weakness; these symptoms are the result of nerve damage (peripheral neuropathy). Blood tests are available to detect vitamin E deficiency.

Vitamin K functions in the synthesis of proteins involved in blood clotting and bone metabolism. Besides being found in green leafy vegetables, vitamin K is synthesized in the body by bacteria in the colon.

Because people depend on bacterial synthesis for vitamin K, deficiency is unlikely except in newborns (whose intestinal tracts are not inhabited by bacteria) and individuals taking antibiotics (which destroy both harmful and helpful intestinal bacteria), anticoagu-

lants, and anticonvulsants. The main symptom of a deficiency is impaired blood clotting and uncontrolled bleeding. Additionally, there are possible negative effects on bone health, such as weakened bones. Newborns are routinely given a vitamin K injection at birth to protect them from hemorrhagic disease. Blood tests to measure clotting function are used to assess vitamin K status.

Treatment consists of vitamin K injections or adjusting the dose of medications.

KEY FACTS: VITAMIN A DEFICIENCY

Description

A deficiency of vitamin A in the body.

Causes

Inadequate intake of preformed vitamin A or the precursor beta-carotene. Disorders involving malabsorption of fat, liver disease, or protein-energy malnutrition (vitamin A requires retinol-binding protein for transport inside the body).

Risk factors

Poor diet, impaired intestinal absorption, liver disease.

Symptoms

Night blindness, xerophthalmia with Bitot's spots (foamy deposits in the whites of the eyes), leading to irreversible blindness. Increase in infections.

Diagnosis

Based on dietary history, symptoms, and low level of vitamin A in the blood.

Treatments

Large oral doses (200,000 IU or 60,000 RE) of vitamin A supplements and correction of protein-energy malnutrition.

Pathogenesis

Low intake leads to depletion of liver stores. Night blindness, xerophthalmia progresses to keratomalacia (softening of the cornea), which leads to irreversible blindness. Accumulation of keratin, a water-insoluble protein, is responsible for the increase in infections.

Prevention

Diets adequate in vitamin A or beta-carotene, protein, and energy.

Epidemiology

Around 3 and 10 million people, mainly infants and preschool children in developing nations, suffer from vitamin A deficiency. About 275 million more children suffer from mild deficiency that impairs immunity and promotes infections. Severe vitamin A deficiency causes more than 500,000 preschool children to become blind each year.

Water-soluble vitamins

Vitamin B$_1$ (thiamine) functions as a coenzyme (thiamine pyrophosphate), a small molecule that promotes enzymatic activity in energy metabolism of the cells. Enzymes are catalysts that allow cellular reactions to take place in a timely fashion. Thiamine is most important in carbohydrate and amino acid metabolism, but it also has a role in nerve function.

A deficiency of thiamine results in beriberi, a disease involving the nervous and cardiovascular systems. Lack of thiamine in the diet is no longer a problem in most developed nations due to the enrichment of flour with B vitamins, but people whose diet consists mostly of polished rice are at risk for deficiency. Alcoholics, who often have a poor food intake, are also at risk. They may develop Wernicke-Korsakoff's syndrome, with memory loss, mental confusion, difficulty walking, and eye problems. Diagnosis of a thiamine deficiency is based on symptoms.

Vitamin B$_2$ (riboflavin), like many B vitamins, functions as a coenzyme (flavine adenine dinucleotide and flavin mononucleotide) in energy metabolism of the cells. Its function is in carbohydrate and fat metabolism, in which it carries hydrogen ions and electrons during various reactions. Riboflavin also serves as an essential component of energy production via the electron transport systems (respiratory chain).

Deficiencies of riboflavin generally occur in concert with other B vitamins. Thus symptoms are often secondary to those arising from other nutrient deficiencies. In the laboratory, an induced lack of riboflavin brings about sensitivity to light, tearing, burning, and itching of the eyes with a loss of visual sharpness, as well as soreness and burning of the lips, mouth, and tongue. Often fissures and cracks develop in the lips and corners of the mouth. Diagnosis is based on the above symptoms and evidence of general malnutrition.

Vitamin B$_3$ (niacin) also functions as a coenzyme (nicotinamide adenine dinucleotide and nicotinamide adenine dinucleotide phosphate) in the energy metabolism of the cells. It is most important in carbohydrate, fat, protein, and alcohol metabolism, DNA replication and repair, and cell differentiation, in which it carries hydrogen ions and electrons during various reactions. Niacin also has an important role in energy production via the electron transport system (respiratory chain).

A lack of niacin leads to pellagra, a deficiency disease with symptoms of diarrhea, dermatitis (a reddened rash similar to sunburn), dementia (confusion, disorientation, hallucinations, and memory loss), and

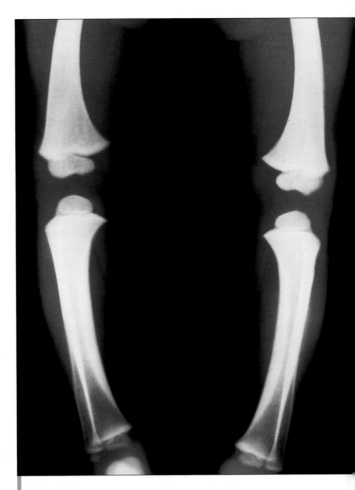

A colored X-ray of a child's legs shows that the long bones are abnormally curved. This severe deformity is a result of rickets, caused by a nutritional deficiency of vitamin D, which is needed for the absorption of calcium from food.

eventually death. In those nations where enrichment of flour with B vitamins occurs, deficiencies are rare. However, in countries where individuals consume a low-protein diet consisting of mostly corn or maize, niacin deficiency may occur. Diagnosis of a deficiency is based on a diet history and symptoms.

Pantothenic acid is part of the chemical structure of coenzyme A (coA), an essential coenzyme involved in the synthesis of fats, neurotransmitters, steroids, and hemoglobin. As coA, it is also an important metabolic intermediate, serving as an entrance point to the tricarboxylic acid (TCA) cycle.

Since pantothenic acid is widespread in foods, deficiency is quite rare. If present, symptoms include fatigue, gastrointestinal problems (nausea, vomiting, cramps), and neurological disturbances.

Pyridoxine (vitamin B_6), in common with a number of other B vitamins, functions as a coenzyme (pyridoxal phosphate) in amino acid, carbohydrate, and fat metabolism. Also, pyridoxine is involved with the synthesis of neurotransmitters and red blood cells.

Dietary deficiencies of pyridoxine are relatively rare; however, a number of drugs interfere with vitamin B_6 metabolism. These include isoniazid (an antibiotic and chemotherapeutuic agent), hydralazine (an antihypertensive), and penicillamin (used to treat arthritis and Wilson's disease). Deficiency symptoms include seizure in infants, microcytic anemia, dermatitis, numbness and prickling in the hands and feet, depression, confusion, and convulsions. Diagnosis of a deficiency is based on symptoms that respond to supplementation.

Biotin functions as a coenzyme in carbohydrate, fat, and protein metabolism. It is involved in the addition or removal of carbon dioxide to and from various compounds. Deficiencies of biotin are rare due to its widespread occurrence in foods and synthesis by intestinal bacteria. Avidin, a protein found in raw egg whites, binds with biotin, making it unavailable. Hence a diet high in raw egg whites (cooking destroys avidin) may precipitate deficiency symptoms, which include dermatitis, hair loss, pallor, nausea, vomiting, and anorexia. Diagnosis of deficiency is based on dietary history.

Folic acid (folate or folacin) functions as a coenzyme in DNA and RNA synthesis and amino acid metabolism. Specifically, it transfers one-carbon compounds in many different reactions, including those involved in formation of red and white blood cells and the metabolism of homocysteine, an amino acid that can build up and may increase the risk of heart disease.

A deficiency of folate leads to changes in DNA and RNA metabolism, leading to poor growth, megaloblastic anemia, neural tube defects in a developing fetus, elevated homocysteine levels, and gastrointestinal tract disturbances. A number of drugs, including antacids, aspirin, oral contraceptive agents, chemotherapeutic agents, and anticonvulsants, have been shown to interfere with the body's use of folate. Pregnant women and alcoholics are at high risk for deficiency. Some researchers suggest that folate deficiency may be the most common vitamin deficiency in humans.

Folate is found in many foods, although brewer's yeast, liver, leafy green vegetables, and legumes have the greatest levels. Recently, flour in the United States has been enriched with folate. Diagnosis of folate deficiency is by a blood test that detects large red blood cells (macrocytic anemia), followed by additional tests that specifically measure folic acid in the blood.

Vitamin B_{12} functions as a coenzyme in the synthesis of new cells. Specifically, it is used to transfer methyl groups in various metabolic reactions. Vitamin B_{12} is necessary for the synthesis of nucleic acids, maturation of red blood cells, normal nerve function, and activation of folic acid.

Vitamin B_{12} is found only in animal products; hence, strict vegetarians (vegans) are at increased risk of deficiency. Since the vitamin requires an acidic environment to be released from food, elderly people whose stomach acidity is low may also be at risk. Intrinsic factor, a protein made in the stomach, is necessary to protect the vitamin until it reaches the end of the small intestine, where it is absorbed. Thus, individuals with stomach injury or an autoimmune disorder that destroys intrinsic factor would also be at risk.

Deficiency symptoms include megaloblastic anemia (called pernicious anemia if it is caused by lack of stomach acid or intrinsic factor); nerve damage, in the form of tingling and numbness of the arms and legs; memory loss; disorientation; and dementia. The anemia develops slowly since the body can store enough vitamin for up to five years. Diagnosing a deficiency can be complicated, since large doses of folic acid will mask symptoms, although nerve damage will proceed unchecked. An anemia with large red blood cells is often the first sign of a deficiency. Blood tests or a Schilling test using a small amount of radioactive vitamin B_{12} can confirm the diagnosis. Treatment of a deficiency is vitamin supplementation by mouth if the deficiency is due to diet, or by injections if it is due to a lack of stomach acid or intrinsic factor.

Vitamin C (ascorbic acid) functions in the synthesis of collagen (a protein necessary for the structure of connective tissue, cartilage, bone matrix, tooth dentin, skin, and tendons) and thyroid hormone; as an antioxidant; in amino acid metabolism; and to increase the absorption of iron. It also promotes resistance to infection.

Vitamin C deficiency causes scurvy, with symptoms that include rough skin, swollen, inflamed, and bleeding gums, loose teeth, dry mouth and eyes, and hair loss. There may also be bleeding under the skin that resembles bruises, poor wound healing, frequent infection, muscle degeneration and pain, and anemia. Diagnosis is based on symptoms followed by a blood test.

Alan Levine

See also
• Anemia • Eating disorders

Wart and verruca

Warts and verrucas are harmless, contagious viral infections of the skin that cause small unsightly growths. Over 80 types of the human papilloma virus (HPV) cause four different types of warts. Verrucas (plantar warts) are warts on the bottom of the feet.

Warts or verrucas are growths that occur on the top layer of skin; the overgrowth of cells develops into a small lump. Warts on the soles of the feet are commonly called verrucas.

Causes and risk factors

Scientists now know that the unsightly but harmless growths are caused when the human papillomavirus (HPV) enters the skin through small cuts. Most common in children and teenagers, the lesions appear on the hands, feet, and face and come in many shapes, colors, and sizes. HPV is passed by direct and indirect contact. For example, if a person touches the damp towel of someone who has warts, the person may pick up HPV. Children who bite their fingernails or pick at hangnails get warts more often than children who do not.

Why some people get warts and others do not is still unknown. One theory is that certain individuals are immune to the virus. Others have recurring warts; those people may harbor the virus, which may lie dormant in underlying skin tissues.

Symptoms and signs

There are several types of warts. Common warts appear most often on tops of fingers, hands, along the cuticles, knees, and elbows. Looking like a rough cauliflower, they may have small black dots, which are tiny blood vessels. The wart may appear alone or with small satellites. Flat or juvenile warts are about the size of a pinhead and have flat tops that are pink, light brown, or yellow. Usually occurring in children, the warts can grow in clusters of as many as 100. Plantar warts or verrucas grow thick calloused areas on the ball of the foot and feel like a stone in the shoe. Filiform warts are those depicted on witches in fairy-tale books. This wart has a fingerlike shape and grows around the mouth, eyes, and nose. Genital warts are lesions that may be sexually transmitted and can extend internally into the reproductive organs. Most are painless, but

some can increase the risk of cervical cancer. A vaccine has been developed to prevent these types of warts.

About 50 percent of warts go away untreated, but others need a doctor's attention. Over-the-counter preparations with salicylic acid may be helpful. Genital warts respond to podophyllin, a topical resin. Cryosurgery freezes warts with liquid nitrogen, and this may get rid of them. Laser treatment is used for stubborn warts, especially plantar warts, which may respond to this treatment. Surgery is not the best treatment because it may leave scars and residual virus. Immunotherapy is now commonly used; a variety of techniques involve painting or injecting a medication at the site of the wart to stimulate immune clearance and to prevent recurrence.

Evelyn B. Kelly

KEY FACTS

Description
Small growths; verrucas are warts on the feet.

Causes
More than 80 types of the human papillomavirus (HPV) cause warts; the virus is passed from person to person.

Risk factors
Virus enters through cracks in the skin; some types are transmitted sexually.

Symptoms
Painless, flesh-colored small cauliflower-like growth with tiny black dots or minute blood vessels.

Diagnosis
Observation.

Treatments
Ranges from no treatment to physical or chemical destruction, or immunotherapy.

Pathogenesis
Warts are generally not harmful; rarely will they become cancerous.

Prevention
Avoid contact with warts or objects that have touched the growths in other people; scratches or cuts on feet or hands may lead to verrucas.

Epidemiology
Most commonly seen in children and teenagers.

See also
• Cold, common • HPV infection

West Nile encephalitis

In 1999, West Nile virus (WNV) was introduced into the Western Hemisphere, perhaps through importation of an infected bird or mosquito, and has since spread rapidly. The emergence of WNV has raised awareness about the introduction of new viruses into naive ecosystems.

West Nile virus (WNV) is a member of the virus family *Flaviviridae*. The virus was first isolated in 1937 from the West Nile district in Uganda. WNV is maintained in birds and transmitted to humans and other vertebrate animals by mosquitoes, primarily *Culex* species. Bird infection is usually benign, although some species, such as crows and jays, have shown mortality rates exceeding 90 percent. Humans and other vertebrates are incidental hosts and may contribute to viral amplification. Transmission of WNV has also occurred through blood transfusions, organ transplants, laboratory exposures, and transplacental passage from mother to child.

Signs and symptoms

Most human infections are asymptomatic or mild. The incubation period is usually around two to six days. People with symptoms experience fever, chills, headache, rash, joint and muscle pains, diarrhea, nausea, and vomiting (West Nile fever). Less than 1 percent of humans infected with WNV, primarily the elderly and immunocompromised, develop neuron-invasive disease (West Nile encephalitis), with signs of meningitis or encephalitis, including muscle weakness, disorientation, tremors, convulsions, paralysis, coma, and death in 3 to 15 percent of cases. Previous infection provides protective immunity.

The infection is diagnosed by tests to detect WNV or antibodies in blood or tissues. Treatment is supportive.

Pathogenesis and prevention

Early infection in the skin and regional lymph nodes seeds the blood, leading to widespread organ infection, including the spleen, liver, lungs, and central nervous system. Viremia normally lasts only a few days and ceases with the onset of symptoms but may be prolonged in the elderly and immunocompromised. Prevention centers on avoiding mosquito bites. Screening blood donations for WNV in the United States in 2003 has greatly reduced the risk of infection via blood products. A vaccine is in clinical trials.

Epidemiology

After WNV was first introduced to the Western Hemisphere in 1999, subsequent migrations of infected birds have resulted in spread of WNV across North America, encroaching further into the Southern Hemisphere of the Americas with each passing year. From 2002 to 2005, annual averages of almost 5,000 cases were reported in the United States.

Ian H. Mendenhall and
Daniel G. Bausch

KEY FACTS

Description
Acute viral infection from an infected mosquito.

Cause
West Nile virus, in birds and transmitted to humans and other vertebrates by mosquitoes.

Risk factors
Spending time outdoors during peak mosquito-biting season. More rarely, blood transfusion or transplantation with infected tissues.

Symptoms
Most infections are asymptomatic or result in mild fever. Elderly and immunocompromised are at risk of central nervous system involvement.

Diagnosis
Test of blood or tissues for antibodies or virus

Treatments
Supportive. No specific antiviral drug available.

Pathogenesis
Combination of direct viral damage from replication in organs and pathologic effects of the immune response.

Prevention
Covering exposed skin and using insect repellants. Monitor mosquito and bird populations for infection. Eliminate mosquito breeding.

Epidemiology
Found in Africa, southern Europe, the Middle East, western Asia, Australia, and North America.

See also
• Lyme disease • Meningitis • Rickettsial infections • Rocky Mountain spotted fever

Whiplash

The term *whiplash* is commonly used to describe a soft tissue injury of the neck caused by hyperextension and hyperflexion of the neck, also called a "neck sprain" or "neck strain." The injury may involve the muscles, nerve roots, intervertebral joints, disks, or ligaments of the neck.

Motor vehicle collisions are the most common cause of whiplash, although the injury may occur with assaults, falls, or with sports activities that cause hyperextension and hyperflexion of the neck. Increasing age and preexisting neck conditions may increase the severity of the condition.

Symptoms

The patient presents with neck pain, stiffness, and tenderness of the neck musculature. The patient may also present with less common symptoms of headache, muscle spasms of the neck, decreased range of motion of the neck, paresthesias (skin sensations) of the upper extremities, pain in the shoulders or between the shoulder blades, dizziness, fatigue, sleep disturbances, or depression. Whiplash is sometimes also associated with memory loss, impaired concentration, irritability, and nervousness. The pain associated with whiplash typically resolves within days to weeks, with complete resolution for most patients within three months. Patients with six weeks or more of pain should have a reevaluation by a physician to determine possible alternate causes for the pain.

Diagnosis

The diagnosis of whiplash is by history and physical exam with a complete neurological exam. X-rays of the cervical spine are done according to the judgment of the physician; if there is pain, palpation of the neck is undertaken to exclude bony injury. In patients with negative X-ray studies who have persistent pain or neurological problems, additional imaging with computed tomography (CT) or magnetic resonance imaging (MRI) may be necessary to further delineate the underlying anatomy and injury.

Treatments and prevention

Treatment of whiplash may include ice or heat application to the affected area. Medications, such as nonsteroidal anti-inflammatory drugs (NSAIDs) or a short course of narcotics or muscle relaxants, may be administered. Additional treatment options include physical therapy, range of motion exercises, traction, massage, local injections, ultrasound, or short-term use of a soft cervical collar. Antidepressants may be prescribed if a patient has associated depression with ongoing pain.

Since motor vehicle collisions are the most common cause of whiplash, prevention has been aimed at the use of head rests on car seats, which, on impact, decrease the range of motion of a person's head.

Joanne L. Oakes

KEY FACTS

Description
Soft-tissue injury of the neck.

Causes
Motor vehicle collisions, falls, and assaults.

Risk factors
Increasing age and prior neck injury.

Symptoms
Localized pain, neck tenderness, decreased range of motion of the neck, headache, paresthesias of the upper extremities, pain in the shoulders or between the shoulder blades, dizziness, fatigue, sleep disturbances, depression, impaired concentration, irritability, and nervousness.

Diagnosis
History and physical exam with a complete neurological exam.

Treatment
Oral pain medications, muscle relaxants, local application of ice or heat, physical therapy, traction, massage, local injections, ultrasound, and temporary use of a soft cervical collar.

Pathogenesis
Hyperextension and hyperflexion of the neck.

Prevention
Use of head rests in cars.

Epidemiology
Common, although actual incidence unknown due to underreporting.

See also

- Depressive disorders • Head injury
- Sleep disorders

Whooping cough

Also called pertussis, whooping cough used to be a common childhood disease in industrialized countries. Thanks to vaccination, it is now much less common in the United States, though outbreaks still occur.

Whooping cough is a sometimes severe respiratory infection caused by the bacterium *Bordetella pertussis*. Young children are particularly at risk from the disease. Today it is most common in less developed countries of the tropics.

Cause and symptoms and signs

Whooping cough results from *B. pertussis* infecting the lining of the upper respiratory system. The incubation time between infection and symptoms appearing is usually around 7 to 10 days. The first symptoms are nonspecific, such as sneezing and a runny nose. Usually it is another week or two before the characteristic coughing fits begin. These fits are often accompanied by a distinctive "whooping" sound, as the sufferer gasps for breath. Coughing fits can go on for 6 to 8 weeks and can be triggered by activities such as laughing or yawning. Adults with whooping cough usually have much milder symptoms than young children.

The disease can be diagnosed either from the symptoms, by taking samples from the sufferer's air tubes and growing the bacteria in culture, or by taking a blood sample to check for antibodies the body has produced against the disease.

Pathogenesis and treatments

Whooping cough bacteria attach to the cells lining the air tubes that lead to the lungs. The more severe symptoms of the disease are caused by toxins that the bacteria produce. Whooping cough also lays the body open to other infections, such as pneumonia. All these effects tend to be more severe in young children. About 1 in 500 young children with whooping cough dies, either from breathing difficulties or from other complications.

Young children with whooping cough need careful attention, especially to make sure they can breathe properly. Children may also be sick after a coughing fit and start to lose weight. Sometimes hospital admission is necessary. Treatment by antibiotics at an early stage, especially before the coughing fits begin, shortens the infection. Treating sufferers and those around them also makes them less infectious to other people.

Epidemiology and prevention

Whooping cough is spread by those infected coughing or sneezing water droplets into the air. Others then breathe in these droplets. The disease is far more common in unvaccinated communities. Because infants and young children are most at risk, vaccination starts at 2 months old, with further vaccinations later in infancy. Vaccination lasts only a few years, so adults can get whooping cough even if they were vaccinated as children. Vaccines are based on whole dead *Bordetella* cells or on the toxins. Cell-free vaccines produce fewer side effects and are the type used in the United States today.

Richard Beatty

KEY FACTS

Description
A bacterial disease of the upper air tubes.

Cause
Infection with the bacterium *Bordetella pertussis*.

Risk factors
Infants are more at risk of severe disease.

Symptoms
Violent coughing fits, usually with a characteristic "whooping" sound when breathing in.

Diagnosis
Usually by the symptoms; also by laboratory investigations.

Treatments
Antibiotics make the sufferers less infectious; symptoms and complications also need treatment.

Pathogenesis
Bacteria release toxins that irritate the respiratory system.

Prevention
Vaccination; avoiding contact with people who have the illness.

Epidemiology
Bacteria spread in air droplets produced by coughing and sneezing.

See also
• Croup

Yeast infection

A yeast infection is a type of fungal infection that can cause a variety of skin infections, including dandruff. The fungus *Candida albicans* is one of the most common yeast infections. It causes vaginal infections in women, but it can also infect the mouth and cause diaper rash in babies.

Although many people think of yeast as just an ingredient for bakers and brewers, there are many yeasts that can cause infections in humans. Under normal, healthy conditions the growth of these microbes goes unnoticed. But when the body gets out of balance, the fungi can quickly grow out of control, causing infections, skin rashes, and even dandruff.

Types of yeast infections

Candida is a fungus that is found almost everywhere, including the digestive system and in the reproductive tract of women. Paronychia is an infection of the skin around the nails that can be caused by candida, bacteria, or other fungi. The infection can be acute or chronic, affecting the nail and cuticle as well as the surrounding skin.

Malassezia furfur (formerly called *Pityrosporum ovale*) is a common yeast that produces dandruff when it grows in abundance on the scalp. It is estimated that one in three people have experienced problems with dandruff. Seborrheic dermatitis is a more severe infection that can occur in infants or adults. In infants, the rash that often occurs on the scalp is commonly called "cradle cap." The rashes can spread to the eyebrows, eyelids, and folds in the skin. In infants, yeasts are one of the causes of diaper rashes.

Causes and risk factors

There are more than 150 species of candida, but only 10 of them can cause disease in humans. More than 90 percent of all infections are caused by a single species: *Candida albicans*. Women are at highest risk, and 75 percent of all women will have a vaginal yeast infection at some point in their life. These often occur when a woman takes antibiotics that destroy the normally beneficial bacteria growing in the vagina. Other risk factors include the use of birth control pills, corticosteroid medications, pregnancy, diabetes, and a depressed immune system. It is rarely transmitted by sexual activity.

Paronychia is common in people whose hands are often in water. Hairdressers and dishwashers are at higher risk. Other risk factors include nail-biting, improper nail care, and exposure to chemical irritants. Women are at higher risk, along with diabetics and patients with compromised immune systems.

The risk of seborrheic dermatitis varies greatly by age. Infants are at risk until about six months of age. After that, the risk is low until puberty. The incidence of dandruff and seborrheic dermatitis appears to peak

KEY FACTS

Description

A fungal infection of the genital tract, mouth, or the skin.

Causes

The fungus *Candida albicans*.

Risk factors

Pregnancy, diabetes, a suppressed immune system, and the use of antibiotics, birth control pills, or steroids. Women are at highest risk.

Symptoms

Vaginal itching, redness, pain while urinating, a thick white discharge from the vagina, or white patches in the mouth.

Diagnosis

Laboratory cultures from swabs of the infected area.

Treatments

Antifungal medicines can be taken orally or applied directly to the infected area.

Pathogenesis

Candida is normally present, but grows out of control during infections. In rare cases, an untreated infection can reach the bloodstream and spread throughout the body.

Prevention

Moist, warm conditions, and nylon underwear should be avoided; cotton is a better choice. Skin should be kept clean and dry.

Epidemiology

Roughly 75 percent of women will have a vaginal infection at least once in their lifetime. Genital infections in men are rare.

around age 40. Hormones appear to play a factor, because men are at greater risk than women. People with weakened immune systems are also at greater risk, as are patients with Parkinson's disease and epilepsy, although it is not clear why the disorders are linked. Dandruff is not caused by dry skin or frequent shampooing. In fact, oily skin is a known risk factor.

Symptoms, diagnosis, and pathogenesis

Vaginal yeast infections produce itching, redness, and a thick white discharge. Infections in the mouth and throat produce patchy white areas. This infection is commonly called "thrush." In babies, the moist damp skin inside a diaper is a prime breeding ground for the fungus. The rash causes weepy, red pustules. Candidemia is an invasive form of the disease. It is one of the most common bloodstream infections found in hospitalized patients and is potentially fatal.

Laboratory tests can identify the candida microbe, but the symptoms are often sufficient for a doctor to make a diagnosis.

Depending on the microbe responsible, paronychia can produce swollen, tender nails with pus-filled abscesses during an acute infection. Chronic infections can spread to include nail discoloration as well as redness and swelling of the nail folds. In rare cases, the infection can spread across the hand and throughout the body as a systemic infection.

Reddish patches with white crusts and oily skin are typical in patients with seborrheic dermatitis. In the milder case of dandruff, the major symptom is an itchy, flaky scalp. The infections can be persistent but are generally mild in nature.

Treatments and prevention

Keeping the skin clean and dry can prevent many yeast infections. Women should use cotton underwear and avoid nylon pantyhose and other tight-fitting clothes. Deodorants, bubble baths, and douches can irritate the vagina and should be avoided.

It is still not clear if eating yogurt can prevent vaginal yeast infections, but yogurt with active cultures does contain lactobacilli, which are beneficial bacteria that can normally be found in the vagina.

If an infection occurs, it can be treated with antifungal ointments or pills. Recurrent infections can be more troublesome if resistance occurs. In the case of candidemia, intravenous medication may be required.

Soaking the infected nails can help to relieve the pressure and infection in paronychia. However, in most cases, an antibacterial or antifungal agent will be

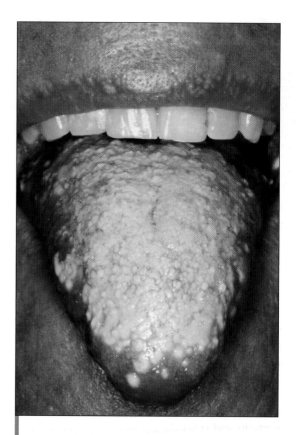

This thick, creamy coating on the tongue is a symptom of severe oral candidiasis (thrush). Candidiasis is an infection caused by a yeastlike fungus, usually Candida albicans.

required to clear up the infection. Chronic cases involving fungal infections can be very difficult to cure and require several weeks or even months of treatment. The best prevention is good nail care. This includes trimming nails regularly, avoiding the use of irritating cuticle removers, and not chewing or biting the nails. Rubber gloves with cotton liners should be used to protect the nails and hands from water and chemical irritants.

Dandruff is best controlled with a medicated shampoo that targets the yeast growing on the scalp. The shampoos need to be left on the scalp for several minutes and should be used regularly until the scalp recovers. Seborrheic dermatitis is usually treated with topical ointments ketoconazole, selenium sulfide, pyrithione zinc, and corticosteroids.

Chris Curran

See also
• Diabetes

Yellow fever

Yellow fever is caused by the yellow fever virus (YFV). The virus is transmitted by mosquitoes. Infection can cause rapid liver failure, hemorrhage, and death within 10 days of onset. In the past, yellow fever occurred in coastal cities of the United States and in many European cities. However, as a result of mosquito eradication programs and the development of an effective live attenuated vaccine in the 1930s, it is now largely restricted to regions of tropical Africa and South America.

Yellow fever is a mosquito-transmitted viral disease occurring in tropical regions of Africa and South America. It may affect both genders equally at any age, although because of a forest cycle involving wild primates, in South America men are more at risk as a result of their occupation as forestry workers. Because of the occurrence of yellow fever in remote locations with poor communications, accurate information is difficult to obtain, and it is believed that official reports may greatly underestimate actual numbers. Between 2000 and 2005 there were 3,309 cases officially reported from Africa and 657 cases from South America. However, the World Health Organization estimates that there may be 200,000 human infections each year with 30,000 deaths, 90 percent occurring in Africa.

Causes and risk factors

The causative agent, yellow fever virus, is transmitted to people via the bite of infected mosquitoes. The most frequent mosquito vector in urban outbreaks is *Aedes aegypti*, a species that breeds in close proximity to humans, laying eggs in any small container that contains water. It feeds preferentially on people and has been responsible for large urban epidemics. Other species are involved in rural and jungle cycles. Not being vaccinated is a significant risk factor, especially for those entering endemic areas and likely to come in contact with infected mosquitoes. The recent development of the ecotourism industry is providing new opportunities for people to visit regions in which yellow fever may occur. Since 1996, at least six travelers (from Belgium, Germany, Switzerland, and the United States) have died of yellow fever virus infections acquired while visiting Africa or South America.

Symptoms, signs, and diagnosis

Symptoms of infection are variable, probably as a result of natural human resistance factors, and perhaps differences between virus strains. Less than 30 percent of people who are infected become sick. The incubation period is 3 to 6 days. Disease can be characterized into three phases. The "period of infection," which lasts 3 to 4 days, presents as mild nonspecific and flulike symptoms, with fever up to 105°F (40.6°C) lasting for three and half days with fatigue, headache, photophobia, back pain and general myalgia, nausea, vomiting, and disorientation and dizziness. In relation to the

---

KEY FACTS

Description
A viral disease that infects the liver.

Cause
Infection with yellow fever virus.

Risk factors
Mosquito bites, mainly in Africa but also in South America. Lack of vaccination.

Symptoms
Flulike symptoms progressing to fatal multi-organ failure. In severe cases, fatality rates range from 20 percent to over 50 percent, with death occurring 8 to 10 days after first symptoms.

Diagnosis
Examination by experienced medical personnel; tests of blood and tissue samples. Protocols for rapid diagnosis using polymerase chain reactions.

Treatments
No specific treatment is available. Where conditions permit, supportive care, including nutritional and fluid maintenance, dialysis, and transfusion, may be administered.

Pathogenesis
Liver damage. Eosinophilic degeneration also occurs in the tubular epithelium of the kidneys.

Prevention
Long-term protection is provided by vaccination with a live vaccine, recommended to travelers visiting areas where the disease is endemic.

Epidemiology
The virus is typically transmitted in a forest cycle between mosquitoes and primates. Although large-scale epidemics are infrequent due to vaccination and mosquito control, yellow fever is regarded as a reemerging disease because of an increasing number of cases over the last 25 years.

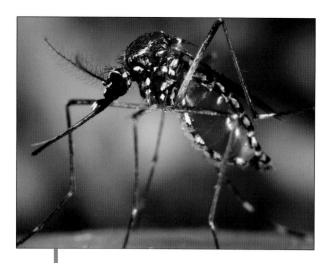

A female A. aegypti *mosquito is about to fly off a host's skin surface after obtaining a blood meal.*

fever, the pulse rate is slow. The tongue is characteristically bright red at the tip and sides, with a central white coating, and the liver may be tender and enlarged. The virus may be isolated from the blood at this stage, and serum transaminase levels are elevated. During the "period of remission" the fever and symptoms wane, and most patients continue to recover. However, after 48 hours, about 15 percent of patients progress to the "period of intoxication." Although anti-YFV antibodies can now be detected, and the virus disappears from the blood, fever and vomiting return, and the patient becomes jaundiced; hence the name *yellow fever*.

Specific diagnosis can now be made based on laboratory detection of viral antigen and specific antibodies using a variety of techniques including enzyme-linked immunosorbent assay (ELISA), hemagglutination inhibition, complement fixation, neutralization tests, immunofluorescence assays, and viral isolation in culture or mice. Polymerase chain reactions (PCR) assays to detect viral nucleic acids in blood and tissues have been developed and will accelerate detection in the future.

About 20 percent of patients with jaundice die as a result of multi-organ failure. Symptoms are complex, but patients can become delirious with convulsions, vomit blood that is blackened as a result of the action of gastric juices (so-called coffee-grounds vomit), and lapse into a coma prior to death. Postmortem diagnosis is based on unique liver pathology, including the detection of "councilman bodies," which are liver cells degenerated by white blood cells. In patients who survive, recovery may take several weeks.

Treatment and prevention

No specific treatment exists, although supportive measures, including nutritional maintenance, fluid replacement, aspiration to prevent gastric swelling, administration of oxygen and vasoactive drugs (affecting dilation or constriction of blood vessels), transfusion of plasma, and dialysis, may all be required to sustain life in severe cases. The live attenuated 17D vaccine, available from travel clinics and hospitals, is regarded as one of the safest and most effective vaccines available. Revaccination is advised at ten-year intervals, although a single dose may provide lifelong protection.

Epidemiology

Yellow fever probably arose in Africa and spread as a result of the slave trade. There is a jungle cycle in Africa that involves *A. africanus* and other mosquito species that feed upon wild primates, and there is a so-called intermediate cycle in moist savanna regions. In South America, a jungle cycle also exists, involving *Haemagogus* and *Sabethes* species of mosquito. The South American primates succumb to fatal infection.

For humans, the most important cycle is the urban cycle, involving transmission between *A. aegypti* and people. In the urban setting, transmission can be intense, and if not controlled can result in massive epidemics. Urban cycles have not been observed in tropical South America since 1942. A few cases have been reported from South American towns and cities, and urban transmission is still reported in Africa, especially in Nigeria. The continuing pattern of increasing numbers of yellow fever cases over recent years may be the result of several factors. In many countries, vaccination programs and mosquito control efforts have not been sustained because of economic reasons. More people are moving from rural areas to urban towns and cities, and most of these people are unvaccinated, so uncontrolled outbreaks occur before emergency vaccination campaigns can be organized. Because the principal mosquito vector, *A. aegypti*, is widely distributed and since the 1970s has become reestablished in many South American cities, the risk of urban transmission of yellow fever virus is also increasing in that continent.

Global warming may represent a new threat, since *A. aegypti* may expand its range into regions in which it has not previously occurred.

Stephen Higgs

See also
• Malaria

Resources for Further Study

General Reference Works

American College of Physicians. 2003. *Complete Home Medical Guide.* New York: DK Publishing, Inc.

American Medical Association. 2006. *Concise Medical Encyclopedia.* New York: Random House Information Group.

American Psychiatric Association (APA). 2000. *Diagnostic and Statistical Manual of Mental Disorders.* 4th ed. Washington, D.C.: APA.

Clayman, Charles, ed. 2005. *The Human Body.* New York: DK Publishing, Inc.

Gray, Henry, and H. V. Carter (illustrator). 2000. *Gray's Anatomy.* New York: Barnes and Noble.

Labrecque, Mary C., Robert Pantell, Harold C. Sox, Timothy B. Walsh, and John H. Wasson. 2002. *Common Symptom Guide.* Columbus, OH: McGraw-Hill.

Marks, Andrea, and Betty Rothbart. 2003. *Healthy Teens, Body and Soul: A Parent's Complete Guide to Adolescent Health.* New York: Simon and Schuster.

Sultz, Harry A., and Kristina M. Young. 2005. *Health Care USA: Understanding Its Organization and Delivery.* Sudbury, MA: Jones and Bartlett Publishers, Inc.

Infections

Bennett, John E., Raphael Dolin, and Gerald L. Mandell. 2004. *Mandell, Douglas, and Bennett's Principles and Practice of Infectious Diseases.* Philadelphia: Elsevier Churchill Livingstone.

Black, Samuel J., Peter J. Krause, Dennis J. Richardson, and Richard J. Seed, eds. 2002. *North American Parasitic Zoonoses.*

Boston, MA: Kluwer Academic Publishers.

Bottone, Edward J. 2003. *An Atlas of Infectious Diseases.* Boca Raton, FL: CRC Press.

Callahan, Gerald N. 2006. *Infection: The Uninvited Universe.* New York: St. Martin's Press.

Chiodini, Jane. 2004. *Atlas of Travel Medicine and Health.* Ontario: B. C. Decker Inc.

Davidson, Robert, Michael Eddleston, Stephen Pierini, and Robert Wilkinson. 2004. *Oxford Handbook of Tropical Medicine.* Oxford, UK: Oxford University Press.

Fauci, Anthony S., John I. Gallin, and Richard Krause, eds. 2000. *Emerging Infections.* Burlington, MA: Elsevier Science.

Freeman-Cook, Kevin, Lisa Freeman-Cook, and Edward Alcamo, eds. 2005. *Staphylococcus Aureus Infections.* New York: Chelsea House Publishers.

Gittleman, Ann Louise, and Omar M. Amin. 2001. *Guess What Came to Dinner: Parasites and Your Health.* Wayne NJ: Avery.

Gualde, Norbert, and Steven Rendall (translator). 2006. *Resistance: The Human Struggle against Infection.* Washington, DC: Dana Press.

Hart, Tony. 2004. *Microterrors: The Complete Guide to Bacterial, Viral, and Fungal Infections That Threaten Our Health.* Toronto: Firefly Books, Ltd.

Heelan, Judith Stephenson. 2004. *Cases in Human Parasitology.* Herndon, VA: ASM Press.

Henderson, Gregory, Allan Warshowsky, and Batya S. Yasgur. 2002. *Women at Risk: The HPV Epidemic and Your Cervical Health.* Wayne, NJ: Avery.

Irving, William L., John W. McCauley, and Dave J. Rowlands, eds. 2001. *New Challenges to Health.* NY: Cambridge University Press.

Martin, Jeanne Marie. 2000. *Complete Candida Yeast Guidebook.* New York: Crown Publishing Group.

Mandell, Gerald L., John E. Bennett, and Raphael Dolin, eds. 2004. *Mandell, Douglas, and Bennett's Principles and Practice of Infectious Diseases,* 6th ed. Philadelphia: Elsevier Churchill Livingstone.

Molyneux, David H., ed. 2006. *Control of Human Parasitic Diseases.* Burlington, MA: Elsevier Science and Technology.

Regush, Nicholas. *The Virus Within.* 2000. New York: Penguin Group.

Richardson, Malcolm D., and David W. Warnock. 2003. *Fungal Infection, Diagnosis and Management.* Malden, MA: Blackwell Publishing.

Sfakianos, Jeffrey N. 2006. *Avian Flu,* edited by I. Edward Alcamo. New York: Chelsea House Publishers.

Sherman, Irwin W. 2006. *Power of Plagues.* Herndon, VA: ASM Press.

Shmaefsky, Brian Robert. 2004. *Meningitis,* edited by I. Edward Alcamo. New York: Chelsea House Publishers.

Superficial Fungal Infections. 2002. UK: Health Press.

Noninfectious disorders
Addiction

Bellenir, Karen, ed. 2002. *Drug Information for Teens: Health Tips about the Physical and Mental Effects of Substance Abuse,* Detroit, MI: Omnigraphics, Inc.

Brick, John, ed. 2004. *Handbook of the Medical Consequences of Alcohol and Drug Abuse.* New York: Haworth Press.

Carson-DeWitt, R., ed. 2001. *Encyclopedia of Drugs, Alcohol, and Addictive Behavior.* 2nd ed. Farmington Hills, MI: Macmillan Reference USA.

Conyers, Beverly. 2003. *Addict in the Family: Stories of Loss, Hope, and Recovery.* Center City, MN: Hazelden.

Ehrlich, Caryl. 2003. *Conquer Your Food Addiction.* New York: The Free Press.

Griffin, Kevin. 2004. *One Breath at a Time: Buddhism and the Twelve Steps.* Emmaus, PA: Rodale.

Nakken, Craig. 1996. *The Addictive Personality: Understanding the Addictive Process and Compulsive Behavior.* Center City, MN: Hazelden.

United Nations Office for Drug Control and Crime Prevention. 2003. *Alcohol and Drug Problems at Work: The Shift to Prevention.* Geneva: ILO.

Aging

Bullen, Timothy, and Anthony Campbell. 2004. *The Directory of Your Back, Your Bones, and Things That Ache.* Secaucus NJ: Chartwell Books, Inc.

Whitbourne, Susan Krauss. 2004. *Adult Development and Aging: Biopsychosocial Perspectives.* New York: John Wiley & Sons, Inc.

AIDS

Greene, Warner C., Merle A.Sande, and Paul Volberding, ed. 2007. *Global HIV/AIDS Medicine.* St. Louis, MO: Saunders Publishing.

Allergies

Mitchell, Dean. 2006. *The Allergy and Asthma Cure: A Revolutionary New Treatment Program for All Airborne Allergies and Asthma.* New York: Marlowe & Company.

Arterial disorders

Gersh, B. J. 2000. *Mayo Clinic Heart Book: The Ultimate Guide to Heart Health.* New York: W. Morrow.

Arthritis

Bruce, Debra Fulgham. 2003. *Pain-Free Arthritis.* New York: Henry Holt & Company, Inc.

O'Driscoll, Erin Rohan. 2004. *Exercises for Arthritis.* New York: Hatherleigh Press.

Vad, Vijay. 2006. *Arthritis Rx.* New York: Penguin Group.

Backache

Freedman, Janet, and Elaine Petrone. 2003. *The Miracle Ball Method.* New York: Workman Publishing Company, Inc.

Katz, Jeffrey N., and Gloria Parkinson. 2007. *Heal Your Aching Back.* Columbus, OH: McGraw-Hill.

Kubey, Craig, and Robin A. McKenzie. 2001. *Seven Steps to a Pain-Free Life.* New York: Penguin Group.

Blood disorders

Sutton, Amy L. 2005. *Blood and Circulatory Disorders Sourcebook.* Detroit, MI: Omnigraphics, Inc.

Cancer

Black, Peter, and Sharon Cloud Hogan. 2006. *Living with a Brain Tumor.* New York: Henry Holt & Company, Inc.

Mayer, Musa. 2003. *After Breast Cancer.* Sebastopol, CA: O'Reilly Media, Inc.

Tsupruk, Pavel. 2005. *Prevent Cancer Today.* Frederick, MD: PublishAmerica.

Weinberg, Robert A. 2006. *Biology of Cancer.* Oxford, UK: Taylor & Francis, Inc.

Chronic fatigue syndrome

Friedberg, Fred, and Jacob Teitelbaum. 2006. *Fibromyalgia and Chronic Fatigue Syndrome.* Oakland, CA: New Harbinger Publications.

Dental disorders

Sutton, Amy. 2003. *Dental Care and Oral Health Sourcebook: Basic Consumer Health Information about Dental Care, including Hygiene, Dental Visits, Pain Management, Cavities, Crowns, Bridges, Dental Implants, and Other Oral Health Concerns.* Detroit MI: Omnigraphics, Inc.

Diabetes

American Diabetes Association. 2000. *Diabetes and Pregnancy: What to Expect.* Alexandria, VA: American Diabetes Association.

Becker, Gretchen E. 2001. *The First Year —Type 2 Diabetes.* New York: Avalon Publishing Group, Inc.

Endocrinology

Gordon, John D., Dan I. Lebovic, and Robert N. Taylor. 2005. *Reproductive Endocrinology and Infertility.* Glen Cove, NY: Scrub Hill Press.

Kronenberg, Henry M., Reed P. Larsen, Shlomo Melmed, and Kenneth S. Polonsky. 2003. *Williams Textbook of Endocrinology.* Philadelphia, PA: Elsevier Health Sciences.

Environmental disorders

Brebbia, C. A., D. Fayzieva, and V. Popov. 2005. *Environmental Health Risk III*, Vol. 9. WIT Press.

Eye disorders

Billig, Michael D., Gary H. Cassel, and Harry G. Randall. 1998. *Eye Book: A Complete Guide to Eye Disorders and Health.* Baltimore, MD: Johns Hopkins University Press.

Mogk, Lylas G., and Daniel L. Roberts. 2006. *Age-Related Macular Degeneration: An Essential Guide to the Newly Diagnosed.* New York: Avalon Publishing Group, Inc.

Shaw, Kimberley Williams, and Amy Sutton. 2003. *Eye Care*

Sourcebook. Detroit, MI: Omnigraphics, Inc.

Genetic disorders and birth defects

Iannucci, Lisa. 2000. *Birth Defects.* Berkeley Heights, NJ: Enslow Publishers Inc.

Wynbrandt, James. 2007. *Encyclopedia of Genetic Disorders and Birth Defects.* New York: Facts on File.

Heart disease

Cohen, B. M., and B. Hasselbring. 2002. *Coronary Heart Disease: A Guide to Diagnosis and Treatment.* Omaha, NE: Addicus Books.

Esselstyn, Caldwell. 2007. *Prevent and Reverse Heart Disease.* New York: Penguin Group.

Gersh, B. J. 2000. *Mayo Clinic Heart Book: The Ultimate Guide to Heart Health.* New York: W. Morrow.

Katzenstein, Larry, and Ileana L. Pina. 2007. *Living with Heart Disease.* New York: Sterling Publishing.

Sheps, Sheldon G. 2003. *Mayo Clinic on High Blood Pressure.* New York: Mayo Foundation for Medical Education & Research.

Hepatitis

Wright, Lloyd. 2002. *Triumph over Hepatitis C.* Malibu, CA: Lloyd Wright Publishing.

Herpes

Connolly, Sean. 2002. *STDs.* Portsmouth, NH: Heinemann.

Stanberry, Lawrence. 2006. *Understanding Herpes.* Jackson, MS: University Press of Mississippi.

Hormonal disorders

Isaacs, Scott, Todd Leopold, and Neil Shulman. 2006. *Hormonal Balance: Understanding Hormones, Weight, and Your Metabolism.* Boulder, CO: Bull Publishing Company.

Immune system

Sompayrac, Lauren. 2003. *How the Immune System Works.* Malden, MA: Blackwell Publishing.

Kidney disorders

Cheung, Alfred K., and Arthur Greenberg, ed. 2005. *Primer of Kidney Diseases.* Philadelphia, PA: Elsevier Health Sciences.

Lupus

Wallace, Daniel J. 2005. *Lupus Book: A Guide for Patients and Their Families.* Oxford, UK: Oxford University Press.

Motor neuron disease

Eisen, Andrew, and Pamela Shaw, eds. 2007. *Motor Neuron Disorders and Related Diseases.* Philadelphia, PA: Elsevier Health Sciences.

Multiple sclerosis

Blackstone, Margaret. 2003. *The First Year—Multiple Sclerosis: An Essential Guide for the Newly Diagnosed.* New York: Avalon.

Hill, Beth, and Joanne Wojcieszek. 2003. *Multiple Sclerosis Q & A: Reassuring Answers to Frequently Asked Questions.* New York: Penguin Group.

Obesity

Brownell, Kelly, and Katherine Horgen. 2004. *Food Fight: The Inside Story of the Food Industry, America's Obesity Crisis, and What We Can Do about It.* Columbus, OH: McGraw-Hill.

Koplan, Jeffrey P., ed. 2005. *Preventing Childhood Obesity: Health in the Balance.* Washington, DC: National Academies Press.

Pain

Abelson, Brian, Kamali Abelson, and Michael P. Leahy. 2005. *Release Your Pain: Resolving Repetitive Strain Injuries with Active Release Techniques.* Berkeley, CA: North Atlantic Books.

Ballantyne, Jane C. 2005. *The Massachusetts General Hospital Handbook of Pain Management.* 2005. Baltimore, MD: Lippincott Williams & Wilkins Publishers.

Egoscue, Pete, and Roger Gittines. 2000. *Pain Free: A Revolutionary Method for Stopping Chronic Pain.* New York: Bantam Books.

Parkinson's disease

Schwarz, Shelley Peterman. 2006. *Parkinson's Disease: 300 Tips for Making Life Easier.* New York: Demos Medical Publishing, LLC.

Prostate disorders

Kelman, Judith, and Peter T. Scardino. 2005. *Dr. Peter Scardino's Prostate Book: The Complete Guide to Overcoming Prostate Cancer, Prostatitis, and BPH.* Wayne, NJ: Avery.

Psychotherapy and psychology

Leszcz, Molyn, and Irvin D. Yalom. 2005. *The Theory and Practice of Group Psychotherapy.* New York: Basic Books.

Reproductive system

DeZarn, Christine (foreword), Milton Hammerly, and Cheryl Kimball. 2003. *What to Do When the Doctor Says It's PCOS.* Gloucester, MA: Rockport Publishers.

Heffner, Linda, and Danny J. Schust. 2006. *Reproductive System at a Glance.* Malden, MA: Blackwell Publishing.

Manassiev, Nikolai, and Malcolm I. Whitehead. 2003. *Female Reproductive Health.* Boca Raton, FL: CRC Press.

Thatcher, Samuel S. 2000. *PCOS (Polycystic Ovarian Syndrome): The Hidden Epidemic.* Indianapolis, IN: Perspectives Press, Inc.

Respiratory disorders

Broaddus, Courtney V., Robert J. Mason, John F. Murray, and Jay A. Nadel. 2005. *Murray and Nadel's Textbook of Respiratory Medicine.* Philadelphia PA: Elsevier Health Sciences.

Sexual and gender identity disorders

Drescher, Jack, and Dan Karasic, eds. 2006. *Sexual and Gender*

Diagnoses of the Diagnostic and Statistical Manual (DSM). New York: Haworth Press, Inc.

Sexually transmitted diseases

Parker, James N., and Philip M. Parker, eds. 2002. *The Official Patient's Sourcebook on Bacterial STDs.* San Diego, CA: ICON Health Publications.

Skin disorders

Goroway, Patricia, and Richard H. Keller. 2006. *Facial Fitness: Daily Exercises and Massage Techniques for a Healthier, Younger Looking You.* New York: Barnes and Noble Books.

Mancini, Anthony J., and Amy S. Paller. 2005. *Hurwitz Clinical Pediatric Dermatology: A Textbook of Skin Disorders of Childhood and Adolescence.* 2005. Orlando, FL: W. B. Saunders Publisher.

SIDS

Byard, Roger W., and Henry F. Krous, eds. 2001. *Sudden Infant Death Syndrome: Problems, Progress, and Possibilities.* London, UK: Hodder Arnold.

Sleep disorders

Breus, Michael. 2006. *Good Night: The Sleep Doctor's 4-Week Program to Better Sleep and Better Health.* New York: Penguin Group USA.

Buysse, Daniel J., ed. 2005. *Sleep Disorders and Psychiatry,* Vol. 24. Arlington, VA: American Psychiatric Publishing, Incorporated.

Urinary system disorders

Datta, Shreelata. 2003. *Crash Course: Renal and Urinary Systems.* Philadelphia, PA: Elsevier Health Sciences.

Mental disorders

Abel, Kathryn M., David Castle, and Jayashri Kulkarni, eds. 2006. *Mood and Anxiety Disorders in Women.* NY: Cambridge University Press.

Andrews, Linda Wasmer, and Dwight L. Evans. 2005. *If Your Adolescent Has Depression or Bipolar Disorder: An Essential Resource for Parents.* 2005. Oxford, UK: Oxford University Press.

Attwood, Tony (foreword), and Isabelle Henault. 2005. *Asperger's Syndrome and Sexuality: From Adolescence through Adulthood.* London, UK: Jessica Kingsley Publishers.

Barkley, Russell A., and Eric J. Mash, eds. 2006. *The Treatment of Childhood Disorders.* New York: Guilford Publications, Inc.

Brown, Thomas. 2005. *Attention Deficit Disorders: The Unfocused Mind in Children and Adults.* New Haven, CT: Yale University Press.

Brownell, Kelly D., and Christopher G. Fairburn. 2005. *Eating Disorders and Obesity: A Comprehensive Handbook.* New York: Guilford Publications, Inc.

Buckman, Dana, and Charlotte Farber. 2006. *A Special Education: One Family's Journey Through the Maze of Learning Disabilities.* New York, NY: Da Capo Press.

Davidson, Larry D. 2003. *Living Outside Mental Illness: Qualitative Studies of Recovery in Schizophrenia.* New York: New York University Press.

Earley, Pete. 2007. *Crazy: A Father's Search through America's Mental Health Madness.* New York: Penguin.

Findling, Robert L., Elena Harlan, and Charles S. Schulz. 2000. *Psychotic Disorders in Children and Adolescents.* Thousand Oaks, CA: Sage Publications.

Guyol, Gracelyn, and Stephen T. Sinatra. 2006. *Healing Depression and Bipolar Disorder without Drugs.* New York: Walker & Company.

Handler, Lowell, and Elkhonon Goldberg (foreword) and Neal R. Swerdlow (afterword). 2004. *Twitch and Shout: A Touretter's Tale.* Minneapolis, MN: University of Minnesota Press.

Kingdon, David G., and Douglas Turkington. 2004. *Cognitive Therapy of Schizophrenia.* 2004. New York: Guilford Publications, Incorporated.

Kreisman, Jerold J., and Hal Straus. 2006. *Sometimes I Act Crazy: Living with Borderline Personality Disorder.* 2006. New York: John Wiley & Sons, Inc.

Le Grange, Daniel, and James Lock. 2004. *Help Your Teenager Beat an Eating Disorder.* New York: Guilford Publications, Inc.

Miklowitz, David J. 2002. *The Bipolar Disorder Survival Guide.* New York: Guilford Publications, Inc.

Nicholl, Malcolm J., and Jacqueline B. Stordy. 2000. *LCP Solution: The Remarkable Nutritional Treatment for ADHD, Dyslexia and Dyspraxia.* New York: Random House Publishing Group.

Notbohm, Ellen. 2005. *Ten Things Every Child with Autism Wishes You Knew.* Arlington, TX: Future Horizons, Inc.

Rosen, Gerald, ed. 2004. *Posttraumatic Stress Disorder.* New York: John Wiley & Sons, Inc.

Sarno, John E. 2006. *Divided Mind: The Epidemic of Mindbody Disorders.* New York: HarperCollins Publishers.

Tammet, Daniel. 2007. *Born on a Blue Day: Inside the Extraordinary Mind of an Autistic Savant.* New York: Simon and Schuster Adult Publishing Group.

Wagner, Aureen. 2004. *Up and Down the Worry Hill: A Children's Book about Obsessive-Compulsive Disorder.* Rochester: Lighthouse Press, Incorporated.

HEALTH HOTLINES

AIDS/HIV Treatment, Prevention, and Research   800-HIV-0440

Alcohol and Drug Abuse
800-729-6686

Alzheimer's Disease
800-438-4380

American Medical Association
312-645-5000

American Public Health Association
202-789-5600

Americans with Disabilities Act Information and Assistance Hotline   800-949-4232

Cancer   800-4-CANCER
800-422-6237

Centers for Disease Control and Prevention
404-639-3311

Child Health and Human Development
800-370-2493

Department of Transportation's Hotline for Air Travelers with Disabilities
1-800-778-4838 (voice)

Diabetes   800-860-8747

Digestive Diseases   800-891-5389

Drug Abuse   301-443-1124

Endocrine and Metabolic Disorders
888-828-0904

Eye Diseases   301-496-5248

Food and Drug Administration (FDA)
301-443-2410

Genetic and Rare Diseases
888-205-2311

Human Genome Research
301-402-0911

Mental Health and Mental Illness
301-443-4513

National Herpes Hotline
919-361-8488

National Mental Health Association
800-969-NHMA (6642)

National Pediatric and Family HIV Resource Center
973-972-0410, 800-362-0071

National Suicide Prevention Lifeline
800-273-TALK (8255)

Neurological Disorders
800-352-9424

Ovulation Research   888-644-8891

Pharmaceutical Research and Manufacturer's Association (drug information)
202–835-3400

Schizophrenia Research
888-674-6464

SIDS (Sudden infant death syndrome)
800-505-CRIB

Smoking Cessation, NCI's Smoking Quitline
877-44U-QUIT

Stroke   800-352-9424

Teens AIDS Hotline   800-283-2473

WE CAN (Ways to Enhance Children's Activity and Nutrition)   866-35-WE-CAN

Weight Control   877-946-4627

Women's Health   301-496-8176

WEB RESOURCES

The following World Wide Web sources feature information useful for students, teachers, and health care professionals. By necessity, this list is only a representative sampling; many government bodies, charities, and professional organizations not listed have websites that are also worth investigating. Other Internet resources, such as newsgroups, also exist and can be explored for further research. Please note that all URLs have a tendency to change; addresses were functional and accurate at the time of publication.

American Academy of Family Physicians
http://familydoctor.org
The website supplies health information and an A–Z index of conditions that can be accessed with links for different groups of people.

American Academy of Orthopaedic Surgeons
www.orthoinfo.aaos.org
Information on growth plate fractures, knee ligament injuries, and impact of osteoarthritis of the knee.

American Cancer Society
www.cancer.org
A self-help website for patients, family, and friends to learn about cancer, treatment options, clinical trials, and coping with the disease. There are links to connect patients with cancer survivors and support programs.

American College Health Association
www.acha.org
ACHA aims to provide advocacy, education, communications, products, and services, as well as to promote research and culturally competent practices to enhance its members' ability to advance the health of all students and the campus community.

American Heart Association
www.heart.org
A comprehensive website including many suggestions for a better lifestyle to reduce the risk of a heart attack; warning signs; and explanations of diseases and conditions.

American Social Health Association
www.ashastd.org
ASHA aims to improve the health of individuals, families, and communities, with emphasis on the prevention of sexually transmitted diseases and infections (STDs/STIs). The website lists information about specific STDs/STIs, tips for reducing risk, and ways to talk with health care providers and partners.

Aurora Health Care
www.aurorahealthcare.org/aboutus/mission.asp
A not-for-profit organization with a mission to promote health, prevent illness, and provide state-of-the-art diagnosis and treatment to meet individual and family needs.

Birth Defect Research for Children
www.birthdefects.org
This resource provides free information about birth defects and details about parent networking and birth defect research through the National Birth Defect Registry.

Centers for Disease Control and Prevention
www.cdc.gov
Government-compiled health information, including health statistics, links to other websites, and research and development.

Childhelp
www.childhelp.org
Childhelp is dedicated to meeting the physical, emotional, and spiritual needs of abused and neglected children by focusing on prevention, intervention, and treatment. The Childhelp National Child Abuse Hotline, 1-800-4-A-CHILD, operates 24 hours a day, 7 days a week.

Mayo Clinic
www.mayoclinic.com
A website produced by a collective of medical experts with the aim of helping people manage their health. Information is up to date and many health issues are discussed.

MedlinePlus
www.nlm.nih.gov/medlineplus
U.S. National Library of Medicine.

National Cancer Institute
www.cancer.gov
Information about cancer.

National Institutes of Health (U.S. Department of Health and Human Services)
www.nih.gov
Health information with an A–Z index of NIH resources, clinical trials, health hotlines, and drug information. Also includes MedlinePlus.

National Institute of Neurological Disorders and Stroke
www.ninds.nih.gov/disorders/stroke/stroke_needtoknow.htm#URGENT
Information about strokes.

National Mental Health Information Center
http://mentalhealth.samhsa.gov
All aspects of mental health are covered on this website, which provides links to a spectrum of topics. A drop-down menu allows users to look for mental health and substance abuse services by state.

Nutrition Source
www.hsph.harvard.edu/ nutritionsource
The website supplies clear tips for healthy eating and dispels nutrition myths. Gives advice on what foods to eat and why.

TeenGrowth
www.teengrowth.com
Health information specifically for teens; debates on relevant topics.

U.S. National AIDS Hotlines and Resources
www.thebody.com/index/hotlines/ national.html
This website supplies hotline numbers for every group of people who are affected by AIDS or HIV.

U.S. National Library of Medicine (National Institutes of Health)
www.nlm.nih.gov
This website provides links to authoritative health information resources on hundreds of diseases, conditions, and health topics.

World Health Organization (WHO)
www.who.int/about/en
WHO is the United Nations' specialized agency for health. WHO's mission is the attainment by all peoples of the highest possible level of health. Health is defined as not just the absence of disease but a positive state of physical, mental, and social well-being.

Specific disorders
Alcohol and Bone Health
www.niams.nih.gov/Health_Info/ Bone/default.asp

Arthritis/Scleroderma Fact Sheet
www.mayoclinic.com/health/ scleroderma/DS00362

Carpal Tunnel Syndrome Fact Sheet
www.ninds.nih.gov/disorders/carpal _tunnel/detail_carpal_tunnel.htm

CDC Emergency Preparedness and Response
www.bt.cdc.gov

CDC Travelers' Health: Yellow Book
wwwnc.cdc.gov/travel/content/ yellowbook/home-2010.aspx

Center for the Evaluation of Risks to Human Reproduction, National Toxicology Program, Department of Health and Human Services
http://cerhr.niehs.nih.gov

Kids and Their Bones
www.niams.nih.gov/Health_Info/ Bone/Bone_Health/Juvenile/ default.asp

Maintain a Healthy Back
http://dohs.ors.od.nih.gov/ spine.htm

National Institute of Diabetes, Digestive, and Kidney Diseases
www2.niddk.nih.gov

North American Spine Society
www.spine.org

Oral and Throat Cancer
www.mayoclinic.com/health/ oral-and-throat-cancer/ DS00349

Peptic Ulcer
www.mayoclinic.com/health/ peptic-ulcer/DS00242

Polio
www.who.int/mediacentre/ factsheets/fs114/en

Polio Eradication
www.polioeradication.org/ history.asp

Public Health Emergencies: Reference Manual
www.in.gov/isdh/files/ Public_Health_Emergencies_ Reference_Manual.pdf

Questions and Answers about Scoliosis in Children and Adolescents
www.niams.nih.gov/Health_Info/ Scoliosis/default.asp

Questions and Answers about Knee Problems
www.niams.nih.gov/Health_Info/ Knee_Problems/default.asp

Radiation Sickness
http://www.mayoclinic.com/ health/radiation-sickness/ DS00432/DSECTION= symptoms

Scleroderma Fact Sheet
www.medicinenet.com/ scleroderma/article.htm

Scleroderma Research Foundation
www.srfcure.org

Sleeping Sickness
www.who.int/mediacentre/ factsheets/fs259/en

Toxoplasmosis Fact Sheet
www.cdc.gov/ncidod/dpd/ parasites/toxoplasmosis/ factsht_toxoplasmosis.htm

Glossary

achondroplasia
Genetic disorder causing severe limitation of skeletal growth.

acromegaly
Abnormal enlargement of face, hands, and feet as a result of a tumor of the pituitary gland.

acute
A term that describes an illness of sudden onset, which may or may not be severe but is usually of short duration.

affective flattening
A lack of emotional response.

AIDS
Acquired immunodeficiency syndrome. Caused by HIV (human immunodeficiency virus), AIDS leads to potentially fatal depression of the immune system.

albinism
A condition characterized by a lack of pigment in the hair, eyes, and skin.

alcoholism
Addiction to alcohol, which can lead to deterioration in physical and psychological health, family life, and social position.

allergen
A substance that causes an allergy.

allergy
Hypersensitive reaction, such as wheezing or a rash, to a foreign substance that stimulates the immune system.

alogia
A lack of appropriate speech. Unless prompted by the questioner, someone with alogia will give minimal responses.

alopecia
A lack or loss of bodily hair that is most obvious on the scalp, which tends to develop patchy hair loss.

alternative medicine
Medical systems, therapies, or techniques that are used in place of conventional medicine.

amebic dysentery
Inflammation of the intestines caused by infestation with the amoeba *Entamoeba histolytica*, characterized by blood-flecked diarrhea.

amenorrhea
Lack of menses (the flow of blood that occurs during menstruation) by age 16 is called primary amenorrhea; the absence of menses for more than three cycles is called secondary amenorrhea.

amniocentesis
A procedure in which a sample of the amniotic fluid around the fetus is removed from the mother's uterus for testing.

amyotrophic lateral sclerosis (ALS)
A form of motor neuron dis-

ease, characterized by weakness in the muscles, caused by degeneration of cells in the spinal cord.

analgesic
A drug that relieves pain.

anaphylactic shock
Severe allergic reaction; often includes respiratory symptoms.

anemia
A disorder of the blood in which there is a deficiency or disorder of hemoglobin, the oxygen-carrying pigment in red blood cells.

aneurysm
A dilatation (stretching) of a blood vessel, often filled with clotting blood, as a result of its wall becoming weakened.

angina
A cramplike pain, often felt in the chest, arms, and legs, resulting from narrowing of the arteries. This narrowing starves the heart muscle of oxygen.

anorexia nervosa
Anorexia nervosa is an eating disorder in which people perceive that they are too heavy, even though they are underweight. This perception results in a refusal or inability to maintain normal body weight.

antibiotic
A drug that selectively attacks microorganisms by breaking down bacteria and prevents

the growth of bacteria. Specific antibiotic drugs will work only against certain bacteria, leaving other bacteria unharmed.

antibody
A protein produced in the blood that inactivates invading organisms (or other foreign substances) and makes them susceptible to destruction by immune system cells such as phagocytes.

anticoagulant
Any drug that delays or prevents coagulation (clotting) of the blood.

antigen
A substance that can trigger the immune system into producing antibodies as a defense against infection and invading organisms.

antipruritic
A drug that relieves persistent itching, or pruritis, by reducing inflammation or numbing nerve impulses.

appendicolith
A calcified deposit within the appendix.

arrhythmia
Any variation in the normal rhythm or rate of the heartbeat.

arteriole
The smallest vessel of the arterial system.

artery
Blood vessels carrying oxygen-rich blood from the heart to the tissues.

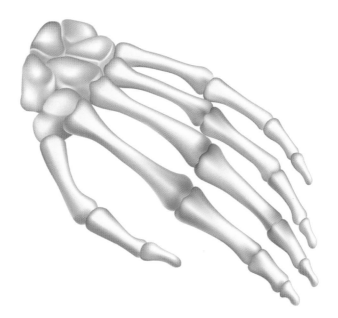

Arthritis has affected the joints of the bones in this hand. The red areas denote swelling and inflammation of the joints.

arthritis
Inflammation leading to pain and swelling of joints.

artificial insemination
The insertion of sperm into the vagina or uterus by mechanical means rather than by sexual intercourse.

astigmatism
A condition that occurs because the cornea (outer lens of the eye) is not the correct spherical shape. As a result, light rays from an object do not focus on the retina but focus either in front of or behind the retina, so that the object appears blurred.

atheroma
Fatty deposit, also called arterial plaque, which is laid

down in the inner lining of the artery walls. Atheroma causes narrowing of the lining of the arteries and reduced blood flow, leading to heart attacks or strokes.

atherosclerosis
Formation of deposits of plaques consisting of cholesterol and lipids in the arteries, causing narrowing of the arteries.

atrophy
Wasting away of tissue or an organ.

autoimmune
The term refers to any disorder caused by the body's immune system reacting against its own tissues and cells.

autonomic nervous system
The part of the nervous system that controls automatic functions, such as heartbeat and sweating.

autosome
Any chromosome that is not a sex chromosome; in each cell, 22 pairs of chromosomes are autosomes.

avolition
Avolition is a condition in which a person lacks energy, spontaneity, and initiative. It is one of the symptoms noted in people who are suffering from schizophrenia.

bacteria
Small unicellular microorganisms. Bacteria exist in many areas in the body, but they are usually restrained by the immune system. Many bacteria cause life-threatening diseases.

benzodiazepine drugs
A class of drugs used as sedatives and mild tranquilizers and for the short-term treatment of insomnia. They have largely replaced barbiturates for these purposes. The advantage of using benzodiazepines is that, at smaller doses, they have a calming effect and allay anxiety, without the sleep-inducing effects of barbiturates.

beta-blockers
A family of drugs that block the effects of epinephrine, beta-blockers are principally used to treat heart disorders and high blood pressure.

bile
Greenish-brown fluid produced by the liver that carries away the liver's waste products and helps to break down fats in the small intestine. Bile enters the duodenum, the first part of the small intestine, through the bile duct.

bipolar disorder
Also called manic depression and manic depressive disorder. Someone with this disorder fluctuates between feeling deep depression and excessive euphoria.

bladder
The hollow, muscular organ situated in the lower abdomen. The bladder is protected by the pelvis and holds urine until it is excreted.

botulism
A dangerous form of food poisoning that is caused by a toxin produced by the bacterium *Clostridium botulinum*. Botulism can occur in preserved food that has been contaminated by the toxin, and can cause paralysis of the muscles.

bradycardia
An abnormally slow heartbeat, below 60 beats per minute.

bronchoscope
Instrument used via the trachea to examine the main airways of the lungs.

calorie
A unit used by dieticians to express the amount of energy taken into the body from digested food. A calorie is defined as the amount of heat that will raise 1 gram of water by 1 degree Celsius.

cancer
A group of diseases in which there is unrestrained growth of abnormal cells in tissues and organs of the body.

carcinoma
A tumor that occurs in the lining membrane of organs, such as the lungs, breasts, and stomach.

cataract
An area of opaque tissue that develops in the internal lens of the eye. If a cataract is not treated, it leads to impaired sight.

celiac disease
A condition caused by sensitivity of the intestinal lining to gluten, that leads to malabsorption of food from the intestines.

central nervous system
The brain and the spinal cord comprise the central nervous system (CNS), which receives sensory information from organs and sensory receptors in the body, analyzes the information, and produces an appropriate response.

cervical smear
A test in which a small sample of cells is removed from the surface of the cervix to detect abnormal changes in the cervix.

cervix
The lower part and neck of the uterus. The cervix separates the uterus from the vagina. The cervix is composed of smooth muscle tissue to form a sphincter or circular muscle that expands during childbirth.

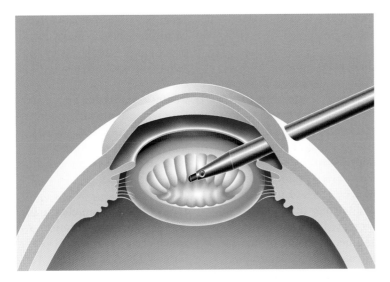

Cataracts can be treated using a simple procedure. A new lens is inserted into a tiny incision, which does not require stitching.

cesarean section
Surgery to remove a baby from the uterus through an incision in the abdominal wall.

chemotherapy
Treatment using anticancer drugs to destroy cancer cells or stop them from multiplying. Normal tissues are also affected; side effects can be severe.

chicken pox
A common infectious disease usually contracted during childhood. The symptoms are mild fever and a rash of fluid-filled spots.

cholesterol
A fatty substance that is essential to the structure of cell walls. However, when cholesterol is present in the blood in excessive quantities (usually owing to a diet too rich in animal fats), there is the risk of

atherosclerosis. Cholesterol can also crystallize as gallstones in the bladder.

chromosomes
Structures in the cell nucleus that carry genetic information. Each human cell has 23 pairs of chromosomes; 22 pairs are autosomal, that is, they are the same in both sexes. The other pair are sex chromosomes, which are either XX (female) or XY (male).

chronic
Term used to describe an illness that persists over a long period of time.

cirrhosis
Long-term damage to the liver that causes scarring and impairment of liver function.

color blindness
Inability to distinguish between colors such as red and green.

coma
A state of profound uncon-

sciousness, as a result of brain damage from head injuries, blood clots, poisoning, or strokes.

complementary medicine
Therapies or treatments used in conjunction with conventional medicine.

compound fracture
A fracture in which a broken bone breaks through the skin.

concussion
A brief loss of consciousness owing to a head injury; often followed by temporarily disturbed vision and loss of memory.

congenital
Term used to describe a disease or abnormality that is present from birth but is not necessarily hereditary.

conjunctiva
The transparent mucous membrane lining the inner surface of the eyelids and the white part of the eyeball.

conjunctivitis
Inflammation of the conjunctiva due to infection or allergy, causing red eyes and a thick discharge.

contrast medium
A radiopaque substance injected into the body in order to enhance detail on X-rays.

cornea
The transparent outer covering of the eye, which is composed of five layers. The

cornea has a dual role in the eye; it protects the eye from damage and foreign bodies, and it also helps focus light rays onto the retina.

coronary thrombosis
A condition in which a clot, or thrombus, blocks one of the coronary arteries, thus preventing oxygen from reaching the heart muscle. When a coronary artery is blocked in this way, the result can be a heart attack.

CT (computed tomography) scan
An X-ray technique that creates detailed pictures of the body's internal structures by producing detailed cross-sectional images of tissue composition.

cystic fibrosis
A genetic disorder that affects the lungs and digestive system. Cystic fibrosis appears in infancy and is characterized by excessive mucus, breathing difficulties, and abnormal secretion and function of many of the other secretory glands of the body. Treatments are available, but so far there is no cure.

cystoscopy
A procedure to examine the urethra and bladder by inserting an instrument called a cystoscope into the urethra. Sometimes the end of the cystocope carries a camera and a small cutting instrument.

cytotoxic drugs
A number of anticancer drugs

that are used to kill cancer cells.

dementia
A set of symptoms that result in impaired intellectual functioning, with loss of memory, confusion, and disorientation.

depression
This state of mind, characterized by a loss of interest in life and feelings of sadness, may be caused by a life event, such as a bereavement, or may be a symptom of a depressive disorder.

diabetes
A disease in which the cells of the body do not get enough insulin, usually because the pancreas is producing too little or no insulin. In other cases, the pancreas produces sufficient insulin, but the cells in the body become resistant to its effects. There are two types of diabetes: type 1, which is insulin dependent, and type 2, which is non-insulin dependent.

Diagnostic and Statistical Manual of Mental Disorders
Also known as the DSM-IV, this reference work is published by the American Psychiatric Association and gives information on mental health disorders affecting children and adults. It also supplies lists of causes of disorders, useful statistics, and

The DNA double helix has a ladder shape; the sides are sugars and phosphates, the rungs are paired complementary bases.

prognoses. The manual is used by professionals to make diagnoses in the United States and other countries.

dilatation (dilation)
A condition in which a body opening is stretched, such as during childbirth, during a medical procedure, or as a result of disease.

DNA (deoxyribonucleic acid)
The genetic material from which chromosomes are formed. DNA is involved in protein synthesis and in inheritance. Because of DNA's structure (a double helix),

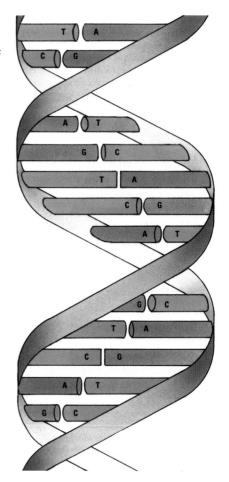

exact replication occurs during cell division.

dysfunction
Any impairment of social, psychological, or physiological function.

ECG (electrocardiogram)
A graph showing the sequence of electrical changes occurring in the heart during a succession of heartbeats. Characteristic changes in the graph can help diagnose heart disorders.

echocardiogram
An ultrasound technique used to build a moving picture of the heart.

eclampsia
An uncommon complication of pregnancy characterized by high blood pressure and seizures.

ECT (electroconvulsive therapy)
An electric shock to the brain given under anesthesia in order to produce a convulsion. Used to relieve symptoms of clinical depression.

ectopic pregnancy
A pregnancy developing outside the uterus, usually in one of the fallopian tubes.

eczema
Superficial dermatitis, characterized by a red, scaly, itchy, and often weeping skin rash.

edema
Any swelling of tissues due to an increase in fluid content.

EEG (electroencephalogram)
A multi-channel recording of electrical activity of the brain.

electrolytes
Soluble mineral compounds that conduct electrical currents; these include sodium, potassium, calcium, magnesium, and chloride, which must be kept within narrow limits for the normal function of cells, especially nerve cells.

elephantiasis
Massive swelling of the legs or areas of the trunk or head due to blockage of the lymph vessels by a tiny worm called *Wuchereria bancrofti*.

embolism
The result of a blood vessel becoming blocked by an embolus.

embolus
A foreign object, usually part of a thrombus, a tumor, or other tissue, or a mass of air, that drifts in the bloodstream until it becomes lodged in a blood vessel. *See also* embolism.

embryo
The early stages of a baby's development in the uterus, from the second week or so after conception until the seventh or eighth week of pregnancy. *Compare with* fetus.

emphysema
A chronic lung disease, resulting from overenlargement of the lung's air spaces, resulting in the destruction of the lung tissue.

encephalitis
Inflammation of the brain.

endemic
Term used to describe a disease that is native to a particular area or population. *Compare with* epidemic, epizootic, *and* pandemic.

endocarditis
Infection on the inner surface of the heart, usually occurring only when there is already some minor abnormality of structure.

endocrine system
The system of endocrine glands (pituitary, thyroid, parathyroid, and adrenal) that produces the body's hormones.

endoscopy
Examination of any part of the interior of the body by a narrow, rigid, or flexible optical viewing device, which is introduced via a natural anatomical opening or through a short incision.

enteritis
Infection of the intestines, leading to diarrhea and abdominal colic.

enzyme
A protein molecule that acts as a catalyst in chemical reactions in the cells of the body, without being altered itself.

epidemic
Term used to describe a widespread outbreak of an infectious disease. *Compare with* endemic, epizootic, *and* pandemic.

epidemiology

The study of the incidence and prevalence of disease among a population. Statistical markers such as the variables of gender, age, race, and occupation are counted. Over a period of time, changes are calculated and information is gathered about the distribution of diseases.

epilepsy

A disease of the nervous system that causes recurrent convulsions due to an overwhelming electrical discharge in the brain.

epinephrine

A hormone produced by the adrenal glands that has many effects. The hormone produces a bodily state appropriate for coping with sudden physical emergency. The hormone is produced synthetically as a treatment for cardiac arrest, anaphylactic shock, and acute asthma. Epinephrine is also known as adrenaline.

epizootic

An outbreak of infectious disease that spreads through an entire species of animal in the same geographic area.

esophagus

The muscular canal that leads from the back of the throat down to the stomach.

estrogen

One of the two important female hormones. Variations in estrogen levels occur during the menstrual cycle and are responsible for many of the changes that occur in the uterus.

fallopian tubes

The two tubes arising out of the uterus and ending near the ovaries, through which eggs produced in the ovaries normally pass on their way to the womb. Also called oviducts.

fertilization

The process whereby a sperm enters an egg and fuses with it to start the process of cell division that may end in the production of an embryo.

fetal alcohol syndrome

Physical and mental abnormalities in a baby as a result of excessive alcohol intake by the mother during pregnancy.

fetus

Human conceptus growing in the uterus—usually called a fetus from the seventh or eighth week of pregnancy. *Compare with* embryo.

fever

A high body temperature, above the normal 98.6°F (37°C). Most infectious illnesses cause fever, which is a sign that the body's temperature-regulating mechanism has been affected by the infection.

fibroids

Benign fibromuscular tumors that grow in the uterus and that may cause heavy menstruation and problems in urination.

fissure

A split in the skin.

fistula

An abnormal channel leading from one body cavity to another, or from an internal organ to the skin.

fomites

Objects that harbor infectious organisms and are able to transmit an infection from one person to another. Examples

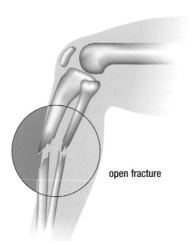

open fracture

The type of fracture depends on the force applied and the injury incurred; stress fractures (right) are caused by unusual stress on a bone. Open fractures (left) are those in which an exterior wound leads to a broken bone.

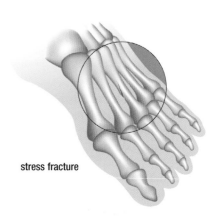

stress fracture

of fomites are books, clothes, handles, telephone receivers, and towels.

forensic medicine
The branch of pathology that investigates unnatural deaths and deaths by criminal injury.

fracture
Term used to describe an injury to a bone in which the continuity of the tissue is broken.

frostbite
Traumatic tissue injury due to cold.

frozen section
Tissue taken during surgery on which a very rapid microscopic examination is carried out in order to determine the course of the operation.

gallbladder
A saclike organ, attached to the liver, that collects bile and then discharges it into the intestine in response to a fatty meal.

gangrene
Death of tissue following a breakdown in the blood supply.

gastrectomy
The surgical removal of the stomach.

gastric ulcer
A break in the inner lining of the stomach, usually resulting from the effects of stomach acid.

gastritis
Inflammation of the mucosa of the stomach, causing pain and vomiting.

gastroenterology
The branch of medicine concerning the stomach, intestines, liver, and pancreas.

gastroscopy
Inspection of the stomach and duodenum using a flexible endoscope that is swallowed through the mouth. On its tip, the endoscope has a camera and a small cutting implement that is used to take a biopsy of tissue.

genes
Biological units that contain hereditary information. A gene is a tiny segment of DNA. The chainlike structure of DNA is composed of intertwined strands; each strand has thousands of pairs of genes, arranged on 23 pairs of chromosomes.

genetics
Genetics is the science of genes, heredity, and the variation of organisms. Modern genetics is based on the understanding of genes at the molecular, or DNA, level.

German measles
A viral infection. Also called rubella.

gerontology
The study of aging from a medical, psychological, and biological perspective.

gingivitis
Painful ulceration of the gums that causes inflammation.

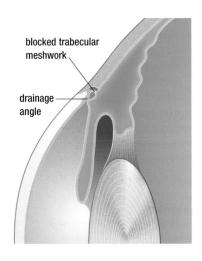

blocked trabecular meshwork

drainage angle

The diagram shows chronic glaucoma, in which the meshwork through which fluid flows out of the eye is blocked.

gland
A group of cells that produce secretions, which may be enzymes or hormones. The adrenal glands, the pituitary, and the thyroid are examples of endocrine glands, which release secretions into the bloodstream. Exocrine glands include salivary and sebaceous glands, which release secretions into the mouth and skin.

glandular fever
See infectious mononucleosis.

glaucoma
An eye disease caused by excessive pressure of fluid in the eye, which may lead to gradual loss of vision.

glucose
A simple sugar produced by the digestion of starch and sucrose. Glucose is the main source of energy for the body's cells.

gluten
A protein constituent of wheat and wheat products. Celiac disease results from sensitivity to gluten.

glycogen
A form of glucose stored in the liver and muscles. Glycogen is released when it is needed for energy.

goiter
A visible swelling of the thyroid gland.

gonorrhea
A sexually transmitted disease that produces a greenish yellow urethral or vaginal discharge.

gout
Swollen painful joints. Gout especially affects the joint at the base of the big toe; it is caused by excessive accumulation of uric acid.

greenstick fracture
A partial fracture of a child's bone, which, because the bone is so pliable, splits rather than breaks.

group therapy
Treatment of psychological problems by discussion within a group of people and under the direction of a trained therapist.

growths
Popularly used to refer to tumors both benign and malignant.

gynecologist
A specialist in the diseases of the female reproductive system.

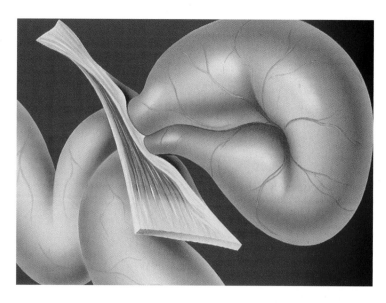

In this strangulated hernia, part of the intestine (orange) has breached the abdominal wall. Swelling may cut off the blood supply, leading to a danger of gangrene.

hallucination
An imaginary sensation perceived through any of the five senses; the result of drug use, alcohol withdrawal, severe illness, or schizophrenia.

hallucinogenic
Term describing a drug that produces hallucinations.

hay fever
Runny nose and coldlike symptoms caused by pollen allergy.

heart attack
A sudden, acutely painful, distressing, and often fatal event in which part of the heart muscle is deprived of its blood supply and dies because of the blockage of a branch of one of the coronary arteries. In those who survive, the dead tissue is replaced by scar tissue, but the pumping power of the heart is usually weakened.

heartburn
A burning sensation behind the sternum, caused by stomach acid in the esophagus.

heart failure
A condition in which the heart can no longer pump enough blood to meet the metabolic requirements of the body.

heart murmur
Any of several sounds heard in addition to the regular heartbeat.

heat exhaustion
Condition caused by loss of body fluids due to prolonged exposure to high temperature, causing cramps, nausea, and finally loss of consciousness. *Compare with* heatstroke.

heatstroke
The medical term for sunstroke. A severe and sometimes fatal condition resulting from the collapse of the body's ability to regulate its temperature, due to prolonged exposure to hot sunshine or high temperatures. Also called heat hyperpyrexia.

hematoma
A trapped mass of blood in the tissues of an organ or in the skin.

hematuria
Blood in the urine.

hemiplegia
Paralysis of one side of the body caused by damage to nerves in the opposite side of the brain.

hemodialysis
The use of a kidney machine to remove waste products from the blood after a patient's kidneys have ceased functioning.

hemoglobin
The oxygen-carrying substance in red blood cells.

hemophilia
An inherited disorder of blood clotting due to absence of one of the factors needed for clotting (factor VIII). Generally only males are affected, but females may be carriers.

hemorrhage
Medical term for bleeding.

hemorrhoids
Varicosity in the blood vessels of the anus that can give rise to bleeding and discomfort. Also called piles.

hemostasis
Arrest of bleeding or hemorrhage.

hepatitis
Inflammation of the liver, usually caused by one of the hepatitis viruses.

hernia
A weakness in the muscular wall of the abdomen that allows tissue (often the small intestine) to push through.

herpes
A group of viruses responsible for cold sores, chicken pox, shingles, and genital sores.

hiatus hernia
Condition in which the stomach pushes up through the diaphragm via the orifice normally occupied by the gullet (esophagus). There may be no symptoms, or the person suffers pain and heartburn.

HIV
The human immunodeficiency virus (a retrovirus), which can lead to AIDS. The immune system makes antibodies in an attempt to combat the virus; the presence of these antibodies in the blood confirms the presence of HIV.

Hodgkin's disease
Cancerlike disease of the lymph nodes.

holistic
An attempt to treat the whole body and mind.

homeopathy
Treatment of disease using tiny doses of a substance that produces symptoms similar to those of the disease itself.

When HIV invades a cell, enzymic action alters the RNA of the virus to DNA. The viral DNA can then invade and infect the chromosomes of the host cell.

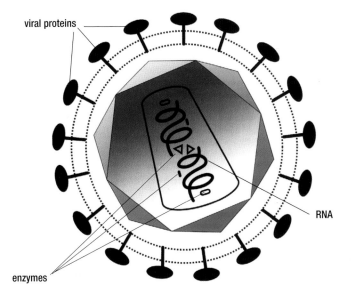

viral proteins

RNA

enzymes

homologue
Any organ that is similar to another organ, for example the hands and feet.

hormone
A chemical messenger released from tissue or a gland to alter the activity of tissues elsewhere in the body. Hormones control processes of metabolism, sexual development, and growth.

hormone replacement therapy (HRT)
Synthetic or natural hormones that are used to counteract hormonal deficiency during menopause. HRT carries a slightly higher risk of heart disease, strokes, breast cancer, and ovarian cancer.

hydatid disease
A disease caused by larval forms of tapeworms, characterized by cysts in the liver and other organs, and sometimes in muscle.

hydrocephalus
Increase in volume of the cerebrospinal fluid within the brain's ventricles. In children hydrocephalus can lead to enlargement of the head, and the condition is often associated with spina bifida.

hyperactivity
A term used to describe excessive activity in children. Associated with brain damage, epilepsy, and psychiatric problems, but only very rarely with food allergy. Also known as attention deficit hyperactivity disorder.

hyperparathyroidism
An excessive production of parathyroid hormone that is often caused by a noncancerous tumor called an adenoma.

hypertension
Raised blood pressure, which puts extra strain on the heart and arteries, thereby increasing the risk of heart attacks, strokes, and kidney damage.

hyperthyroidism
Overactivity of the thyroid gland that can lead to weight loss, tremor, protrusion of the eyes, hyperactivity, moist skin, and jumpiness.

hypertrophy
Abnormal enlargement of an organ or tissue in order to meet extra demands made on it by the body.

hyperventilation
Abnormally rapid breathing, leading to dizziness, tingling in the hands, or even sometimes loss of consciousness. Hyperventilation can be caused by anxiety.

hypochondria
Neurotic preoccupation with one's own health and with disease.

hypoglycemia
An abnormally low level of sugar in the blood, which can cause such symptoms as confusion, coma, trembling, sweating, and even death.

hypotension
Low blood pressure.

hypothalamus
The area at the base of the brain that coordinates part of the nervous and endocrine (hormonal) systems.

hypothermia
Abnormally low body temperature—below 95°F (35°C)—usually caused by prolonged exposure to cold, leading to a faint heart rate, pallor, and eventual collapse.

hypothyroidism
Underactivity of the thyroid gland, leading to fatigue, weight gain, and thick, dry skin.

hypoxia
A low level of oxygen in the tissues as a result of lung or heart disease.

hysterectomy
Removal of the uterus.

iatrogenic
A disorder caused by medical treatment.

ichthyosis
A skin condition in which the skin is abnormally thick and scaly.

idiopathic
Denoting a disease or symptom for which the cause is unknown.

immune system
The complex system by which the body defends itself against infection.

immunization
Preparing the body to fight

and prevent an infection through the injection of material from the infecting organism, or by using an attenuated (non–disease-causing) strain of the organism itself.

immunoglobulin
See antibody.

immunomodulatory
An agent that can stimulate or reduce immune responses.

immunosuppressive drugs
Drugs that suppress the immune system. They are used to treat autoimmune disorders such as rheumatoid arthritis, and after transplant surgery.

impetigo
An acute staphylococcal skin infection characterized by pustules with yellowish crusts.

impotence
Failure to achieve or sustain an erection of the penis.

incontinence
Failure to control the bladder or bowel movements, or both.

incubation period
The period between exposure to a contagious or similar infection and the first appearance of any symptoms of the disease.

infectious mononucleosis
Viral infection that causes swollen lymph nodes and a sore throat. Also called glandular fever.

infertility
Inability of a couple to conceive and reproduce after a reasonable period of time (about 1 year to 18 months).

inflammation
A reaction of the body's tissues to injury or illness, characterized by redness, heat, swelling, and pain. A mechanism of defense and repair.

inoculation
Administration of a vaccine in order to stimulate the immune system to produce antibodies and, hence, immunity to disease.

insulin
A hormone, secreted in the pancreas, that regulates blood sugar levels.

interferon
A protein produced by the body cells when triggered by a virus infection. The activity of killer cells is increased by interferon. It is also produced artificially as a drug to treat certain diseases.

intrauterine device (IUD)
A small device inserted into the uterus in order to prevent pregnancy.

intravenous (IV)
Within or into a vein. The term describes a procedure by which drugs, or fluids such as blood, can be introduced into the body either by injection or by infusion.

in vitro fertilization (IVF)
A method of enabling women who are unable to conceive to bear children; egg cells are fertilized with sperm outside the body ("in vitro" literally means "in glass," that is, in an artificial environment), and then some of the fertilized eggs are inserted in the uterus.

irradiation
Exposure to any form of radiant energy, such as light, heat, and X rays, for therapeutic or diagnostic purposes.

irritable bowel syndrome
A common condition that is characterized by episodes of abdominal pain and disturbance of the intestines (constipation or diarrhea). Also called irritable or spastic colon.

ischemia
Condition in which tissues receive an inadequate blood supply.

isotope scanning
A diagnostic technique based on the detection of radiation emitted by radioactive isotopes introduced into the body. Also called radionuclide scanning.

keyhole surgery
Surgery performed via an endoscope through small incisions rather than one large incision. Also known as minimally invasive surgery.

kwashiorkor
A disease in children, caused by a protein-deficient diet, resulting in retarded growth, edema, lassitude, and diarrhea. It is common in many parts of Africa.

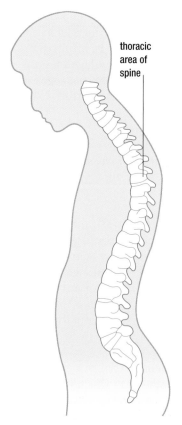

thoracic
area of
spine

The thoracic area of the spine has an exaggerated curve, giving a stooped appearance. The condition, called kyphosis, has a number of causes, including tuberculosis of the spine, poor posture, and rickets.

kyphosis
Outward curvature of the thoracic part of the spine, which can be caused by a congenital abnormality.

laparoscopy
The use of a special endoscope that is passed through the abdominal wall in order to view the abdominal organs.

laparotomy
Surgical incision to open the abdominal cavity for diagnostic purposes or surgical treatment.

laryngitis
Inflammation of the mucous membrane lining the larynx, caused by an infection or irritation, and accompanied by hoarseness or loss of voice.

lassa fever
A frequently fatal viral disease occurring in sub-Saharan Africa.

leptospirosis
Acute infectious disease caused by the organism *Leptospira interrogans*, which is transmitted to humans via the urine of rats and dogs. Symptoms include jaundice and fever. The most serious form is Weil's disease.

lesion
An area of tissue in which the structure and function are altered or impaired owing to injury or disease.

leukemia
A blood disease in which cancerous changes in the bone marrow produce abnormal numbers and forms of immature white blood cells.

leukocytosis
An excess of white cells in the blood, often due to infection.

leukopenia
Lack of white blood cells, often the result of blood disease or a side effect of anti-cancer drugs, causing a reduced resistance to infection.

leukoplakia
A condition featuring white patches of thickened mucous membrane, especially in the mouth. Leukoplakia can proceed to cancer.

lupus erythematosus
A chronic inflammatory autoimmune disease of the connective tissue, affecting the skin and internal organs.

lymphatic system
A network of vessels that transfer lymph from the tissue fluids to the bloodstream. Lymph nodes occur along the lymphatic vessels.

lymph node
A small structure that filters infection; part of the lymphatic system.

lymphocyte
A type of white blood cell that is produced in bone marrow and is present mainly in lymph and blood. Lymphocytes are part of the immune system and fight infection and cancer.

malabsorption
Failure of the small intestine to absorb nutrients properly.

malaria
Serious infectious illness that is common in the tropics. It is caused by four species of the organism *Plasmodium*, which is passed to humans via an infected anopheles mosquito. Typical symptoms are fever and an enlarged spleen.

malignant
Term used to describe tumors that spread into surrounding

tissues and elsewhere in the body. The term is also used to describe other dangerous diseases or states.

malnutrition
A nutritional deficiency, usually brought on by a severe food shortage, but which can also be caused by inadequate absorption of food or an intake of inappropriate food. The term *malnutrition* increasingly refers to the type of excessive eating that causes obesity.

malocclusion
Improper alignment of the upper and lower teeth, which affects the bite and the appearance of the teeth.

mammography
X-ray of the breast, used to help detect tumors.

mania
A state of excessive excitement, in which patients lack insight into their behavior.

manic depression
See bipolar disorder.

Mantoux test
A skin test used to determine exposure to infection with tuberculosis.

Marfan's syndrome
A genetic disorder of the connective tissue that causes elongation of the bones. It is often accompanied by heart, eye, and spinal abnormalities.

mastoiditis
Inflammation of the air cells in the bone behind the ear.

measles
An acute, highly contagious viral disease that occurs principally in childhood, characterized by red eyes, fever, and a rash. Also called morbilli and rubeola.

melanin
The black or dark brown pigment that is present in the skin, hair, and eyes.

membrane
Any thin layer of tissue.

Ménière's disease
A chronic disease of the inner ear, found in older people who have recurrent deafness, buzzing in the ears, and vertigo.

meninges
This is composed of three membranes that surround the brain and spinal cord.

meningitis
Any infection of the meninges.

meningocele
A hernial protrusion of the meninges or covering of the spinal cord.

menopause
The cessation of ovulation and menses, which in the majority of women occurs between the ages of 45 and 55.

menorrhagia
Excessive bleeding during menstrual periods.

menses
The flow of blood that occurs during menstruation.

menstruation
Periodic bleeding as the uterus sheds its lining each month during a woman's reproductive years. Menstruation begins at puberty and ends at menopause.

mental retardation
A low level of mental ability, which is usually congenital.

metabolism
The various vital processes that are necessary for bodily functions. These processes include the breakdown of complex molecules to produce energy (catabolism) and building up complex molecules, such as proteins, from simpler components (anabolism).

metastasis
The process by which cancerous cells spread from a tumor to remote sites in the body. *Metastasis* also refers to a secondary tumor.

microsurgery
Surgery on tiny structures, such as blood vessels or eyes, using a microscope and miniature instruments.

migraine
Recurrent severe headaches that are associated with nausea and visual disturbance.

minerals
Metallic elements, such as sodium, that are vital to many bodily functions.

miscarriage
Loss of an embryo or fetus from the uterus before 28

weeks of pregnancy, but usually occurring during the first 16 weeks. The medical term is *spontaneous abortion*.

mitogen
A chemical that triggers a cell to commence mitosis (cell division).

mitral stenosis
An obstructive lesion in the valve between the left atrium and ventricle, usually as a result of rheumatic fever.

MMR vaccine
A combined vaccine that protects children against measles, mumps, and rubella. The MMR vaccine is first given to a child between 12 and 15 months. Follow-up booster doses occur when the child is between 3 and 5 years old. Large-scale administration of the vaccine in the developed world has greatly reduced the occurrence of mumps.

mole
A pigmented spot on the skin.

MRSA (methicillin-resistant *Staphylococcus aureus*)
A bacterium that is difficult to treat, particularly in hospitals, where it may be fatal for already ill patients.

mumps
An acute viral disease that primarily affects the parotid glands in the cheeks.

narcotic
A drug that dulls the senses. Used to induce sleep or as a painkiller.

naturopathy
A system of health care or therapies that relies on natural substances, exercise in water, and a natural environment to maintain health and attempt to effect cures.

nausea
The sensation of wanting to vomit.

necrosis
Death of tissue.

neurology
Branch of medicine concerned with the treatment of diseases of the nervous system.

neuron
A nerve cell. The nervous system is made up of billions of neurons, each comprising a cell body, a long fiber called an axon, and shorter projections, or dendrites. There are three main types of neurons: sensory neurons that transmit information from sense receptors toward the brain; motor neurons that transmit signals toward the muscles and glands; and interneurons that transmit signals within the central nervous system.

neurosis
An emotional disorder such as mild depression, anxiety, or any of the phobias.

over-the-counter (OTC) drug
A drug sold lawfully without a prescription in a pharmacy or drugstore. Painkillers, such as acetaminophen and aspirin, are available in this way.

pandemic
Any disease that spreads over a very wide area, sometimes worldwide. *Compare with* epidemic.

pap smear
A simple method of detecting cervical cancer. The test involves the staining of a sample of exfoliated cells taken from the cervix. Also called Papanicolaou smear.

pediatrics
The branch of medicine concerned with the treatment of children and childhood diseases.

phocomelia
A defect in which the legs or hands are joined to the body by short stumps. Phocomelia occurred in many children as a result of their mothers taking the drug thalidomide during pregnancy.

prophylaxis
Any procedure to prevent a disease from developing or from becoming worse.

psychosis
Any psychiatric disorder, such as schizophrenia or bipolar disorder, in which the person has distorted beliefs that are inappropriate and disconnected from reality. Delusions or hallucinations can occur.

retrovirus
A type of virus that has RNA (ribonucleic acid) as its genetic material and that uses an enzyme (reverse transcriptase) to produce DNA from the RNA.

The viral DNA thus produced is then incorporated into the DNA of the host cell. HIV is an example of a retrovirus.

RNA (ribonucleic acid)
Genetic material in animal and plant cells that transmits the coded instructions held in DNA to the protein-synthesizing system of the cell. In some viruses, RNA is the genetic material, not DNA.

sarcoma
A malignant tumor arising in muscle, bone, or other connective tissue.

scabies
Skin infection caused by mites that burrow into the skin.

schistosomiasis
A tropical parasitic infestation, afflicting over 200 million people worldwide. The disease can damage the bladder and liver. Also called bilharzia.

schizophrenia
A group of psychiatric disorders in which thinking, emotions, and behavior are disrupted and the person is often delusional. Symptoms are hallucinations, which are often auditory (a person "hears voices") rather than visual.

septicemia
A condition in which bacteria multiply in the bloodstream. Also called blood poisoning.

side effect
An unwanted result that occurs as a consequence of a medication or therapy.

syncope
The medical term for fainting.

syndrome
A collection of symptoms or signs that occur together to indicate a specific disorder.

synthesize
To produce a substance by building it from smaller components. Proteins are synthesized in the body from smaller units called amino acids.

tachycardia
An abnormally fast heartbeat of more than 100 beats per minute, which can be experienced by a healthy person during exercise. If someone is resting and experiences tachycardia, it can indicate hyperthyroidism, fever, anxiety, or coronary artery disease.

tachypnea
An abnormally fast rate of breathing, induced by exertion, anxiety, or heart or lung problems.

tamponade
Breathlessness and sometimes collapse as a result of fluid buildup and pressure in the double membrane surrounding the heart (pericardium). It can occur after heart surgery, from inflammation of the pericardium, or after a chest injury.

teratogen
Any agent that causes abnormalities in a fetus. The agent may be a virus, a drug (for example, thalidomide), or an environmental factor such as radiation.

trisomy
The condition of having three of a certain chromosome instead of just two.

The diagram below shows the life cycle of schistosomiasis.

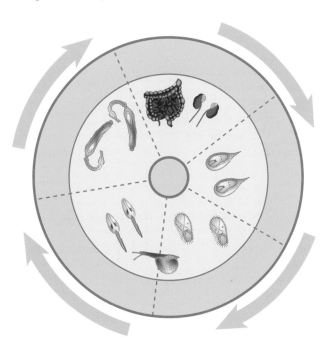

Index